Praise for

YOGA THERAPY & INTEGRATIVE MEDICINE

"*Yoga Therapy & Integrative Medicine* brings together some of the world's leading health professionals, researchers, and renowned yoga therapists to share clinical experiences, effective uses of yoga therapies, and knowledge to help redefine how we can integrate and use yoga therapy as an essential modality within healthcare. I recommend this book wholeheartedly."

—DEAN ORNISH, M.D.
Founder & President, Preventive Medicine Research Institute
Clinical Professor of Medicine, University of California, San Francisco
Author, *The Spectrum* and *Dr. Dean Ornish's Program for Reversing Heart Disease*

"This is the first scientifically backed book on integrating yoga therapy with conventional medicine. Exceptionally written by authorities in both fields and beautifully illustrated. Highly recommended for anyone interested in the future of yoga therapy and the future of medicine."

—DILIP SARKAR, M.D., F.A.C.S., C.A.P.
President, International Association of Yoga Therapists
Fellow of the American Association of Integrative Medicine
Certified Ayurvedic Practitioner and Yoga Teacher

"The emerging field of yoga therapy is finding its footing in the West, and this book will be a major contribution to that success. Not only is the content broad and engaging, it is thorough and relevant. I recommend this book very enthusiastically to both yoga teachers and yoga therapists, but additionally to those in the medical field."

—JUDITH HANSON LASATER, PH.D., P.T.
Author of eight books and Yoga Teacher since 1971

YOGA THERAPY & INTEGRATIVE MEDICINE

Where Ancient Science Meets Modern Medicine

Larry Payne, Ph.D., E-RYT500, YTRX
Terra Gold, M.A., L.Ac., E-RYT500, YTRX
Eden Goldman, D.C., E-RYT500, YTRX

Foreword by Lilias Folan,
PBS's "First Lady of Yoga" in America

Basic Health
PUBLICATIONS, INC.

DISCLAIMER: The information provided in this book is strictly for reference and is not a substitute for medical advice or direct guidance from a qualified Yoga instructor, therapist, or healthcare provider. Always consult your healthcare provider and obtain full medical clearance before practicing Yoga or any other exercise, dietary, and/or lifestyle-modification program. All forms of Yoga, Yoga Therapy, physical activity, and exercise carry with them a small inherent risk of injury that includes, but is not limited to: strains, sprains, intervertebral disc compromise, neurologic compromise, dislocations, skin irritation, fractures, disc trauma, and/or cardiovascular accidents and insufficiencies—and even death. Not all Yoga practices and poses are suitable for all practitioners and a qualified instructor and/or therapist may be able to help determine what poses are suitable for your particular situation and case. While results are not guaranteed, evaluation by a qualified therapist or health professional is always advised if pain, numbness, and/or tingling exist. Moreover, practicing Yoga under the direct supervision and guidance of a qualified instructor and at the direction of your healthcare provider may reduce the risk of injuries and potential complications. The authors, illustrators, editors, publishers, and distributors assume no responsibility or liability for any injuries or losses that might result from practicing Yoga, Yoga Therapy, or engaging in any other exercise or program contained within this book.

The information contained in this book is based upon the research and personal and professional experiences of the authors. It is not intended as a substitute for consulting with your physician or other healthcare provider. Any attempt to diagnose and treat an illness should be done under the direction of a healthcare professional.

The publisher does not advocate the use of any particular healthcare protocol but believes the information in this book should be available to the public. The publisher and authors are not responsible for any adverse effects or consequences resulting from the use of the suggestions, preparations, or procedures discussed in this book. Should the reader have any questions concerning the appropriateness of any procedures or preparation mentioned, the authors and the publisher strongly suggest consulting a professional healthcare advisor.

Library of Congress Cataloging-in-Publication Data

Payne, Larry.
Yoga therapy and integrative medicine : where ancient science meets modern medicine / Larry Payne, Terra Gold, Eden Goldman; foreword by Lilias Folan.
pages cm
Includes bibliographical references and index.
ISBN 978-1-59120-366-7 (paperback) —ISBN 978-1-59120-390-2 (hardcover) 1. Yoga—Therapeutic use. 2. Integrative medicine. I. Gold, Terra II. Goldman, Eden III. Title.
RM727.Y64P39 2014
613.7'046—dc23

2014030191

Editor: Carol Killman Rosenberg
Cover and Illustrations: Albert Soratorio
Interior design and layout: Gary A. Rosenberg

Contents

PART TWO DIVERSE APPROACHES TO YOGA THERAPY

PART THREE THE EVOLUTION OF YOGA THERAPY

ACKNOWLEDGMENTS

I would like to thank Eden Goldman and Terra Gold for bringing the idea for this book to me and for their tireless efforts. My personal editor, Deborah Myers, who is grand and my counsel of advisors who are always there for me: Zhou-Yi Qiu, L.Ac., Richard Usatine, M.D., David Allen, M.D., Art Brownstein, M.D., Christopher Chapple, Ph.D., Richard Miller, Ph.D., Rick Morris, D.C., the staff of Basic Health Publications, especially Norman Goldfind, Carol Killman Rosenberg, and Gary Rosenberg, and the love of my life, Merry Aronson, without whom none of this would be possible.

—Larry Payne, Ph.D.

I give my heartfelt thanks to Larry Payne for his endless inspiration and genuine love and mentorship through so many aspects of my life's path in Yoga Therapy, to Eden Goldman for his steadfast determination to see a dream through to fruition, and for the many ways we continue to grow knowing each other in our lives. I thank the incredible team of Norman Goldfind, Carol Killman Rosenberg, and Gary Rosenberg at Basic Health Publications for guiding the creative process of this book with impeccable leadership, collaboration, and for graciously empowering us to bring our best. Thank you to Albert Soratorio for his brilliance in capturing spirit through his artistry, John Casey for personally helping me with research and for sharing his wisdom of Sanskrit for the benefit of us all, and all the amazing authors who dedicated their writing efforts and ultimately their life's passion into this text. Most of all, I thank my beloved family that have always encouraged me to live authentically, however that may be, and for teaching me to trust the innate wisdom that guides my expressions. They have been a constant inspiration and supported me in countless ways as this book came into being, and I adore them. With heart and soul, I dedicate this book to my family and to my son, River, for teaching me more about the essence of Yoga than anyone throughout the creation of this book. He reminds me daily what is possible through Love.

—Terra Gold, L.Ac.

I would like to thank my satguru, whose eyes are always on me, whose wisdom always guides me, and whose heart is always with me. My friend and teacher, Larry Payne, whose kind heart brought together the amazing people in this book and whose example of living an honorable life very few could follow. My friend and colleague, Terra Gold, whose hard work and dedication to this project brought it into existence and whose passion for Yoga is always inspiring. My teacher, Chet Alexander, who taught me "there's no such thing as a free lunch" and to always strive to do my best. My amazing publishing team at Basic Health Publications, including Norm Goldfind, Carol Killman Rosenberg, and Gary Rosenberg and our brilliant illustrator, Albert Soratorio. My rehabilitation mentor, Craig Liebenson, and my early teachers Gaia Buddhai, Devi Hart, John Leeds, Duncan Wong, and Ira Schneider. My late grandmother, Bosh, who offered me the space to open my first Yoga studio, and my late uncle Ed, who encouraged me to get my doctorate and do something that's never been done before. My parents, Paul and Arlene, who introduced me to the world, to Spirit, and to Yoga and who have always been there for me when I needed them. My sister Joy, my little Eva, my soul brother Michael Brandwajn, and my family for always encouraging me in my spiritual endeavors and, most important, my Beloved, soon-to-be wife, Paula, who I fall in love with more and more every day and whose love for Yoga was expressed in her support, her understanding, her beautiful heart, and her truly unconditional love for me.

—Eden Goldman, D.C.

FOREWORD

by Lilias Folan

•••••••

Namasté. "The light in me greets the light in thee." I'm Lilias Folan, and chances are we have connected in some way walking through this sacred journey called life. Perhaps, it was in the late 1970s or early 1980s, when you were sitting in front of your television set tuned to the Public Broadcasting Station (PBS), patiently waiting for *Sesame Street* to begin. There was this lady who came on in a pink leotard and long braid and maybe you and/or your mom sat on the floor and did some stretching with *Lilias! Yoga and You.*

Lilias! Yoga and You aired nationally on most PBS stations, but it was incredibly challenging for me to "teach" to the red light on the TV camera. I couldn't "see" you, my students. So, I had to teach Haṭha Yoga and yogic breathing with great caution and created lots of modifications for cranky knees, tight shoulders, and sore backs. Looking back on it today, I realize that these moments on PBS were where the seeds of Yoga Therapy in the West were born. Phrases like "If you can't do it this way, try it the other way," "Listen to your body," and "Go to your edge of sweet discomfort, no pain" became popular sayings on the show and helped provide encouragement for people to adapt the poses to *their* bodies.

Teaching Yoga in this way on PBS opened up many opportunities to travel and teach in other cities and meet new Yoga friends. On one of my early Yoga teaching trips to California, I met experienced Yoga teachers and Yoga Therapists, Richard Miller, Ph.D., Larry Payne, Ph.D., Michael Lee, M.A., and Jnani Chapman, R.N. These endearing friendships provided a forum where we were able to share our concerns about working with people with injuries. We voiced questions like "Which Yoga postures can cause more injuries?" "How can we modify the poses and practices to keep people safer?" and "What are the qualifications for official Yoga teachers or Yoga Therapists?" We all agreed that no matter how long you've been teaching, continuing one's study of Yoga is vital. Then, in the early 1980s, sitting around a kitchen table in San Francisco with the founders of the International Association of Yoga Therapists (IAYT), I was named Honorary President of the IAYT. My how far we've come!

Understandably, writing this foreword is a considerable honor to me. This book, *Yoga Therapy & Integrative Medicine: Where Ancient Science Meets Modern Medicine,* provides us all with new and fascinating information to study and share with others about Yoga. Eden Goldman, D.C., Terra Gold, L.Ac., Lorin Roche, Ph.D., and so many others write with such skill and eloquence while sharing about Yoga, Yoga Therapy, and integrative medicine. It is in the essence of the yogic traditions that the authors take the whole person into consideration in body, mind, and spirit and strive to bring balance to modern medicine.

It is with a deep bow and a smile of gratitude for the ancient Yoga teachings, the medical doctors, Yoga Therapists, and Yoga teachers, past, present, and to come that I offer this foreword to you. May the stories, ideas, techniques, and information that you're about to explore serve you well in your life, your health, and your Yoga practice.

Namasté,
Lilias Folan

Recognized as the "First Lady of Yoga" since her groundbreaking 1972 PBS television series, "Lilias! Yoga and You," Lilias Folan is regarded as one of America's most knowledgeable and beloved Master Yoga teachers.

Introduction

by Larry Payne, Ph.D., Terra Gold, L.Ac., and Eden Goldman, D.C., with Shrikant Mishra, M.D., A.B.M.S.

This publication, *Yoga Therapy & Integrative Medicine: Where Ancient Science Meets Modern Medicine,* brings together a world-class collection of Yoga-oriented health professionals and therapists and represents the first integrative medical textbook in history to link modern medicine and alternative therapies with Yoga. Uniting respected doctors, licensed healthcare professionals, scholars, researchers, Yoga Therapists, and Yoga practitioners, who represent the respective traditions of many disciplines, this book is offered as a guide and reference to all. We dedicate it to medical and healthcare professionals helping others attain a greater sense of well-being, to practitioners and teachers of Yoga who want to know more about the healing potential of Yoga Therapy, to academia and the research community who are committed to the advancement of complementary and alternative medicine (CAM) therapies, and to the general public who are always seeking alternative ways of living healthier and happier lives.

Within this book, you'll discover historical stories about the lineages, teachers, and practices that have helped develop, evolve, and shape Yoga and Yoga Therapy from time immemorial to today. It is said that people begin the practice of Yoga when they are experiencing dukha (suffering) of some sort and need assistance in finding freedom from it, whether it is from physical suffering (as pain), mental suffering (as disorder), emotional suffering (as stress), and/or spiritual suffering (as separation). The term *Yoga Therapy* is a relatively contemporary description for a system of practices that, as observed through the varied definitions in this book, is still being clearly defined. It is generally agreed upon that Yoga Therapy consists of therapeutically natured practices from Yoga that may or may not include āsanas (postures), prāṇāyāma (breathing practices), dhyāna (meditation), bhāvana (imagery), philosophical training, lifestyle modification techniques, and experiential and foundational elements of Ayurveda.

As a discipline of health and wellness, Yoga Therapy takes into consideration the complete state of one's health in terms of physical conditioning, emotional state, energetic balance, attitude, dietary and behavioral patterns, personal associations and relationships, and the environment. Moreover, what the many modern interpretations of Yoga Therapy have in common is an understanding of the vital integration of mind, body, and spirit to heal the whole person. Additionally, it can be accurately claimed that both Yoga and Yoga Therapy can be used to promote health and prevent disease. The difference between the two is that, while Yoga is generally shared as a physical group practice in the Western world, Yoga Therapy is designed for the individual and is applied according to that particular person's constitution. It is generally sought out by those who cannot take a class with others due to lifestyle needs, injuries caused by chronic pain, physical limitations, social disorders, and/or compromised immunity as in the case of diseases, such as cancer.

The history and systemization of Yoga as a therapy in India can be traced back to the *Yoga Sūtras of Patañjali,* which is a compilation of yogic knowledge intended to end suffering and lead to mokṣa (freedom) written in the second century C.E. In America, Yoga and Yoga Therapy date as far back as 1893 when Swami Vivekananda introduced Yoga, Vedanta, and Hinduism to the West at the Parliament of World Religions in Chicago. In the 1920s, Paramahansa Yogananda, author of the spiritual classic *Autobiography of a Yogi,* followed from India and came to the United States introducing millions of westerners to Kriyā Yoga and meditation before he took mahāsamādhi (consciously leaving the body for the final time) in 1952. In the 1950s, Dr. Ram Murthy spread Yoga teaching throughout the New York area, and Selvarajan Yesudian launched a series of books, including *Yoga and Health and Sport + Yoga,* which has sold about two million copies since its publication. By the 1960s, the influence of The Beatles launched Maharishi Mahesh Yogi and Yoga, itself, onto the world stage while Swami Sivananda, who was an Indian trained physician, created a modern Yoga boom that began with his disciples, Swami Vishnudevananda (who coined the term *Sivananda Yoga* out of respect for his teacher) and Swami Satchitananda (who founded Integral Yoga and gave the opening speech at Woodstock). Satchitananda's teachings inspired several of the next generation's leaders in Yoga Therapy like Dean Ornish, M.D. (whose Yoga-based program for reversing heart disease has been heavily researched and approved by Medicare) and Michael Lerner, Ph.D. (who founded the Commonweal cancer treatment center in Northern California).

Soon after the expansion of Sivananda Yoga, teachers who studied with Professor Tirumalai Krishnamacharya, now regarded as the "Father of Modern Yoga," began coming to the West in the 1970s. Krishnamacharya was a scholar, philosopher, and Yoga master who held equivalent knowledge and training for what would be considered as multiple doctorates in Western studies and his students, B. K. S. Iyengar (named by *Time Magazine* as one of the 100 most influential people in the twentieth century), Indra Devi (the first-ever First Lady of Yoga), Pattabhi Jois (founder of Ashtanga Vinyasa Yoga), T. K. V. Desikachar (Krishnamacharya's son), and A. G. Mohan (cofounder of Svastha Yoga and Ayurveda), among others, inspired tens of millions of Yoga practitioners in the Americas alone, including many of today's most popular teachers and advocates of the yogic path. Out of the foundational teachings of these great yogis and countless others, Yoga shifted its role in the late twentieth century into a scientific healing modality and books on Yoga as a therapy became readily available, such as Tim McCall, M.D.'s *Yoga as Medicine; Yoga Rx* by Larry Payne, Ph.D., and Richard Usatine, M.D.; Leslie Kaminoff's bestselling book *Yoga Anatomy; Yoga for Wellness* by Gary Kraftsow; Ray Long M.D.'s *The Key Muscles of Yoga;* T. K. V. Desikachar's *The Heart of Yoga: Developing a Personal Practice;* and *Yoga Therapy: A Guide to the Therapeutic Use of Yoga and Ayurveda for Health and Fitness* by A. G. Mohan, Indra Mohan, Ganesh Mohan, and Nitya Mohan.

Furthering Yoga's role as a therapeutic intervention, numerous chapters in this book include holistic, wellness-based Yoga Therapy techniques and approaches that can be used collaboratively for a variety of medical and humanistic conditions to provide the best possible care for each individual. Whether you are a Yoga practitioner, therapist, or healthcare professional with an interest in the therapeutic potential of Yoga, there is tremendous diversity, depth, and breadth of knowledge in this book that can be used to expand your understanding of Yoga and assist you in honoring your own personal health and well-being and that of your clients/patients. For example, Art Brownstein, M.D., offers his years of insight into why he gives śavāsana to cardiac patients for 20 minutes per day; Richard Miller, Ph.D., shares the practices and results of his scientifically backed iRest system of Yoga Nidrā that has been used in the military for posttraumatic stress disorder (PTSD); Matthew Taylor, P.T., lends his reflections on how Yoga Therapy can be integrated into physical rehabilitation practices; Shanti Shanti Kaur Khalsa, Ph.D., explains the energetic psycho-emotional approach in the Kundalini tradition; Jnani Chapman, R.N., proposes ways in which Yoga Therapy can be applied in cancer treatment; and sports scientist, LeRoy Perry, D.C., describes yogic practices that he has used with great success while training Olympic athletes and championship sports teams. And the list of respected authors and topics goes on and on.

Meanwhile, this book also features chapters representing the views, insights, and research from many of the first generation of modern Yoga Therapists while detailing the public rise in interest for Yoga Therapy as a field, which has grown significantly in recent times. In their chapter "Scientific Research on Yoga Therapy," renowned Harvard Yoga scholar and researcher, Sat Bir Singh Khalsa, Ph.D., and Heather Mason, M.A., remind us, "Evidence revealing Yoga's role as a preventive strategy is supported by both surveys of long-term practitioners and prospective studies," and they document findings of the most up-to-date research regarding the efficacy of Yoga practices for specific health issues.

At the same time, this book highlights where Yoga Therapy still has to be better defined both for the sake of recognizing it as a profession and for the sake of gaining accurate and relevant data on the effectiveness of its application. The National Institutes of Health (NIH) has funded some research on Yoga Therapy and other research has received funding from nonprofit organizations such as the Bill & Melinda Gates Foundation and the Bernard Osher Foundation. Yet, like other CAM therapies, creating Yoga Therapy studies that account for placebo effect, a large enough cohort/body of testable people, scientific mechanisms of action, and a documentable effectiveness of improvement are incredibly challenging to design, test, and fund. As the current executive director of the International Association of Yoga Therapists (IAYT), John Kepner, M.A., says in his chapter on the development and the future of Yoga Therapy, "Evidence based [research] is slowly developing but funds for Yoga, as well as all CAM practices that cannot be patented, are severely limited. Conventional research is expensive and emerging fields cannot support such research directly." Nonetheless, it is vital that this research continues and includes reputable institutions working alongside these groups using a more comprehensive model for assessment within the studies.

The Yoga Therapy model supports, enables, and empowers the *whole* individual and his/her health using therapeutically natured practices and yogic modalities that have withstood the test of time and outlived other systems, the diversity of cultures, and economic realities. Integration of this ancient model with the most current scientific, evidence-based medicine ensures the wisdom of Yoga Therapy will continue to advance on its own and, as such, is the perfect complement to any other system of medicine seeking a more natural and holistic approach. All in all, Yoga Therapy can transform lives, change people's perspectives on life, positively influence habits, improve health, and end suffering. When applied as a modality for healing, wellness, and prevention, Yoga Therapy's use in modern medicine is powerful and limitless. With this being the case, it is our intention as Yoga practitioners and therapists, integrative healthcare professionals, authors, and pioneers that this book inspire a whole new generation of medical doctors, scholars, researchers, and yogins. The future of Yoga Therapy depends on it.

Oṁ Shanti Shanti Shanti.

In dedication,

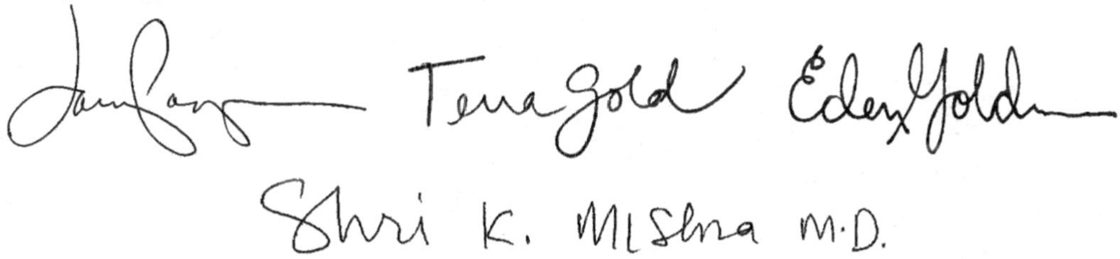

Larry Payne, Ph.D. ~ Terra Gold, L.Ac. ~ Eden Goldman, D.C.
Shrikant Mishra, M.D., A.B.M.S.

PART ONE

YOGA THERAPY AND INTEGRATIVE MEDICINE

ACUPUNCTURE, CHINESE MEDICINE, AND YOGA THERAPY

Terra Gold, M.A., L.Ac., C.Y.T., Y.T.R.X., E-RYT500

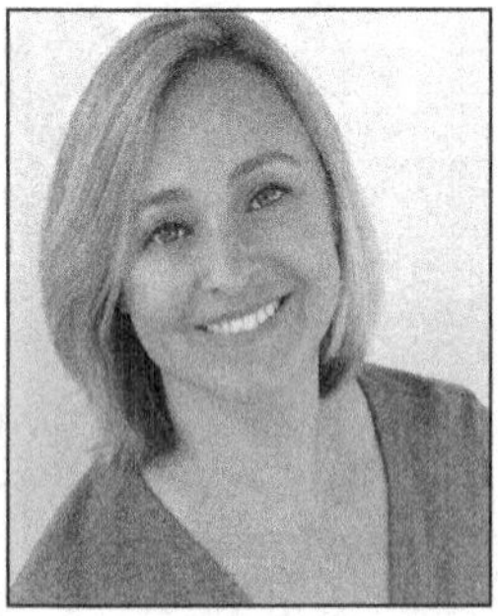

Terra Gold is a certified Yoga Therapist, licensed acupuncturist and Chinese Medicine practitioner, clinical nutritionist, and an allied health professional in integrative body psychotherapy (IBP). Graduating *summa cum laude* from UCLA with a B.A. in world arts and cultures, and from Emperor's College with an M.A. in Traditional Chinese Medicine, Terra has been helping to improve clients' health in the Los Angeles area for over twenty years. She is the founder of Terra Wellness, cofounder of Yoga Doctors, and codirector of Loyola Marymount University's Yoga and the Healing Sciences Yoga Teacher Training Program. Terra is also a Bhakti Kirtan musician with a self-released album entitled *Sun and Moon,* and she has been featured in the widely acclaimed books *Yoga for Dummies* and *Shakti: The Feminine Power of Yoga*.

INTRODUCTION

en·light·en·ment *noun* \in-'lī-t^{ə}n-mənt, en-\ : the state of having knowledge or understanding; the act of giving someone knowledge or understanding (*Merriam-Webster Dictionary,* 2014)

The path to enlightenment is unique to each individual. A myriad of practices exist in the philosophy and science of Yoga Therapy and through other cultural philosophies and sciences—both Eastern and Western—that can provide the inspiration for a practitioner to find equanimity, improved health, awakened consciousness, and enlightenment. The word *enlightenment* was defined by the late yogic scholar Georg Feuerstein as "that condition of the body and mind in which it is perfectly synchronized with the transcendental Reality." It is identical to self-realization and ātma-jñāna (self-knowledge) in the yogic traditions and is synonymous with mokṣa (liberation) (Feuerstein, 1997).

Many traditions have spoken about pathways to enlightenment for the sake of spiritual wisdom, secular knowledge, and to bring about a better understanding of the human condition. Born in Scotland's holistically minded Findhorn commune and raised between the San Francisco Bay Area and Hawaii, I was introduced to many healing modalities early on. The most impactful were two varying practices for healing that have become complementary fields that I now offer in my daily medical practice to patients and in university training programs: the merging of acupuncture, Chinese Medicine, and Yoga Therapy.

In the health fields, our objective is to create powerful and integrated options for healing and self-care, and our goal is to assist people in finding balance, freedom from pain, and physical and/or emotional enlightenment.

This chapter is dedicated to the therapeutic potential that can be universally utilized by acupuncturists, Chinese Medicine professionals, Yoga Therapists, and those interested in the healing modalities offered through the healing traditions of India and China. We begin by exploring the roots, timeline, and philosophical influences of Indic medicine, yogic therapies, and Chinese Medicine. Next, we explore some of the traditionally private practice modalities used in Chinese Medicine, Ayurveda, and other yogic therapies that can be used as a blended model for Yoga Therapy practice, including patient assessment and treatment considerations. This leads to a discussion about the modern-day rise in the popularity of these healing modalities and the methods for training in each profession. The chapter concludes with a vision for the future of Chinese Medicine and Yoga Therapy as a collective of knowledge that can be used to benefit many conditions and people all over the world.

THE HISTORICAL ROOTS OF YOGA THERAPY AND CHINESE MEDICINE

The roots of Ayurveda and early practices of Yoga in India, and the roots of acupuncture and Chinese Medicine in China, stem from two different world cultures that were evolving simultaneously. Historically, they had little overlap in their ancient origins, yet moments in history exist where Yoga and its "sister science" of Ayurveda had shared philosophies and practices with Qi Gong, acupuncture, and/or Chinese Medicine for health and healing that were mutually influential.

Yoga Therapy consists of, but is not limited to, Yoga and Ayurveda. Early Indic sources of healing modalities define Ayurveda as "the knowledge or science of life, health, and longevity," or in other words, "health science" (Casey, 2014). Ancient yogic and Ayurvedic practices for health, as well as Chinese Medicine practices, look at an individual as being influenced by nature as well as being a unique part of it. This individualized view applied to modern health translates to each person and each treatment being different according to the circumstances presenting in that particular person at the time of his/her treatment.

Cultures throughout history have faced the challenge of staying healthy and fighting disease, thus "the origin of health science must be thought of as being co-emergent with human civilization itself" (Casey, 2014). The Ayurvedic traditions of India and Chinese Medicine of China loosely resemble each other as both have principles and practices that have withstood the test of time. It is impossible to define a true starting point for any of the healing traditions based solely on texts given that the modalities surely existed orally for a long time before the texts came into existence.

Sources differ in dating the origin of Chinese Medicine as anywhere between 3,000 and 5,000 years ago. This is partly due to the fact that like Yoga and Ayurveda, Chinese Medicine is not a completely unified system of medicine with defined origins. Instead, China's medical history has included both "official doctors" that were educated through government-run medical colleges and unofficial "folk doctors" who were trained by family teachers or through spiritual mentors. Both branches of medicine have produced medical texts and oral traditions that have been valuable to the evolving practices known as Chinese Medicine (Vercammen, 1997).

There also seems to be a wide gap in agreement among scholars and practitioners of Ayurveda and Yoga regarding the beginnings of traditional practices we call "medicine" or "yogic therapies." Feuerstein stated, "Ayurveda and Yoga have influenced each other during their long history, starting in Vedic times" (*The Shambhala Encyclopedia of Yoga*, 1997), and the oral tradition undoubtedly was in existence before the actual writing of the Vedas. The Vedas are the earliest known Indian documents that contain the history of health practices that may be referred to as "therapies." The most relevant and helpful Veda on the topic of health is known as the *Atharva Veda* (Feuerstein, 1997). The treatment for health and healing appears primarily in Kanda 19, which is "widely considered by scholars to be a late addition to a collection, whose core contents were probably in place by around 1200–1000 BCE" (Casey, 2014). This Veda can be thought of as a "proto-Ayurveda approach" to Yoga therapies, given that the core principles of Ayurveda emphasize the philosophy of tri-doṣa theory (three bodily humors), which is entirely absent from the *Atharva Veda* text. Even so, within the *Atharva Veda* there are "herb-based remedies and the use of mantras" (Casey, 2014). There are also hymns with a "medical or healing intent," "speculations about breath and breath control (prāṇāyāma), and within the fifteenth book, known as the '*Vratya-Kanda*,' there exists information about the Vratya brotherhoods, in which early yogic practices were developed" (Feuerstein, 1997).

As is found in the historical timeline of Indic medicines and therapies, diverse opinions exist regarding the inception period of Chinese Medicine. There are few historical sources describing the historical origins of Chinese Medicine. However, there are generally two sources that are regarded as the "legendary founders": The Yellow Emperor (Huang Di) and the Divine Farmer (Shen Nong) (Vercammen, 1997). Scholars agree that the earliest written source of all early Chinese medical theory is the *Huang-di Nei-Jing* (Inner Classic of the Yellow Emperor), referred to as *Nei-Jing* for short, dating back 300 to 100 BCE (Kaptchuck, 2000). Compiled by unknown authors, it is primarily a dialogue between the Yellow Emperor and his advisors, discussing the origin and theory of diseases. It refers to prior theories and practices, thus alluding to a tradition that began long before. Moreover, it is the earliest work available to explain some of the foundational theories that are still used in Chinese Medicine today, including the *Wu Xing* (five agents) and *Yin-Yang*, the famous unity of opposites.

When considering the first Yoga Therapy texts, we must take into account the first known textbooks of Ayurveda. "The earliest attestable compendiums, or *saṁhitās*, of what can clearly be identified as a matured system of Ayurveda are the

Caraka Saṁhitā and the *Sushruta Samhita*" (Casey, 2014). In terms of their relevance to Yoga Therapy and its history, both texts feature the philosophy of tri-doṣa theory and, similar to Chinese Medicine's *Nei-Jing*, Ayurveda's *Caraka Saṁhitā* specifically covers medical topics like "pharmacology, dietetics, pathology, anatomy, embryology, diagnosis, prognosis, toxicology, and general therapy"(Feuerstein, 1997). Still, Yoga's focus on mokṣa (spiritual liberation), which can be described as "an eventual radical release from the cycle of living incarnation in the physical world," is distinctly different from Ayurveda's focus on the "health sciences." In other words, "Ayurveda concerns itself with the health of *the physical body*, while Yoga's essential focus is ultimately transcendental" (Casey, 2014).

HAṬHA YOGA AND QI GONG

Where Yoga and Ayurveda most succinctly intersect and support each other is in the practice of Haṭha Yoga. The primary assertion of Haṭha Yoga is that "it is possible, through the application of intensive physical techniques, to transform the body into an ideal instrument for the practice of deep meditation, thus making possible the achievement of profound and liberating samādhi (bliss) experiences" (Casey, 2014). The earliest writings connecting the teachings of Ayurveda and Haṭha Yoga is said to be the *Ayur-Veda-Sūtra* (Aphorisms on the Life Science), "a 16th C.C.E. text that sought to connect Patañjali's eightfold path to enlightenment with Indian medicine" (Feuerstein, 1997). Written traces of practices that are considered to be a part of modern Yoga Therapy date back as early as the mid-fourteenth century C.E. in the most widely used manual on Haṭha Yoga, the *Haṭha Yoga Pradīpikā* (Light on the Forceful Yoga) (Feuerstein, 1997). The *Haṭha Yoga Pradīpikā* was authored by Svatmarama Yogin and has received many Sanskrit translations and commentaries over the years to try to clarify its meanings and uses. Haṭha Yoga dates back before the time of the *Haṭha Yoga Pradīpikā*, but how far back, scholars don't exactly know. Feuerstein stated in his research that the historical roots of this eclectic Yoga are varied. One thing that is certain is that, although Haṭha Yoga is focused on attaining samādhi and was not originally intended as a "health regimen," the Haṭha Yoga system postulates that physical illness impedes the practice of samādhi and must be addressed within the context of the practice (Casey, 2014). Some further assertions within the *Haṭha Yoga Pradīpikā* that could serve as a starting point for a system of Yoga Therapy are listed in the chart below.

	I.28–29	*pascimottanasana*	(back stretch pose)	increases digestive fire, flattens abdomen, render one free from disease
	I.30–31	*mayurasana*	(peackock pose)	alleviates enlargement of the glands, dropsy, other stomach disorders, rectifies imbalances of the doshas, kindles gastric fire
	II.16–17	*pranayama*	(extension of breath)	alleviates hiccups, asthma, cough, headache, earache, eye pain
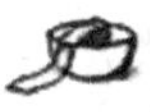	II.24–25	*dhauti*	(swallowing, churning, and retrieval of cloth strip for cleansing of the stomach lining)	alleviates cough, asthma, diseases of the spleen, leprosy, and twenty kinds of disease brought about by excess mucus (kapha)
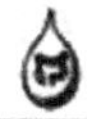	II.26–27	*basti*	(yogic enema)	alleviates enlargement of glands and spleen, all diseases arising from excess of the doshas
	II.29–30	*neti*	(nasal cleansing with thread or water)	destroys diseases which manifest above the throat
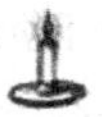	II.31–32	*trataka*	(staring at a point with open eyes until tears are produced)	eradicates all eye diseases and fatigue
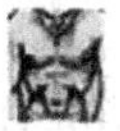	II.33–34	*nauli*	(rhythmic churning of the abdominal muscles)	kindles digestive fire, removes indigestion, remedies slow digestion
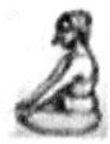	II.35–36	*kapalabhati*	("skull-shining"- bellows breath with emphasis on the exhale)	destroys all mucus disorders
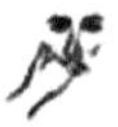	II.48–50	*suryabhedana*	("opening the flow of the sun" – inhale thru right nostril, exhale thru left)	destroys imbalances in vāta (wind dosha), eliminates worms
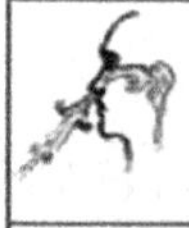	II.51–53	*ujjayi*	("victorious" - audible breathing with constricted throat)	removes phlegm from the throat, stimulates digestive fire, removes dropsy
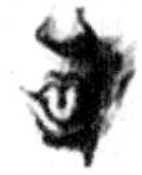	II.57–58	*shitali*	("cooling" – inhaling through curled tongue)	cures enlarged stomach or spleen & other related disorders, reduces fever & excess bile (pitta)

In the Chinese tradition, the *Wu Qin Xi* movements were the earliest-known written examples found in a text describing exercises that are akin to Yoga āsanas (postures) for physical health. They held that distinction until the 1973 discovery of texts named the *Mawangdui,* which include illustrations of the practices Daoyin (Guiding [the Qi] and Stretching [the muscles and joints]). Currently, *Mawangdui* is considered "the most important collection of ancient [Chinese] texts, medical or otherwise" and covers "therapeutic exercises comparable to the exercises practiced

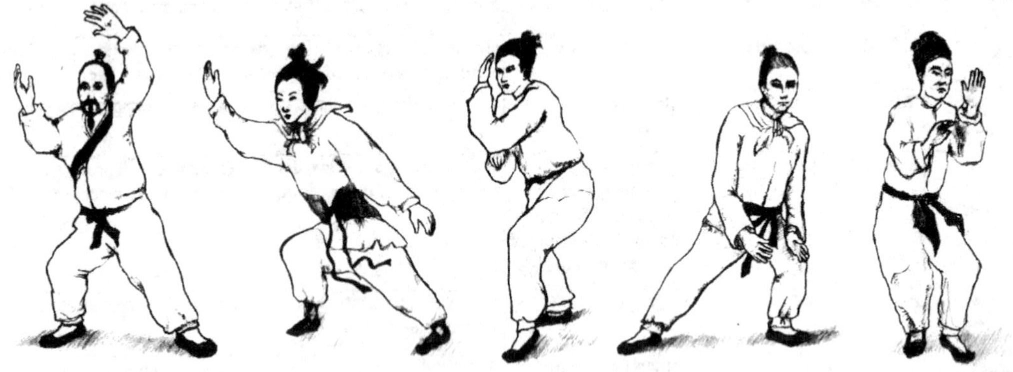

by Taoists of later times," illustrating that the author, Hua Tuo, likely described physical health practices that were "extant before his time" (Vercammen, 1996).

Finally, another important text commonly used by philosophers and everyday practitioners as a tool for health and healing in Chinese Medicine is the *Yijing* (I Ching, or Book of Changes), whose origins date back to the third and second millennia BCE (Stamps, 1980). The *Yijing* "reduces the complex manifestations of change to the simple observation that any change is created by the interplay of two 'forces,' *Yin* and *Yang*" (Vercammen, 1997).

LIFE FORCE, QI, AND PRANA

Taoist thought and Chinese Medicine hold that we are a microcosm of the macrocosm. To understand how our bodies function, rather than thinking in terms of "organs" and biomechanical function, we must think beyond these microcosmic concepts and include "phenomena we know from the world around us" (Vercammen, 1996). This view overlaps with the Indian yogic traditions in that they both share the view that "all manifest reality stems from an unseen universal force of infinite, expansiveness that is without beginning or end, a singular pulsation or unmoving center from which all action springs" (Powers, 2008). Though given different names, this idea is called *Brahman* by the Hindus, *Tao* (or *Dao*) by the Taoists, and *Śūnyatā* by the Buddhists. All three agree (more or less) that the dimension of infinite energy is the genesis of creation itself and is often expressed as being seated in the human heart (Powers, 2008).

Both Taoist thought and ancient yogic thought purports that moderation in all areas of life is essential to a long and fruitful life. To understand moderation at the level at which it is intended in these traditions, one must consider what is known as Qi (or chi) in the Chinese tradition and what is known as prāṇa in yogic and Ayurvedic therapies. *Prana* can be described as "the energy that flows through creation," and after a series of processes, it lastly becomes "the organic and inorganic universe" (Lad and Durve, 2008). To all of these systems, everything in the universe, organic and inorganic, is composed of Qi or prāṇa.

In one of the great Chinese Medicine books of the twentieth century, *The Web That Has No Weaver*, which covers the fundamental philosophies and schools of thought in Chinese Medicine including Qi, Ted Kaptchuck writes:

> Qi is the thread connecting all being. Qi is the common denominator of all things—from mineral to human. Qi allows any phenomenon to maintain its cohesiveness, grow, and transform into other forms. Metamorphosis is possible because Qi takes myriad forms. Qi is the potential and actualization of transformation. The universe moves—ceaselessly manifests and engenders because of Qi. Qi is the fundamental quality of being and becoming. (Kaptchuck, 2000)

Qi has no beginning and no end, but, within a lifetime, it is believed that we have a limited amount of certain kinds of Qi. In Taoism, it can be found as a common definition to equate Qi as "the energy, or vital substance," that links mind, body, and spirit. A more complete definition states, "*Qi* is not some primordial, immutable material, nor is it merely vital energy, although the word is occasionally so translated. Chinese thought does not easily distinguish between matter and energy. We might think that Qi is somewhere in between, a kind of matter on the verge of becoming energy, or energy at the point of materializing" (Kaptchuck, 2000). Even the process of life, itself, is explained in terms of Qi. An ancient Chinese text known as *The Simple Questions* states, "A human being results from the Qi of Heaven and Earth . . . The union of the Qi of Heaven and Earth is called human being" (Maciocia, 1989).

When referring to diagnostic techniques used in Chinese Medicine, Qi is not the only consideration for sustaining a long and healthy life. Qi is considered one of the "three treasures" along with Shen (spirit) and Jing (essence) as the substances that collectively fuel us. Shen, like "spirit," is sometimes compared to the concept of "soul." It is the "domain of human life that defies the limitations of time and space. It is the human capacity for relationships that are not restricted by physical or temporal contact" (Kaptchuck, 2000). Within the individual, Shen manifests personality, thought, sensory perception, self-awareness, and the impetus for "self-transformation." As Kaptchuck puts it, "It is also what allows for humans to insert or interject their 'authentic self' into their mundane lives and be participants in shaping their fate," (Kaptchuck, 2000) which is also a yogic concept by nature.

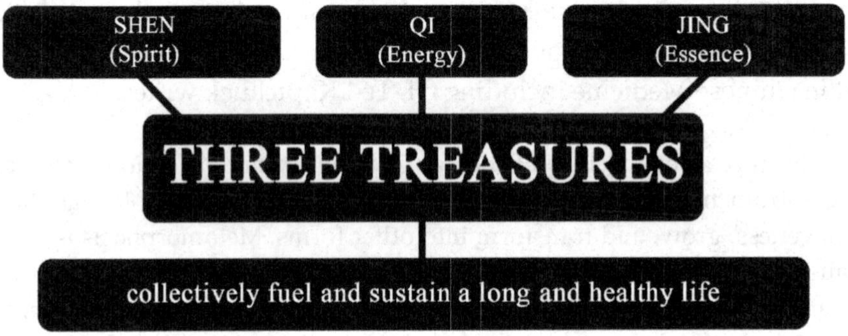

As opposed to Shen, Jing is what "distinguishes organic life from inorganic material." Jing is that which is responsible for growth, development, and reproduction. There are two sources to Jing. One source is limited and could be considered what we genetically inherit. It is called xian-tian-zhi-jing (or Prenatal Essence) and determines how we grow and develop. The amount of Prenatal Essence is "fixed at birth and, together with Original Qi, determines an individual's basic makeup and constitution" (Kaptchuck, 2000). The other source of Jing is called hou-tian-zhi-jing (or Postnatal Essence). This type of essence is derived from the refined parts of "ingested food and continuous exercise, emotional, and mental stimulation from a person's environment" (Kaptchuck, 2000). Some of the actions that deplete Jing are living a life of excess, drinking too much, excessive emotional reactions, working too hard, and inappropriate sexual behavior. Together, the Prenatal and Postnatal essences that constitute Jing are sustained by living in moderation to help preserve the finite Jing we have as individuals. Yoga has similar practices to conserve our essences known as the yamas (restraints) and niyamas (adherences) that are found in Patañjali's eight-limbed approach to Rāja Yoga.

Much like the "three treasures" from Chinese Medicine, it is said in Ayurveda

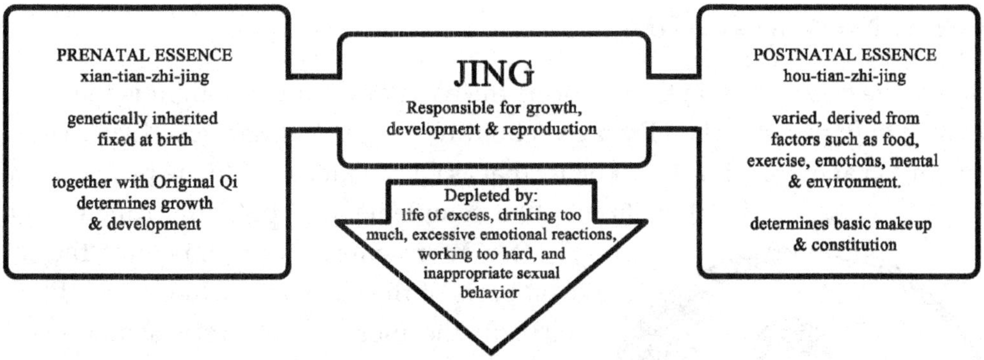

that prāṇa "exists in conjunction with *'ojas'* and *'tejas,'* forming a trinity within the microcosm of the body and the macrocosm of the universe" (Lad and Durve, 2008). Within a human being, *prāṇa* is defined as "cellular awareness," *tejas* is defined as "cellular digestion and intelligence," and *ojas* is referred to as responsible for "cellular immunity." Though these concepts are not an exact translation, they are similar enough to compare in a useful way for health considerations (Lad and Durve, 2008).

In the philosophy of Traditional Chinese Medicine, some of the diagnostic methods currently used include: 1) sensing quality of pulse, 2) visual tongue assessment, 3) observation of the eyes, 4) appearance of skin (texture and color), 5) observation of voice (tone and dynamic quality), and 6) smell of the patient. In other words, within these diagnostic techniques, one uses his/her own senses to observe the qualities of how Qi, Shen, and Jing are manifesting within the person being observed. These diagnostics were used in the most ancient Chinese texts in conjunction with the principles of Wu Xing (five agents/elements), which are covered in greater detail later in this chapter.

While Ayurveda uses similar, yet different means of making these kinds of observations, it wasn't until the beginning of the sixteenth century that there was a Sanskrit text that mentions a diagnostic technique called aṣṭa-sthāna-parikṣa ("examination of the eight bases"). A routine was described in this set of diagnostic practices for "examining the pulse, urine, feces, tongue, eyes, general appearance, voice, and skin of the patient" (Wujastyk, 1996). This, along with "pulse taking," which likely crossed over as a modality due to cultural exchanges between Indic traders or Buddhist monastics interacting with Chinese traders during the time of Emperor Ashoka (269–232 BCE), marked significant historical overlaps between Indic yogic therapies and Chinese diagnostic therapies (Casey, 2014).

YIN YANG AND HA-THA

One of the central concepts that forms the basis of Chinese thought is the *Yin* and *Yang* dating from the Zhou Dynasty (about 1000–770 BC) (Maciocia, 1989). The concept of Yin and Yang is a Taoist belief that as Qi "condenses into the physical realm, it splits into two complementary polarities called Yin and Yang," often represented as the image of the interwoven parts of the black and white circle (Powers, 2008). In the most ancient representations, Yin and Yang are referred to as "two faces of a single mountain, one face bright and sunny (Yang), and the other cloudy and dark (Yin)" (Vercammen, 1997). In ancient times, the Chinese characters for Yin represented the moon and Yang represented the sun. These terms extended to include Yin as night and Yang as day, Yin as winter and Yang as summer, and Yin as female and Yang as male. Ultimately, everything was viewed as the dynamic interplay of Yin and Yang. They are constantly influencing and determining each other, and there is always some measure of Yin within Yang and Yang within Yin (Powers, 2008).

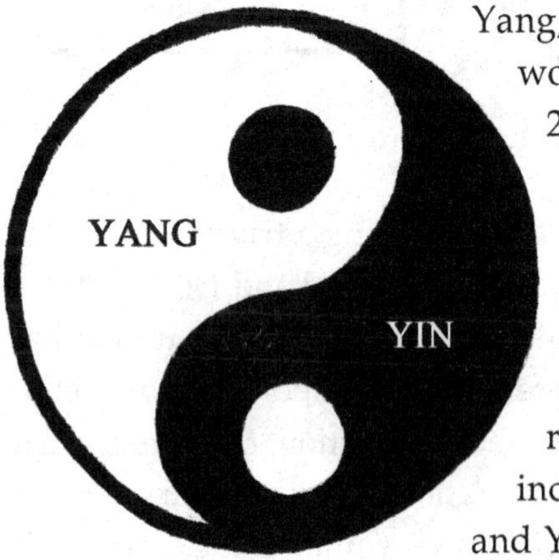

Not unlike Yin and Yang, the Sanskrit word *Haṭha,* from Haṭha Yoga, can be broken into two parts: *Ha,* meaning "the warming, sun-like manifestations (from the sun god, Surya)" and *Tha,* meaning "the cooling or moon elements (from the moon goddess, Chandra)." Thus, Haṭha Yoga, like Yin and Yang, represent the "marriage" of these two forces that are always in relationship with each other and together can be either in or out of harmony (Powers, 2008). The two forces mutually generate and sustain each other, and we can use various treatment strategies with the concepts of Yin and Yang/Ha and Tha to assist the body's innate ability to maintain health and defend itself from disease.

THE FIVE ELEMENTS

A foundational theory for assessment and treatment in Chinese Medicine practices is *Wu Xing,* also known as five phases, five elements, five steps/stage, or five agents. The word *Wu* means "five" and *Xing* means "movement," referring to the five elements not as "basic constituents of Nature, but [as] five basic processes, qualities, phases of a cycle, or inherent capabilities of change of phenomena" (Maciocia, 1989). Beyond Chinese Medicine, the elemental concept of the Wu Xing is present in Ayurveda, Tibetan medicine, and in ancient Greek medicine. The earliest known Chinese reference to the use of Wu Xing "dates back to the Warring States Period (476–221 BCE) (Maciocia, 1989). For the sake of comparing Indic use and Chinese use of the five elements as a therapeutic model, there is some diversity in the elemental correspondence properties between the two traditions, but either model can be used to further assist an individual in understanding the relationship between aspects of his/her body and the attributes of the elements. A simple definition of the respective elements of these traditions would be defined as: "the five-fold *mahābhūtas*, or great elements, of Indian cosmology, which are earth, water, fire, wind, and space, while the Wu Xing are understood as earth, water, fire, metal, and wood" (Casey, 2014).

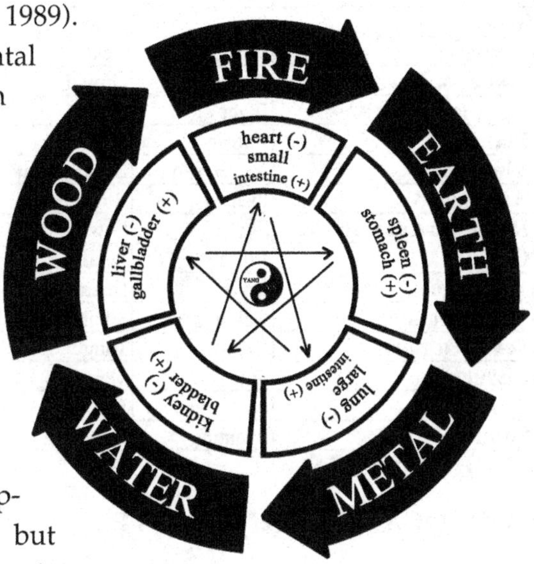

The same school that is largely credited with developing the Yin-Yang theory, the Naturalist School (third century BCE), also advanced the theory of the five elements. This Wu Xing theory had times throughout history where it was used as a predominant means of diagnosis and treatment, and periods where it fell out of favor for a time due to being considered too simplistic. As philosopher Wang Chong (AD 27–97) described, it was "too rigid to interpret *all* natural phenomenon correctly" (Maciocia, 1989). Thus, Wu Xing is currently taught as one of several essential theoretical models for diagnosis and treatment, yet it is commonly overlaid with other approaches. In the chart on page 20, the Wu Xing system is further broken down in accordance with describing the relationship between the organs.

	Wood	Fire	Earth	Metal	Water
Seasons	Spring	Summer	None	Autumn	Winter
Directions	East	South	Center	West	North
Colors	Green	Red	Yellow	White	Black
Tastes	Sour	Bitter	Sweet	Pungent	Salty
Climates	Wind	Heat	Dampness	Dryness	Cold
Stages of Development	Birth	Growth	Transformation	Harvest	Storage
Numbers	Eight	Seven	Five	Nine	Six
Planets	Jupiter	Mars	Saturn	Venus	Mercury
Yin-Yang	Lesser Yang	Utmost Yang	Center	Lesser Yin	Utmost Yin
Animals	Fish	Birds	Human	Mammals	Shell Covered
Domestic Animals	Sheep	Fowl	Ox	Dog	Pig
Grains	Wheat	Beans	Rice	Hemp	Millet
Yin Organs	Liver	Heart	Spleen	Lungs	Kidneys
Yang Organs	Gallbladder	Small Intestine	Stomach	Large Intestine	Bladder
Sense Organs	Eyes	Tongue	Mouth	Nose	Ears
Tissues	Sinews	Vessels	Muscles	Skin	Bones
Emotions	Anger	Joy	Pensiveness	Sadness	Fear
Sounds	Shouting	Laughing	Singing	Crying	Groaning

HOW QI AND PRĀṆA MOVE

In Chinese medicine and Ayurveda, Qi and prāṇa, respectively, flow through subtle energy pathways known as jing luo (channels, or meridians) in Chinese medicine and nāḍīs (channels, or conduits) in Ayurveda. How they move involves an intimate relationship between Qi and blood, or, as is stated in Ayurveda, between prāṇa (energy) and rakta (blood). In Chinese Medicine "*Qi* is *Yang* in nature and blood is *Yin*" (Lad and Durve, 2008). A saying that is instilled in Chinese Medicine practitioners to help understand the relationship between blood and Qi is, "*Qi* is the commander of the Blood. . . . Blood is the Mother of *Qi*" (Kaptchuk, 2000). Similar to this, we find that in Ayurveda, blood is known as *rakta* and it is expressed *"prāṇa raktanu dhavati,"* translated as "prāṇa moves with the blood" (Lad and Durve, 2008).

ACUPUNCTURE POINTS VERSUS MARMA POINTS

Energy channels exist in the body in both Yoga Therapy and Ayurvedic medicine, as well as in Chinese Medicine. In Ayurveda, points along the trajectories of the channels are known as marmani, or marma (mortal, or vulnerable point) points, and in Chinese Medicine they are known as acupuncture points. In both traditions, the points are located on the surface but can penetrate the deepest depths of the body, including one's consciousness. While Indian medicine texts differ in their claims, the principle marma point is said to be the heart, and there are as many as 117 and as few as 107 marma points in total (Lad and Durve, 2008).

The Yoga scriptures mention eighteen marmani. "The *Shandilya-Upanishad* (1.8lf.) names the feet, big toes, ankles, shanks, knees, thighs, anus, penis, navel, heart, throat, the "well" (kupa—the "throat well" or jugular notch), the palate (talu), nose, eyes, the middle of the eyebrows (bhru-madhya), forehead, and head" (Feuerstein, 1997). These are all based on locations that can be used for therapeutic purposes as well as for inflicting injury (such as in martial arts) (Lad and Durve, 2008). It is stated in the *Kṣurikā Upaniṣad,* "one should cut through these vital spots by means of the mind's sharp blade." Then, place "attention and breath on each marmani to free it from the tensions so that the life force (prāṇa) can flow freely through the subtle channels (nāḍī)" (Feuerstein, 1997). Though not intended for needling, focusing on these points such as one might in a Yoga nidrā meditation is intended to free up tensions. (For more information on Yoga nidrā techniques, please see Dr. Richard Miller's chapter "Integrative Restoration iRest® Yoga Nidrā: Healing in Wholeness" in this text.)

Chinese Medicine initially referenced 365 points on the body. However, many acupuncture points are bilateral, making the actual total 670. By the second century CE, China collectively recognized 649 points making up the trajectory of "The Twelve Principle Meridians" and the "Eight Extraordinary Channels" (Needham and Gwei-Djen, 1980). The twelve principle meridians are divided into Yin and Yang groups and are named according to their associated internal organs and other related internal structures, including Lung Channel (Tai Yin), Heart Channel (Shaoyin), Pericardium Channel (Jueyin), San Jiao Channel (Shaoyang), Small Intestine Channel (Taiyang), Large Intestine Channel (Yangming), Spleen Channel (Taiyin), Kidney Channel (Shaoyin), Liver Channel (Jueyin), Gall Bladder Channel (Shaoyang), Bladder Channel (Taiyang), and Stomach Channel (Yangming). The therapeutic use behind the "Eight Extraordinary Channels" is intended to "act like reservoirs of energy" to the primary channels, which are referred to as "rivers" (Needham and Gwei-Djen, 1980).

Whether using an awareness of the marma points, or acupoints with needles, essential oils, tuning forks, or high-powered tiny magnets, understanding the intention behind these points is an important part of the healing session for a client coming in for treatment. These are access points for consciousness that, with the client's and practitioner's combined intentions, can assist the physical treatment.

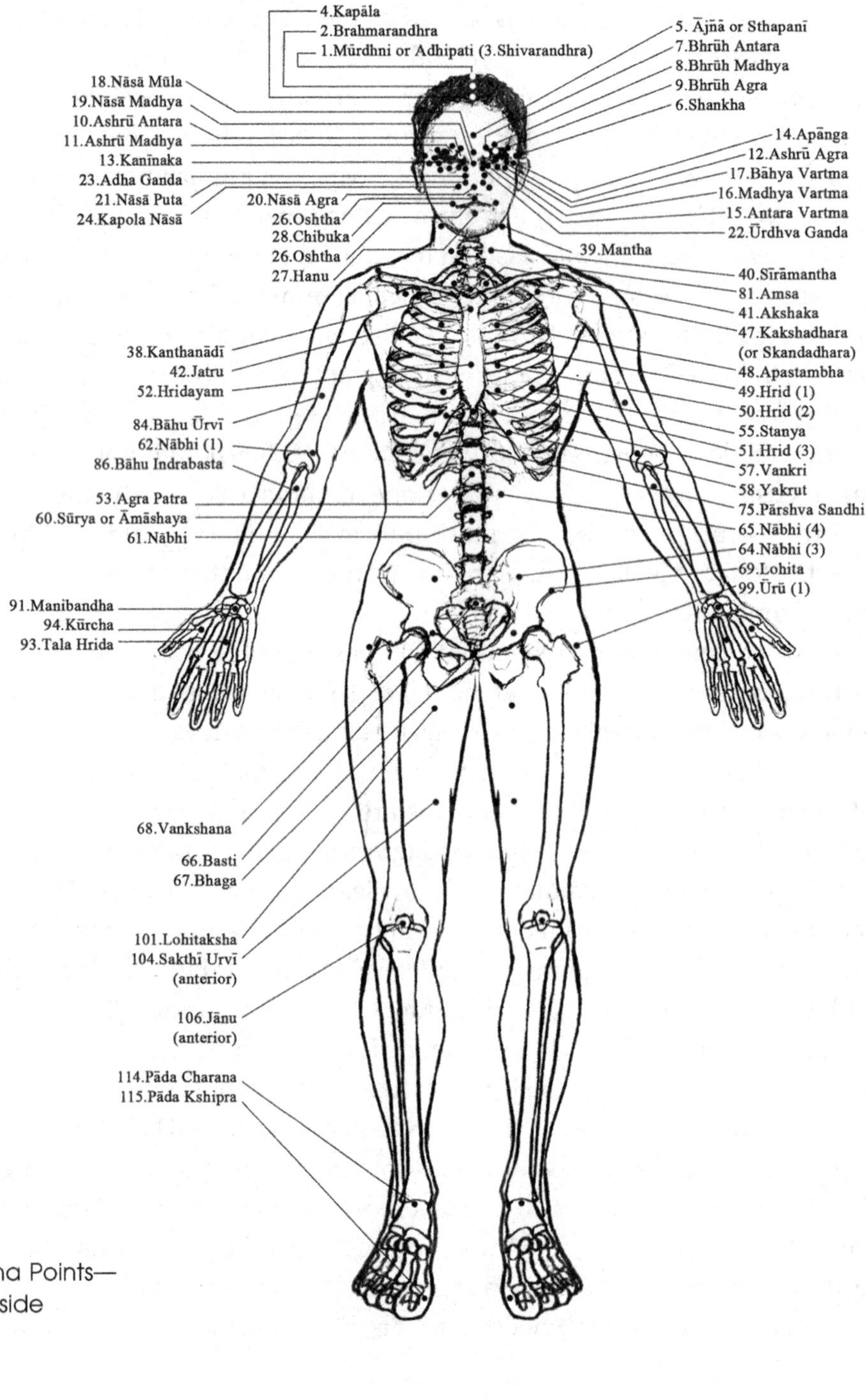
4.Kapāla
2.Brahmarandhra
1.Mūrdhni or Adhipati (3.Shivarandhra)
5. Ājñā or Sthapanī
7.Bhrūh Antara
8.Bhrūh Madhya
9.Bhrūh Agra
6.Shankha
18.Nāsā Mūla
19.Nāsā Madhya
10.Ashrū Antara
11.Ashrū Madhya
13.Kanīnaka
23.Adha Ganda
21.Nāsā Puta
24.Kapola Nāsā
20.Nāsā Agra
26.Oshtha
28.Chibuka
26.Oshtha
27.Hanu
14.Apānga
12.Ashrū Agra
17.Bāhya Vartma
16.Madhya Vartma
15.Antara Vartma
22.Ūrdhva Ganda
39.Mantha
40.Sīrāmantha
81.Amsa
41.Akshaka
47.Kakshadhara
(or Skandadhara)
48.Apastambha
49.Hrid (1)
50.Hrid (2)
55.Stanya
51.Hrid (3)
57.Vankri
58.Yakrut
75.Pārshva Sandhi
65.Nābhi (4)
64.Nābhi (3)
69.Lohita
99.Ūrū (1)
38.Kanthanādī
42.Jatru
52.Hridayam
84.Bāhu Ūrvī
62.Nābhi (1)
86.Bāhu Indrabasta
53.Agra Patra
60.Sūrya or Āmāshaya
61.Nābhi
91.Manibandha
94.Kūrcha
93.Tala Hrida
68.Vankshana
66.Basti
67.Bhaga
101.Lohitaksha
104.Sakthī Urvī
(anterior)
106.Jānu
(anterior)
114.Pāda Charana
115.Pāda Kshipra

Marma Points—
front side

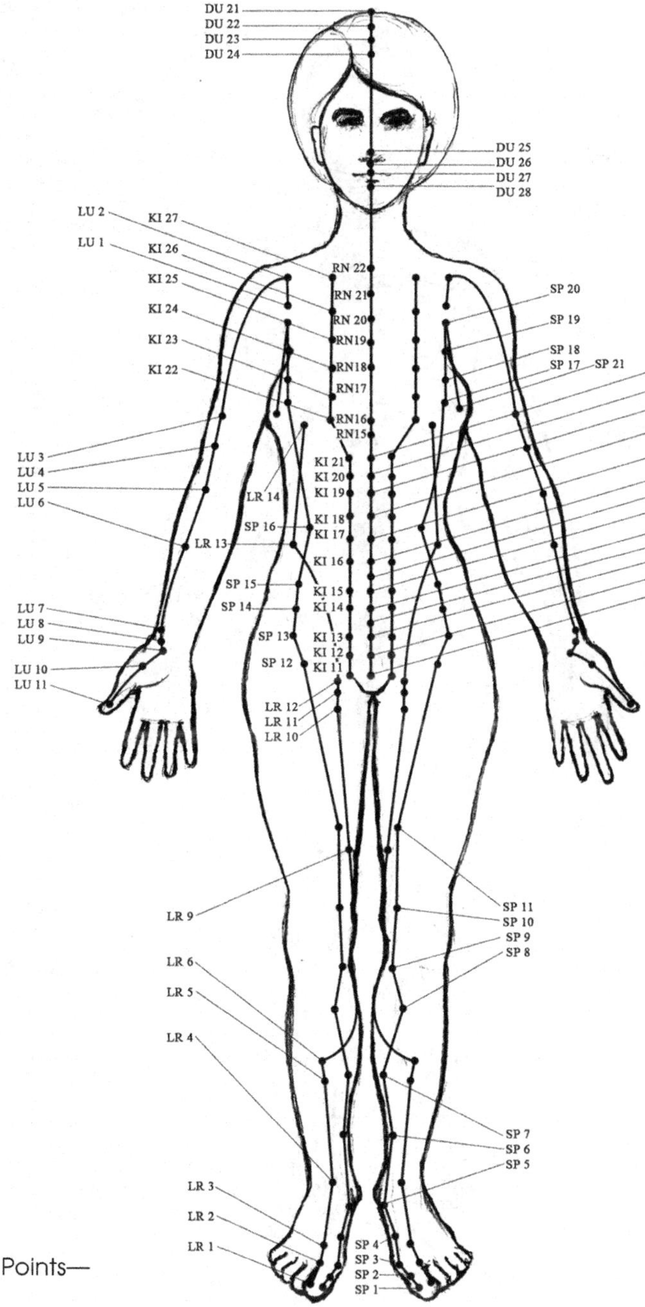

Acupuncture Points—
front side

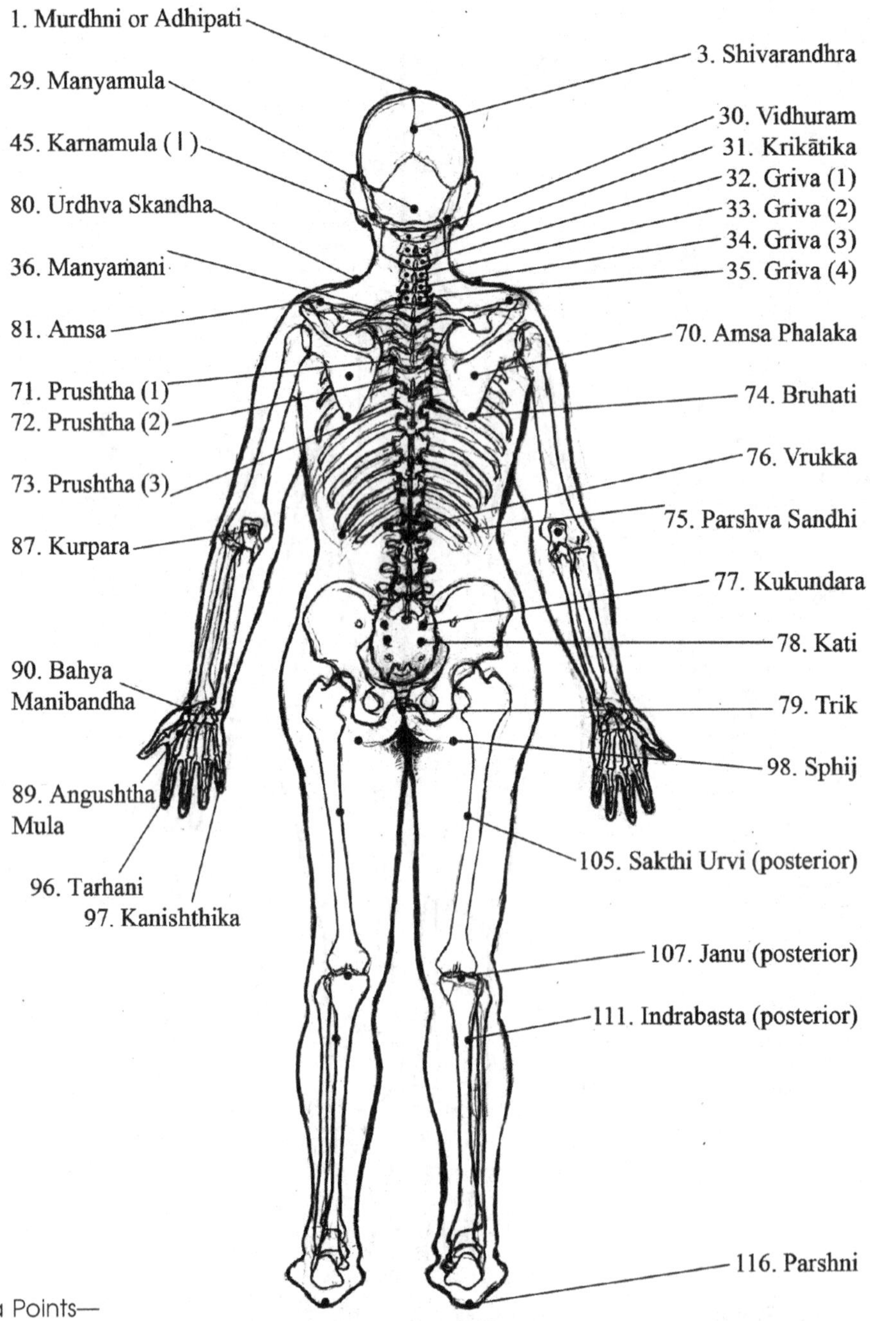
1. Murdhni or Adhipati
29. Manyamula
45. Karnamula (1)
80. Urdhva Skandha
36. Manyamani
81. Amsa
71. Prushtha (1)
72. Prushtha (2)
73. Prushtha (3)
87. Kurpara
90. Bahya Manibandha
89. Angushtha Mula
96. Tarhani
97. Kanishthika
3. Shivarandhra
30. Vidhuram
31. Krikātika
32. Griva (1)
33. Griva (2)
34. Griva (3)
35. Griva (4)
70. Amsa Phalaka
74. Bruhati
76. Vrukka
75. Parshva Sandhi
77. Kukundara
78. Kati
79. Trik
98. Sphij
105. Sakthi Urvi (posterior)
107. Janu (posterior)
111. Indrabasta (posterior)
116. Parshni

Marma Points—
back side

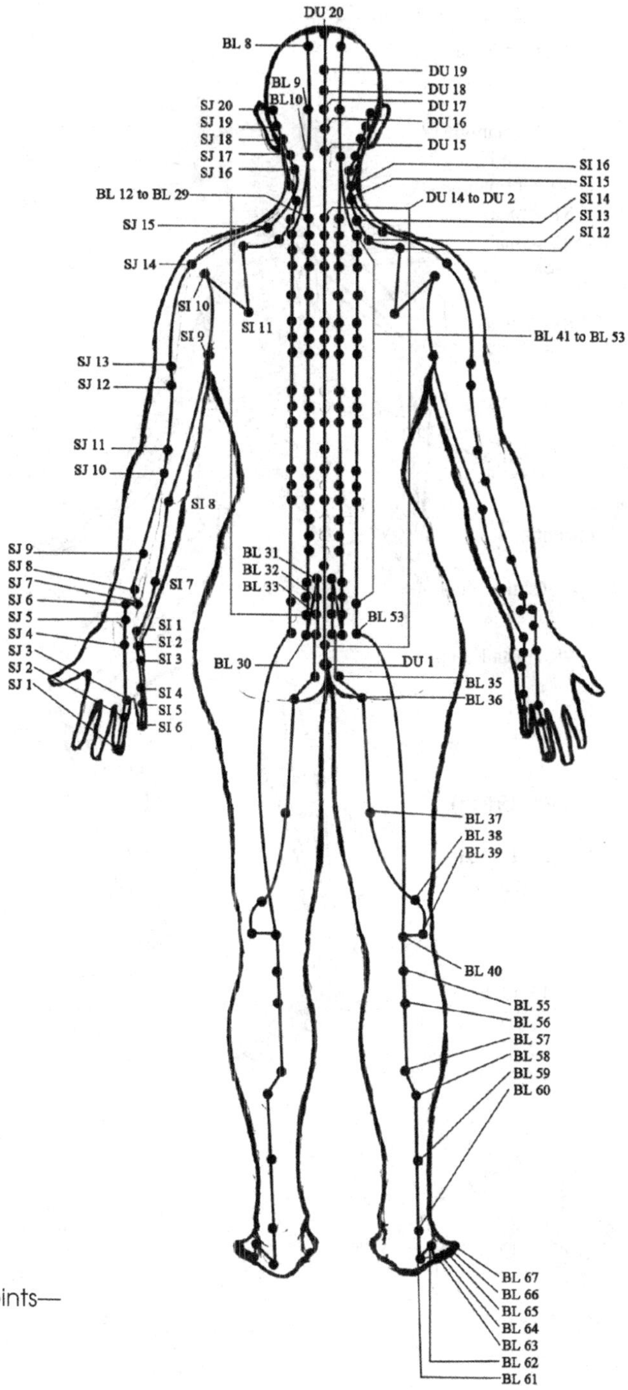

Acupuncture Points—
back side

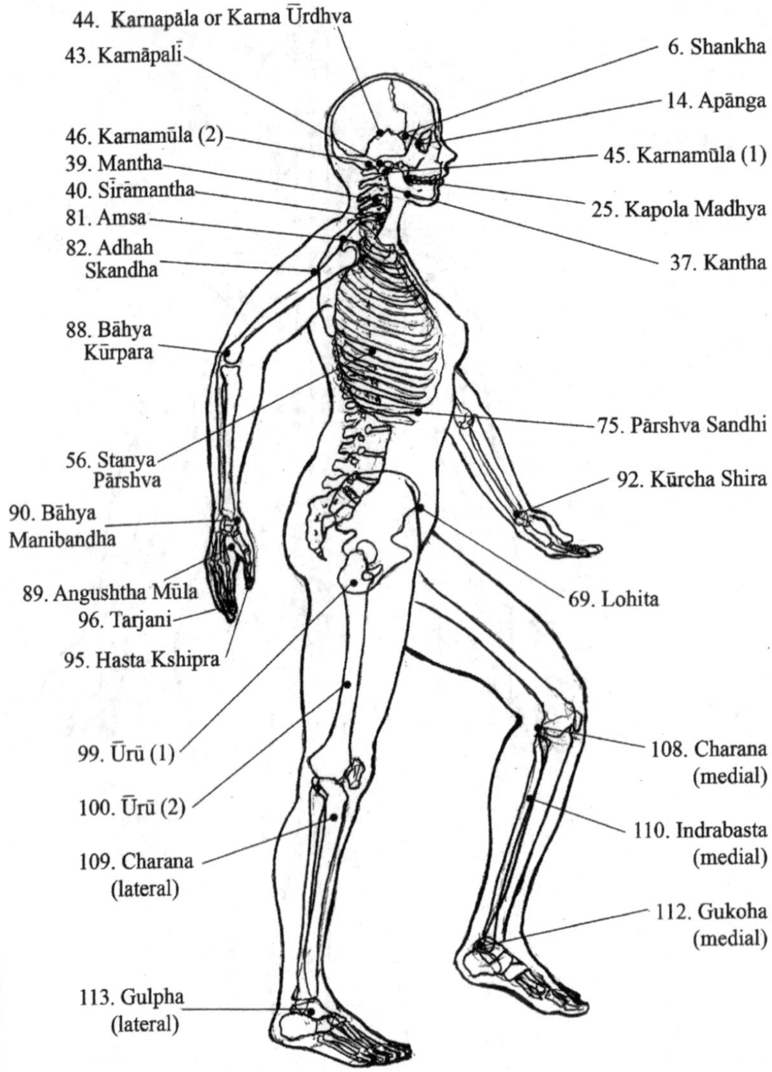
44. Karnapāla or Karna Ūrdhva
43. Karnāpalī
46. Karnamūla (2)
39. Mantha
40. Sīrāmantha
81. Amsa
82. Adhah Skandha
88. Bāhya Kūrpara
56. Stanya Pārshva
90. Bāhya Manibandha
89. Angushtha Mūla
96. Tarjani
95. Hasta Kshipra
99. Ūrū (1)
100. Ūrū (2)
109. Charana (lateral)
113. Gulpha (lateral)
6. Shankha
14. Apānga
45. Karnamūla (1)
25. Kapola Madhya
37. Kantha
75. Pārshva Sandhi
92. Kūrcha Shira
69. Lohita
108. Charana (medial)
110. Indrabasta (medial)
112. Gukoha (medial)

Marma Points—profile

Marma Points—intimate

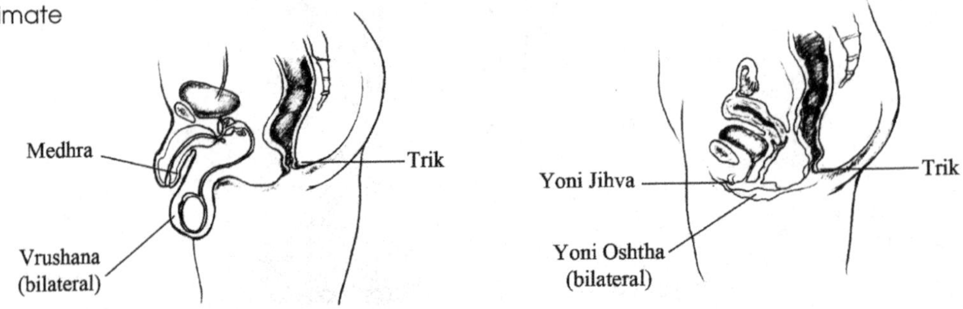
Medhra
Trik
Vrushana (bilateral)
Yoni Jihva
Trik
Yoni Oshtha (bilateral)

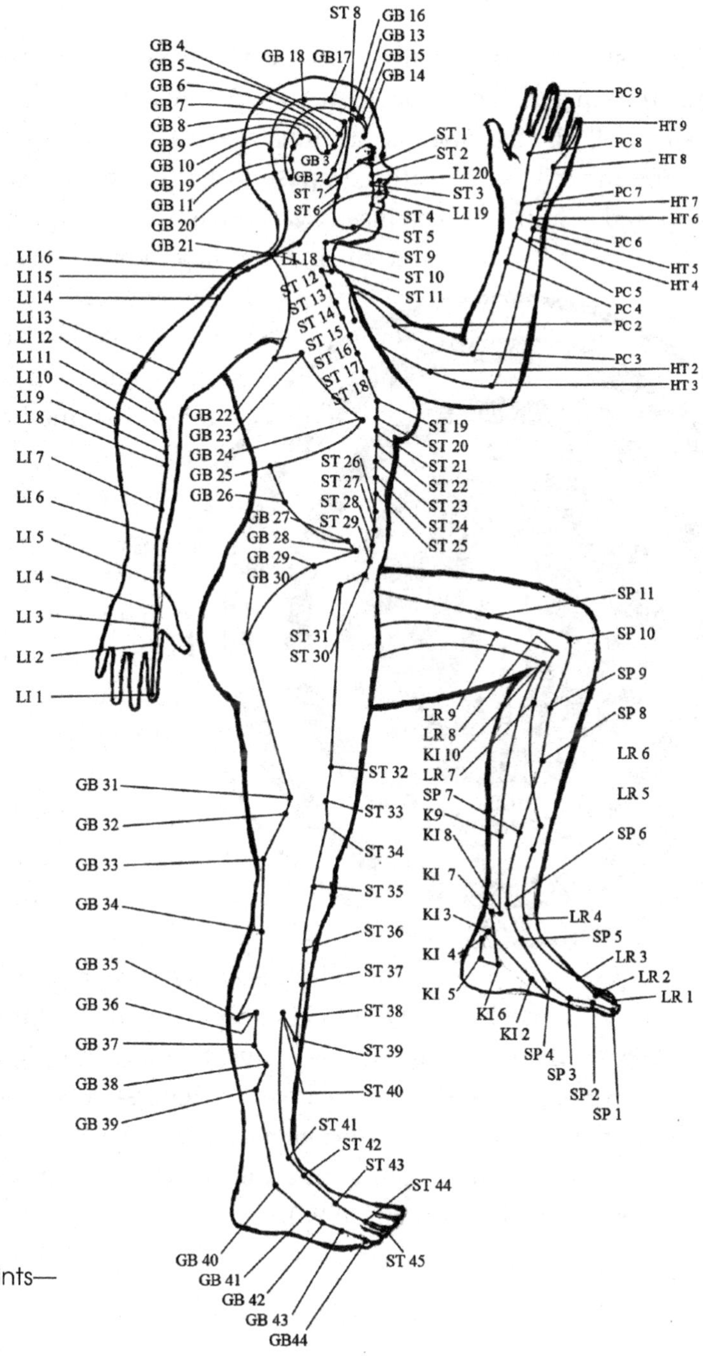

Acupuncture Points—
profile

THE KOŚAS

The kośas are "sheaths" or "casings." The earliest mention of the kośas in Yoga comes from the ancient *Taittirīya Upaniṣad* (2.7) where "the pure light of the transcendental Self" is described as: 1) anna-maya-kośa (the sheath composed of food); 2) prāṇa-maya-kośa (sheath composed of life force); 3) mano-maya-kośa (sheath composed of mind); 4) vijñāna-maya-kośa (sheath composed of awareness); and 5) ānanda-maya-kośa (sheath composed of bliss) (Feuerstein, 1997).

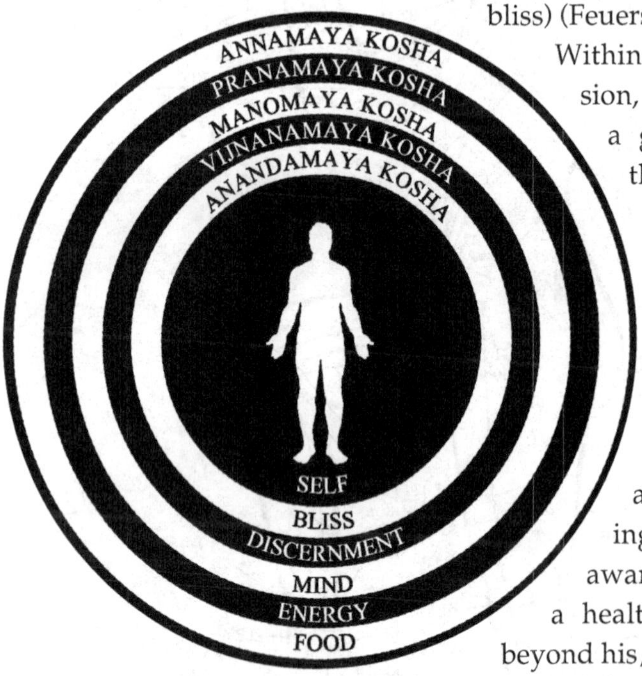

Within the context of a private session, I sometimes invite a client into a guided meditation involving the five kośas used in both Ayurveda and Indic Yoga therapies. This can be done before or at the end of an acupuncture session, Yoga Therapy āsana session, and/or prāṇāyāma practice. We often begin with the first kośa and end with the last, visualizing their existence to instill one's awareness of himself or herself as a healthy, vital individual existing beyond his/her biophysical and biochemical self. It is an effective reminder that the body is not just an object to mechanically *fix*. This deeper awareness provides the soil in which we help plant the seed of greater self-investigation and self-compassion and a doorway into experiencing greater self-love. As Feuerstein said, "All major spiritual traditions of the world sanction the belief that the physical body is not the only vehicle in which consciousness can express itself or in which the Spirit, or Self (ātman), manifests itself" (Feuerstein, 1997).

CAKRAS

Another option for guided meditation that can be used in the context of an acupuncture treatment is the awareness of *cakras*. The word *cakra*, meaning "wheel," or "to move," refers to "the psychoenergetic vortices forming the major 'organs' of the body composed of life energy (*prāṇa*)" (Feuerstein, 1997). Schools of "Yoga and Tantrism propose six principle centers (*shat-cara*), with a seventh center being thought of as transcending bodily existence" (Feuerstein, 1997). Although some books suggest that cakras have a direct correlation to nerve plexuses in Western science, many yogis have disagreed (Feuerstein, 1997).

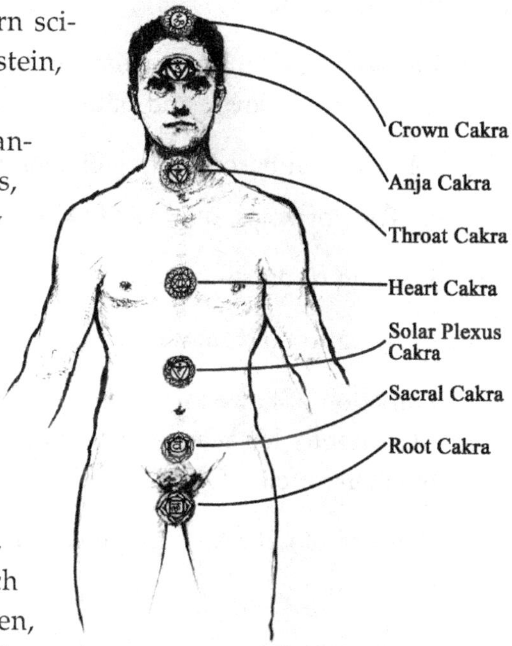

Within the "Eight Extraordinary Channels" used in acupuncture treatments, there are two channels that I commonly use to influence the cakras. The Ren Mai, which exists along the central axis of the front side of the body, and the Du Mai, which predominantly resides along the central axis of the backside of the body, both have points along their trajectories that can be utilized to influence the organ function, blood flow, or Qi, associated with each specific cakra (Needham and Gwei-Djen, 1980). One of my teachers, Dr. Mikio Sankey, Ph.D., founder of Esoteric Acupuncture, has written several wonderful books on the topic of blending acupuncture treatments with visualization exercises based on the understanding of the cakras and the importance of using sacred geometry in treatment protocols. Engaging a client to use visualization and meditative awareness on the cakras while they receive acupuncture treatment can not only enhance the treatment but is something that can then be used as an ongoing home practice, assisting the client in finding an inner tranquility and energetic sense of balance. This is one of many ways that my patient treatments integrate Yoga Therapy and Chinese Medicine practices.

PATIENT ASSESSMENTS AND TREATMENTS

Each practitioner of Chinese Medicine and/or of Yoga Therapy comes with a unique blend of practices stemming from the tradition(s) he/she follows. In my personal assessment and treatment examples below, the outlines for care are based on what I have found most effective, while treating each session and individual uniquely.

I. Patient assessments

  a. Questions about family history, lifestyle, occupation, relationships, diet, sleep, energy level, and pain scale (if relevant)

  b. Observation based on five elements

    i. Tone of voice, quality of skin, smell, and body type

  c. Reading of pulse

  d. Observation of tongue

  e. Palpation of key acupressure points (based on the teachings of Kiiko Matsumoto, her teacher Nagano, and handed down to me by my teacher, Stephen Stiteler, O.M.D., N.D.)

  f. Western blood tests, urinalysis, or referral to other practitioners for x-rays and MRIs

II. Evaluation of the three most common dysfunctions that impede treatment

  a. Excessive sympathetic nervous system (SNS) stress observed through pulse, quality of breathing, and/or symptoms of an overactive SNS that include possible insomnia, high blood pressure, and symptoms of inflammation in the system

  b. Digestive imbalances and the compromised ability to assimilate foods and take in nourishment

    i. Encourage balanced blood sugar levels through altering the person's dietary habits

ii. Support proper removal/release of toxins through eating high-fiber foods and/or using enzyme supportive food supplements

iii. Maintain hydration through drinking adequate amounts of water and eating essential fats

c. Other symptoms of disharmony that may be either acute or chronic

i. structural/postural

ii. organ function related

iii. emotional in nature

III. My personal treatment techniques utilizing both Chinese Medicine and Yoga Therapy

a. Acupuncture on the body utilizing the Twelve Primary Meridians and the Eight Extraordinary Meridians, or other known extra points; or the use of small powerful magnets on the hands that correlate to the acupuncture points on the body (based on the Korean hand system developed by Tae-Woo Yoo).

b. Acupressure, cupping, and massage techniques known as *gua sha* used to assist the movement of blocked *Qi*

c. Dietary recommendations and usually food-based nutritional supplements or ancient Chinese formulated herbal remedies

d. Suggestions for prāṇāyāma and/or Haṭha Yoga āsanas that the patient can do at home such as restorative postures to encourage more parasympathetic nervous system response for clients with adrenal stress or fatigue; or modifications of setu bandha sarvāṅgāsana (bridge pose) for clients with low back pain, to help strengthen underused hamstrings, adductors, and glutes.

e. A meditation practice that might involve bhāvana (guided imagery and meditation), an affirmation, or a mantra for the client to continue as a self-care practice at home

f. It is a common practice of mine to refer clients out for Western blood tests and urinalysis, or to refer them to other practitioners for x-rays and MRIs, using the best of what Eastern and Western assessment measures can offer

IV. Understanding outcome measures and ways to gauge if the healing is beneficial

a. Observing breathing patterns for signs of deep relaxation (steady, slow, unimpeded diaphragmatic breathing)
b. An increased quality of calm in client's nervous system and/or less awareness of anxiety or depression
c. A decline in pain scale (when relevant)
d. Results are often noticed by the client as a perceived change in the way he/she experiences his/her relationship to his/her own body or to the world outside, mainly with less strain, or a sense of resistance to what had ailed him/her when he/she first came in for treatment

---

RESEARCH STUDIES IN THE FIELDS OF YOGA THERAPY AND ACUPUNCTURE

Few exist, but the horizon is rich with published studies where both an acupuncture treatment and Yoga Therapy practices were observed, recorded with blind study, and outcomes measured, but I have observed positive results from the blending of these modalities with the majority of clients I have treated. In the contemporary medicine practices of China, and as is being taught in the current standards of practice within the U.S.-regulated Chinese Medicine schools, it is common practice to mix therapies founded on dissimilar Chinese and Western theories. The challenge is that it creates paradoxical ways of explaining and treating diseases, which does not work well for gaining well-established outcome measures in Western-based scientific research methods.

Currently, much of the data that exists to support the beneficial properties and outcomes of Chinese Medicine and Yoga Therapy has been derived from observational studies, and it is not considered empirical evidence. There are many more empirical studies that have been done on the positive effects on acupuncture alone than on Yoga Therapy. At the same time, many feasibility studies are emerging that justify and warrant further blind scientific study for both traditions of healing. Of all forms of studies, the least found are blind-controlled studies that control for sham or placebo effect, but there are more coming and more called for because existing empirical evidence suggests that these practices do in fact have a beneficial effect.

PARALLELED MODERN-DAY RISE IN POPULARITY

While we await additional studies to provide empirical evidence of positive outcome measures in both Chinese Medicine and Yoga Therapy, it is impressive to witness the rise in public popularity in the use of both modalities as a means of self-care. Acupuncture is currently licensed in most states within the United States. To date, more than 3,000 U.S. physicians have integrated acupuncture into their clinical practice and there are 20,000 licensed acupuncturists working in the United States overall (McMillen, 2011). According to the NIH's National Center for Complementary and Alternative Medicine (NCCAM), "3.1 million people tried acupuncture [in 2007], a million more than in 2002, to relieve discomfort caused by fibromyalgia, chemotherapy-induced nausea and vomiting, low back pain, and other ailments" (McMillen, 2011). This data also suggests up to "25% of people, regardless of nationality or ethnicity, will at some time try acupuncture, mostly for some kind of musculoskeletal pain" (McMillen, 2011).

In comparison, at the time of this publication, the most recent and reputable survey study on Yoga in 2012 was still focusing on Yoga as a practice rather than as a health science or treatment methodology. The study observed the number of Yoga practitioners in the United States and found that "8.7 percent of U.S. adults, or 20.4 million people, practice yoga, while 44.4 percent of non-practitioners were interested in trying Yoga (Sports Marketing Surveys USA, Yoga in America Study 2012). The top-five reasons for starting Yoga were: flexibility (78.3 percent), general conditioning (62.2 percent), stress relief (59.6 percent), improved overall health (58.5 percent), and physical fitness (55.1 percent).

Although we do not know how many physicians and healthcare practitioners have integrated Yoga Therapy as part of complementary care, the International Association of Yoga Therapists (IAYT) has reported approximately 3,400 members spanning over fifty countries worldwide (Kepner, 2014). There is a strong increase in interest for using Yoga within the context of other integrative medicines, but, as of yet, no specific demographic information exists documenting people who are using Yoga as a therapy and healing modality.

CONCLUSION

The respective integrative practices of what constitutes Chinese Medicine and Yoga Therapy are both intended to be used for health care, not sick care. Both are intended to optimize health of the individual on the levels of the physical body, biochemical constitution, and organ levels of the body, as well as emotionally and spiritually. Both models for wellness also shift one's relationship to his/her environment and the world at large. They are not intended to be strictly pathology-based models, and, yet, the statistics and research generally minimize the findings and effectiveness based on specific pathologies.

On a global level, medicine, traditions, and modalities continue to evolve. The majority of people in the field of Yoga Therapy are offering one-on-one care for a variety of issues beyond what is commonly offered in a group āsana class setting. The future of Yoga Therapy in application will likely take on a path similar to that of acupuncture and other Eastern health/clinical sciences. As is stated by Chinese Medicine scholar Dan Vercammen, "People who still practice medicine in an ancient way are fewer all the time, and certain traditions have disappeared or are officially discouraged or condemned as superstition. Chinese medicine—as it is practiced today—is no longer based on Chinese fundaments alone; changes and adaptations through history have made it more cosmopolitan" (Vercammen, 1997). Thus, will Yoga Therapy become regulated and pieces of the practices become utilized separately from other facets of Yoga Therapy, such as acupuncture getting utilized as a separate component of Western practice, separate from its parent science of Chinese Medicine? Only time will tell.

Enough healers and skilled practitioners in the ancient traditions inherent to Yoga Therapy exist to keep the practices alive. It is up to us, who care about the evolution of medicine, science, and education, to give honor to those traditions that are ancient while simultaneously embracing those that are emerging, mutually supportive, and effective. It is my hope that this publication and its collective wisdom will aid in achieving that goal.

REFERENCES

Balkin, J. M. *The Laws of Change: I Ching and the Philosophy of Life.* New York: Schocken Books, 2002. Print.

Burke, A., et al. "Acupuncture: An Introduction." National Center for Complimentary and Alternative Medicine (NCCAM). NCCAM Pub No.: D404. Created Dec. 2007. Web. 1 Nov. 2013. http://nccam.nih.gov/health/acupuncture/introduction.htm.

Casey, J. Select Historical Notes Concerning Ayurveda, Yoga Therapy, and Chinese Medicine. Los Angeles, CA. 2 Feb. 2014. Interview.

Chinese Health Qigong Association. "Wu Qin Xi." Public Physical Exercise Press, 2007. Web. http://classicqigong.com/wu-qin-xi/.

Deife, J. "Is Yoga Medicine?" *LA Yoga* (March 2007). Print.

Dupuis, C. "Introduction to Acupuncture and Chinese Medicine." 3 May 2006. Web. 22 April 2014. http://www.yinyanghouse.com/basics/introduction_to_acupuncture.

Feuerstein, G. *The Shambhala Encyclopedia of Yoga.* Boston: Shambhala, 1997. Print.

Kaptchuck, T. *The Web That Has No Weaver.* New York: McGraw-Hill, 2000. Print.

Lad, V., and A. Durve. *Marma Points of Ayurveda.* Albuquerque, NM: Ayurvedic Press, 2008. Print.

Macioca, G. *The Foundations of Chinese Medicine: A Comprehensive Text for Acupuncturists and Herbalists.* Edinburgh: Churchill Livingstone, 1989. Print.

McMillen, M. "Acupuncture Goes Mainstream: Why Doctors Are Increasingly Turning to Acupuncture to Help Their Patients." WebMD. 4 Jan. 2011. Web. 22 April 2014. http://www.webmd.com/balance/features/acupuncture-goes-mainstream.

Meriam-Webster Dictionary (online). "Enlightenment" (definition). 2014. Web. http://www.merriam-webster.com/dictionary/enlightenment.

Needham, J., and L. Gwei-Djen. *Celestial Lancets.* New York: Cambridge University Press, 1980. Print.

Powers, S. *Insight Yoga.* Boston: Shambhala Press, 2008. Print.

Stamps, J. *Holonomy: A Human Systems Theory, Systems Inquiry Series.* Salinas, CA: Intersystems Publications, 1980. Print.

Vercammen, D. "Traditional Chinese Medicine Today," *Oriental Medicine: An Illustrated Guide to the Asian Arts of Healing.* Editors: Jan Van Alphen, Anthony Aris. Boston: Shambhala, 1997. Print.

Wujastyk, D. "Theory and Practice of Ayurvedic Medicine," *Oriental Medicine: An Illustrated Guide to the Asian Arts of Healing.* Editors: Jan Van Alphen, Anthony Aris. Boston: Shambhala, 1997. Print.

Yoga Journal. "Yoga in America" study. Study conducted by Harris Interactive Service Bureau on behalf of Yoga Journal. 2012. Web. http://www.yogajournal.com/press/yoga_in_america.

AN INSTINCTIVE APPROACH TO MEDITATION THERAPY

Lorin Roche, Ph.D.

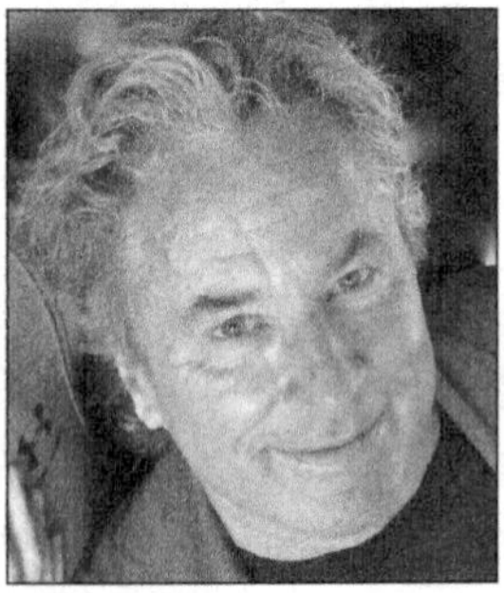

Lorin Roche began meditating in 1968 as part of a research project on the physiology of meditation at the University of California at Irvine. It was love at first sight—and touch and sound. He began training as a meditation teacher in 1969 and taught for the Transcendental Meditation organization from 1970 to 1975. Since 1976, he has been in private practice, developing and teaching meditation methods that accommodate individual uniqueness, so that people can customize everything to suit their nature. Lorin is the author of *Meditation Made Easy* and *The Radiance Sutras*, and, with his wife, Camille Maurine, *Meditation Secrets for Women*. He lives in Los Angeles and teaches worldwide.

OVERVIEW

Meditation is a catchall term that refers to innumerable techniques that can be done sitting quietly with the eyes closed. According to government statistics, more than 20 million people in the United States practice meditation, which is almost 10 percent of the adult population (Barnes, Bloom, and Nahin, 2008). Yet, because of the internal nature of meditation, no one specifically knows what these millions of people are actually doing in their meditations. Moreover, it can be difficult for individuals to find meditation techniques that are suitable for their individual constitution. Quite often people select practices that go against their nature and perpetuate or exacerbate preexisting imbalances on the physical, emotional, and mental levels. Since meditation is invisible internal behavior, it can be challenging

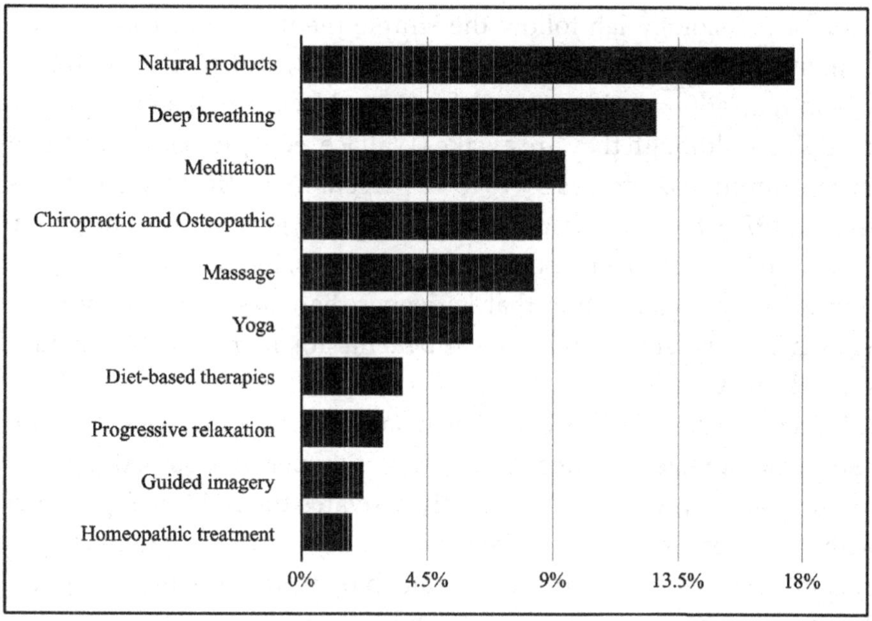

to detect what an individual meditator is doing and if it is good for his/her health. When meditators present themselves to alternative health practitioners with aches, pains, anxiety, digestive problems, and fatigue, occasionally their approach to meditation is part of the problem. With a few adjustments, however, their meditation practice can become part of the solution. This chapter highlights some points to keep in mind about meditation as a form of Yoga Therapy and provides a checklist of skills that meditators and practitioners may find useful in their practice.

SIMPLE, POWERFUL, INSTINCTIVE

Meditation can be simple. Select something you enjoy repeating—a word, sound, phrase, prayer, mental image, breath-counting sequence, or a muscular motion such as breathing or a mudrā (gesture). Attend to this in the same effortless way you attend to anything that attracts you. When your attention wanders off, return to your repetition without trying to block out thoughts (Beary and Benson, 1974; Roche, 1998).

Meditation can be powerful. In a series of studies at Harvard Medical School throughout the 1970s, Herbert Benson and his associates found that when experimental subjects in a physiology lab follow the simple meditation instructions described above, an integrated full-body response is activated, which creates profound restfulness and relaxation; within a few minutes, subjects are in a state of rest deeper than deep sleep, although they are awake (Wallace, et al., 1971). During meditation, oxygen consumption decreases by 10 to 17 percent in the first 3 to 5 minutes (Beary and Benson, 1974). By comparison, during sleep, oxygen consumption drops gradually by about 8 percent over a period of hours. Thus, meditation gives quick access to a kind of rest and relaxation that is deeper than sleep, and daily practice has been shown to have significant clinical benefits for many stress-related illnesses (Benson and Proctor, 2010).

Meditation is instinctive. The body has wonderful responsiveness built in, as part of our survival intelligence (Sapolsky, 1994). If you perceive something frightening in your environment, your body instantly activates the fight-or-flight response to deal with the emergency. If you even *think* of something frightening, your body responds in the same way—your heart rate, blood pressure, breathing, digestion, and blood chemistry are all immediately affected. Conversely, if you think of something peaceful and wonderful, the body responds by activating the parasympathetic, "rest and digest," relaxation response. Ultimately, we all have this built-in ability to activate the relaxation response, and it is as natural and instinctive as the stress response. Meditation can be considered a powerful, reliable, and efficient way of activating this relaxation and healing response, which is the mirror opposite of the stress response.

CASE REVIEWS: WHEN MEDITATION NEEDS THERAPEUTIC SUPPORT

■ Julianne

Julianne is forty-five, a Yoga teacher, and the mother of a teenage boy. Her Yoga studio is thriving, and, as the demands on her increase, she has been finding great relief in meditation sessions of 40 minutes to an hour. One morning she realized that she had been so deep in meditation for so long that she was late to leave the house and go teach Yoga. She got up quickly, not realizing that her legs had fallen asleep. She took a step and then . . . CRACK! She broke her ankle.

Julianne was practicing a svabhāva style of meditation. In Sanskrit, *svabhāva* means, "[one's] native place, own condition or state of being, natural state or constitution, innate or inherent disposition, nature, impulse, spontaneity." The Transcendental Meditation (TM) Technique, The Relaxation Response, Deepak Chopra's Primordial Sound Meditation, and The Art of Living's Sahaj Samādhi Meditation are all examples of this approach, each with its own variations and modifications to the basic formula. The universal technique is to be natural with yourself and accept the desire to instinctively go into meditation as a spontaneous impulse. Unfortunately, Julianne did not realize how deep she was going in her svabhāva state because it just felt normal, and it led to some pretty drastic consequences.

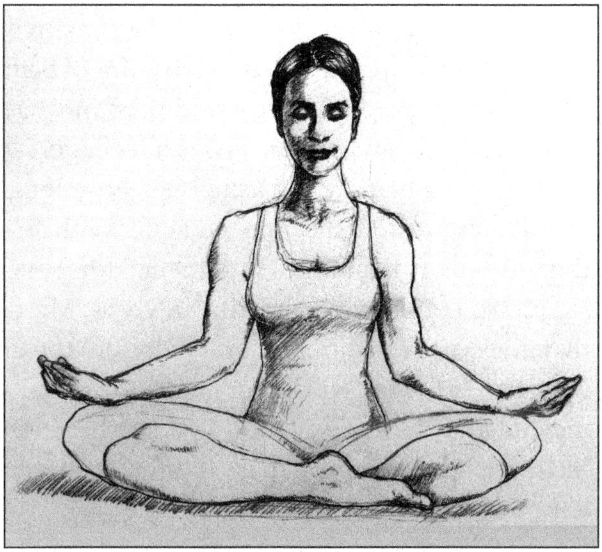

Ankle injuries—sprains and breaks—related to meditation are not uncommon in female Yoga practitioners and teachers, who tend to sit cross-legged and almost cannot conceive of meditating in any other position than being on the floor. I suggested Julianne sit in a chair to meditate, with her feet on the ground to additionally ground her, but she refused. Finally, with some resistance, Julianne agreed to meditate with back support and her legs extended, at least part of the time. It is often a matter of pride with Yoga practitioners, wanting to fit the body into the stereotypical cross-legged pose. The solution is to apply a simple hamstring stretch or ankle rolls, before getting up, to wake up the legs and ankles and make sure the transition to being more physical and active is comfortable.

Marcy

Marcy is twenty-four and a Yoga teacher. She came for a session complaining that meditation makes her feel "spacey" and "unfocused." She said that, on days when she meditates, she does not function well and feels as if she is "stoned." And yet, on days when she does not meditate, she feels that she is missing out on an important part of her life. This struggle had been going on for several years.

When we sat together, it seemed as if her meditation practice was natural and beautiful. Marcy is one of those rare individuals that, when she closes her eyes, is immediately in a vast and peaceful inner world. When I inquired into more detail, I was surprised to hear that, when she meditates, she stays there for about 45 minutes. I said, "That is too much for you, for your body. Where did you get the idea that you should meditate for that long?" I knew from my own personal experience of starting meditation at age 18, that, with young people, too many minutes of meditation per day can make one overly sensitive—touch, hearing, vision, and even taste and smell are amplified to the point of being distracting. Marcy then explained that both her parents were Buddhists and had been meditating since before she was born. One day when she was a teenager, she told her father that she had been exploring meditation. He asked her how long she meditated each time, and she said 20 minutes. He then looked at her with an expression of scorn and said, "Anything less than 45 minutes is pathetic, don't even bother unless you are going to go for it." So that became her rule. In years, Marcy had not even considered the idea that all bodies are different and therefore the dosage of meditation time should be adjusted for what works for that individual with his/her lifestyle. She experimented and ultimately found that she functions the best with 15 to 20 minutes of meditation in the morning, in a seated pose, and a 10-minute napping style of meditation in the late afternoon.

Matthew

Matthew is twenty-eight and works in finance. He came in for a session with me a few months after returning from India, where he had been on a long meditation retreat. He had been doing a technique that involved concentrating on the third eye, the Ajna center in the forehead. In India, he was closely supervised by a teacher, who kept saying, "Be one-pointed!" and encouraged him to try harder and concentrate intensely. Matthew now complained that, whenever he meditated, he got a headache. If he continued the practice, the headache just got worse. Even by mentioning meditation, he said he could feel a headache coming on.

Matthew and I explored a variety of different meditation styles involving breathing and movement, but nothing worked. The habit of straining to concentrate was too firmly embedded in him. The only thing that seemed to give him relief was to go outside and take a slow, meditative walk with his eyes open. So, I assigned him walking meditations and invited him to come back and see me again in the future. Nine months later Matthew returned and was much improved. He was not getting headaches anymore; however, if he did a sitting meditation with eyes closed, a slight headache began to return. The style of meditation he had been practicing when he first came to me was simply not suitable for his constitution and straining to make it work just gave him somewhat of a "sprained third eye."

Jake

Jake is thirty-nine and a policeman in a large metropolitan area. Previously, he was in the military and saw combat in Iraq and Afghanistan. He began the practice of Transcendental Meditation (TM) several years ago, and liked the relaxation, but found that the TM left him in an unpleasant state of being "loose and anxious." He went to his meditation teacher several times to be "checked," and the teacher told him to continue with the practice, that the unpleasant symptoms would pass. Jake could tell that he "was being fed the party line," and that the teacher was not really listening to him. It is part of the central system of TM teachers that the practice of TM cannot have any negative effects and that it is a universally beneficial technique for all people of every type. Jake continued doing TM for several months and only felt himself getting worse. He reported to me that practicing TM in the morning left him feeling slightly dissociated all day. He contacted me to see if I had any ideas that could help him adjust his meditation practice so that he could still go function as a policeman after doing it. We explored a variety of different practices but nothing clicked for him, except for one technique that Jake invented on his own: a breathing meditation in which he focused on the rhythm and sensations of touch. When he practices this instinctive breathing and touch meditation in the morning for 20 minutes, Jake said he feels nicely relaxed and alert all day.

Olivia

Olivia is twenty and in college. She had been practicing meditation for nine months, using an approach she learned at the Yoga classes she regularly attends. She came for a session and reported that she loves meditation, but that she suspects it is somehow making her depressed. Her best friend pointed out to her that, since she began meditating, she was calmer, but she was also lacking in vitality and seemed to be a bit out of touch with reality. When I asked Olivia to describe her meditation procedure, essentially what she thinks the rules of meditation are, she emphasized blocking out thoughts to quiet her mind and she made a warding off gesture with her hands. Olivia had internalized the often-repeated suggestion that, in meditation, you are supposed to push away distractions and concentrate on your object of attraction like a mantra. For some people, this "blocking" approach to meditation does not have much of a negative effect. However, in Olivia's case, her meditation practice was actively creating blockage of her enthusiasm for life. Metaphorically speaking, if her cakras were flowers, they immediately wilted in the stultifying atmosphere she was creating in herself.

I asked Olivia to tell me about a typical morning before she began meditating. She described her routine of getting ready, selecting clothes, doing her hair, and feeling excited about all the people she was going to talk to and hang out with during the day. In short, in the mornings, Olivia mentally choreographed her day and mobilized her excited prāṇa (life force) to be ready for each meeting, each event, each person. This was a natural part of her healthy approach to her life. When she began meditating, what she began doing was taking 20 minutes out of her morning to practice blocking this very excitement that was so central to her individual human style. When I explained to Olivia that it is okay to just sit there in meditation, simmering with excitement and wiggling with joy at the thought of the upcoming day, she was incredulous and looked at me as if I were putting her on. "But I have *never* heard *anyone* say *anything* like that," she replied. I said, "Meditation is infinitely customizable. We each have to modify the practice so that it suits our character and daily life. You have been practicing a style of meditation that perhaps goes with someone else's character and daily life, but it's not yours." That was all Olivia needed, just a small adjustment of her attitude, to welcome her own impulses of life and prāṇa flowing through her.

Violet

Violet is thirty-five and has been divorced for two years. She began meditating soon after the divorce and has had some beneficial effects, but she is bothered by intrusive thoughts and memories of abuse she suffered in childhood and the fights that led to her divorce. In our first session, we spent a lot of time with Violet just talking about the thoughts and emotions that were "intruding" on her meditations and disturbing her. In the second session, I explained to Violet that, when a person relaxes, he/she naturally becomes aware of what he/she is tense about. Fear and distressing emotions can arise in meditation only to be soothed and released. Gradually over time, the painful memories are healed by the ease and relaxation of meditation. This is how the inner healing happens. Violet and I did several sessions in which I invited her to enter a relaxed state and then welcome her feelings, her memories, and the story of how she came to be here. In this way, Violet learned to accept this "unstressing" as part of meditation and experienced significant benefits from her meditation practice.

Riley

Riley is twenty-five and a gourmet chef. She had been meditating on her own for four months and came for a session because she thought she was doing something wrong in her meditation. We meditated together, and she described sensations of "melting, falling, expanding, spinning, electric, pins and needles, achy, clammy, alert, sleepy, alive, buzzing with excitement, dizzy, dull, blocked, and breathless." You could say that Riley brings to the experience of her body during meditation the same kind of intense aesthetic she brings to tasting food: everything is vibrantly alive. I explained to her that we are usually not aware when we are this deeply restful, and relaxation can be very intense. Meditators often report feeling, "bubbly, burning, faint, buzzy, speedy, prickly, tender, intolerably vulnerable, pulsing, radiating, tense, thick, tingly, shivery, and tremulous" (Roche, 1987). All Riley needed was the knowledge that when she meditated she was awake and in a state of rest deeper than sleep and that whatever sensations came to her were okay.

Logan

Logan is fifteen and decided on his own to come for a session and pay with his own money. His presenting problems, which he stated as a kind of complaint against himself, were that he was always restless and his mind wandered a lot during class. In essence, he didn't like school, but he realized he was doomed to spend a couple more years in it. I asked him to give me an example of a time when his mind was wandering, and he mentioned that afternoon's math class. I then asked him to tell me about the particular math problem he was working on and to describe what happens in his mind, second by second, as he focuses on the numbers. Logan closed his eyes for a while and then opened them and reported with surprise, "The numbers turn to colors, like multicolored neon, and start moving around." I asked him if this was new, or if it seemed like his mind always was that way. He said he thought that his mind was always doing this, and he just now noticed. Being a teenager, he was slightly ashamed of the way his mind was functioning and thought maybe something was wrong with him.

As a way of getting him to lighten up, I grabbed a copy of the *Bhagavad Gītā* and read to him from the section in which Krishna is listing the Yoga siddhis (supernatural powers, skills), including aṇima (smallness, minuteness, fineness, atomic nature) and mahimat (greatness, largeness). "Numbers are an indication of small or large," I informed him, "and the ability to close your eyes and think in numbers is a kind of Yoga. And it is a form of play—there are whole meditations in which you pretend you are smaller than an atom, and then you let your awareness extend to being infinitely large." We explored some more and developed a meditation for him to practice for 5 minutes before doing his homework, in which he visualizes a series of numbers and gives them permission to be as vivid and energetic as they want. As the numbers are dancing around, lighting up his inner world, he is to enjoy his breathing and let it be smooth, regular, and even. "Let your breathing remind you to be relaxed."

Logan gave the overall sense of being a very healthy teenage boy, with wild impulses that were distracting him from being able to function well at school. In terms of a prescription, he needed just a taste of detachment—the ability to step back from the compelling intensity of his ideas and sensations, and practice calmness—but not so much that he would suppress his natural excitement. For Logan, meditation became a kind of video game he could play in his mind, with his eyes closed, in which he could witness the desires that seemed to be continually jumping out of all of his cakras, and then decide which ones to act on and which ones to simply enjoy as internal movies. Logan took to meditation quickly and practiced every day before doing his homework, and he found that his ability to focus was much improved.

A CHECKLIST OF SKILLS

If we consider meditation as antar-yoga (internal Yoga), then, unlike āsana practice, we must realize that very few meditators ever get skilled "corrections" to their practice. The knowledge of how to modify a practice to suit an individual's constitution is not widespread and interviews show that most people who practice meditation at some point experience negative side effects (Otis, 1984).

If a meditation practitioner comes to you for a session or you're looking at your own practice, here is a checklist you may find useful for developing the micro-skills of a seated practice that are suitable to the person's nature and may help correct any tendencies that are putting him/her out of balance:

- ❑ **Acceptance of needs.** The first thing to check is the initial attitude the person has in approaching meditation: "Are you accepting your need for rest, time to sort yourself out, and a time and space to feel your emotions?" Communicate in some way, "Meditation is a place where you can just be yourself."
- ❑ **Posture.** Check the person's posture for meditation and make sure it is suitable for his/her body given that he/she may be sitting that way in a deep hypometabolic state every day for a significant amount of time. It is important to make sure he/she is not defaulting to the cross-legged pose because "it how one is supposed to meditate." Remember too that sitting meditation is only appropriate for some people; whereas, walking meditations may be more appropriate for others.
- ❑ **Naturalness.** In a svabhāva type of meditation, the student selects a mantra or focus they are attracted to and enjoy. This makes the process of thinking it, and returning to it, effortless. When people make up their own mantras, they are often more effective than anything they can get from one of the meditation schools; Sanskrit mantras are beautiful, but many Americans feel uncomfortable using the name of a Hindu goddess, for example.
- ❑ **Effort.** Make sure the meditator is not using any extra effort in his/her technique, unless that truly is part of the practice. In an instinctive style of meditation, there is no straining, and it is enough to just "be" with one's object of attraction.
- ❑ **Closing the eyes.** People tend to close their eyes too soon. Encourage and allow the eyes to close naturally when they are ready and know that it is okay to just sit there with the eyes open until they do.

- ❑ **Take a welcoming attitude toward all thoughts, emotions, and "distractions."** With the eyes closed, notice thoughts coming and going. Some thoughts will have tension, urgency, and/or other unsettling emotions. Other thoughts will be your to-do list, your brain's way of organizing the flow of your day. Welcome all these thoughts, feelings, and sensations. This is just your brain doing its housecleaning. Afterward, if you allow the thoughts to flow through you, you will feel clearer. But during the practice, the brain is busy. Doing the dishes. Cleaning the closet. Polishing the valuables.
- ❑ **Accept the rhythms of experience.** When the body enters the restorative parasympathetic state, it is not a flat state; there is usually a continuous cycling of sensations of relaxation and stress release. When the body begins to relax, muscles relax and let go of chronic tension. When the muscles let go, whatever fears made the meditator tense will sometimes come to the foreground of one's awareness in order to be felt and healed. This is a natural process. This is how the body and mind heal.
- ❑ **Exit gradually.** Make sure to spend 3 to 5 minutes gently, gradually, and progressively activating the body after meditations of 10 minutes or more. Sit there, aware that you are going to exit the meditation, but just stay there with the eyes closed for at least 3 minutes. Then, open the eyes a bit and close them. Breathe a few deeper breaths. Again, open the eyes. Then, close them. Make sure you have caught up with yourself on all levels before getting up.

CONCLUSION

Millions of people are out there practicing a variety of techniques that go by the name meditation. Yet, almost all meditators are completely unsupervised in their practice and do not have access to someone who can help them adapt the standard practices to suit their individual constitution. Meditation teachers tend to give group instruction and are usually not oriented to think in terms of adapting the techniques to suit an individual.

Professor Tirumalai Krishnamacharya emphasized that a Yoga teacher must always consider his/her students and ask, "Is this practice that I am teaching appropriate for this particular student?" (Mohan, 2010). Specifically, the practices are to be appropriate for that individual's deha (body, shape, appearance, mass), vṛttibheda (differences in mental modifications), and mārga (path, route, way, passage). Thus, Yoga Therapists and alternative healthcare providers who understand how to adapt treatments to individuals may be the only available resource for a meditator to get "corrections" to their practice.

Meditators are often practicing in a way that gives mixed blessings. They develop some inner peace and relaxation but also can harm themselves by applying a technique that does not quite fit with their nature and/or daily life. The more every aspect of meditation practice is tailored to suit the needs of the individual, the better it will work. A daily meditation practice in accord with one's body, mind, and way of life has the potential to produce measurable enhancements to physical and emotional health: blood pressure is normalized, inflammation is reduced, indications of heart disease are reduced, and the stress hormones circulating in the blood tend to be reduced (Benson and Proctor, 2010). Subjectively, meditators report an increased sense of energy, joy, and ease in life. When a person's meditation does not seem to be working, sometimes it is enough to simply suggest a tiny change in the practice; other times it may be necessary to point out that they may have outgrown the particular technique they are using and it is time to move on and find a different approach.

Whenever a person is in a nicely balanced state as a result of a treatment, you can invite him/her to sit for 5 or 10 minutes and memorize the sensations. Have them remember the feeling of being in a state of balance. Help them to bond with the balanced state, give it permission to continue, and have it become an inspiration for their technique, so that when they practice meditation, they are practicing being in a state of health and flow, all the elements of their being functioning in harmony. In the Yoga tradition, one of the words for meditation technique is *yukti,* which has many meanings: union, conjunction, connection, practice, and application. In medical treatment, *yukti* has the meaning, "rational application of reason to diagnose and treat" (Roche, 2014). Alternative health practitioners have a profound role to play in helping meditators move from an irrational imposition of techniques that go against their nature to skillful application of just those practices that serve their individual *mārga,* their path through life. In this way, when meditation is employed as part of an integrated mind-body approach to healing, the ancient tradition is brought alive, refreshed, and integrated into the pulse of modern life in the Western world.

REFERENCES

Barnes, P. M., B. Bloom, and R. Nahin *CDC National Health Statistics Report #12.* "Complementary and Alternative Medicine Use Among Adults and Children: United States, 2007." 24 pp. 10 Dec. 2008. Web. PDF, press release, and graphics available at http://nccam.nih.gov/news/camstats/2007.

Beary, J. F., and H. Benson. "A Simple Psychophysiologic Technique Which Elicits the Hypometabolic Changes of the Relaxation Response." *Psychosomatic Medicine* 36 (1974): 115–20. Print.

Benson, H., and W. Proctor. *Relaxation Revolution.* New York: Scribner, 2010. Print.

Maurine, C., and L. Roche. *Meditation Secrets for Women.* San Francisco: HarperOne, 2001. Print.

Mohan, A. G. *Krishnamacharya: His Life and His Teachings.* Boston: Shambhala, 2010. Print.

Monier-Williams Sanskrit-English Dictionary, p. 1276. Print.

Otis, L. "Adverse Effects of Transcendental Meditation." *Meditation: Classic and Contemporary Perspectives.* Eds. D. Shapiro, and R. Walsh. New York: Aldine, 1984. Print.

Roche, L. *The Semantic Structure of Meditative Experience.* Ph.D. Dissertation, University of California at Irvine, Social Sciences Department, 1987. Print.

——. *Meditation Made Easy.* San Francisco: HarperOne, 1998. Print.

——. *The Radiance Sutras: 112 Gateways to the Yoga of Wonder & Delight.* Boulder: Sounds True, 2014. Print.

Sapolsky, R. *Why Zebras Don't Get Ulcers.* New York: St. Martin's Press, 1994. Print.

Wenger, D., A. Broome, and S. Blumberg. "Ironic Effects of Trying to Relax Under Stress." *Behavior Research and Therapy* 35.1 (1997): 11–21. Print.

AYURVEDA AND YOGA: COMPLEMENTARY THERAPEUTICS

Vasant Lad, M.A.Sc., B.A.M.S.

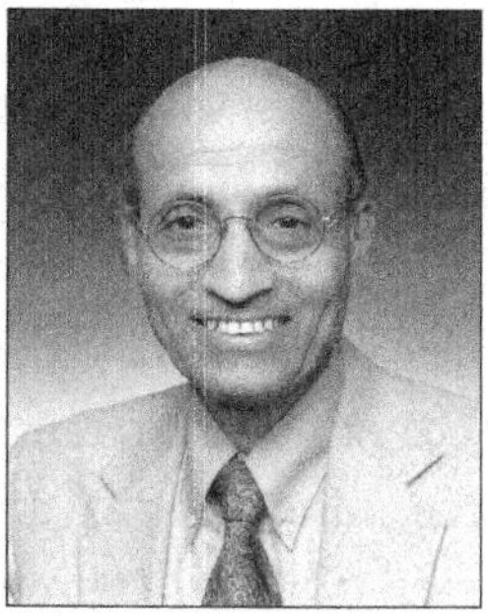

A native of India, **Vasant Lad** is one of the current global leaders in the field of Ayurvedic Medicine. Dr. Lad served as the medical director of the Ayurveda Hospital in Pune, India, after serving as a professor of clinical Ayurvedic Medicine for fifteen years. He holds a B.A. in Ayurvedic medicine and surgery from the University of Pune and a M.A. in Ayurvedic science from Tilak Ayurved Mahavidyalaya. Dr. Lad's academic and practical training include the study of allopathy (Western medicine) and surgery as well as traditional Ayurveda. He has more than 500,000 copies of his books in print in the United States alone, and his work has been translated into more than twenty languages. Currently, Dr. Lad is the chief director of the famed Ayurvedic Institute in Albuquerque, New Mexico, and he travels around the world teaching workshops and trainings.

OVERVIEW AND DEFINITION OF AYURVEDA

Ayurveda is considered by many scholars to be the oldest healing science. In Sanskrit, *Ayurveda* means "the science of life." Ayurvedic knowledge originated in India more than 5,000 years ago and is often called the "Mother of All Healing." It stems from the ancient Vedic culture and was taught for many thousands of years in an oral tradition from accomplished masters to their disciples. Some of this knowledge was set to print a few thousand years ago, but much of it is inaccessible. The principles of many of the natural healing systems now familiar in the West have their roots in Ayurveda, including homeopathy, naturopathy, allopathy, and Polarity Therapy. Hence, Ayurveda encompasses the whole of life.

A SHARED HISTORY BETWEEN YOGA AND AYURVEDA

Yoga and Ayurveda have their roots in the six ancient systems of Indian philosophy: Sāṁkhya, Nyāya, Vaiśeṣika, Mimāṁsā (Pūrva-mimāṁsā), Vedānta (Uttara-mīmāṁsa), and Yoga. According to Vedic philosophy at the time of the Vedas, an expert yogī was a good Ayurvedic physician and an Ayurvedic physician was also a good yogi. Thus, Yoga and Ayurveda are and always have been concurrent and inherent within each other, and, when practiced together, they form a great spiritual discipline.

The yogic system of philosophy as well as the Ayurvedic system of medicine both accept that śarīra (body), sattva (mind), and ātman (consciousness) are the holy trinity, or foundation of life. But, the overlapping of the traditions does not stop there. The languages are similar too. Yoga talks about the seven dhātus (tissues of the body): rasa (plasma), rakta (blood), māṁsa (muscle), meda (adipose), asthi (bone and cartilage), majjas (nerve, marrow, and connective), and śukra/ ārtava (male/female reproductive), and Ayurveda speaks of all seven dhātus. Yoga highlights the doṣas—vata, pitta, and kapha—and Ayurveda also highlights the doṣas. Yoga says to do Yoga to enhance prāṇa (life force, breath, circulation), tejas (essence of life, flame of intelligence), and ojas (vitality, immunity, well-being), and so does Ayurveda. Even the goals of Ayurveda and Yoga are very similar, and they are represented as the four pillars of life: dharma, artha, kāma, and mokṣa. Dharma is righteous duty; artha is monetary success; kāma is the fulfillment of positive desire;

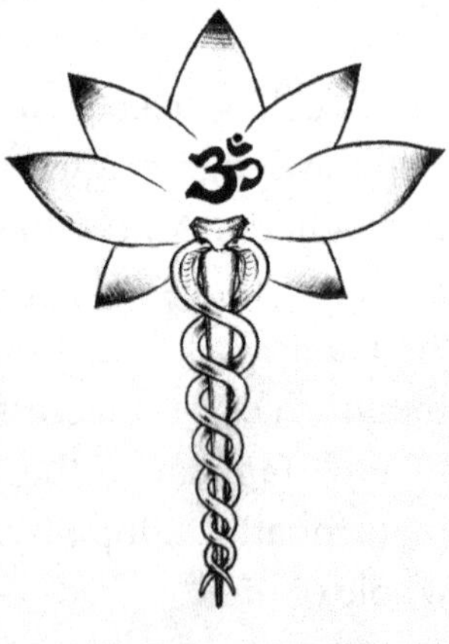

A Definition of Ayurveda

hitāhitaṁ sukhaṁ duḥkhaṁ āyustasya hitāhitaṁ mānaṁ ca tat ca yatroktaṁ āyurvedaḥ sa ucyate.

That (science) is designated as Ayurveda where advantageous and disadvantageous as well as happy and unhappy (states of) life along with what is good and bad for life, its measures and life itself are described.

***Caraka Saṁhitā, Sūtrasthānaṁ*, Chapter 1, verse 41**

and mokṣa is enlightenment or self-realization. Keeping these four pillars in balance in both systems leads one to perfect health in the physical, mental, and spiritual realms. Altogether, these two parallel systems of Yoga and Ayurveda support, enhance, and share with each other in many ways in order to bring radical changes in the lives of practitioners and clients.

THE DOṢAS

Just as everyone has a unique fingerprint, each person has a particular pattern of energy—an individual combination of physical, mental, and emotional characteristics—which comprises their own constitution. This constitution is determined right at the time of fertilization by a number of factors and remains the same throughout one's life. It is the blueprint of an individual's life recorded as genetic code.

Many factors, both internal and external, act upon us to alter this balance and reflect as changes in one's constitution from the balanced state. Examples of these emotional and physical stresses include one's emotional state, diet and food choices, lifestyle, seasons and weather, physical trauma, work, and family relationships. Once these factors are understood, one can take appropriate actions to nullify or minimize their effects or eliminate the causes of imbalance and reestablish one's original constitution. Balance is the natural order; imbalance is disorder. Health is order; disease is disorder. Therefore, the potential for order lies within disorder. Inside the body, there is a constant interaction between order and disorder. When one understands the nature and structure of disorder, one can reestablish order.

The ancient texts of Ayurveda identify three basic types of energy or functional principles that are present in everyone and everything. Since there are no single words in English that convey these concepts, we use the original Sanskrit words *vāta, pitta,* and *kapha.* These principles can be related to the basic biology of the body.

Energy is required to create movement so that fluids and nutrients get to the cells, enabling the body to function. Energy is also required to metabolize the nutrients in the cells and is called for to lubricate and maintain the structure of the cell. Vāta is the energy of movement, both voluntary and involuntary; pitta is the energy of digestion or metabolism and the transformation of food into microchyle or ahar rasa (digested food); and, kapha is the energy of lubrication and structure, the building block materials. All people have the qualities of vāta, pitta, and kapha, but one is usually primary, and one is secondary, while the third is usually the least prominent. The cause of disease in Ayurveda is viewed as a lack of proper cellular function due to an excess or deficiency of vāta, pitta, or kapha at the cellular level. Disease can also be caused by the presence of toxins.

In Ayurveda, body, mind, and consciousness work together in maintaining balance. They are simply viewed as different facets of one's being. To learn how to balance the body, mind, and consciousness requires an understanding of how vāta, pitta, and kapha work together. According to Ayurvedic philosophy, the entire cosmos is an interplay of the energies of the five great elements of Space, Air, Fire, Water, and Earth. Vāta, pitta, and kapha are combinations and permutations of these five elements that manifest as patterns present in all creation.

Vāta is the subtle energy associated with movement composed of Space and Air. It governs breathing, blinking, coughing, muscle and tissue movement, yawning, pulsation of the heart, and all movements in the cytoplasm and cell membranes. It is responsible for elimination of urine, feces, and sweat. In balance, vāta promotes creativity and flexibility. Out of balance, vāta produces fear and anxiety.

Pitta expresses as the body's metabolic system and is made up of Fire and Water. It governs digestion, absorption, assimilation, nutrition, metabolism, and body temperature. It is responsible for color and complexion of the skin, luster of the eyes, and absorption of sensory information into cognitive knowledge. In balance, pitta promotes understanding and intelligence. Out of balance, pitta arouses anger, hatred, and jealousy.

Kapha is the energy that forms the body's structure (bones, muscles, and tendons) and provides the "glue" that holds the cells together. It is formed from Earth and Water and supplies the water for all bodily parts and systems. Kapha lubricates joints, moisturizes the skin, and maintains immunity. It heals irritation, inflammation, and ulceration by replacing them with scar tissue. Healthy kapha gives long life. In balance, kapha is expressed as love, calmness, and forgiveness. Out of balance, it leads to attachment, greed, and envy.

THE PURIFICATION METHODS OF YOGA THERAPY AND AYURVEDA

The aims and objectives of the discipline of Yoga Therapy are practical and spiritually motivated and are designed to help the practitioner achieve enlightenment. The approach of Ayurveda is to understand the individual's prakṛti (constitution) and vikṛti (current state), the doṣa that is affected, the dhatu that is involved, and the srotas (bodily channels) and organs that may have a pathological lesion or disease. By knowing these things, the complex network of symptoms coming from the pathology can be relieved and, in Ayurvedic terms, the aggravated doṣa that is attacking the dhatu can be stopped. Freeing the dhatu from the clutches of the doṣa thereby restores balance to the overall system and brings optimal health.

To help accomplish these aims and objectives both systems offer several purification methods. Yoga Therapy traditionally offers the ṣaṭkarmas (six actions) whereas Ayurveda provides the method of pañca karma (five actions). In Yoga Therapy, even while a yogī is doing āsana, prāṇāyāma, and/or meditation, his/her unresolved emotions can come up in the form of toxins disguised as emotions of happiness and unhappiness because yogic practice stirs up the consciousness. The practice itself, while healing in nature, sometimes brings up unresolved, subconscious emotions that may disturb the doṣas. Alternatively, the Ayurvedic cleansing program, pañca karma, can cause a lot of unresolved emotions to come out. With both of these systems, the language of the purifications is the same and their concepts are the same, only the applications of technique are different.

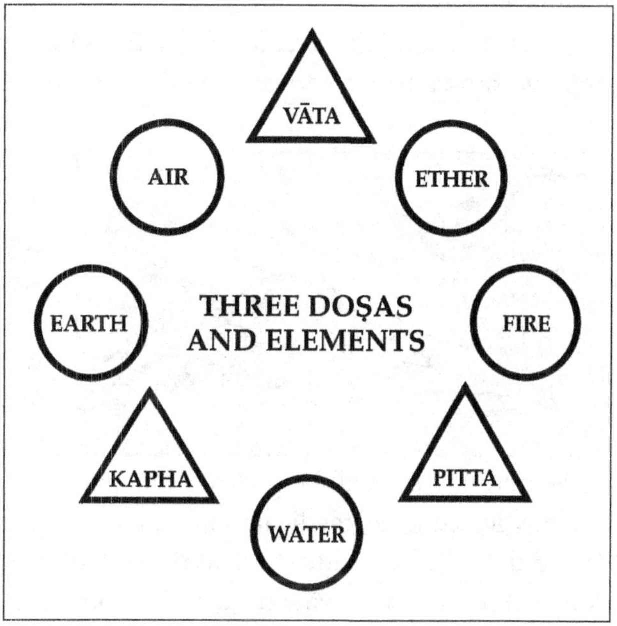

Yoga Therapy's ṣaṭkarmas consist of dhautī, basti, neti, trāṭaka, nauli, and kapālabhāti, according to modern books written in the West.

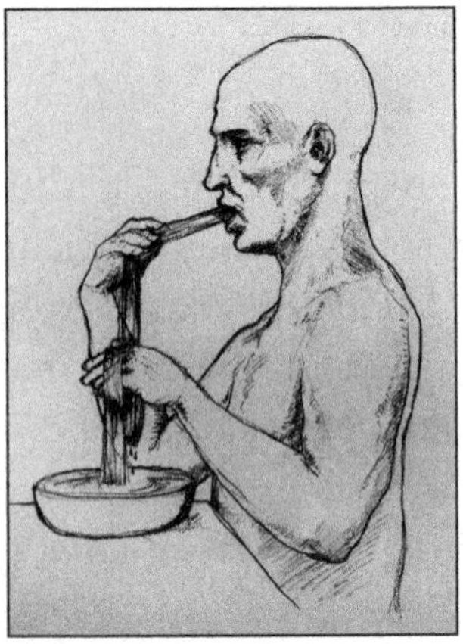

1. Dhautī is the first and most difficult shat karma. It involves swallowing a piece of muslin cloth into the stomach. One has to soak the cloth in a little salted water, then swallow about 12 feet of it and then slowly and carefully pull that cloth back up and out the mouth. It takes a great deal of guidance and discipline. Few of us can swallow that long ribbon of cloth, 3 inches wide and 12 feet long. To do that a person must be relatively healthy. A patient with asthma, emphysema, or tuberculosis could not do this. Therefore, this yogic discipline is appropriate for a normal, healthy person.

Dhautī is the yogic way of removing kapha from the stomach. To remove kapha from the stomach in Ayurveda, vamana (therapeutic vomiting) is done after strictly following a pre-pañca karma preparation that ripens kapha. It is easier to express the juice from a ripe fruit than from a green one. This "ripening" process is not required for dhautī. We then give Ayurvedic herbs like licorice tea, vacha tea, or salt water and have the person induce vomiting by rubbing the back of the tongue, creating a gag reflex that stimulates vomiting. This is followed by gently rubbing the person's back in an upward motion to complete the act of vomiting. This is a more gentle way.

Dhautī essentially accomplishes the same thing as vamana, but vamana can remove kapha from a very sick person and requires less skill.

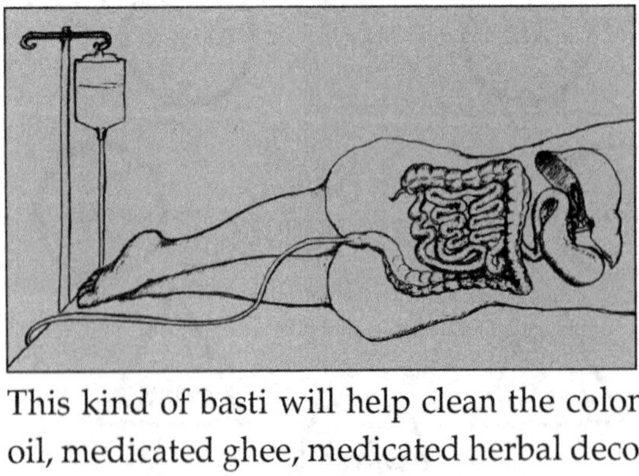

2. Basti is the second shat karma and is the ancient Indian version of an enema. Basti in Yoga Therapy and in Ayurveda are quite similar. In Yoga Therapy, basti is done with plain water because yogis are relatively healthy people; they may have a little elevated vāta doṣa and constipation. This kind of basti will help clean the colon. Ayurveda uses herbal tea, medicated oil, medicated ghee, medicated herbal decoction, and concoction. These choices are based upon the individual's prakṛti (constitution) and vikṛti (current state). These kinds of basti remove vāta doṣa and chronic ama (toxins) from the system.

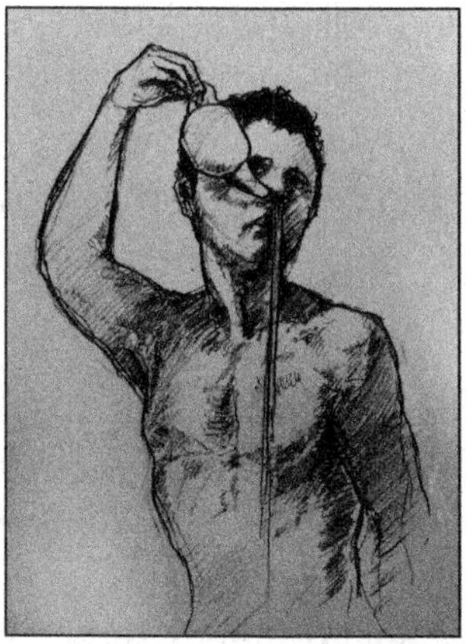

3. **Neti** is the third shat karma. This practice involves cleansing of the nasal passage as well as the throat. It can be done with jala neti (water neti) or with sūtra neti (a big wick dipped into salty water). Sūtra neti is put into one nostril, moving it back and down to the throat then swallowed into the mouth. Once in the mouth, the thread or string is grasped with the fingers and brought out of the mouth. Then, the yogī starts the cleansing by drawing the thread back and forth, pulling forward through the nose and then downward through the mouth. This is a quite powerful cleansing process and can be intense. This kind of neti requires guidance from a teacher.

The Ayurvedic parallel cleansing is nasya, which is an easy process. The person lies on his/her back with a pillow under the scapula and the head facing in the sky. Five drops of sesame oil, ghee, vacha medicated oil, or any other medicated ghee is then put into each nostril. These drops pass into the nose and down into the pharynx and the sinuses. After lying down for a minute or two, the person sits up and has the upper back and neck gently massaged. This method is a wonderful cleansing of doṣa from the upper part of the prāṇa vāha srotas (air channel).

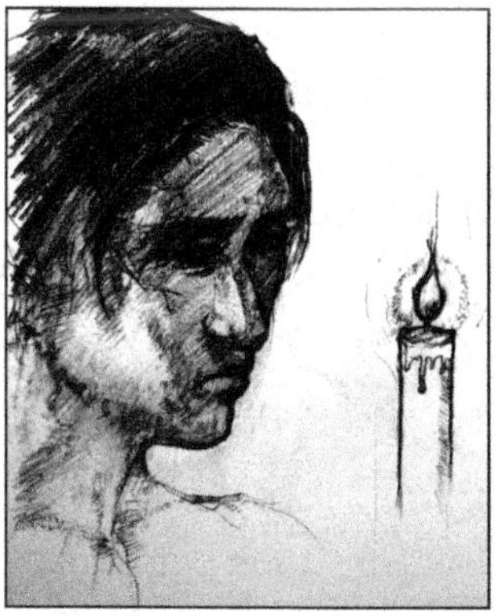

4. **Trāṭaka** is the fourth shat karma and is cleansing and strengthening to the eye. Trāṭaka is practiced by gazing at a flame or gazing at a star in the sky. While gazing at the object, one is not supposed to blink. By gazing without blinking, the cornea is exposed to the air, causing irritation to the eye and tears are formed. Once tears arise, the eyes are closed and the image of the flame persists. Seeing this image will improve the function of ālocaka pitta (the subdoṣa of pitta responsible for vision and color perception), and the eyes will look more charming, attractive, and full of luster. As the great yogic texts state, you will mesmerize others with your look. Trāṭaka heals ālocaka pitta.

An Ayurvedic technique that is similar to trāṭaka is netra basti. To do this cleansing, a whole-wheat dough of wheat flour and water is made in the form of a doughnut. It is placed around the orbit of the eye and sealed with a little water on the inside and outside of the dough. This creates a little pool around the eye. Finally, lukewarm ghee is poured into this pool over the eye. Be cautious that the ghee is not too hot; it should be just liquid. With the ghee covering the eye, open and close it repeatedly until tears occur in the other eye as well. Netra basti has the same benefit as trāṭaka. It also benefits ālocaka pitta, improving eyesight and any strain of the eye muscle.

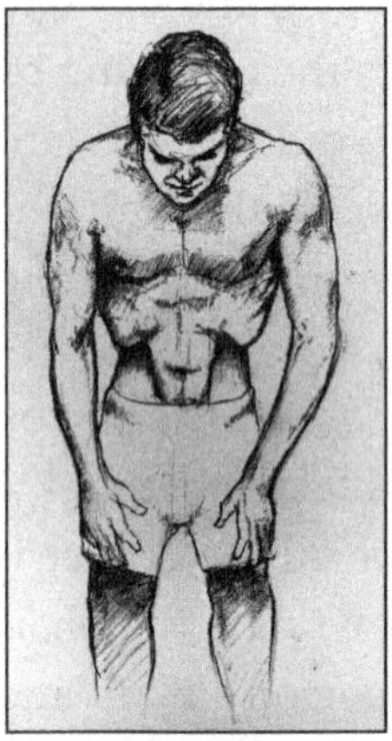

5. Nauli kriyā (navel cleansing) is the fifth shat karma. The rectus abdominus muscle is contracted on an exhale breath while standing upright and leaning forward with the knees slightly bent. The hands are placed on each thigh for support, and, after a full exhalation, the abdomen is drawn in and contracted so that a center, vertical pillar of abdominal muscle is formed. Pressing on the right thigh will help the right rectus muscle to shift to the right side. The same happens with the left. Pressing back and forth—left to right and right to left—causes a "churning" of the whole gastrointestinal (GI) tract. This is a very difficult practice. Nauli kindles a heat in the abdominal area and helps to improve a practitioner's digestion of food. Nauli awakens kundalini śakti and performs cleansing of kledaka kapha, samāna vāyu, pacaka pitta, and apāna vāyu.

Ayurveda can accomplish a similar effect with nabhi basti. The same doughnut shape described above in netra basti is created, but this time, it is put on the abdomen around the navel. The doughnut is sealed as above and a medicated oil, according to the disorder, is poured into the pool. This oil will penetrate through the skin, superficial fascia, and deep fascia. It stimulates the peritoneum and omentum and balances kledaka kapha, samāna vāyu, pacaka pitta, and apāna vāyu.

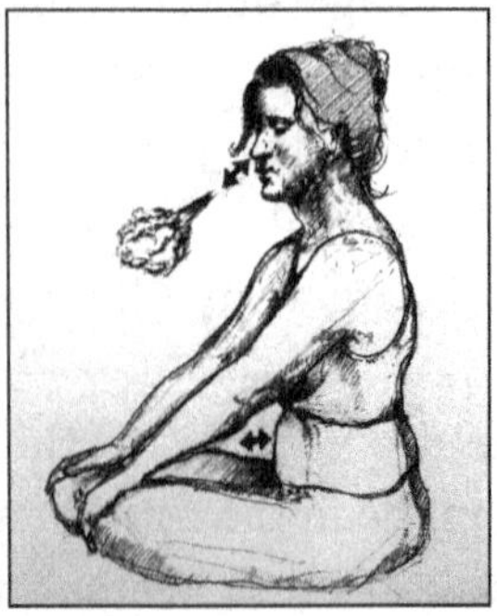

6. Kapālabhātī is the last shat karma. Kapālabhātī is a prāṇāyāma (breathing technique) where one performs a repeated series of forceful exhalations and passive inhalations. It cleanses the respiratory passages, sinuses, and the mind. Kapālabhātī is jivān sañjīvanī (life promoting). In Ayurveda, there is nothing like kapālabhāti.

OVERVIEW OF PANCHAKARMA IN AYURVEDA

The chief purification method of Ayurveda is pañca karma. Panchakarma teaches that the doṣas are at home in the gastrointestinal (GI) tract. The stomach is the seat of kapha, the small intestines are the seat of pitta, and the colon is the seat of vāta. Because of changes in the season, changes in diet, changes in emotions, and changes in the environment, these doṣas move out of the GI tract. They undergo saṁcaya (accumulation), prakopa (provocation), and prasāra (spread) into the tissues of the body, where they are *not* at home. Even if we maintain balance in our lives, the external environment will cause this to happen. Kapha accumulates during winter and melts during the spring season, thereby moving into the periphery. It shows up as congestion, allergies, and mucus. Whatever pitta has accumulated in the late spring becomes aggravated in the summer. This manifests as hives, rash, or urticaria. In the late summer whatever vāta has accumulated in the colon becomes provoked during the fall season and spreads, creating arthritis, sciatica, and muscle twitching.

This is a normal vector of the doṣas. Although the doṣas belong in the GI tract, they can leave it. As long as they are at home, we can control them in a healthy way. Once they leave the GI tract, they create pathological changes. Therefore, Ayurveda says the root cause of all disease is entry of the doṣa into the peripheral tissue.

Ayurveda asks, "How we can bring the doṣas back to the GI tract?"

For that, there is snehana (application of oil, oleation), svedana (sudation or medicated sweat), and abhyanga (oil massage). We start with internal and external snehana and this lubricates the srotas. Once the srotas is lubricated, the doṣa and ama will loosen their grip on the tissue and start moving back to the GI tract. Snehana performs many actions; it pacifies vāta doṣa, lubricates the srotas, and removes stiffness. Svedana serves to cause perspiration, dilation of the tissues, improve circulation, reduce pain, and relax the muscles. This opens the channels to the flow of the doṣa and ama back to the GI tract.

When doṣas come back to the GI tract, we remove them by the nearest pathway. If the doṣas are in the stomach, kapha doṣa, we remove them by vamana. If the doṣas are in the small intestine, pitta doṣa, then we remove them by virecana (purgation). Vāta doṣa returns to the colon and its nearest pathway is basti. If there is doṣa in the hematopoietic system, then its nearest pathway is rakta mokṣa (bloodletting). This can be done by application of leeches, venous section (traditional bloodletting), aspiration of the blood through a syringe, or donating blood to a blood bank. Residual doṣa can remain in the neuromuscular cleft or the nervous system and is removed by nasya through the sinuses.

REJUVENATION THERAPY

The therapies that are exceptional about Ayurveda are rasāyana (rejuvenation) and vājī-karaṇa (virilization) therapies. These are performed after doing pañca karma. Just as when you want to dye your shirt, you wash the cloth first, the same applies with pañca karma. If you wash it and then dye it, the color will shine. This cleansing is pañca karma; the body is our cloth. We have to wash it through pañca karma, then dye it and color it by rasāyana. You could say that ironing and pressing the cloth is similar to vājī-karaṇa.

Ayurveda speaks of rasa, vīrya, vipāka, and prabhāva and the action of the plant and how we can use that plant for healing. Generally, yogis need the rejuvenation of rasāyana; they can get a weakness in a particular tissue and need rasāyana. A yogī who does a lot of prāṇāyāma may need a prāṇa rasāyana because the lungs become dry or congested. Pippali rasāyana is generally used for this. When a yogī does āsana that kindles agni (internal fire), they can use shatavari rasāyana to calm down that agni if too much pitta is burning the stomach and making digestion uncomfortable. A Yoga practitioner may develop aches and pain in the muscle because vāta in māṁsa dhatu has increased. For this, they can use dashamula rasāyana. After a certain age, age and fatigue may cause problems with premature ejaculation and debilitated sexual activity, and this may affect one's life and relationship. To bring harmony, happiness, and perfume into the life of that relationship, Ayurveda recommends rejuvenation strategies. For rejuvenation of all seven dhātus, chayvanprasha rasāyana is excellent. If pitta is increased by too many inverted poses in Yoga Therapy, they can use shatavari, or gudduchi rasāyana, and gulwel sattva or kumari (aloe vera) to cool down the pitta. In the past, there was integration between Ayurveda and Yoga Therapy rejuvenation practices as both systems are timeless disciplines of healing the body, mind, and spirit.

rasa—the first experience of food stuff in the mouth, e.g., taste. There are six tastes in our diet. Each of these tastes is perceived by different groups of taste buds in the oral cavity.

vīrya—The energy or potency of a substance; the secondary action of an ingested substance, experienced after taste; two primary kinds: hot or cold.

vipāka—The final postdigestive effect of food that occurs in the colon and has an action on the excreta: urine, feces, and sweat. Vipāka is described as sweet, sour, or pungent.

prabhāva—The dynamic, electro-magnetic action of a substance that cannot be explained by the logic of its taste, energy, and postdigestive effects (rasa, vīrya, and vipāka).

Subtle Benefits of Padmāsana

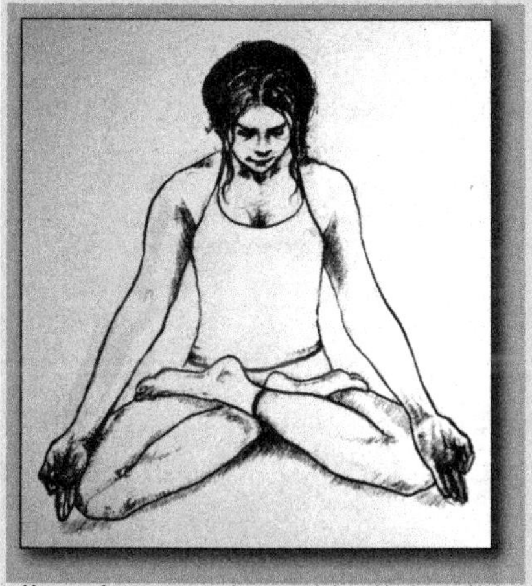

In padmāsana (lotus pose), we put the right foot on the left thigh, left foot on the right thigh. In this pose, we are actually pressing the femoral artery, femoral vein, and femoral nerve. A man who sits in lotus pose for a considerable amount of time will rarely have prostate problems or premature ejaculation problems. This pressure on the thighs slows down the blood supply to the lower extremity and enhances blood supply to the pelvic floor organs. Lotus pose is effective in strengthening the rectum, anal orifice, pelvic floor, prostate, cervix, and vagina as well as the glans penis and testicles. It is great for people who suffer from hypersomnia since you cannot sleep in lotus pose because you must remain alert and aware. Additionally, lotus pose has the spiritual benefits of isolation, liberation, and enlightenment.

Why is it called lotus pose? The lotus flower has petals, and we could say that the right thigh is a petal, left thigh is another petal, and the nose creates a third petal. Additionally, if you look from above, the head forms a petal and each thigh forms two more petals. The person looks like a lotus. A lotus is born out of the mud, yet the lotus is far away from the mud. We are born in the mud of this world, but, if we practice lotus pose, we will be far away from the world. We are in the world, but we are not of the world. That is a real vacation, to vacate the mind. That is the principal benefit of lotus pose.

CAKRAS

Cosmic prāṇa goes in every individual at the bottom of the spine and becomes the dormant coil that is kundalini. Yoga discipline helps to awaken this kundalini through posture, gesture, and breathing and to bring it from the root of the spine, from mūladhāra cakra (root cakra) at the base of the pelvis to sahasrāra cakra (crown cakra) at the top of the head. By bringing the prāṇa from the root to the crown, a person obtains physical health as well as mental and pranic health. This is the whole purpose of Yoga Therapy through the yogic disciplines of āsana (posture), mudrā (gestures), and prāṇāyāma (breathing techniques).

Ayurveda uses the same model of the cakra system as Yoga Therapy and explains its unique psychophysiology with each cakra. It discusses how each cakra is connected to the glandular system, to the physiological system, to the elements—ether, air, fire, water, and earth—and to their respective deities. Together, Yoga Therapy and Ayurveda both bring about radical mutation and radical transformation of the human being by creating balance between the seven dhātus, three malas, three doṣas, and the cakras.

THE AYURVEDIC VIEW OF ĀSANA

Āsana is defined as a stable, steady, comfortable, quiet posture without any pain, without any strain, without any discomfort. Sitting in that posture and watching the breath is the real definition of āsana. Every posture has a unique healing power, a unique psychophysiology, and a unique energy flow.

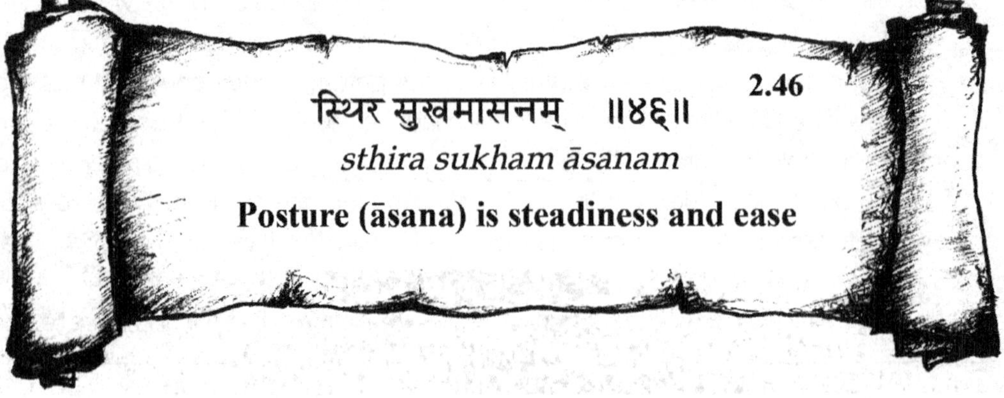
2.46
स्थिर सुखमासनम् ॥४६॥
sthira sukham āsanam
Posture (āsana) is steadiness and ease

Yogāsana is not just muscular exercise. Yogis do not look like macho, muscular guys; they look slim and supple. They tend to look strong and healthy when a balance of agni (digestive fire), a balance of the metabolism, and a balance of the hormones are maintained. They have good coordination and their muscular tone, power, and coordination are perfected. Therefore, a yogī is bright and light. Although we are using the muscles, Yoga exercise is not only muscular exercise. It is an exercise of the glandular system, nervous system, and hormonal system. Yoga Therapy brings harmony to these systems, and that harmony is very important.

Śamana cikitsā are treatments that lead to palliation, pacification, or neutralization of the doṣas. Śamana cikitsā is done in Ayurveda when a person is not strong enough to bear the strain of pañca karma. It is good for older people, children, and the debilitated patient. There are a number of therapies to strengthen the client. One of them is vyāyāma (exercise).

Exercise has incredible therapeutic value. Nevertheless, exercise should be done according to the age, illness, and/or pathological disorder. *Vyāyāma* means to induce stress in the body, specifically physical stress, to enhance the tone, power, and coordination of the muscle so that the muscles that are hardly used by an individual are brought back into action. When these unused muscles are used, they burn cholesterol, triglycerides, and sugar and bring the blood chemistry back to normal. Vyāyāma improves circulation, elimination, stimulates perspiration, and cleanses. Its aim is to provide the same benefit as Yogāsana.

The beauty of Ayurveda is that it uses the Yoga Therapy model according to an individual's prakṛti/vikṛti paradigm. That is the exceptional quality of Ayurveda. Not every āsana is good for every person. If everyone were to do a headstand for 15 minutes, the pitta predominant person could be in danger of cerebral aneurisms or hemorrhage. In addition, the increase in pitta can lead to being judgmental and critical. Therefore, a pitta person should spend only a minute or two in inverted poses. It is okay for kapha people; it is okay for vāta people. Simply knowing a person's constitution, one is able to introduce incredible Ayurvedic wisdom into applied Yoga Therapy. Ultimately, this more specific care can help treat the whole person more precisely and bring about perfect health.

We can also avoid injuries that are involved in Yoga. Some people do Yoga in a way that is not right for them because they do not know what diet or lifestyle to follow, not knowing their prakṛti. We should be aware of the person's constitution when using Yoga as a therapy.

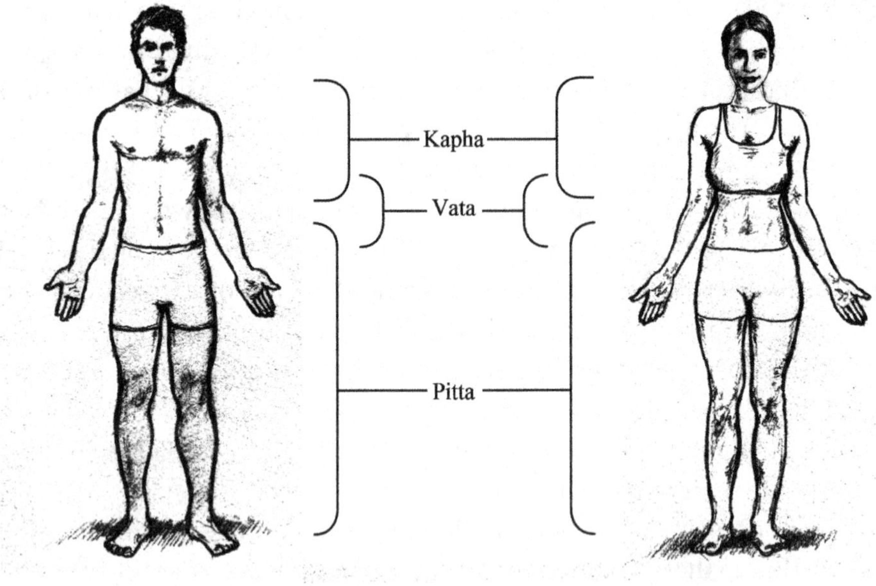

Ayurveda recommends āsana according to the person's constitutional need. It tells you which āsanas are good for vāta, pitta, or kapha prakṛti. The thorax and upper stomach are related to kapha. The navel area is related to pitta and below the belly button is vāta, including the lower extremities. Therefore, āsanas that stretch the chest and the throat help reduce kapha. Āsanas that cause more stretching of the belly button and abdominal muscles help to relieve pitta. And āsanas that help to stretch the pelvic floor and lower extremities will calm down vāta. The basic principle behind Yoga's classification as vāta, pitta, and kapha is based upon how that particular Yoga posture stretches a part of the body. Certain āsanas, like cakrāsana (wheel pose), are tri-doshic and stretch all three areas. Uṣṭrāsana (camel pose) is good for vāta. Mayurāsana (peacock pose) is good for pitta because it directly exerts pressure on the liver and the gallbladder. Ayurveda classifies āsanas depending upon the part of the body that is most stretched and/or most affected.

Another factor Ayurveda considers is the doṣa gati (movement of doṣa) of a posture. The movement of the doṣa is directed by the movement of the posture. Upward doṣa gati can create hiccough, breathlessness, nausea, and migraine headache. We have to bring the doṣas downward by doing Yoga postures that use gravitational force as a vector to change the direction of the doṣa. In cases like this, headstand, reverse, and inverted poses are not recommended. Perform standing poses like taḍāsana (palm tree pose), garuḍāsana (eagle pose), or vīrabhadrāsana (warrior pose) so that the doṣa will calm down. When the doṣa gati is moving downward, creating diarrhea, dysentery, or prolapsed rectum, then one should do inverted poses such as sarvaṅgāsana (shoulderstand), śīrṣāsana (headstand), or halāsana (plow pose).

Every Yoga posture has a specific psychophysiology and therapeutic value. In each posture, we are changing the gravitational imprints of the gravitational force. Therefore, blood flows in a different direction to the brain and to the heart. In Yoga, we use unused muscles, and there is no muscle atrophy, no muscle dystrophy, no muscle stiffness, and no muscle rigidity. These can be completely eradicated by Yoga.

Most of the postures have the name of the animals: cobra pose, camel pose, cat pose, dog pose, elephant pose, etc. That means these animals have a distinct physiology and anatomy. Because of that, they have a specific strength in a particular organ. The cobra has a very nice spine, a flexible spine. If we do cobra pose, we can obtain a flexible spine. Spinal disorders can be easily controlled and balanced by cobra pose. The camel has a hump, but a camel also has a strong stomach. A camel can eat thorns and digest them. Performing camel pose assists your stomach. Your stomach will digest any raw food because camel pose kindles agni in the stomach. It stretches the stomach wall and celiac plexus and controls hydrochloric acid secretion. It is beneficial for hiatal hernia. In addition, it is good for kidney disorders. Another example is cakrāsana (wheel pose). It stretches all the cakras and releases any blockage in the cakras. Wheel pose brings a beautiful blending of the seven rainbow colors into the life of the individual. Wheel pose is good for awakening kundalini energy, which is supreme intelligence, cellular intelligence. It helps to bring happiness, bliss, and enlightenment.

PRĀṆĀYĀMA

Prāṇāyāma offers great benefits to body, mind, and consciousness. As it is said in India, even if you cannot do your Yoga practice one day, that is acceptable, but never, ever miss your prāṇāyāma. Prāṇāyāma should be done daily. It is totally accepted by Ayurveda as coming from Yoga. Surprisingly, there is quite a bit of exercise involved in prāṇāyāma. The abdominal muscles move in and out as you breathe.

Prāṇāyāma can cure all diseases . . . this is not an exaggeration! It is a fact. I have seen the miracle of prāṇāyāma in my clinical practice. Prāṇāyāma can eradicate asthma, help obesity, benefit a person with hyperthyroidism, even high blood pressure, asthma, and emphysema. So many disorders can be improved just by prāṇāyāma. It changes your neurochemistry, your blood chemistry, and it brings your blood chemistry back to your prakṛti. That is the beauty of prāṇāyāma. Prāṇāyāma is the ultimate medicine.

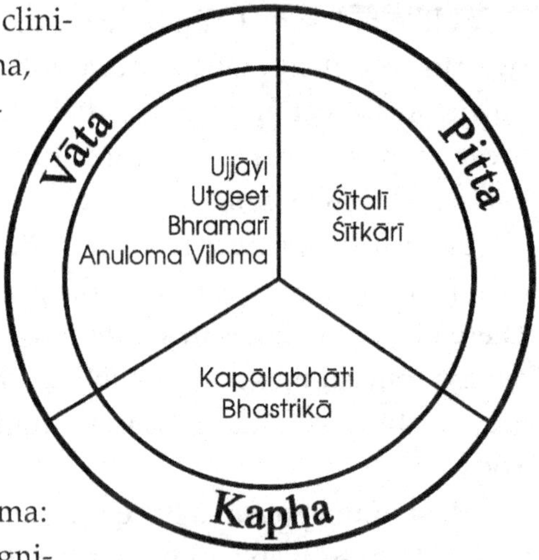

Board Classification of prāṇāyāma by doṣa

There is a package of eight prāṇāyāma: bhastrikā, kapālabhāti, anuloma viloma, agnisāra, bhramarī, ujjāyi, and śītalī. Śītkārī and udgīta prāṇāyāma are also very important. It takes only 35 to 40 minutes to do this whole set of prāṇāyāma. Doing this set of breathing exercises each day brings freshness, alertness, cleansing, and detoxification. From these, a person can work the whole day without fatigue.

AYURVEDIC YOGA THERAPY AND DISEASE CONDITIONS

The purpose of Yoga Therapy is to maintain the health of the healthy person. Ayurveda cures the disease of the diseased person while concurrently maintaining the health of the healthy person. This is the biggest difference between an Ayurvedic approach and a yogic approach. Yoga āsana, pañca karma, and shat karma are for relatively healthy people. Ayurveda is really for sick people. People with conditions like Parkinson's disease, paralysis, lumbago, multiple sclerosis, diabetes, or obesity can seek relief from modern medicine and need modified Yoga—simplified, modified Yoga stretching so that the person starts to move some of his/her organs beneficially and balances the body's biochemistry. When we use Yoga as a form of therapy, we have to mold the Yoga practice according to Ayurvedic principles. Realistically, not everyone can do a headstand or a peacock pose. So Ayurveda says we can mold the Yoga practice. Modify it according to the prakṛti and vikṛti of the client. This is the unique approach of Ayurveda. No one else has done that.

MOKṢA: THE ENLIGHTENED STATE

Finally, the last aim of Ayurveda and Yoga Therapy is mokṣa (enlightenment). Enlightenment is the birthright of every individual. Irrespective of one's caste, creed, color, or country, it does not matter. Your birthright is to become enlightened, to enjoy your life fully and completely. Human life is unique, and we are fortunate to have human body, human consciousness, and human brain. "Hu" means light. Man who is a light to himself is human. Unfortunately, we have only human form, human shape. We are not yet human beings. We will become human beings—if we really follow Yoga and Ayurvedic discipline. Yoga Therapy and Ayurveda are sister systems; they go together and they love the human being. They hug the human being completely. Yoga Therapy and Ayurveda heal the human being and the goal of each is to be enlightened, to realize God. God is satyam shivam sundaram: God is truth, God is holy, sacred, and God is beauty. There is so much beauty around us and within us. We never appreciate that beauty. Just by doing Yoga and Ayurveda, we realize that beauty, that ecstasy, that joy, so that our life will become whole. A whole life is holy; therefore, Yoga and Ayurveda make every human life whole. By doing Yoga and Ayurveda, you will realize that you are the temple of God and that your heart is the altar of divinity.

CONCLUSION

Yoga Therapy is not acrobatics; Yoga is not a circus. It is a discipline to bring harmony between body, mind, and consciousness by maintaining one's posture. The real definition of *asana* is to stay in a posture comfortably and breathe quietly. Then, you gain the benefit of what Yoga has to offer. Ultimately, the goal of Yoga Therapy and the goal of Ayurveda are the same: to balance ojas, tejas, and prāṇa. Yoga Therapy and Ayurveda are two sides of the same coin. They bring perfect health, happiness, peace, and bliss.

Family Medicine and Yoga Therapy

Richard P. Usatine, M.D.

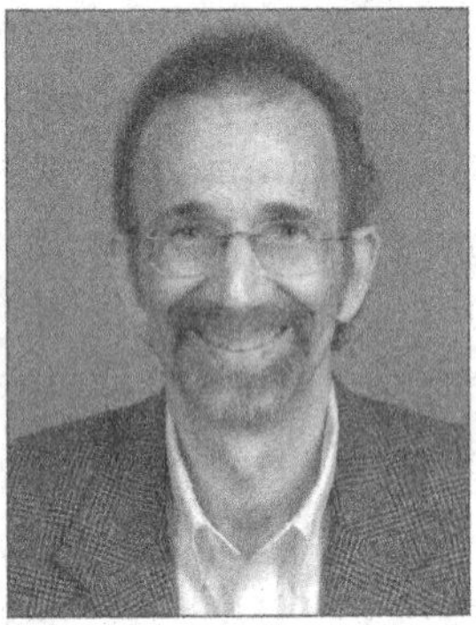

Richard P. Usatine is a full professor in the Department of Family and Community Medicine at the University of Texas Health Science Center at San Antonio. He received his M.D. from Columbia University and completed his family medicine residency at UCLA Medical Center. He is a coauthor of *Yoga Rx,* five medical textbooks, and over one hundred articles. In the 1990s, Dr. Usatine cofounded the first Yoga in Medicine course at a U.S. medical school with Larry Payne, Ph.D. He has won numerous teaching and community service awards throughout his career and was the recipient of a National Humanism in Medicine award from the Association of American Medical Colleges in the year 2000. Since then, he has been chosen yearly by his peers to be included in "The Best Doctors in America" list. Dr. Usatine loves teaching medical students to become compassionate doctors through his work with them in free clinics and in global health work where people live in areas of extreme poverty.

INTRODUCTION TO FAMILY MEDICINE

Family medicine has its roots in general practice and was started as a specialty in the 1970s in the United States. The founders of family medicine wanted to create a specialty that was patient-centered and humanistic. They believed that doctors must listen to their patients, show empathy, and provide clear information to help patients become partners in their own health care. Family physicians put preventive care first and are advocates for healthy lifestyles, encouraging good diet and regular exercise. In many ways, they were a counterculture movement against the high technology and big business side of medicine. Many family physicians have embraced complementary and alternative methods of health care like Yoga and Yoga Therapy for their patients over the years. Even to this day, family doctors strive to create homes for their patients that combine comprehensive preventive care with medical disease management, and Yoga Therapy can be a great resource in cultivating this balance.

YOGA THERAPY'S ROLE IN FAMILY MEDICINE

If healthcare reform is going to work, every person in America will need a family physician or primary-care doctor. Studies by Barbara Starfield, M.D., M.P.H., and others have shown that access to family physicians keeps the cost of medical care down and the quality of health care up (Starfield, Shi, and Macinko, 2005; Starfield, 2005). Primary-care access prevents unnecessary testing and invasive procedures. In areas with well-developed healthcare systems like North America and Europe, family medicine is the foundation of the health system. Educating family physicians about the value of Yoga Therapy is one way to elevate the role of Yoga Therapy in the health of our population.

While most family physicians are familiar with Yoga, most do not know about the existence of Yoga Therapy. Publications like this and *Yoga Rx* can help open the eyes of family physicians to this important field. Yoga and Yoga Therapy classes within medical schools are important to alert doctors in training about the role Yoga Therapy can play in healthcare delivery.

MY PERSONAL EXPERIENCES WITH YOGA THERAPY

I took my first Yoga class when I was in college at Columbia University. In 1990, I began teaching doctors how to help their patients cope with the stress and anxiety of quitting smoking through abdominal breathing, which was the same Yoga breathing I had learned years before. After an auto accident where I was the passenger in 1996, I developed chronic low back pain. I had x-rays, a CAT scan, a MRI scan, and a bone scan, but nothing structural was found to explain the pain. Like so many other patients out there, there was no "evidence" of my pain from the Western medical model. Eventually, my physiatrist referred me to Larry Payne, Ph.D., for Yoga Therapy. Larry developed a Yoga program specifically for me, and, within a few short weeks, I was essentially pain-free for the first time in more than a year since the accident. To this day, I use elements from the program Larry developed for me to keep my back strong, flexible, and pain-free. As a family physician, I continue to practice Yoga and prescribe it to my patients for enhancing their health and for treating many common ailments.

As Larry and I continued to work together, we began to discuss how valuable it would be for medical students to be exposed to Yoga, both for their own well-being and to provide them with noninvasive techniques for their patients. Together, we created an elective class in Yoga and Medicine at the UCLA School of Medicine, and it became a regular part of the school's elective curriculum in 1998—a first for a U.S. medical school.

BENEFITS OF YOGA THERAPY

Why should a physician prescribe Yoga or Yoga Therapy to patients? It is clear that there is a high quality of scientific evidence showing that exercise enhances health and prevents illness. Additionally, exercise leads to:

- Increases in muscle and bone strength to prevent falls and osteoporosis
- Preventing and/or treating obesity and cardiovascular disease
- Better controlling one's weight and symptoms of diabetes
- Enhancements in psychological well-being and general mood
- Reductions in symptoms of anxiety and depression
- Improvements in lipid profile, including decreasing total cholesterol and increasing HDL
- Decreases in high blood pressure
- Prevents cardiovascular disease

Yoga can offer all of the aforementioned benefits of exercise while also providing a deeper spiritual relationship for the individual, a greater sense of purpose, and an improved quality of life. As a therapy, Yoga maintains and enhances flexibility, strengthens muscles without putting too much stress on the joints, and can be used by all age groups and populations. It is safe and gentle and can be enjoyed late into life to counteract the normal aging process, which causes loss of flexibility and strength. Advocates of the "no pain no gain" mentality are not in synch with Yoga's underlying philosophy. It is essential that patients avoid going beyond their limit and observe the Sanskrit concept of ahiṁsa (nonviolence) since injuries occur when people try to force the body to do something it is not prepared to do. A sensible, noncompetitive, and individualistic approach to Yoga Therapy can help patients improve their health in a myriad of ways.

STRESS AND YOGA

There is overwhelming scientific evidence that the severity of most medical problems increases with stress. Virtually all types of pain worsen when a person is under great stress. Essentially, we feel pain when our body sends pain messages to the brain through pain receptors in the spinal cord called nociceptors. When the brain is performing optimally, it sends blocking signals (utilizing endogenous opioids and serotonin) down the spinal cord to decrease the transmission of pain messages through the central nervous system. When the brain is under stress, these blocking signals don't work as well, and the pain signals from the nociceptors become more intense.

In addition to all of the advantages and benefits of exercise, Yoga Therapy has the wonderful added feature of reducing stress. Yoga breathing calms the mind and relaxes the body by stimulating the parasympathetic nervous system to reduce the heart rate and pump intensity, thereby lowering blood pressure and perceived stress. The slow and measured breathing is sufficient therapy for some patients, while others who still need medication still find additional benefits.

EVIDENCE FOR YOGA AND YOGA THERAPY FROM THE MEDICAL LITERATURE

There are numerous studies in medicine that now support the use of Yoga and Yoga Therapy as part of the therapeutic options available to family physicians. The best evidence is found for the treatment of chronic low back pain and other musculoskeletal disorders. However, there is some evidence for the use of Yoga Therapy in other lifestyle-based family medicine afflictions like hypertension, obesity, stroke rehabilitation, anxiety, and depression.

Chronic Low Back Pain and Other Musculoskeletal Disorders

A systematic review and meta-analysis of Yoga for low back pain found strong evidence for short-term effectiveness and moderate evidence for long-term effectiveness of Yoga for chronic low back pain (Cramer, et al., 2013). The authors concluded that Yoga can be recommended as an additional therapy to chronic low back pain patients. A joint clinical practice guideline from the American College of Physicians and the American Pain Society states that for patients who do not improve with self-care options, clinicians should consider the addition of nonpharmacologic therapy with proven benefits for low back pain, including Yoga among other exercise therapies (Chou, et al., 2007).

Evidence from another systematic review suggests that Yoga is an acceptable and safe intervention to decrease pain and improve functional outcomes associated with a range of musculoskeletal conditions (Ward, et al., 2013). In this meta-analysis, Yoga interventions resulted in a clinically significant improvement in functional outcomes in mild to moderate low back pain and fibromyalgia. Yoga significantly improved pain in osteoarthritis, rheumatoid arthritis, and mild to severe low back pain. Psychosocial outcomes were significantly improved in mild to moderate low back pain and osteoarthritis. (Ward, et al., 2013). In one evaluation of a Yoga-based regimen for treatment of osteoarthritis of the hands, Yoga was effective in providing relief in hand osteoarthritis (Garfinkel, et al., 1994). A randomized control trial published in the *Journal of the American Medical Association* and confirmed in a Cochrane review showed significant short-term benefit for carpal tunnel syndrome from Yoga (Garfinkel, et al., 1998; O'Connor, Marshall, and Massy-Westropp, 2003).

As a family physician, I regularly teach my patients Yoga breathing mixed with various gentle exercises for their chronic back pain like Williams flexion exercises and McKenzie extension exercises, which are discussed in this text in the chapter "Yoga Therapy and the Spine" by Eden Goldman, D.C. These exercises are similar to what physical therapists prescribe but become more powerful when conscious breathing and relaxation are added to address the mind-body issues that influence chronic back pain. In a given case for musculoskeletal problems, referring patients for Yoga Therapy may be the single most important and helpful adjunct to other treatments that a family doctor can prescribe.

Hypertension

One recent systematic review found seventeen studies on Yoga for hypertension (all had unclear or high risk of bias). Yoga had a modest, yet significant effect on systolic blood pressure (SBP) (–4.17 mmHg) and diastolic blood pressure (DBP) (–3.62 mmHg). For interventions including three basic elements of Yoga practice (postures, meditation, and breathing), the results were better (SBP: –8.17 mmHg; DBP: –6.14 mmHg) than for more limited Yoga interventions (Wang, Xiong, and Liu, 2013). As a trainer of family physicians, I do believe that Yoga can help reduce blood pressure, though it is best recommended as part of healthy lifestyle changes. All patients with high blood pressure should be counseled to quit smoking, drink alcohol only in moderation, lose weight when needed, and exercise regularly. The Yoga lifestyle can encourage good diet and avoidance of tobacco and alcohol and it thus can be part of an overall wellness program as it can also assist with stress reduction. On the whole, family physicians are unlikely to use Yoga Therapy *instead of* antihypertensive medications, but surely could use Yoga Therapy *in addition to* pharmacotherapy. Patients with mild hypertension may even be able to avoid medication completely with appropriate weight loss, exercise, and Yoga-lifestyle training.

Obesity

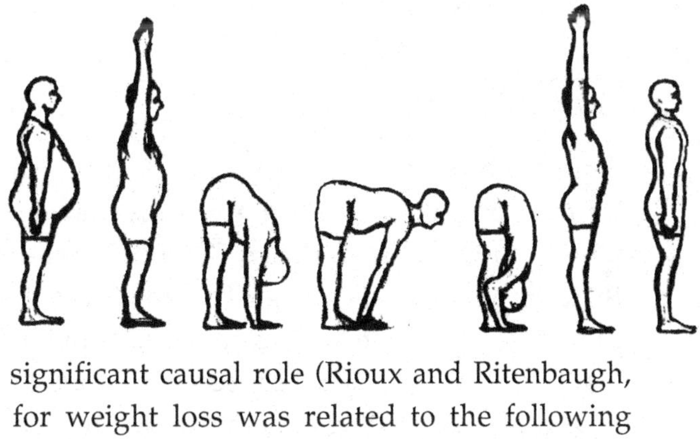

One recent review of the literature concluded that Yoga appears to be an appropriate and potentially successful intervention for weight maintenance, prevention of obesity, and risk reduction for diseases in which obesity plays a significant causal role (Rioux and Ritenbaugh, 2013). The effectiveness of Yoga for weight loss was related to the following features: 1) an increased frequency of practice; 2) a longer intervention duration; 3) a yogic dietary component; 4) the comprehensive inclusion of yogic components; 5) and a home-practice component (Rioux and Ritenbaugh, 2013). As a family physician, I am always looking to help patients lose weight, and a Yoga lifestyle is now a good and valid evidence-based method that can be recommended.

Stroke Rehabilitation

In a systematic review on the effectiveness of Yoga and mindfulness practices for stroke rehabilitation, nine studies were found of sufficient quality to include in the review (Lazaridou, Philbrook, and Tzika, 2013). These studies reported positive results, including improvements in cognition, mood, balance, and reductions in stress. Modifications to different Yoga practices made comparison between the studies difficult and a lack of controlled studies precluded firm conclusions on the benefits. However, the authors concluded that Yoga could be a valuable option for stroke rehabilitation (Lazaridou, Philbrook, and Tzika, 2013). Family physicians would be wise then to keep Yoga Therapy in mind when suggesting treatment options for stroke rehabilitation.

Anxiety and Depression

The evidence for the use of Yoga Therapy to treat anxiety and depression is well documented in the chapter "Psychiatry and Yoga Therapy" by Elizabeth Visceglia, M.D., in this text. As a family physician, I see patients suffering from anxiety and depression on a daily basis, and Yoga Therapy can be a valuable adjunct to psychological analysis, supportive counseling, and pharmacotherapy (Gill, Womack, and Safranck, 2010).

CONCLUSION

Family physicians need to know about the value that Yoga Therapy can provide for their patients. Yoga Therapists give one-on-one attention to patients similar to a physical therapist, yet the difference separating the former from the latter is that the core philosophy of Yoga Therapists centers on breathing and stress reduction in addition to whatever treatment is provided, which helps the patient manage his/her psychoemotional aspects of treatment. Greater collaboration between family physicians and Yoga Therapists is now at the forefront of family medicine, and some insurance companies are even paying for Yoga Therapy and offering clients discounts on Yoga classes. This is a trend that is increasing across the country and does not seem to be going away. All in all, it can only be helpful for our patients and our healthcare system to have Yoga Therapy as an additional methodology of care available in family medicine.

REFERENCES

Chou, R., et al. "Diagnosis and Treatment of Low Back Pain: A Joint Clinical Practice Guideline from the American College of Physicians and the American Pain Society." *Annals of Internal Medicine* 147 (2007): 478–491. Print.

Cramer, H., et al. "A Systematic Review and Meta-Analysis of Yoga for Low Back Pain." *Clinical Journal of Pain* 29 (2013): 450–460. Print.

Garfinkel, M. S., et al. "Evaluation of a Yoga-Based Regimen for Treatment of Osteoarthritis of the Hands." *Journal of Rheumatology* 21 (1994): 2341–2343. Print.

Garfinkel, M. S., et al. "Yoga–Based Intervention for Carpal Tunnel Syndrome: a Randomized Trial." *JAMA* 280 (1998): 1601–1603. Print.

Gill, A., R. Womack, and S. Safranek. "Clinical Inquiries: Does Exercise Alleviate Symptoms of Depression?" *Journal of Family Practice* 59 (2010): 530–531. Print.

Lazaridou, A., P. Philbrook, and A. A. Tzika. (2013). "Yoga and Mindfulness as Therapeutic Interventions for Stroke Rehabilitation: A Systematic Review." *Evidence-Based Complementary and Alternative Medicine* (2013): Article ID 357108. http://dx.doi.org/10.1155/2013/357108. Web.

O'Connor, D., S. Marshall, and N. Massy-Westropp. "Non-Surgical Treatment (Other Than Steroid Injection) for Carpal Tunnel Syndrome." *Cochrane Database Systematic Review* 1 (2003): CD003219. Web.

Page, M. J., et al. "Exercise and Mobilisation Interventions for Carpal Tunnel Syndrome." *Cochrane Database Systematic Review* 6 (2012): CD009899. Web.

Rioux, J. G., and C. Ritenbaugh. "Narrative Review of Yoga Intervention Clinical Trials Including Weight–Related Outcomes." *Alternative Therapies in Health and Medicine* 19 (2013): 32–46. Print.

Starfield, B. "Insurance and the U.S. Health Care System." *New England Journal of Medicine* 353 (2005): 418–419. Print.

Starfield, B., L. Shi, and J. Macinko. "Contribution of Primary Care to Health Systems and Health." *Milbank Quarterly* 83.3 (2005): 457–502. Print.

Wang, J., X. Xiong, and W. Liu. "Yoga for Essential Hypertension: A Systematic Review." *PLOS ONE* (2013). DOI: 10.1371/journal.pone.0076357. Web.

Ward, L., et al. "Yoga for Functional Ability, Pain and Psychosocial Outcomes in Musculoskeletal Conditions: A Systematic Review and Meta-Analysis." *Musculoskeletal Care* 11.4 (2013): 203–217. doi: 10.1002/msc.1042. Epub 9 Jan. 2013. Web.

Mastering Clinical Assessments and Observation in Yoga Therapy

Rick Morris D.C., C.C.S.P., Q.M.E., C.Y.T.

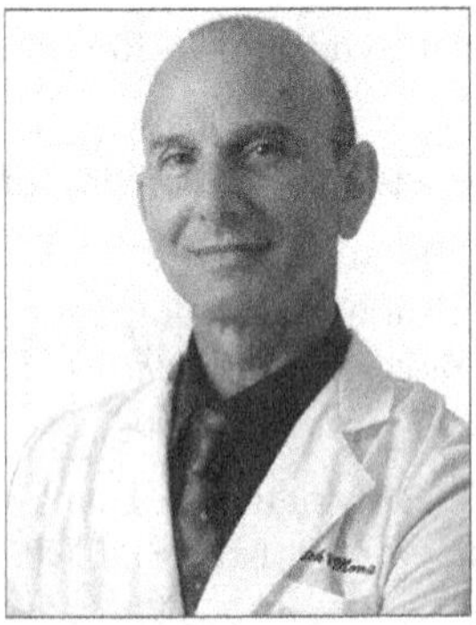

Rick Morris has been the team doctor for various athletic events and teams, including the U.S. Olympic track and field trials, University of California–Los Angeles (UCLA), California State University–Northridge (CSUN), the L.A. Track Club, and the NBA's Los Angeles Clippers. He has presented and published original research in the fields of sports medicine, spinal cord compression, and failed back surgery syndrome and has advanced certifications in sports medicine (CCSP), antiaging medicine (ABAAHP), accident reconstruction (certification from Texas A&M University), and is a qualified medical examiner for the State of California (QME). Dr. Morris runs an internationally known center for the treatment of severe back disorders, the Morris Spinal Stenosis and Disc Center (www.SpinalStenosisandDisc.com), and is an associate director and teacher for the Yoga Therapy RX program at Loyola Marymount University in Los Angeles, California.

INTRODUCTION

Not only does our frame of mind and mental state of well-being affect our body, but the health of our body also affects our mind. The yogic saying, "As above, so below," only tells half of the story and would be better written as, "As above, so below *and* as below, so above," if we apply it to this relationship between the mind and the body. Most people want to get well as quickly as possible, so it's essential the therapist and the client both look at these aspects of well-being and collaborate on their goals and treatments. It is equally important that they both understand

and agree on the benefits of that treatment program. This is especially important since we all tend to lose our objectivity when in chronic pain, when using less traditional treatments, and when paying for services out of our own pocket (rather than through insurance). Thus, properly evaluating, assessing, observing, and communicating with clients in Yoga Therapy is vital to its effectiveness as these skills create the foundation of all therapeutic treatments and take time to master since they are based on scientific knowledge, art, and insight.

TAKING A CASE HISTORY

Taking a case history is a vital part of the clinical assessment process, both in Yoga Therapy and in conventional Western medicine. It is obvious that a poor understanding of the problem leads to an equally poor understanding of a solution. One who is gifted at asking the relevant questions and listening carefully to the answers will help far more people than those who are not. While Yoga Therapists do not diagnose, gathering information is the key first step for all healthcare providers.

A typical shorthand way to gather information taught in medical and professional schools is through this twisted piece of alphabet—LMOPPQRST, which can be broken down as:

1. L—Location: Where does it hurt?
2. M –Mechanism of Injury: How did it get hurt?
3. O—Onset: When did it start hurting?
4. P—Provocative: What makes it hurt more?
5. P—Palliative: What makes it hurt less?
6. Q—Quality: Describe the hurt . . . is it sharp, dull, achy, electric, numb, etc.?
7. R—Radiation: Does the discomfort radiate anywhere, like to an arm or leg?
8. S—Severity: On a scale of 0–10, how bad is it?
9. T—Time of Day: When does it hurt the most?

In a detailed case history (possibly in a questionnaire the patient fills out before you speak to them face to face), one would also ask about past accidents, injuries, hospitalizations, surgeries, family history, and diet. But, most important, functional questions need to be asked (probably in person) such as:

How does this problem affect your life?

How long can you sit before you want to stand up?

How long can you stand before you want to sit down?

How far can you walk before you want to sit down?

What are the top two or three things you want most from our program?

This information is important in helping you to develop a treatment plan and measuring the success of your program. It also has a subtle but most important effect of focusing the client on the seriousness of their condition and the need for following through with a treatment program.

TAḌĀSANA ASSESSMENT

One of the most common ways that doctors and therapists evaluate clients is through static observation of the client's posture. The client is asked to stand in a position that is similar to taḍāsana (mountain pose). The Yoga Therapist scans the person's body, looking from different angles, to see if harmony or disharmony exists between a variety of structural relationships.

When looking from back-to-front and front-to-back in taḍāsana, some major areas to evaluate on a person's body include, but are not limited to:

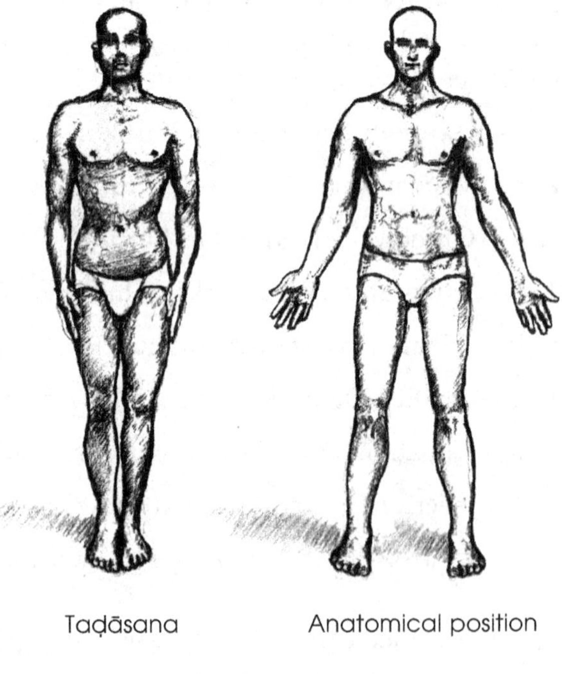

Taḍāsana — Anatomical position

1. Head tilt: Does it tilt laterally to one side?
2. Trapezius symmetry: Is one more developed than the other?

3. Shoulder height: Is one higher than the other?
4. The scapulas: Are they level, angling, and/or rotated?
5. Lordosis and kyphosis: Do the natural posterior curves of the thoracic and sacral spine and anterior curves of the neck and low back appear symmetrical and neither excessive nor insufficient.
6. Spinal alignment . . . does there appear to be a scoliosis. Is there rib symmetry?
7. Iliac crest symmetry: Are the tops of the hips even in height?
8. Gluteal muscles: Is one glute over- or underdeveloped and are the gluteal folds level or does one appear higher or lower than the other. How about the line between the left and right glutes; is it perpendicular to the ground or does it tilt to one side?
9. Inward/outward rotation or favoring of the knees: Are the kneecaps facing excessively inward or outward and are they symmetrical in their position?
10. Pronation and supination of the feet/ankles: How are the feet positioned on the floor? Are they symmetric in their appearance or does one ankle/foot appear to be more pronated or supinated than the other.

Studying and observing one's posture in taḍāsana is a useful first step in a Yoga Therapy exam. For example, when the head is tilted, and/or the upper body is not lined up with the lower body and pelvis, bad postural habits like sleeping on the stomach with one hip brought up and rotated outward, working on a computer monitor that far off to the side of the torso, and carrying a heavy purse repeatedly on the same shoulder must be sought out. Forward bending may seem to improve the postural deviations in most people since the spine is stretched out, but severe spinal curvatures will not change much when bending and deserve special attention from a spine specialist. Forward bends that cause pain and are guarded or people who feel that their back may "go out" at any moment may indicate an unstable or herniated disc and require a spine consult as well. Yoga Therapists are usually not the primary practitioners for acute conditions and in this chapter we focus on the conditions where Yoga Therapy is most beneficial and the areas where most of our clients seek assistance—the spine and the hip.

THE SPINE

While proper exercises and Yoga āsanas are powerful tools in countering pain, the forces of gravity and age continually conspire against us to compress our spines. Most people over the age of forty move away from compression sports such as running and jumping and naturally gravitate toward activities like Yoga that lengthen and decompress their bodies. The more we fight this inner wisdom, the more serious the problems can become.

Since we are bipeds, to achieve our most stable posture, we would ideally be designed with each vertebra positioned and fused directly above the other. But, in fact, our spines are twenty-six moveable segments positioned in a gentle "S-like" forward to backward curve. Admittedly less stable, the curved structure of the spine is far more effective at absorbing the impact and wear caused by gravity and compression, since the spine needs a combination of both strength and flexibility.

Excessive forward-to-backward or side-to-side curvatures strain the supporting ligaments, muscles, and discs of the spine. Think of the effort that would be required to hold a watermelon close to the center of your body. Next, think of the increased strength that would be required to hold it slightly off to your side or at arm's length in front of you. This example provides illustration to the strength that is required to support the spine from within when the curves are extreme levels.

Interestingly, different races, sexes, and body types all have slight variations in spinal curvature and have proclivities toward certain activities. If the spinal changes are slight and not associated with pain or decreased function, the practitioner might correctly accept these as normal variations that do not require treatment (Ohran, Sagir, and Zorba, 2013).

Let me give you an example. When I worked as a doctor for many of the U.S. Olympic Track and Field athletes, it was well known that the fastest woman in the world (the name must be omitted due to HIPPA privacy regulations) had a running style with a much greater forward lean and a higher back kick than did the other women. Of course, the others tried to imitate her but never performed as well. When she came to my office as a patient, I discovered why she ran that way: she had a 54-degree forward tilt to her tailbone. This was about 20 degrees more than the typical person. Of course she ran tilted forward, she had no other choice.

Eventually, one of the other runners with a normal pelvic angle (I knew this as she was also a patient of mine), who had been trying to emulate the world record holder for years, changed her technique and began running far more upright and with a longer stride . . . and she set a new world record. Of course, the other runners then started emulating her. Neither pelvic angle needed to be changed, nor should everyone's running or walking style be identical. We see this in Yoga Therapy all the time. No two poses will be exactly the same, sometimes even in the same body from one side to the other. The job of a Yoga Therapist is to help our clients be as healthy and pain-free as they can, which rarely means they will be identical to the person next to them.

So when do we attempt to change a person's structure? Of course, there isn't universal agreement on the answer. However, most will agree that, if increased pain and degeneration is associated with your posture, then it needs to be changed. But there are a few postures that lead to excessive wear and degeneration and should be modified without waiting for pain and limitation. These structural dysfunctions include:

1. Anatomical leg length discrepancies (Sharpe, 1983; Knutson, 2005). I personally believe 9 mm of leg length inequality is the limit one should be allowed without using a lift, and many will need it starting at 6–7 mm.
2. Scoliosis (de Vries, 2010)
3. Excessive kyphotic and lordotic curves
4. Excessive genu valgus (knock knees) (Sharma, 2010)
5. Ankle pronation (Sharma, 2010)

THE NECK

Beginning with the top of the spine, the neck, let's observe its alignment from the side. The ears should be near the front-center of their shoulders (Schafer, 1986). If the head is notably forward, it is called an anterior head carriage and puts increased strain on the muscles in the back of the neck.

As mentioned in the "carrying a watermelon" example earlier, greater neck strength is required to hold the head in front of the spine, rather than directly over it (Peollson, et al., 2013). Anterior head carriage commonly appears in the long-necked, slender body type known as an ectomorph. This body type inherently requires more neck strength. But faulty postures are possibly the leading cause of cervical dysfunc-

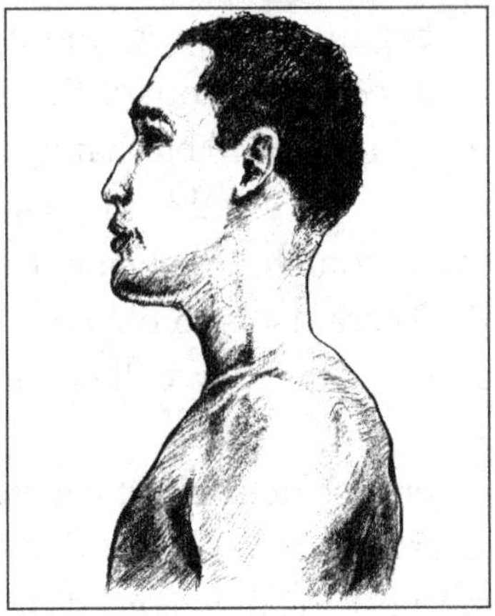

Normal head carriage

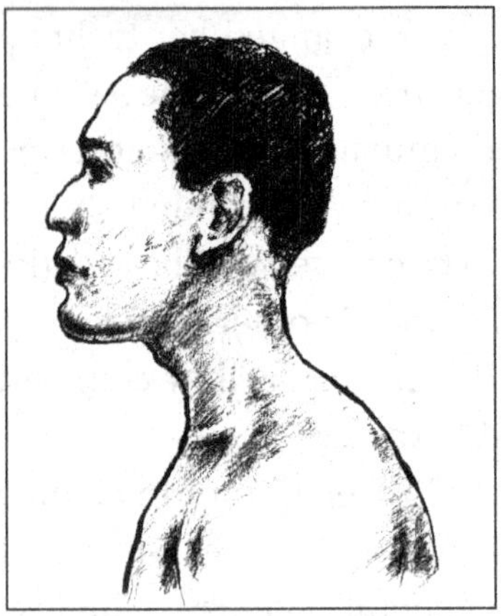

Anterior head carriage

tion, for example, spending too many hours looking at a computer screen that's too far away, requiring one's head to reach forward for optimal viewing, having shoulders that are allowed to slump forward, and, probably most often, from just being unaware or lazy. As the neck muscles strain trying to hold the head in this posture, they usually shorten, pulling downward on the base of the skull where the neck muscles insert, compressing and irritating the upper cervical nerves. This is a common cause of upper neck pain and headaches called suboccipital neuralgia, which causes pain to run from the base of the skull, over the top of the head, to the forehead and eyes (NIH, 2013). Of course, the middle and lower neck vertebrae, discs, and nerves can compress as well in this position. And while finding and changing the postural cause sounds obvious, it is often the least focused on aspect of treatment by today's busy healthcare practitioners who may have only 10 minutes to provide in-office treatments like medication, adjustment, and/or physical therapy. Ultimately, changing one's posture and correcting faulty spinal habits are important Yoga Therapy treatment modalities that get to the root of many chronic problems.

From the front, we look for uneven head tilt and asymmetry in shoulder heights. Both of these structural misalignments often start lower in the spine. It may be a result of a scoliosis, leg length discrepancy or asymmetrical daily activity. Signs of scoliosis and leg length discrepancy will be discussed later in this chapter, but postures that lead to such bad neck alignment include holding a bag on just one shoulder, sleeping on one's stomach with the head turned to one side, prolonged talking on the phone without a headset, unilateral occupations with one arm such as ceiling painting or construction and unilateral sports such as pitching or tennis. Treatment will not only include stretches that lengthen the shortened, overworked side but also modifications of those faulty mechanics wherever possible. This again is perfectly situated for the Yoga Therapist to use their time, biomechanical knowledge, and creativity in finding workable, necessary solutions.

THE MIDDLE BACK

Looking at the middle back, we notice from the side if the chest is properly positioned and directed straight ahead. We observe whether the shoulders are rolled excessively forward and/or if the shoulder blades are relaxed and not squeezed tightly together.

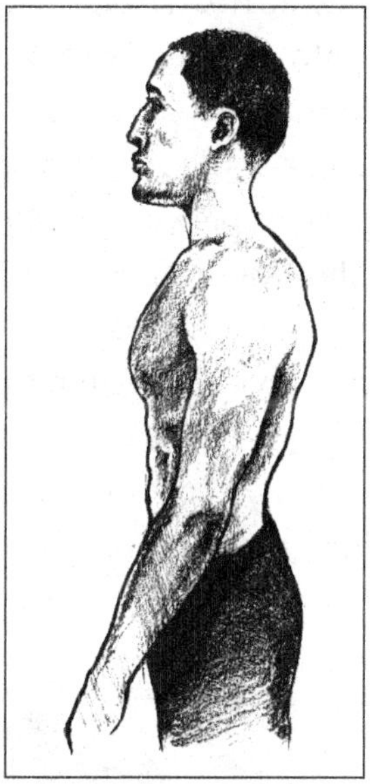

Normal thoracic/chest posture. The shoulders are not rolled forward and the chest is directed straight ahead

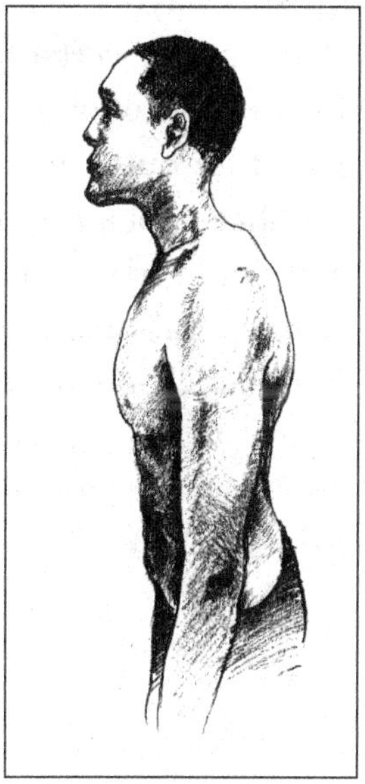

Rounded shoulders and chest pointing downward

Rotational alignment of the thoracic spine is best seen from behind when the client bends forward (with knees straight, if possible, to keep the leg lengths level) (Schafer, 1986). An asymmetric rotation can be observed and even palpated with a little bit of practice. When investigating the causes of thoracic rotational asymmetry, it is necessary to ask about asymmetrical sports like soccer (where players have a dominant leg), tennis (where players overdevelop or overuse one arm), golf (a one-sided swing sport), surfing (where surfers usually look behind themselves in just one direction), and swimming (where most people breathe only to one side). Many sporting activities, especially when performed repeatedly or excessively, are inherently asymmetric and create structural imbalances. Some creative modifications should be made during the Yoga Therapy treatment, such as breathing on both sides while swimming and taking practice swings in the opposite direction during golf, tennis, and baseball, and asymmetrical Yoga āsanas can be effective at "unwinding" the "twisted" spine. For example, I've found sukhāsana (easy pose) with a forward fold, while the shoulder and arm on the side of the posterior thoracic spine is pulled across the body with the torso turning to the opposite side, is helpful in correcting the rotational deviations of the upper back.

Aging, low computer monitors, large breasts, overdeveloped chest muscles, and lanky torsos are all common culprits of excessive thoracic rounding called thoracic hyperkyphosis. Keep in mind that when a kyphosis appears extreme, occurs suddenly, or is especially painful, less common causes may need to be ruled out such as compression fractures, ankylosing spondylitis, Schmorl's nodes, and osteochondrosis (Mayo Clinic Staff, 2010). These disorders change the normal rectangular shape of the vertebrae into one that's more triangular, forcing the spine to bend forward. Moreover, a thoracic hyperkyphosis is not only caused by compression fractures, but it also increases the likelihood of getting one (Kebaish, et al., 2013). But that's not all, a thoracic hyperkyphosis leads to other problems as well, such as anterior head carriage, shoulder impingement (Nagarajan and Vijayakumar, 2013), and low back pain (Snijders, et al., 2008).

Some clients have excessive straightening of the normal thoracic curve. This is visible when observing from the side and back. Just bring the chin down to the chest and pay attention to any senses of pain or tightness in the upper back due to excessive flattening. Often, the spinous processes, or little "bumps" on the backs of

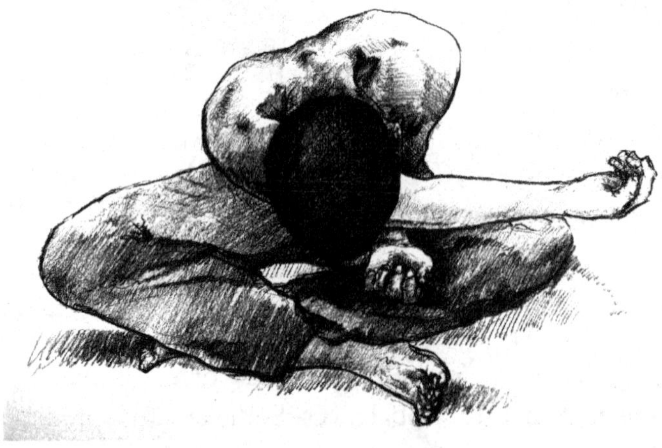

those with reduced thoracic curves, are abnormally tender to touch as they are excessively pulled downward and resistant to neck flexion. For some this lack of curvature is normal, while others may self-create this posture by "pulling their shoulders back" or "squeezing their shoulder blades together" as is improperly taught in some ballet, Yoga, and some fitness classes, or when performing deep, bench presses with heavy weights.

When trying to correct excessive thoracic rounding, the Yoga practitioner would best be taught to lift from the breastbone or sternum, rather than pulling the shoulders back. The desired stretch in the front of the shoulders and chest can be attained with chest opening stretches of the pectoralis muscles, without losing the normal thoracic curve. Āsanas, correction of postures, and changes to asymmetric activities are answers uniquely suited to the practice of Yoga Therapy.

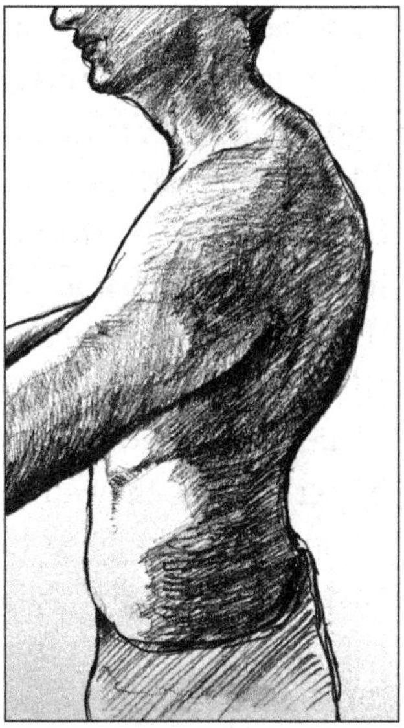

Excessive thoracic kyphosis due to vertebral malformation

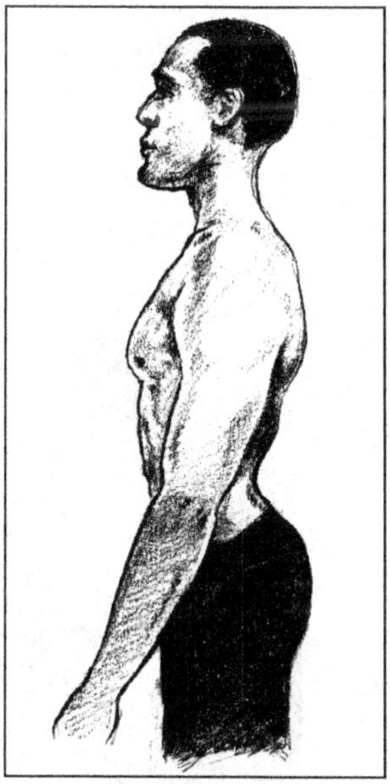

Hyperlordosis of the lumbar spine

THE LOW BACK

As already described in the neck and middle back sections, the low back can be excessively arched, flattened, or rotated as well. Excessive arching, known as hyperlordosis, can "jam" the back of the spine together, compressing the facets and nerves. Hyperlordosis of the lumbar spine usually causes the buttocks to be elevated and the back excessively arched (Shafer, 1986) as seen in the illustration to the left. Not only may the hyperlordosis be visible, but accentuating it by having the client perform a backward bend, at the waist, increases the lordosis and usually aggravates his/her low back or leg pain. This gives the therapist the useful information that low back extension exercises may not be helpful or should be done with caution.

Flattening or loss of the normal low back curve, or

hypolordosis, can be caused by excessive sitting, especially in a soft, deep seat, or without proper lumbar support. Tight hamstrings as well as a posteriorly bulged lumbar disc herniations can also flatten the normal lordosis (McCarthy and Betz, 2000). Hypolordosis often leads to the low back feeling "unstable" upon forward bends and lumbar rounding. Of course, there are many other conditions that create lumbar instability as well (e.g., spondylolisthesis, hyperelastic joint syndromes) (Penning and Blickman, 1980). If hypolordosis is a symptomatic problem for your client, flexion-based postures like forward bends and downward dogs may be irritating and not advisable or should, at least, be used with caution; whereas in hyperlordosis they stretch the low back and may be most helpful. Yoga practitioners and teachers need to understand that postures that increase the lumbar curve, such as cobra pose, wheel pose, and locust pose, may be better in hypolordotic conditions, even if it initially feels a bit compressive to the client. Of course all postures need to initially be viewed skeptically and watched to see the response over the first few sessions. There are clients with a generous lordosis who do well with extension exercises and those with a straightened lumbar curve who enjoy forward bends. Remember the story of the Olympic sprinters. The athlete with the increased pelvic angle did not need to be fixed—in fact, she was the best in the world. Watch for the reactions to the postures; that may be the most important indicator of the sequences and āsanas the patient will best respond to.

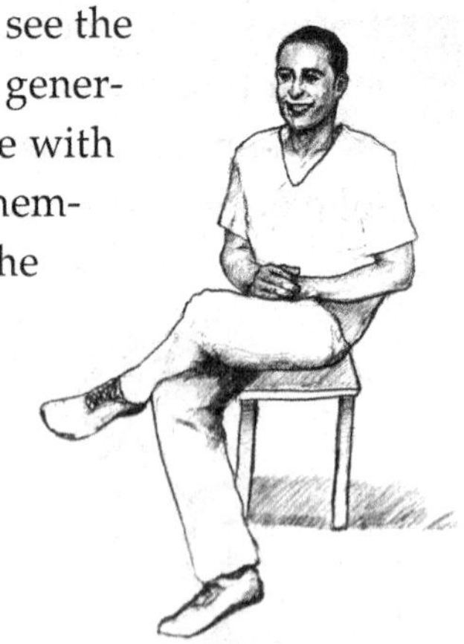

The causes of rotational malpositions in the low back are similar to those already mentioned in the middle back. Additionally, there are a few postural and structural causes that may be especially important for the lumbar spine:

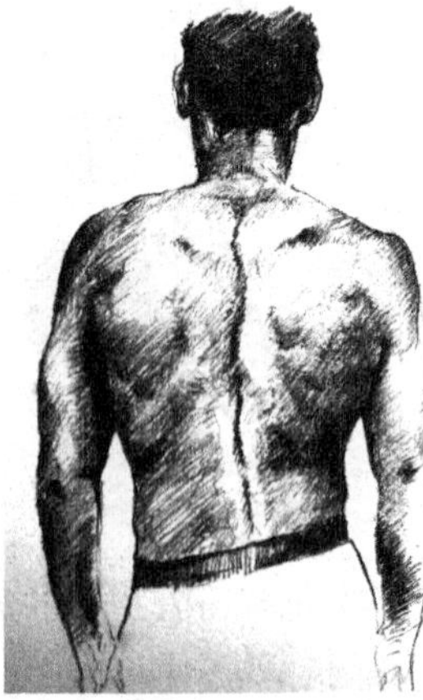

1. Sleeping on one's stomach with one leg brought up or hip rotated to the side.
2. Sitting on one's leg or with one leg crossed over the other (see figure above right), especially when they are not lined up with the spine, can cause rotational malpositions in the spine.
3. An anatomical leg discrepancy (below right) highlighting rotational spinal malpositions due to leg length discrep-

ancy when bending and leg length inequality's appearance when standing straight.

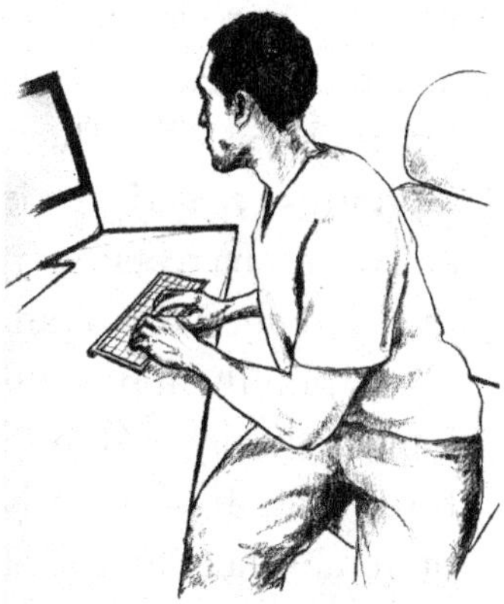

4. Sitting twisted on a chair due to faulty ergonomics (top right). Is the shoulder facing forward while the legs are directed to the side?
5. Sacral malformation and transitional vertebrae (congenital malformations in the tail bone) that abnormally curve the spine.
6. Asymmetry of the right and left ankles in either pronation or supination (right). The ankle that is most rolled out (supination) will make that leg functionally longer (Rothbart, 2006). In the image to the right, asymmetrical pronation/supination of the ankles can be seen, which creates a functional leg length discrepancy that will not be corrected until the foot alignment is balanced. In this case, the right foot is pronated, or turned inward, in relationship to the left. This person needs a foot insert or orthotic.

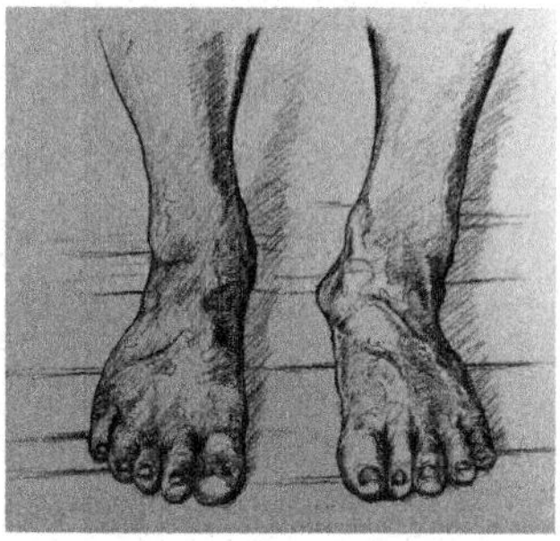

THE HIP

Many patients I see in my clinic don't know whether their pain is coming from their hips or their lower back. While doctors sometimes tell patients conflicting diagnoses (or no diagnosis at all), surprisingly most cases are pretty easy to differentiate. Pain from the hip usually starts in the groin, runs down the front of the thigh, and stops above the knee (Mayo Clinic Staff, 2013). It almost never causes posterior thigh pain or radiates below the knee.

In Yoga, hip pain is especially aggravated by postures that rotate the hip, such as lotus or crossed-legged poses, and sometimes simply by bringing a knee to the chest. Occasionally, hip flexors are not just tight, but significantly shortened. We call this a hip flexure contracture, and, if it is fairly significant, it will be evident upon a simple, single knee to chest posture (Shimada, 1996) known orthopedically as a positive Thomas test. In this position, the hip flexor of the nonflexed hip is so tight it can't stay flat on the ground, causing that hip to flex. Unilateral contractures can lead to rotational misalignments in the hips and spine. When they are bilaterally tight, it causes the lumbar spine to be pulled forward and excessively arch. Obviously, a Yoga Therapy program in this situation would be helpful in including a progressive series of hip flexor stretches for the iliopsoas and rectus femoris like añjaneyāsana (crescent pose) and naṭarājāsana (dancer's pose). If the back is arched, then care should be taken to avoid further arching the low back during the stretches.

Typically, in patients with hip arthritis or bursitis, the first few steps after prolonged sitting are the most painful causing the client to limp (AAOS, 2007). Postures that stretch the hip open and extend the hip, like lunge poses, are often preferable here to those that compress and close the joint, such as pigeon pose (flexion with rotation) and hero's pose (internal rotation). Modifications of these hip extensions can be done while sitting on a chair with one thigh pointing down toward the floor, while the other knee is in the normal chair-sitting position.

If the hip doesn't flex more than 90 degrees and doesn't substantially improve with gentle stretching, the individual may need a consultation with a hip surgeon. Hip surgeries today are far more successful than they were just ten years ago. Be sure to note if the individual already has a hip replacement and be careful stretching their hips excessively as they may dislocate (especially the older hip replacements). Eventually, postures that lightly stretch the hip into external rotation are gently introduced and can be quite beneficial in restoring normal range of motion and full function in the hip.

THE BREATH

Yogis understand the importance of the breath in balancing the sympathetic and parasympathetic nervous systems and the breath's role in our sense of well-being (Raghavendra, 2012). Observance of the breath is probably the single ingredient that most separates Yoga from basic stretching and calisthenics (Lakkireddy, et al., 2013). So what should we observe in breathing, and how do we know what's healthy and what isn't?

Yogic breathing for balance is usually relaxed, without notable wheezing or distress. When we are trying to relax and center ourselves, we visibly and slowly expand the abdomen and chest as we breathe in (inspiration) and we breathe out (expiration) even more slowly. The normal resting rate varies between 12–16 breaths per minute (Johns Hopkins University), but per my observation, many students of Yoga have rates that are significantly slower than that. The Ohm Test (Morris, 2013), originally described in the Morris-Payne Yoga Therapy Exam, is a simple yogic tool to measure lung capacity changes before and after a series of treatments. The Yoga practitioner is instructed to take in as deep of a breath as he/she can and make the longest, continuous sound possible, vocalizing *oṁ, āḥ, ma,* or *sa* during the exhalation. Use a pitch tool to replicate the sound (when possible) and time with a watch. Record the best of three tries. Breathing that increases neck tension or shows recruitment of the neck muscles is counterproductive and is discussed in detail in Dr. Eden's Goldman's chapter "Yoga Therapy and the Spine" in this text. Yoga Therapy can benefit students by teaching them to break this habit. For in Yoga Therapy, good assessments lead to effective treatments in balancing the mind, body, and breath.

OBSERVING AND UNDERSTANDING THE DIFFERENT KINDS OF CLIENTS

Ms. Branson, your 10 a.m. Yoga Therapy patient, arrives 20 minutes late, seems harried, and chatters with little focus while you are taking her case history. She records her pain level as a 12, on a 0–10 pain scale. When asked about the location of her pain, she leaves few places unmentioned, and most are above a 7. You notice the discrepancy between her complaints and your initial observations: "How could someone with a 12 pain rating (out of a possible 10) easily get up from a chair, walk at full speed, and comfortably bend and twist?" Ms. Branson didn't seem very peaceful or focused and her subjective factors, such as pain, didn't seem to match her objective findings, i.e., ability to stand, move, and walk. While there may be some distinguishing physical reason that's not immediately apparent, in Yoga Therapy we look more deeply into the elements of well-being and people in general.

As humans, we all deal with fear, anxiety, denial, anger, and narcissism, and attempt to balance these emotions and traits with the insights we learn as we grow and mature. However, when these emotions become imbalanced or excessive, they create a special challenge to the healthcare practitioner. These clients need our help, possibly more than the others who have greater mental balance. But, today's patients are rushed through a busy healthcare system that either ignores or doesn't have the time to address their underlying factors of well-being, which are critical to their healing.

Depression

It is not unusual after prolonged periods of pain or disability to be depressed. Waking up each morning to another day of suffering, combined with the fear of losing your financial security, personal relationships, and the daily activities you enjoy wears on even the sunniest of dispositions. Yet, many of us (including several doctors) assume that depression is the *cause* of their pain rather than its effect. Even if an underlying depression predisposes the patient to increased pain, the depression needs to be effectively treated and not viewed as a self-indulgent choice the patient made. Those who assume the client receives a secondary benefit from being sick and depressed are rarely correct, and this shows the naivety of those with that opinion.

Clients will often admit to their depression when asked how their condition affects their lives. They will stop, think deeply, and often break into tears. Once they know you understand and will not judge them negatively, they will usually be quite open to you about it and be willing to listen to your suggestions.

Fear/Anxiety

Many with "subjective-objective incongruency," as seen with Ms. Branson, have complaints that don't seem to match their physical findings. It is intellectually lazy and often incorrect to assume she is exaggerating her symptoms just to get attention or because she enjoys being sick (Hassed, 2013). While this is occasionally the case, in my experience, it's more often brought on by their fear of being unable to work, find love, and/or be physically active.

Taking a good case history is essential for those with severe anxiety. When anxiety or fear is excessive, bothersome annoyances can turn into intolerable pain and mental preoccupation (Castillo, et al., 2013). Even as the pain and function begin to improve, the fear and anxiety persist, so the client doesn't feel relieved and the natural ups and downs that normally occur as we heal from chronic pain seem too slow, insufficient, or even nonexistent. It's often difficult to keep these patients in treatment long enough for them to fully recover, as they continually search and try multiple approaches simultaneously, making it impossible to know which therapies are helping and hurting their progress. The reexamination comparing pre and post ranges of motion, strength, and function helps the client recognize his/her improvement and assists him/her in following through with the therapy. Yoga breathing techniques and daily practice are helpful in balancing the sympathetic and parasympathetic nervous systems (Mourya, 2009) and quiet some of the mind chatter that goes along with fear and anxiety. Of course, professional counseling may be needed and encouraged by their trusted Yoga Therapist.

Denial

Denial needs to be recognized and addressed and presents itself in an opposite manner to those with anxiety disorders. Often, Yoga Therapy clients may choose a Yoga Therapist over a doctor just to avoid recognizing the seriousness of their problem. The hallmark presentation of "the denier" is an unrealistically low pain level that belies the painful grimaces and slow, awkward movements observed by the therapist during normal, daily activities (e.g., getting out of a chair, standing, walking and performing simple postures) (Fox, et al., 1989). When you ask how their condition impacts their life, the denier's responses seriously challenge your believability. How can a client that grimaces as they rise from a chair in the waiting room and limps to the examining room not be more severely impacted by his/her condition? The denier will not only need to be correctly assessed but may also need support in facing his/her problems.

Anger

Anger is an outlet for anxiety-laden feelings in those who have not developed the emotional resources—or ego strength—to successfully cope with them in other ways (Seltzer, 2013). In clients, anger issues affect their health and, in turn, many of the important personal relationships in their lives.

The angry client characteristically spends the first 15 minutes of each visit complaining about life and the treatment not working. While it is not unusual to have a patient concerned about the effectiveness of their treatment program, the angry person seems to enjoy the confrontation and feels entitled to extra time, emails, and phone calls. Even the therapist is often made uncomfortable by these individuals and may secretly smile when they miss their appointments. I've found the only hope in gaining their confidence is to not get mad back or show irritation, but to be very direct. Explain what their condition was originally, show the signs of improvement, and the direction and measurements that will be used to mark their progress in the future. The patient usually minimizes this angered approach after he/she sees that it's not working, allowing him/her to follow your recommendations and get the help that is really desired.

Narcissism

The narcissistic client has an inflated sense of him/herself and therefore demands lots of your time listening to stories, which are often quite dramatic and filled with heroes and villains (Mayo Clinic Staff, 2011). There are usually many doctors who saved his/her life and many incompetents who missed crucial diagnoses. One animated story runs into the next and most rarely pertain to the topic. Trying to get the information you need is a real act of focus and direction by the practitioner, often requiring you to interrupt him/her in midsentence to extract the necessary

What was the hardest physical activity you could do for at least 2 minutes?				
1	2	3	4	5
Very heavy (for example)	**Heavy** (for example)	**Moderate** (for example)	**Light** (for example)	**Very light** (for example)
• Run, fast pace • Carry a heavy load upstairs or uphill (25lbs/10kgs)	• Jog, slow pace • Climb stairs or a hill moderate pace	• Walk, fast paced • Carry a heavy load on level ground (25lbs/10kgs)	• Walk, medium pace • Carry light load on level ground (10lbs/10kgs)	• Walk, slow-paced • Wash dishes

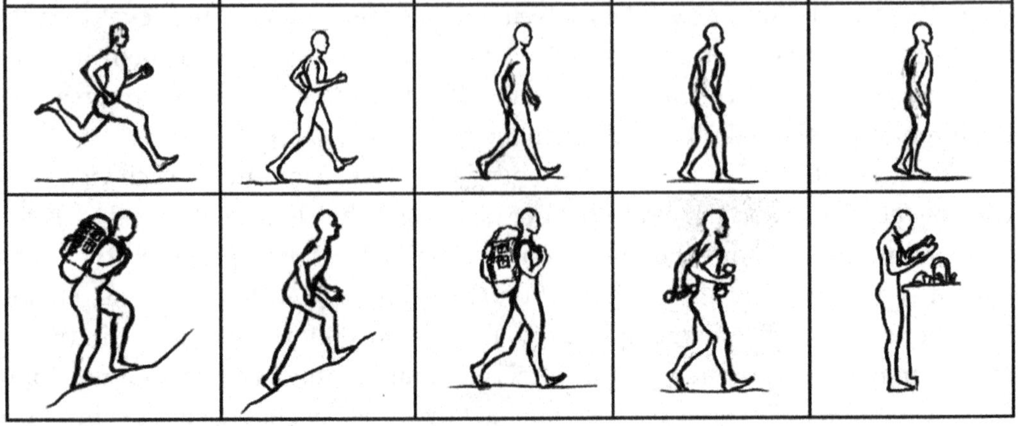

Dartmouth-Coop Test

information within the time allotted. In my experience, the narcissistic patient can turn from being your most adoring client to the one that feels most betrayed. You can go from being a hero to a villain rather easily (Hyphantis, et al., 2009).

Narcissistic clients often lack deep, personal relationships though they may know many people (Kaufman, 2013). They may have severe health conditions that need attention but generally require a lot of direction from the Yoga Therapist to keep them focused so they can be helped. Yoga Therapy can support this individual if the relationship aspect of the practice is emphasized.

Mental health assessment tools, like the Dartmouth-Coop Test (see figure on previous page), measure the client's state of well-being and is performed by having the client fill out a brief questionnaire. It assesses nine quality of life issues such as the patient's perception of his/her health, level of pain, social support, and emotional functioning. This can lead to several good discussions between you and your client that help forge a partnership in finding help together (de Azevedo-Marques and Zuardi, 2011).

CONCLUSION

Yoga Therapy is the evaluation of the individual's mind, body, and breath. It's an assessment of his/her physical health and mental well-being. This assessment begins with observation, using all of one's senses to detect structural and physical abnormalities and emotional challenges that prevent this person from living his/her life more fully and with greater peace and happiness. We then take the practice of Yoga, in its most comprehensive sense, to help the individual achieve his/her goals.

I have found that understanding and empathizing with my clients' situations are essential in earning their trust (Borigini, 2013). In fact, when appropriate, I share my personal journey as it relates to theirs. It often breaks down barriers and helps them to trust me as a guide on their journey.

Of course, this trust should be deserved and earned by the Yoga Therapist. We do this by being well trained in both the Eastern arts of Yoga and the Western sciences of anatomy, physiology, and diagnosis. Although we are all tempted to simplify and accept what we already know as enough, the best healers I've known haven't fallen into this trap and see knowledge as an endless adventure and seeming failures as the avenue of their future growth.

REFERENCES

American Academy of Orthopaedic Surgeons (AAOS). "Hip Bursitis." OrthoInfo, 2007. Web. 9 Nov. 2013. http://orthoinfo.aaos.org/topic.cfm?topic=a00409.

Arsenault, M., et al. "Pain Modulation Induced by Respiration: Phase and Frequency Effects." *Neuroscience* 252 (2013): 501–511. Print.

Back, M. D., et al. "Narcissistic Admiration and Rivalry: Disentangling the Bright and Dark Sides of Narcissism." *Journal of Personality and Social Psychology* 105 (Dec. 2013): 1013–1037. Epub ahead of print. doi: 10.1037/a0034431. Web. 14 Oct. 2013.

Bale, P., S. Rowell, and E. Colley. "Anthropometric and Training Characteristics of Female Marathon Runners as Determinants of Distance Running Performance." *Journal of Sports Sciences* 3.2 (Summer 1985): 115–126. Print.

Baykara, R. A., et al. "Low Back Pain in Patients with Rheumatoid Arthritis: Clinical Characteristics and Impact of Low Back Pain on Functional Ability and Health-Related Quality of Life." *Journal of Back* and *Musculoskeletal Rehabilitation* 26.4 (1 Jan. 2013): 367–374. Print.

Beazell, J. R., M. Mullins, and T. Grindstaff. "Lumbar Instability: An Evolving and Challenging Concept." *Journal of Manual and Manipulative Therapy* 18.1 (18 Mar. 2010): 9–14. Print.

Borigini, M. "So You Feel My Pain?" *Psychology Today.* Web. 5 Nov. 2013. http://www.psychology today.com/blog/overcoming–pain/201301/so–you–feel–my–pain.

Brewer, J. A., et al. "Meditation Experience Is Associated with Differences in Default Mode Network Activity and Connectivity." *Proceedings of the National Academy of Sciences* 108.50 (2011): 20254–20259. Print.

Castillo, R. C., et al. "Longitudinal Relationships Between Anxiety, Depression, and Pain: Results from a Two–Year Cohort Study of Lower Extremity Trauma Patients." *Pain* 154.12 (Dec. 2013): 474–480. Print.

Castro, M. M., et al. "Cognitive Behavioral Therapy Causes an Improvement in Quality of Life in Patients with Chronic Musculoskeletal Pain." *Arquivos de Neuro-Psiquiatria* 70.11 (2012): 864–868. Print.

de Vries, A. A. Benjamin, et al. "Spinal Decomposition in Degenerative Lumbar Scoliosis." *European Spine Journal* 19(9) (2010): 1540–1544.

de Azevedo-Marques, J. M., and A. W. Zuardi. "COOP/WONCA Charts as a Screen for Mental Disorders in Primary Care." *Annals of Family Medicine* 9.4 (2011): 359–365. Print.

Fox, E., et al. "Repressive Coping Style and Anxiety in Stressful Dental Surgery." *British Journal of Medical Psychology* 62 (Dec. 1989; Pt. 4): 371–380. Print.

Garrison, K. A., et al. "Real-Time fMRI Links Subjective Experience with Brain Activity During Focused Attention." *NeuroImage* 81 (Nov. 2013): 110–118. Print.

Hanada, E., et al. "Measuring Leg-Length Discrepancy by the 'Iliac Crest Palpation and Book Correction' Method: Reliability and Validity." *Archives of Physical Medicine and Rehabilitation* 82.7 (2001): 938–942. Print.

Hassed, C. "Mind-Body Therapies: Use in Chronic Pain Management." *Australian Family Physician* 42.3 (2013): 112–117. Print.

Hyphantis, T., et al. "Narcissistic Rage: The Achilles' Heel of the Patient with Chronic Physical Illness." *Patient Preference and Adherence* 3 (2009): 239–250. Print.

Jenkinson, C., et al. "Evaluation of the Dartmouth COOP Charts in a Large–Scale Community Survey in the United Kingdom." *Journal of Public Health Medicine* 24.2 (2002): 106–111. Print.

Jensen, M. P., et al. "Effects of Non-Pharmacological Pain Treatments on Brain States." *Journal of Clinical Neurophysiology* 10 (2013): 2016–2024. Print.

Johns Hopkins University. "Vital Signs (Body Temperature, Pulse Rate, Respiration Rate, Blood Pressure)." Health Library, n.d. Web. http://www.hopkinsmedicine.org/healthlibrary/conditions/cardiovascular_diseases/vital_signs_body_temperature_pulse_rate_respiration_rate_blood_pressure_85,P00866/.

Kaufman, S. B. "How to Spot a Narcissist." *Psychology Today*. Web. 11 November 2013. http://www.psychologytoday.com/articles/201106/how–spot–narcissist.

Kebaish, K. M., et al. "Use of Vertebroplasty to Prevent Proximal Junctional Fractures in Adult Deformity Surgery: A Biomechanical Cadaveric Study." *Spine Journal* 13.12 (Dec. 2013): 1897–1903. Epub 2013 Oct 4. DOI: 10.1016/j.spinee.2013.06.039. Web.

Knutson G. A. "Anatomic and Functional Leg-Length Inequality: A Review and Recommendation for Clinical Decision-Making. Part I, Anatomic Leg-Length Inequality: Prevalence, Magnitude, Effects and Clinical Significance." *Chiropractic and Osteopathy* 13 (2005): 11. 20 Jul. 2005. Web. http://www.chiroandosteo.com/content/13/1/11.

Lakkireddy, D., et al. "Effect of Yoga on Arrhythmia Burden, Anxiety, Depression, and Quality of Life in ParoxysmalAatrial Fibrillation: The YOGA My Heart Study." *Journal of the American College of Cardiology* 61.11 (2013): 1177–1182. Print.

Liiv, H., et al. "Anthropometry and Somatotypes of Competitive Dance Sport Participants: A Comparison of Three Different Styles." *HOMO–Journal of Comparative Human Biology*. 21 Sep 2013. Epub ahead of print. doi: 10.1016/j.jchb.2013.09.003. Web.

Lindquist, K. A., et al. "Authors' Response: What Are Emotions and How Are They Created in the Brain?" *Behavioral and Brain Sciences* 35.3 (2012): 172–202. Print.

Lovejoy, C. O. "The Natural History of Human Gait and Posture." *Gait & Posture* 21 (2005): 95–112. Print.

Mannello, D. M. "Leg Length Inequality." Journal of Manipulative and Physiological Therapies 15.9 (1992): 576–90. Print.

Mayo Clinic Staff. "Narcissistic Personality Disorder." *Psychology Today*. Jan. 2010. Web. 8 Nov. 2013. http://www.mayoclinic.com/health/narcissistic–personality–disorder/DS00652.

——. "Kyphosis." Mayo Foundation for Medical Education and Research. 2012. Web. 7 Nov. 2013. http://www.mayoclinic.com/health/kyphosis/DS00681/DSECTION=causes.

——. "Hip Pain." Mayo Foundation for Medical Education and Research. 2013. Web. 1 Nov. 2013. http://www.mayoclinic.com/health/hip–pain/MY00257.

McCarthy, J. J., and R. R. Betz. "The Relationship Between Tight Hamstrings and Lumbar Hypolordosis in Children with Cerebral Palsy." *Spine* 25.2 (2000): 211–213. Print.

Moore, D. J., C. Eccleston, and E. Keogh. "Does Sex Moderate the Relationship Between Anxiety and Pain?" *Psychology & Health* 28.7 (2013): 746–764. Print.

Mourya, M., et al. "Effect of Slow—and Fast—Breathing Exercises on Autonomic Functions in Patients with Essential Hypertension." *Journal of Alternative and Complement Medicine* 15.7 (2009): 711–717. Print.

Mullender, M. G., et al. "Spinal Decompensation in Degenerative Lumbar Scoliosis." *European Spine Journal* 19.9 (2010): 1540–1544. Print.

Nagarajan, M., and P. Vijayakumar. "Functional Thoracic Hyperkyphosis Model for Chronic Subacromial Impingement Syndrome: An Insight on Evidence-Based 'Treat the Cause' Concept—a Case Study and Literature Review." *Journal of Back and Musculoskeletal Rehabilitation* 26.3 (2013): 227–242. Print.

Orhan, O., M. Sagir, and E. Zorba. "Comparison of Somatotype Values of Football Players in Two Professional League Football Teams According to the Positions." *Collegium Antropologicum* 37.3 (2013): 401–405. Print.

Pawl, R. "When the Pain Won't Wane It's Mainly in the Brain." *Surgical Neurology International* 13.4 (2013; Suppl 5): S330–S333. Print.

Peleg, S., et al. "Sacral Orientation Revisited." *Spine* 32.15 (2007): E397–E404. Print.

Penning, L., and J. R. Blickman. "Instability in Lumbar Spondylolisthesis: A Radiologic Study of Several Concepts." *American Journal of Roentgenology* 134.2 (1980): 293–301. Print.

Peolsson, A., et al. "Does Posture of the Cervical Spine Influence Dorsal Neck Muscle Activity When Lifting?" *Manual Therapy*. 20 Jul. 2013. Epub ahead of print. doi:10.1016/j.math.2013.06.003. Web.

Rausa, M., et al. "Personality Traits in Chronic Daily Headache Patients with and Without Psychiatric Comorbidity: An Observational Study in a Tertiary Care Headache Center." *Journal of Headache Pain* 14.1 (2013): 22. Print.

Rothbart, B. A. Relationship of Functional Leg-Length Discrepancy to Abnormal Pronation. *Journal of the American Podiatric Medical Association* 96.6 (2006): 499–507. Print.

Schafer, R. C. *Symptomatology and Differential Diagnosis: A Conspectus of Clinical Semeiographies*. Arlington, VA: Associated Chiropractic Academic Press, 1986. Print.

Seltzer, L. F. "Anger—How We Transfer Feelings of Guilt, Hurt, and Fear." *Psychology Today*. 14 Jun. 2013. Web. 11 Nov. 2013. http://www.psychologytoday.com/blog/evolution–the–self/201306/anger–how–we–transfer–feelings–guilt–hurt–and–fear.

Sharma, L., et al. "Varus and Valgus Alignment and Incident and Progressive Knee Osteoarthritis." *Annals of the Rheumatic Diseases*. 69.11 (2010): 1940–1945. Print.

Sharpe, C. R. "Leg-Length Inequality." *Canāḍīan Family Physician* 29 (1983): 332–336. Print.

Shimada, T. "Factors Affecting Appearance Patterns of Hip-Flexion Contractures and Their Effects on Postural and Gait Abnormalities." *Kobe Journal of Medical Sciences* 42.4 (1996): 271–290. Print.

Snijders, C. J., et al. "Changes in Autonomic Variables Following Two Meditative States Described in Yoga Texts." *Journal of Alternative and Complementary Medicine* 91.1 (2012): 35–42. Print.

Snijders, C. J., et al. "Effects of Slouching and Muscle Contraction on the Strain of the Iliolumbar Ligament." *Manual Therapy* 13.4 (2008): 325–333. Epub 5 Jun 2007. Web.

Woby, S. R., et al. "Coping Strategy Use: Does It Predict Adjustment to Chronic Back Pain After Controlling for Catastrophic Thinking and Self-Efficacy for Pain Control?" *Journal of Rehabilitative Medicine* 37.2 (2005): 100–107. Print.

Wood, B. M., et al. "Catastrophizing Mediates the Relationship Between Pain Intensity and Depressed Mood in Older Adults with Persistent Pain." *Journal of Pain* 14.2 (2013): 149–57. Print.

Zurowski, M., et al. "Psychiatric Comorbidities in Dystonia: Emerging Concepts." *Movement Disorders* 28.7 (2013): 914–20. Print.

NATUROPATHIC MEDICINE AND YOGA THERAPY

Sarah Murphy, N.D., L.Ac., R.Y.T.

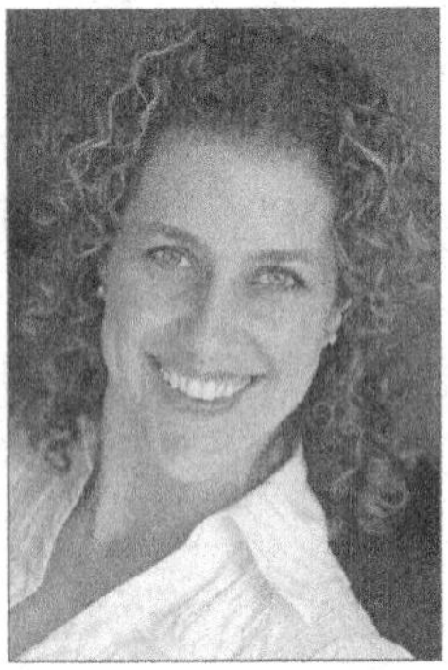

Sarah Murphy is a licensed naturopathic doctor and acupuncturist with an additional healing arts background in massage and Yoga Therapy. Her introduction to Yoga practice began in college and was part of a turning point that led her to pursue the path of becoming a holistic doctor. She completed her doctorate at the National College of Naturopathic Medicine in naturopathy, her master's at the Academy for Five Element Acupuncture in acupuncture and Chinese herbs, and her Yoga certification at Kripalu Center for Yoga and Health in Stockbridge, Massachusetts. Professionally, Dr. Murphy currently runs a private naturopathic clinic practice in Malibu, CA.

"The doctor of the future will give no medicine, but will interest his patients in the care of the human frame, in diet, and in the cause and prevention of disease."

—THOMAS EDISON

INTRODUCTION

It is a basic part of human evolution to pursue things that keep us healthy and prevent illness and death. Just like animals in the wild, we instinctively seek out medicines from plants and nature that aid us in healing if we are diseased or injured. At the same time, it is in our basic nature to develop lifestyle behaviors that promote survival. As complements to these basic tendencies, the body is constantly seeking homeostasis on a cellular level through a variety of physiological processes. Mirroring this search for equilibrium and working on both the subtle and gross levels, Yoga and naturopathic medicine are practices that assist people in consciously engaging in natural techniques and healthy lifestyle practices to reestablish homeostasis when out of balance.

Naturopathic doctors are trained at accredited, four-year, postgraduate naturopathic medical schools and are licensed primary-care doctors. Naturopathic medicine is a holistic medical system that provides a framework for approaching the treatment of illness and the promotion of health in a comprehensive and natural way. Naturopathic philosophy teaches that illness is best remedied by identifying and treating the underlying causes of disease and by strengthening the inherent homeostatic mechanisms of the body using natural therapies. The naturopathic medical paradigm serves as an umbrella for a full spectrum of natural therapies that can be used by a naturopathic doctor in clinical practice. Therapies including dietary nutrition and nutritional supplements, intravenous (IV) nutrients, lifestyle counseling, botanical medicine, homeopathy, hydrotherapy, naturopathic manipulation therapy (musculoskeletal bodywork techniques), and therapeutic exercise may be employed in an individualized combination for the optimal healing of each person. Other natural therapeutics not currently taught in naturopathic medical school, such as Yoga Therapy, may be incorporated too—depending on the doctor's additional background, experience, and licensing in the healing arts.

At their essence, Yoga and Yoga Therapy are ideal therapies to include in the naturopathic doctor's toolbox since they have a similar holistic-based philosophy and their own personal set of therapeutic practices. The principles of Yoga align with the naturopathic mind-set and the benefits of Yoga make it a valuable resource for those interested in healing via the naturopathic healthcare model.

HISTORY

The practice of Yoga originated in India over 5,000 years ago as an oral tradition before the written word (Dhyansky, 1987). Yoga positions have been identified in ancient stone carvings at various archaeological sites (Possehl, 2002). Approximately 2,000 years ago, Patañjali's *Yoga Sūtras* appeared in written form and became the foundation for modern Raja and Haṭha Yoga. With a likewise long history, naturopathic medical philosophy and treatments originated long before the use of the term *naturopathy*. The use of herbs and foods for medicine, exposure to fresh air and sunlight, and hydrotherapy (the use of hot and cold water applications) have been in use for many thousands of years. The rationale behind Naturopathic healing can be traced back to Ancient Greece and great influential medical thinkers like Hippocrates (the father of Western medicine) circa 400 BCE (Pizzorno, 2011).

The term naturopathy was coined by Dr. John Scheel and purchased by Dr. Benedict Lust, a German immigrant, who established naturopathic medicine as a distinct profession in North America at the turn of the twentieth century. Lust's teacher, Father Sebastian Kneipp, was famous in Europe for being involved with a movement known as "Nature Cure." The Nature Cure movement promoted a healing system of utilizing clean food, water, air, sun, exercise, and hydrotherapy to restore health. Lust began using the term *naturopathy* to describe the mixture of disciplines and therapies he used to treat illness. He opened Yungborn "health sanitariums" or "health resorts" (modeled after clinic resorts in Germany) in New Jersey and Florida. Patients visited these health clinics (in-patient style) and underwent naturopathic treatment methods for their woes. In 1902, Lust founded the first school of naturopathic medicine in New York. Dr. Benedict Lust also had a fifty-yearlong prolific writing and publishing career on naturopathic medicine via his *Kneipp Water Cure Monthly, The Naturopath and Herald of Health, Natures Path Magazine*, and the *Universal Naturopathic Encyclopedia Directory and Buyer's Guide: Year Book of Drugless Therapy*.

However, naturopathy quickly decreased in visibility in the early to mid-twentieth century with the advent and professionalization of modern conventional medicine (drugs and surgery), but, similar to Yoga, it began to flourish as a practice in the West again during the 1960s and 1970s. Since then, the continued growing interest in these ancient practices shows that Yoga and naturopathic medicine share lifestyle guidelines and healing principles that are cross-cultural and timeless.

THE SYNERGISTIC PRINCIPLES OF YOGA AND NATUROPATHY

Naturopathic medicine is defined by six principles and a holistic way of looking at health and illness. Many varieties of natural therapeutics are free to be utilized as long as they can be performed in a way that fits within the overarching holistic medical philosophy. In my experience of utilizing both, the principles of Yoga and naturopathy overlap like waves in the ocean. Naturopathy is a container for natural healing modalities and Yoga Therapy is a perfect addition that aids in manifesting these naturopathic principles.

PRINCIPLE 1. First Do No Harm (*Primum Non Nocere*)

"I will prescribe regimen for the good of my patients according to my judgment and ability and never do harm to anyone."

—Hippocratic Oath

The first principle of naturopathic medicine and Yoga Therapy is one and the same: "First do no harm." This is a commonsense guideline for healing and a foundational medical ethics concept that applies to all medical modalities. Step one in practicing medicine is to avoid doing anything that will further hurt or injure the patient while performing the treatment or therapy. This aligns with the first principle of Yoga philosophy, ahiṁsa (nonviolence), which means to act without harm.

The principle of ahiṁsa, moreover, means to have compassion toward all living beings and is part of the first limb of Yoga, the *yamas*—a code of ethics about how to behave toward the world in a nonharmful way. The five yamas listed by Patañjali in Chapter II, Sūtra 30 are as follows:

1. Ahiṁsa (nonviolence, compassion)
2. Satya (truthfulness, honesty)
3. Asteya (nonstealing, generosity)
4. Brahmacarya (continence, moderation)
5. Aparigraha (noncoveting, satisfaction)

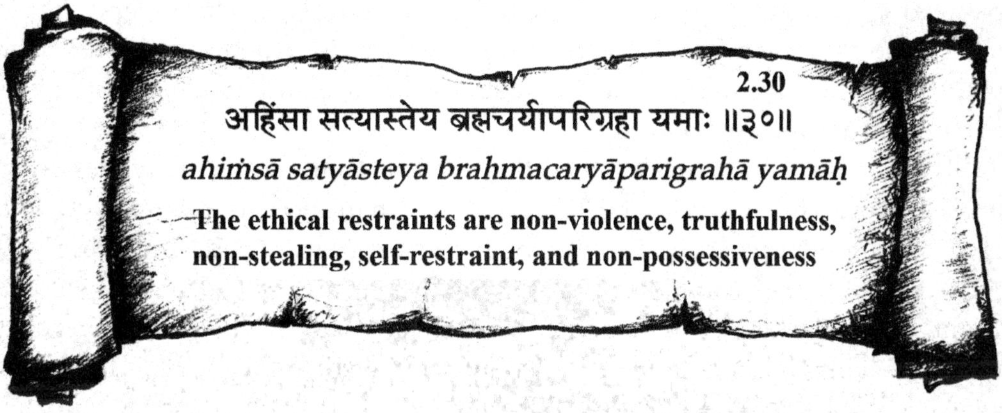
2.30
अहिंसा सत्यास्तेय ब्रह्मचर्यापरिग्रहा यमाः ॥३०॥
ahiṁsā satyāsteya brahmacaryāparigrahā yamāḥ
The ethical restraints are non-violence, truthfulness, non-stealing, self-restraint, and non-possessiveness

Along these same lines, my goal as a good holistic doctor is to meet my patient with love and compassion, speak to him/her in an honest way, and develop a professional relationship based on balance and generosity. I aim to see the patient in his/her highest spiritual potential from the very start, viewing the patient above and beyond his/her ill state of being while focusing on his/her whole, truest, and best self. The healing process, then, becomes about supporting the creation of a physical, mental, emotional, and spiritual state from which the patient can live from his/her greatest self. Following the *yamas* and maximizing their intent within our relations and ourselves heals on a level deeper than any pill can go.

PRINCIPLE 2. The Healing Power of Nature (*Vis Medicatrix Naturae*)

"The natural healing force within each of us
is the greatest force in getting well."

—HIPPOCRATES

The body has an ordered intelligence or "vitality" to it and wants to be well. It has inherent, built-in physiological mechanisms that, in health, maintain homeostatic balance and function consistently to keep us alive. The body sustains a normal blood pressure, body temperature, blood pH balance, mineral balance, etc. It can mount a fever to kill off infections, induce vomiting or diarrhea to get rid of something harmfully ingested, and clears out toxins through liver, kidney, and intestinal pathways. We become ill when this natural healing force is overrun and the systems of the body have difficulty recovering homeostasis. In naturopathic medicine, natural remedies are implemented that stimulate this natural vitality of the body to reorient back toward balance.

The Yoga path also speaks about this natural vitality in the body and calls it *prāṇa*. In Yoga Therapy, this vital force, or prāṇa, in the body is cleansed and nourished through the practice of *āsanas* (body postures), *prāṇāyāma* (breathing practices), and *dhyāna* (meditation). These techniques help to self-regulate the body's innate natural healing force and teach the prāṇa how to flow with greater ease to the places in the body where it is needed most for healing.

PRINCIPLE 3. Identify and Treat the Causes (*Tolle Causum*)

"It is far more important to know what sort of person the disease has than what sort of disease the person has."

—HIPPOCRATES

This principle highlights the art of medicine. While certain medical protocols may exist for many disease processes, these should never be blindly followed without regard for the person who has walked into the door. Why did *this* person contract this illness? What is the general constitution and tendencies for imbalance in *this* person? Does he/she have other health conditions and how are they all connected? What does *this* person require to heal? For example, if he/she has chronic headaches, are they being caused by an environmental toxicity, nutritional deficiency, emotional stress, blood circulation problem, or some other factor(s)? For true healing and cure to occur, each person (even if they have the same diagnosis as someone else) requires an individualized treatment plan that addresses the specific reasons and problems that are causing his/her imbalances and illness.

Yoga philosophy also lays out guidelines regarding how to remove the causes of disharmony or disease and restore balance. It identifies the three guṇas (qualities of nature) that must be balanced in each individual for good health: rajas, tamas, and sattva. Essentially, an overabundance of *rajas* (activity, greed, passions) and/or *tamas* (darkness, inertia, laziness) causes suffering as it leads one away from *sattva* (a state of purity, harmony, balance, health, and contentment that is free from sickness). Various Yoga techniques may be chosen or emphasized to reduce and modify rajas and/or tamas depending on what the individual requires. Several specific Yoga Therapy techniques to improve the balance between the guṇas are discussed in "Ayurveda and Yoga: Complementary Therapeutics" by Vasant Lad and "Structural Yoga Therapy and Ayurvedic Yoga Therapy" by Mukunda and Chinnamasta Stiles in this text.

PRINCIPLE 4. Treat the Whole Person (Mind, Body, and Spirit)

"The whole is greater than the sum of its parts."

—ARISTOTLE

Our bodies are not just physical machines. A person's health and well-being is affected by mental, emotional, physical, social, environmental, and spiritual factors. According to holistic medicine, all of these factors are interconnected and must be assessed and treated for healing to occur. Every level and aspect of a person must be considered and nurtured in naturopathic medicine in order to maintain health.

The Yoga system also works on the full human being. Yoga Therapy teachings describe the wholeness of a person using the five pancha kośas (soul sheaths or layers). The five kośas are the anna-maya-kośa (physical sheath), the prāṇa-maya-kośa (energy sheath), the mano-maya-kośa (mental-emotional sheath), the vijñāna-maya-kośa (wisdom or higher-mind sheath), and the ānanda-maya-kośa (universal consciousness or bliss sheath). Disturbances to any layer of a person can have a ripple effect and disturb other parts of his/her being. Yoga Therapy is designed to bring these sheaths back into healthy alignment through therapeutic techniques found in the classical eight limbs of Yoga like āsana, prāṇāyāma, sense withdrawal, concentration, and meditation.

PRINCIPLE 5. Doctor as Guide or Teacher (*Docere*)

Docere means "to teach" and is the origin of the word *doctor* in Latin. This naturopathic principle says the doctor is a guide who helps the patient connect with his/her own inherent healing abilities. Doctors are knowledgeable and trained in what a person can do to heal, but ultimately the individual must take charge and do his/her part. The doctor can only provide guidance, support, and encouragement. When a patient does heal, per the doctor's guidance and therapy, the doctor has not healed the person. The doctor nudges and the therapy nourishes, but the person ultimately does the work; and his/her body's vital force restores the balance.

Akin to this concept, Yoga Therapy empowers people to honor the wisdom and power of their own body. Through Yoga āsana practice, people increase body awareness, alignment, strength, and flexibility and come to understand the mind and human spirit in a deeper way. A Yoga Therapist can guide a person in the practice of Yoga techniques, but all of the benefits of Yoga Therapy can only come through direct experience of actually doing the Yoga. It is an experiential practice and therapy. As Pattabhi Jois, the founder of Ashtanga Vinyasa Yoga, says, "Do your practice and all is coming" (Donahaye and Stern, 2010).

PRINCIPLE 6. Prevention Is the Best Medicine

"Let food be thy medicine and medicine be thy food."

—HIPPOCRATES

Naturopathic medicine emphasizes that quality air, sunlight, food, water, exercise, recreational time, and natural therapies are necessary, not only when we are sick, but also when we are healthy in order to maintain health. The Yoga path teaches that when we live in an ethical way with the world around us, train and enhance the basic movements of our bodies, learn to advance our breath capacity, and teach ourselves to calm our minds through the wisdom of Yoga techniques—we enhance our health and quality of life.

In living the healthy lifestyle guidelines set forth by naturopathic philosophy and the *Yoga Sūtras of Patañjali,* we lower our risk factors for developing illnesses. In Chapter II, Verse 16 of the *Yoga Sūtras,* Patañjali says, "Heyam Dukham Anagatam" (Suffering that is not yet experienced is avoidable) (Iyengar, 2002). "Chronic diseases such as heart disease, stroke, cancer, diabetes, and arthritis are among the most common, costly, and preventable of all health problems in the U.S." (CDC, 2012). "Modifiable health risk behaviors [such as lack of physical activity and poor nutrition] are responsible for much of the illness, suffering, and early death related to chronic diseases" (CDC, 2012). Studies show that Yoga has many beneficial health effects—it decreases stress and anxiety, lowers blood pressure, improves cholesterol levels, enhances cardiovascular endurance, balances blood sugar, improves respiratory fitness, and improves mood, quality of life, and general functioning (Sengupta, 2012).

All in all, just like naturopathic medicine, Yoga Therapy is a compassionate practice that stimulates the natural vitality of the body to heal, addresses the wholeness of our being (mind, body, and spirit), and develops self-awareness and strength to maintain health and prevent illness.

KRIPALU YOGA THERAPY

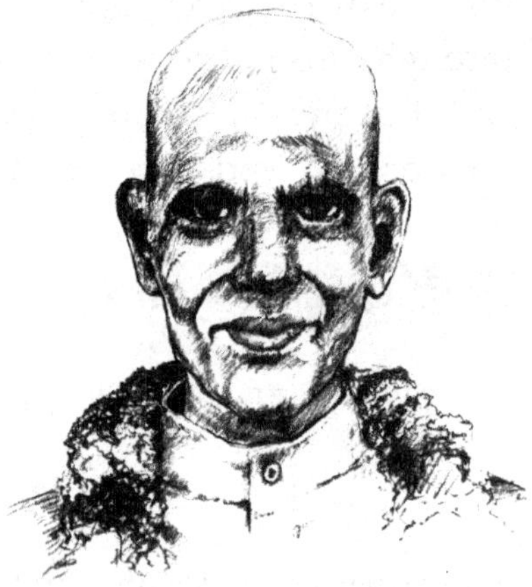

Swami Kripalvananda (1913–1981)

One of the great Yoga styles brought to and made popular in the West during the twentieth century was Kripalu Yoga as developed by Swami Kripalvananda (1913–1981) from Gujarat, India. A dancer at heart, I became attracted to Kripalu Yoga because of its focus on how awakened prāṇa can spontaneously dance us into motion. This essence of Kripalu Yoga nicely exemplifies the crossover between Yoga and naturopathic philosophy. Just as naturopathic medicine is about stimulating the vital force, or prāṇa, of a patient to heal from within, Kripalu Yoga also encourages one to feel inside oneself and move, discover, and heal from this pure, uninhibited pranic (vital) force. Along with learning the foundational Yoga philosophy and proper alignment of Yoga poses, the Kripalu Yoga student is encouraged to tap into internal logic and intuition and create an individualized Yoga practice organically, in the moment, motivated from the inside. Yoga becomes like an improvisational dance where we are guided through Yoga poses by our own natural knowing and flow of prāṇa into how we need to move for further opening, healing, and awakening. Being in touch with life force in this way, we become our own healer.

YOGA AS A THERAPEUTIC PRESCRIPTION IN NATUROPATHIC MEDICINE

Creating an individualized Yoga prescription specific for the patient's particular condition, as an adjunct to nutritional and other lifestyle changes, is very supportive of the healing process. Naturopathic doctors are already versed in the implementation of patient homework with instructions for diet and lifestyle practices. Prescribed sets of Yoga poses can provide problem-specific corrections and empower patients to take healing into their own hands. As patient homework, Yoga Therapy creates an avenue for healing to extend beyond the treatment room. It is a therapy to keep a patient on a healthy track and serves as a healing reminder on a daily basis.

Let us take insomnia as an example. For a patient who is anxious and has trouble winding down to go to sleep at night, a sedating Yoga combination may be a key prescription for him/her along with a full sleep hygiene makeover. In my practice, I make several recommendations to achieve this goal of improved rest. The patient must go to bed at a routine time, before 11 p.m. is best, each night. In the hours before bed, dimmed lights and quiet activities are crucial. A nightly relaxing Yoga routine is beneficial. Examples of calming Yoga āsanas that may be included are:

1. Paśćimottanāsana (Seated Forward Bend Pose)

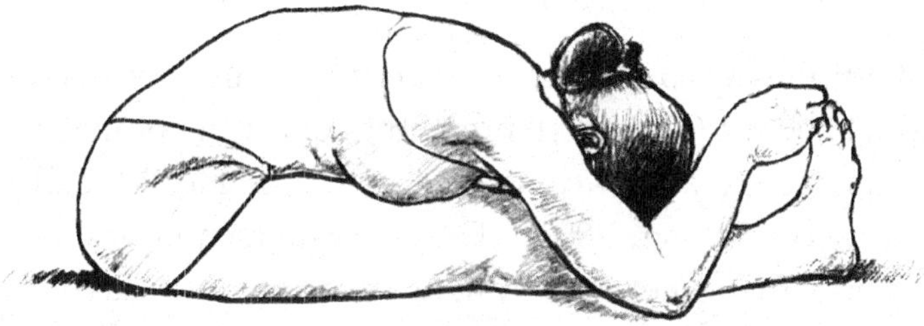

2. Bālāsana (Child's Pose)

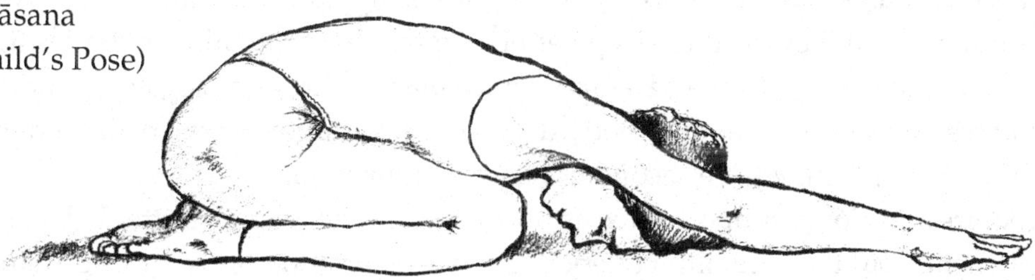

3. Viparīta Karaṇī (Legs Up the Wall Pose)

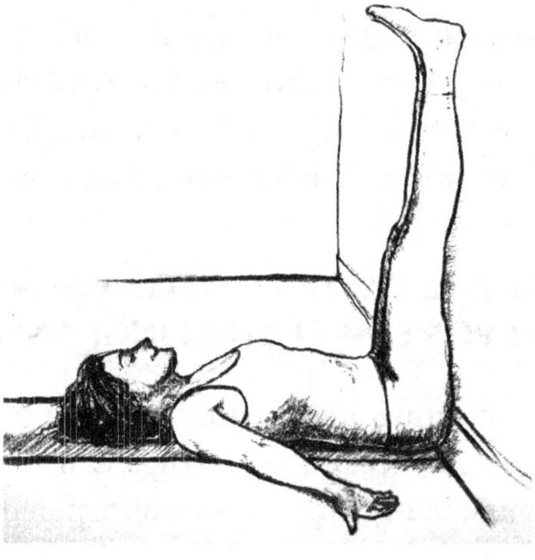

4. Śavāsana (Corpse Pose)

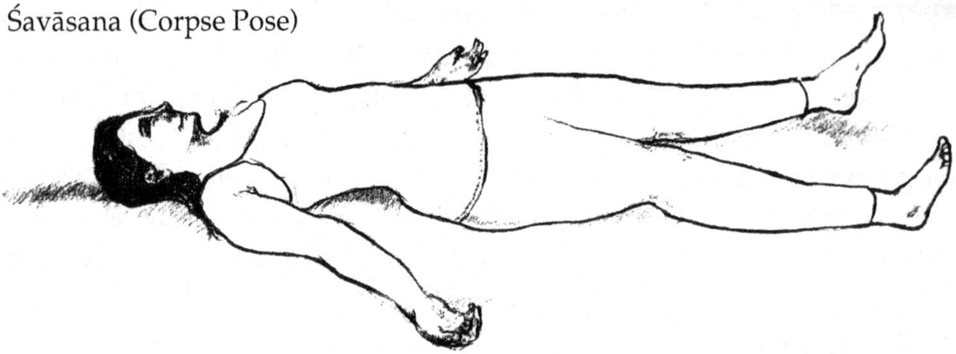

Additionally, prāṇāyāma breathing techniques can be beneficial for rest like candra bhedana (left nostril breathing) or dīrgha prāṇāyāma (deep breathing) with an extended exhale twice as long as the inhale (McCall and Yoga Journal, 2007; Payne and Usatine, 2002). These Yoga techniques regulate cortisol, enhance parasympathetic nervous system function, and have an overall calming effect (McCall and Yoga Journal, 2007). For many patients, these simple nighttime lifestyle changes, with a short nightly Yoga Therapy practice, and regularity in their routine are all they need to sleep better. It removes stimulating activities that may be an obstacle to sleep and empowers patients, through Yoga's scientific techniques, to learn to calm their body down in preparation for sleep all on their own. Other patients may have secondary causes of insomnia that must be addressed or require additional support, such as hormonal and neurotransmitter balancing supplements, but the regulation of good lifestyle activity patterns for improving sleep lays a great foundation.

Integrating Yoga and Yoga Therapy into our daily lives doesn't have to mean finding time to go to a Yoga studio for a full Yoga class. Adding specific daily Yoga prescriptions helps patients form a deeper understanding of their treatment and brings awareness to areas of their life where they can take a more proactive approach.

EMPOWERING THE PATIENT WITH YOGA: FOR HEALTHY LIFESTYLE SUPPORT, SELF-HEALING, AND SELF-DISCOVERY

In healing, we are creating a new patterned way of being that must be reinforced by healthy lifestyle practices such as Yoga. Our in-office discussion and in-office therapies (e.g., acupuncture, intravenous nutrition therapy) are aimed at balancing the body, and this balance must be maintained by what the patients do in their day-to-day lives. The work and healing transformation in the office can be supported or sabotaged by what patients do when they leave the office. It is common to see great improvements in how patients feel when they are following the prescribed diet/lifestyle/exercise plan. It is likewise common to see a slip backward in symptoms and well-being when they go off the treatment plan. Yoga Therapy prescriptions that result in a daily or even weekly Yoga practice will support the in-office therapies and empower self-healing and self-discovery.

YOGA AS GENERAL EXERCISE AND AS MIND-BODY EXERCISE

Due to the broad spectrum of effects, Yoga is one of the top exercises that I recommend to my patients. Exercise, in general, has a multitude of extremely well-established healthy influences. For example, it helps with weight loss, builds body strength and functionality, aids bone health, and improves mood and sleep (HHS, 2008). Regular exercise lowers risk for premature death, heart disease, stroke, diabetes, and some cancers (HHS, 2008). It improves brain function and prevents Alzheimer's disease and dementia (Ahlskog, et al., 2011). Moreover, "The studies comparing the effects of Yoga and general exercise seem to indicate that, in both healthy and diseased populations, Yoga may be as effective as or better than exercise at improving a variety of health-related outcome measures" (Ross and Thomas, 2010). There is also a growing body of scientific research exhibiting the healthy effects of Yoga āsana itself (Field, 2011).

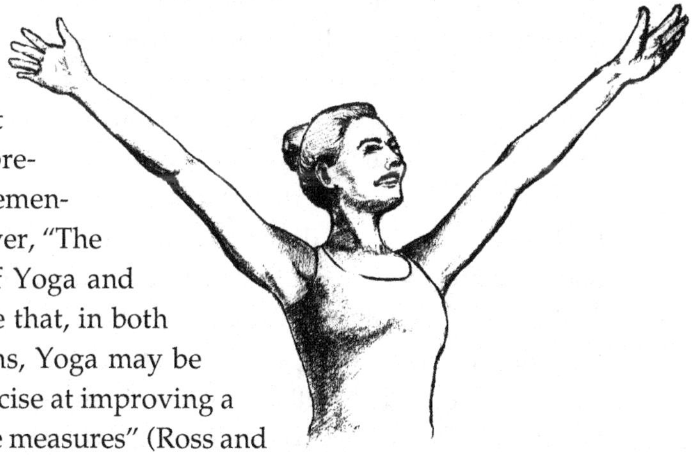

What sets Yoga apart from other exercise forms is the wisdom behind the specific Yoga postures and their effects on the body and the fact that it is a mindful physical exercise. There is a definite, yet complex, interactive circuit between our mind and body upon which Yoga postures act. Our minds change our bodies, and our bodies change our minds. For example, "power posing," standing in a confident pose (for as little as 2 minutes), raises testosterone and lowers cortisol levels, and makes us feel more powerful (Cuddy, 2012). Furthermore, Yoga āsana as a moving meditation or mindful exercise encourages the engagement of mental awareness in the exercise. Meditation on its own has researched health benefits (Arias, 2006), and mindful movement exercise may exert enhanced healing influences over general exercise via the power of the mind-body connection and the extra relaxation response incurred. Evidence shows a reduction in stress, pain, depression, anxiety, high blood pressure, and insulin resistance with mindful exercise practices such as Yoga (Howley and Thompson, 2012).

YOGA FOR EFFICIENCY AND PERFORMANCE

Sickness often occurs when we forget to take care of ourselves in some way, when our life demands become overwhelming, and when we run out of time to nurture ourselves. For healing to occur, our health and well-being must become a top priority again. It is common for patients to object to this, saying they don't have time to work on their health and make all the required diet and lifestyle adjustments. Many patients claim that their life has many stresses and demands and that they have no control over or power to change this situation—"That's just the way it is." It is commonly expressed that "My life is too busy, I don't have time to get the right foods, take these supplements, or do Yoga." These are viparyayas (misperceptions) according to Patañjali and unconscious defense mechanisms holding us back from change. We do have a choice: How we react to the stressors in our life and if we are going to make time to take care of ourselves are completely up to us. It literally takes only a few minutes a day to take supplements and another 3 minutes for a Yoga breathing exercise midday that can make an exponential difference in stress level and overall well-being. In my experience, when we take care of our health and well-being, we are smarter, clearer, more productive, more effective, and more efficient in the rest of our lives.

For example, there was a point in naturopathic medical school when the workload got very heavy and I started to sacrifice my sleep and Yoga/exercise routine in exchange for more study time. I was getting decent grades, but feeling lousy. The cold, dark, rainy wintertime in Portland, Oregon, also didn't help my mood. I cashed in on a special deal for a hot Yoga studio membership thinking that the heat in the Yoga room would be a great balance to offset the cold winter. I started doing lots of Yoga classes at the sacrifice of my school study time. So now I had much less time to study for my exams. And guess what? My school grades went up! I did more Yoga, studied less, and with less effort in the classroom and more focus on my practice and myself I performed better in school.

I see this in clinical practice with my patients too. I often encourage and inspire my patients by sharing the above personal story with them. I have supported many patients who were stressed, tired, overworked, and overwhelmed. They often put up a fight at first saying they don't have the time for Yoga. It is sometimes hard to get them out of the mind-set that the harder they work and the busier they are, the more they will achieve. As I learned, sometimes the opposite is true—if they do the Yoga and other healing work, they will function more efficaciously in their lives with far less effort and hardship. The net result is decreased stress and increased energy, focus, creativity, and productivity, which is everything they wanted in the first place.

HOLISTIC PRACTICES, SCIENCE, AND THEIR MODERN RELEVANCE

The modern Yoga and naturopathic landscapes are moving in two directions as they get assimilated into our current cultural reality. One direction is the adoption of these therapies into the dominant reductionism paradigm. For instance, Yoga has gained a lot of interest in the West primarily as a means of exercise. Similarly, naturopathic therapies are often oversimplified and used in a "green allopathic" method where an herbal pill is taken instead of a drug medication pill—treating the symptoms rather than the whole person. In these styles, not much attention is paid to the holistic way of thinking that defines these paradigms and systems.

The other influence that these therapies have as we assimilate them into modern times is that they invite us to examine our standard way of thinking and being. The deeper yogic and naturopathic philosophies synergistically challenge us to learn, grow, and heal by expanding our way of being, observing the larger patterns at play, and acknowledging the interconnectedness of all things. On a personal level, Yoga has transformed from being an interesting college exercise class into a pivotal tool for evolving my way of being in and relating to the world. It seems impossible to engage in these types of holistic practices without becoming rooted in an expanded, holistic worldview.

The viewpoint and goals of naturopathic medicine and Yoga Therapy are consistent. The holistic paradigm that underlies both naturopathy and Yoga teaches us to look at things with an open mind and tap into internal logic. In these holistic practices, science becomes just a part of the picture of how we know what we know. Rather than ignore the scientifically unquantifiable variables in life, holistic thinking allows us to incorporate personal experiences and other sensory methods of understanding the world into our paradigm. We begin to use a whole being awareness and approach. For this reason, above and beyond the scientific studies, there are certain wisdoms and benefits to be obtained through naturopathic and Yoga healing that may only be understood by stepping into their world and experiencing them firsthand.

CONCLUSION

Discovering Yoga and naturopathic medicine were wonderful *aha* moments for me. I knew I had found invaluable practices that would teach me about myself and the nature of life that books, in and of themselves, could not. The practices were a turning point for me on my own healing journey. Yoga helped me live with grace through some very tough times, and it has been a source for uncloaking the beauty and magic of life at other times. At moments when I was a student and couldn't afford regular health insurance or healthcare visits, I regarded Yoga as my health insurance and as a way of balancing my health on my own. It alleviated accumulated stress in my body and mind, energized and nourished, and has been the perfect therapy for me to embody the "physician heal thyself" concept. Fundamentally, our bodies must be healthy and balanced if we want to be able to help others achieve the same.

One of the highlights of the naturopathic medicine tradition is its skill at mixing and blending a variety of therapies in an artful way in order to address an individual's health concerns from multiple angles. Yoga provides a strong foundation for the development of the body, mind, and soul and as a therapy. Yoga can be a powerful tool for self-healing and transformation. Naturopathic medicine and Yoga Therapy serve the same purpose: to awaken and stimulate a person's natural capacity for self-healing and vitality. For naturopathic doctors, Yoga Therapy is a vital therapy to have a basic awareness of and, moreover, a professional responsibility to understand. Together, Yoga Therapy and naturopathic medicine are beneficial tools for evolving a powerful holistic healthcare model for modern times.

REFERENCES

Ahlskog, J. E., et al. "Physical Exercise as a Preventive or Disease-Modifying Treatment of Dementia and Brain Aging." *Mayo Clinic Proceedings* 86.9 (2011): 876–884. Print.

Arias, A. J., et al. "Systematic Review of Meditation Techniques as Treatments for Medical Illness." *Journal of Complementary and Alternative Medicine* 12.8 (2006): 817–832.

CDC. "Chronic Diseases and Health Promotion." CDC: 2012. Web. 8 Jan. 2013. http://www.cdc.gov/chronicdisease/overview/index.htm?s_cid=ostltsdyk_govd_203.

Cuddy, A. (2012). "Your Body Language Shapes Who You Are." TED.com Jun. 2012. Web. 8 Jan. 2013. http://www.ted.com/talks/amy_cuddy_your_body_language_shapes_who_you_are.

Dhyansky, Y. "The Indus Valley Origin of a Yoga Practice." *Artibus Asiae* 48.1–2 (1987): 89–108. Print.

Donahaye, G., and E. Stern, *Guriji: A Portrait of Sri. K. Pattabhi Jois Through the Eyes of His Students.* New York: North Point Press, 2010. Print.

Field, T. "Yoga Clinical Research Review." *Complementary Therapies in Clinical Practice* 17 (2011): 1–8. Print.

Howley, E., and D. Thompson. "Mindful Exercise for Fitness Professionals." *Fitness Professional's Handbook, Sixth Edition.* Eds. E. Howley and D. Thompson. Champaign, IL: Human Kinetics, 2012. 439–457. Print.

Iyengar, B. K. S. *Light on the Yoga Sutras of Patanjali.* London: Thorsons, 1993; Harper Collins, 2002. Print.

McCall, T., and Yoga Journal. *Yoga as Medicine: The Yogic Prescription for Health and Healing.* New York: Bantam, 2007. Print.

Payne, L., and R. P. Usatine. *Yoga Rx: A Step-by-Step Program to Promote Health, Wellness, and Healing for Common Ailments.* New York: Broadway, 2002. Print.

Pizzorno, J., et al. "Naturopathic Medicine." *Fundamentals of Complementary and Alternative Medicine.* Ed. M. Micozzi. St. Louis, MO: Elsevier, 1996; Saunders, 2011. 292–321. Print.

Possehl, G. *The Indus Civilization: A Contemporary Perspective.* Walnut Creek, CA: Rowman & Little-field Publishers; AltaMira Press, 2002. Print.

Ross, A., and S. Thomas. "The Health Benefits of Yoga and Exercise: A Review of Comparison Studies." *Journal of Alternative and Complementary Medicine* 16.1 (2010): 3–12. Print.

Sengupta, P. "Health Impacts of Yoga and Pranayama: A State-of-the-Art Review." *International Journal of Preventive Medicine* 3.7 (2012): 444–458. Print.

U.S. Dept. of Health and Human Services. *2008 Physical Activity Guidelines for Americans.* 2008. Web. 8 Jan. 2013. http://www.health.gov/paguidelines/guidelines/chapter2.

NEUROLOGY AND YOGA THERAPY

Acharya Pandit Shri Kant Mishra, M.D., M.S., A.B.M.S., B.H.U., F.A.A.N.,

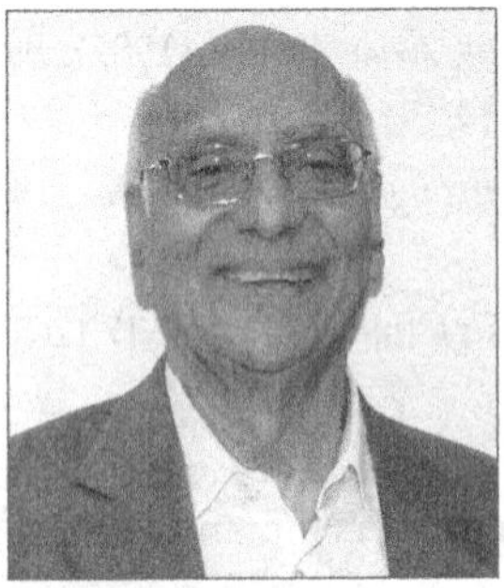

Acharya Pandit Shri Kant Mishra is a gold medalist in Ayurvedacharya and has a bachelor of medicine and surgery (A.B.M.S.) degree, with a diploma in Yoga, from India's Banaras Hindu University in Varanasi, Uttar Pradesh, one of the most prestigious universities in the region. He is currently a professor of neurology at the David Geffen School of Medicine at UCLA, Los Angeles and the Keck School of Medicine at the University of Southern California (USC), where he was the director (and one of the founders) of the Integrative Medicine program. Dr. Mishra serves as the director of neuromuscular disorders at the VA in greater Los Angeles and at Olive View–UCLA Medical Center. He has been a valuable resource in promoting scientific collaboration between the National Institutes of Health's (NIH) National Center of Complementary and Alternative Medicine (NCCAM) and the Department of Ayurveda, Yoga, and Naturopathy, Unani, Siddha and Homeopathy (AYUSH) in India. He founded and served as president of the American Academy of Ayurveda (AAAM) and organized meetings in the United States and India for evidence-based work on the Indian system of medicine, including Yoga and Ayurveda. An expert in the concepts of Patañjali Yoga and a firm believer in the principles of Aṣṭāṅga Yoga, which he teaches and practices, Dr. Mishra has published several evidence-based articles in peer-reviewed journals on Yoga and Ayurveda and their influence on human well-being.

INTRODUCTION

Yoga started roughly 5,000 years ago in the Indian subcontinent as part of the Ayurvedic healing science. The word *Yoga* is derived from the Sanskrit word *yukti* meaning "union," aiming to unify spirit (consciousness) with super spirit (God). The ancient yogis recognized that a healthy body is essential to accomplish the highest states of Yoga. As a spiritual practice, Yoga utilizes mind (meditation) and body (exercises) to balance our systems and explores the mind's abilities to affect the senses and the body. An estimated 15.8 million Americans practice Yoga today for various medical purposes. "Yoga is a mind and body practice with origins in ancient Indian philosophy" reports the National Center for Complementary and Alternative Medicine (Mishra, et al., 2012).

TYPES OF YOGA

Yoga is one of the six systems of Indian Vedic philosophy known as the Six Darśanas along with Sāṁkhya, Nyāya, Vaiśeṣika, Mimāṁsā, and Vedanta. Maharishi Patañjali, rightly known as the "Father of Yoga," compiled and formulated the various aspects of Yoga systematically in his compilation of *Yoga Sūtras* (aphorisms). In the *Yoga Sūtras,* he advocated the eight-fold path known as Aṣṭāṅga Yoga for an all-round development of human personality. These include yamas (moral codes), niyamas (self-purification and study), āsana (posture), prāṇāyāma (breath control), pratyāhāra (sense control), dhāraṇā (concentration), dhyāna (meditation), and samādhi (super contemplation). These are articulated on the basis of diverse psychological understanding of human personality (Mishra, 1999). Patañjali defined *Yoga* in Sanskrit as *citta-vṛtti-nirodha,* meaning "Yoga is the inhibition (nirodha) of the modifications (vṛtti) of the mind (citta)." The yogic values are broadly classified into four categories: Work, Worship, Philosophy, and Psychic control. Karma Yoga, the path of work, promotes pleasure in labor without indulging in thoughts of success or failure, which aids in performing tasks in a skillful manner. Bhakti Yoga, the path of worship, is a systematic method of engaging the mind in the practice of divine love to soften our emotions and tranquilize our minds. Jñāna Yoga, the path of philosophy, is a systematic way of enlightening the mind about the realities of life by contemplation. It strips off the garb of avidyā (ignorance) from our mind as it goes to its natural state of rest. And finally, Rāja

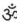

Yoga, the path of psychic control, is a systematic process of culturing the mind. It is based on the eight-fold path set by Patañjali (Mishra, 1999). Together, these paths of Yoga can be used for health promotion and disease prevention and for the treatment of various physical, mental, and spiritual disorders.

OVERVIEW OF INTRODUCTORY NEUROANATOMY AND NEUROPHYSIOLOGY AS IT RELATES TO YOGA

The nervous system is broadly classified into the central nervous system (CNS) comprised of the brain and spinal cord and the peripheral nervous system (PNS), which in itself contains the peripheral nerves, neuromuscular junction, and muscles. The practice of Yoga involves coordination between all these structures at various levels. The PNS is further divided into the somatic nervous system and autonomic nervous system (ANS). The somatic nervous system is responsible for voluntary functions of the body, and ANS is responsible for involuntary functions. The ANS is also known as visceral nervous system, or involuntary nervous system, and is further classified into sympathetic nervous system (SNS) and parasympathetic nervous systems (PSNS).

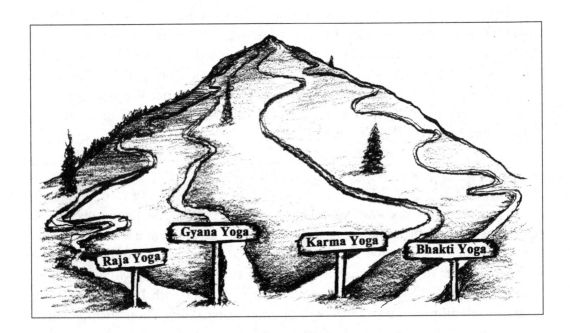

The SNS controls involuntary stress response; hence it is called the fight-or-flight response. The PSNS controls vegetative functions and is referred to as "feed or breed" or "rest and repose." It works as an opposition response to SNS. Both SNS and PSNS control involuntary functions of vital organs of the body like heart, lungs, glands, etc. While generally referred to as "involuntary," the ANS can be controlled by proper meditation and yogic practices, particularly those that increase parasympathetic input, which leads to decreased sympathetic nervous system activities. This is how the practice of Yoga neurologically stimulates the nervous system and aids in the normal function of the mind and body.

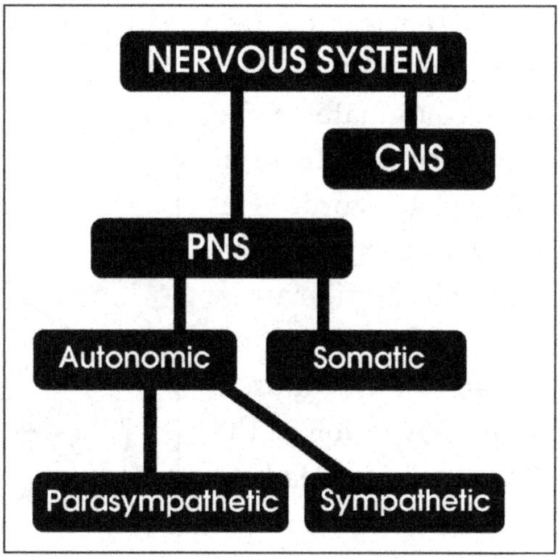

Classification of the Nervous System

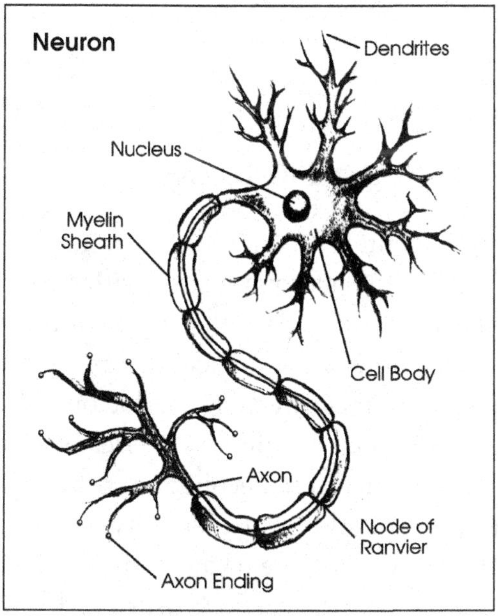

The central and peripheral nervous systems are composed of millions of neurons (nerve cells) connected by axons and dendrites as seen in the illustration at left. Information is transmitted across the nervous system from one axon to another via nerve terminals that are connected by synapses. The electrical stimulus is transmitted across the synapse through chemicals referred to as neurotransmitters. Norepinephrine is the neurotransmitter for SNS and acetylcholine is the neurotransmitter for PSNS.

There are two types of neurons. Sensory neurons (afferent neurons) transmit information from the peripheral nervous system (skin, muscles) to central nervous system (brain). Motor neurons (efferent neurons), on the other hand, transmit information from the central nervous system to peripheral nervous system to perform voluntary movements.

The efferent pathway is further divided into upper motor neuron (UMN) pathway and lower motor neuron (LMN) pathway. The UMN consists of neurons, which originate in the brain and terminate in the spinal cord. The LMN consists of neurons, which originate in the spinal cord and terminate on the muscle surface. A lesion in the UMN pathway leads to spastic weakness in the limbs, and a lesion of LMN pathway results in flaccid weakness of the limbs. Regular Yoga not only helps in relaxing the spastic limbs but also provides strength to the flaccid muscles.

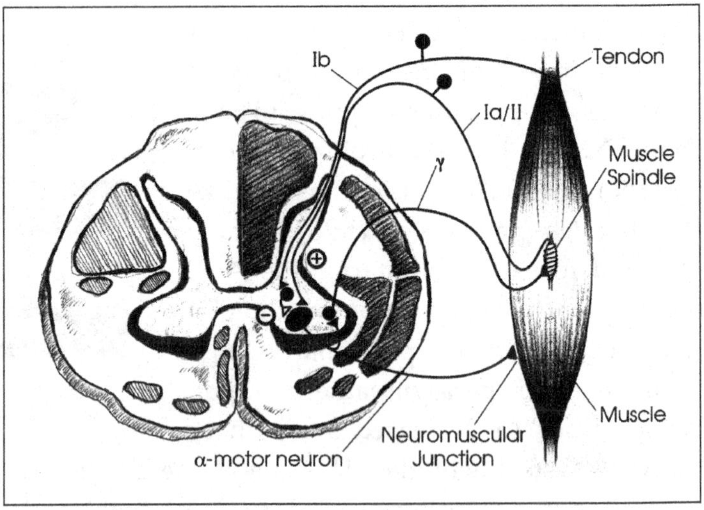

Motor Neuron Pathways

UTILIZATION OF YOGA IN NEUROLOGICAL DISORDERS

Yoga has been used for prevention and complementary treatment of various neurological disorders. More than 600 disorders afflict the nervous system with stroke, epilepsy, Parkinson's disease, headache, and dementia being the most common conditions (Mishra and Vinjamury, 2001) Many other neurological disorders are rare and are known only to the individuals and families affected, the doctors, and the scientists. Neurological disorders affect an estimated 50 million Americans each year, resulting in an incalculable personal toll and an annual economic cost in the hundreds of billions of dollars in medical expenses and lost productivity. Numerous studies have been performed to validate the use of Yoga as a complementary alternative treatment modality in various neurological disorders (Mishra and Vinjamury, 2001). Yoga has been used successfully as an adjuvant to health promotion and disease prevention for various physical and mental disorders, particularly neurological health (Mishra and Vinjamury, 1999).

Epilepsy

About 50 million people worldwide have epilepsy, and nearly 80 percent of epilepsy occurs in developing countries. Epilepsy is usually controlled, but not cured, with medication. More than 30 percent of people with epilepsy do not have seizure control even with the best available medications. Patients with epilepsy who do not respond to conventional antiseizure medications may find results in alternative treatment modalities, such as Yoga Therapy. In a group of twenty patients with drug-resistant epilepsy, the practice of Yoga meditation twice daily showed an overall decrease in seizure frequency (Rajesh, et al., 2006). Panjwani demonstrated that patients with epilepsy responded to Sahaja Yoga in reducing stress, in a randomized controlled study (Panjwani, et al., 2000). This provides hope to patients with refractory epilepsy that nonpharmaceutical techniques may be successful in reducing seizure frequency.

Furthermore, Sirven surveyed the use of complementary and alternative medicine (CAM) treatments, including Yoga, among Epilepsy Foundation of Arizona (EFAZ) members (Sirven, et al., 2003). Yoga was reported as effective in seizure control in 57 percent of participants. All CAM modalities were partly perceived to be beneficial; however, botanicals, stress reduction, and Yoga were reported as being the most helpful. In a study involving eighteen patients with EEG-diagnosed epilepsy, Yoga showed therapeutic effects of decreasing seizure index along with an improvement in quality of life (Lundgren, et al., 2008). Augmenting Yoga to help people with epilepsy presents an inexpensive, noninvasive, enjoyable, and potentially cross-cultural supplementation to epilepsy control and quality of life improvement (Lundgren, et al., 2008).

Stroke Prevention and Rehabilitation

According to the World Health Organization (WHO), stroke is currently the second most common cause of adult mortality in the United States and is responsible for almost 5.8 million deaths each year worldwide. About 795,000 people annually have strokes in the United States, and, of these, 137,000 are fatal. Roughly 610,000 of these cases are first strokes, and 185,000 people who survive a stroke will have another stroke within five years (CDC, 2012). Since strokes occur suddenly with effects lasting a lifetime, approaches for prevention and rehabilitation are essential, and the practice of Yoga is gaining significance in this arena. Upon review of numerous studies employing Yoga in patients with stroke, it was found that eliciting relaxation through meditation was useful in both stroke prevention and post-stroke rehabilitation. Relaxation promotes positive effects on carotid atherosclerosis (Castillo-Richmond, et al., 2000), hypertension (Benson, et al., 1974), diabetes (Jain, et al., 1993), and coronary artery diseases (Ornish, et al., 1998), which are all identified risk factors associated with stroke occurrence or reoccurrence. Bell and Seyfer have described specific adaptations of Yoga postures that can be utilized by people with limited mobility due to neurological conditions such as multiple sclerosis and stroke (Seyfer and Bell, 1990).

Additionally, Bastille investigated the effects of a Yoga-based exercise program on balance, mobility, and quality of life for people with chronic poststroke weakness or hemiparesis (Bastille and Gill-Body, 2004). A single-subject study design assessed the primary outcome variables of balance on the Berg Balance Scale [BBS] (Berg, et al., 1989) and timed mobility on the Timed Movement Battery [TMB] (Creel, Light, and Thigpen, 2001) while a secondary outcome variable to the research was perceived quality of life on the Stroke Impact Scale [SIS], Version 2.0 (Duncan, et al., 1999). All subjects demonstrated some positive effects in the primary and secondary outcome variables. Improvements in aphasia (inability to speak, read, or write) and coordination among limbs in poststroke patients was noted after a twelve-week regime of Kundalini Yoga (Lynton, Kilgler, and Shiflett, 2007). In a recent preliminary study involving a ten-week Yoga program comprising of āsanas (physical practices) and prāṇāyāma (breathing practices), the Yoga group showed improvements in bio-psychosocial health when compared to the control group. Emerging trends included greater sensation, feeling calmer, and becoming connected with mind and body, as well as improvements in perceived physical strength, range of movement, body awareness, gait, balance, energy, concentration, confidence, and stress (Garrett, Immink, and Hillier, 2011). These findings illustrate the positive physical and psychosocial impact Yoga can instill in stroke victims and lend support to the growing evidence that improvements in impairments and mobility limitations can be achieved, in people with chronic poststroke hemiparesis, through Yoga based practices (Dean, Richards, and Malouin, 2000).

Multiple Sclerosis

Multiple sclerosis (MS) is a debilitating and demyelinating disease that damages the myelin sheath surrounding the spinal cord. The disease presents with varying degrees of severity affecting cognitive, motor, and sensory functions. MS is thought to affect more than 2.3 million people worldwide. While the disease is not contagious or directly inherited, certain factors such as female gender, genetics, adult age groups, geography, and ethnic background influence this disorder. There is no cure, yet therapies exist with the goal of slowing the progression of the disease to control symptoms and maintain or regain an appropriate quality of life. Some medications result in adverse side effects and poor toleration, leading many patients to seek alternative methods of management, one of which is Yoga. In 1997, an anonymous poll sent to 129 MS-diagnosed patients in Germany reported that 63 percent of patients used some form of alternative therapy, nearly half of these being some form of Yoga meditation (Winterholler, Erbguth, and Neundtrfer, 1997). This was an astounding finding! Patients were taking an active part in their treatment and having positive outcomes in managing their chronic MS. In another study, a 17 percent improvement in selective attention was demonstrated using Yoga, although it did not have significant reductions in fatigue (Velikonja, et al., 2010). The findings suggested that Yoga as well as other forms of aerobic exercise can play a role in improving mobility, activity, and mental function in people with MS. Several studies suggest that Yoga may be comparable to other forms of exercise in relieving symptoms of fatigue; however, there are different types of Yoga, and more specific investigations are needed to determine the effects of Yoga Therapy's various approaches to MS symptoms and mechanisms.

Alzheimer's Disease and Other Dementia

Alzheimer's disease is the most common form of dementia, a general term for memory loss and other intellectual abilities serious enough to interfere with daily life. Alzheimer's disease accounts for 50 to 80 percent of dementia cases, and an estimated 5.2 million Americans of all ages reported cases of Alzheimer's disease in 2013. Of these, an estimated 5 million people are sixty-five years and older, and approximately 200,000 are under the age of sixty-five. Meditation has shown great potential for preventing cognitive and memory decline because of its stress-reducing effects (Kabat-Zinn, et al., 1992). Stress is related directly to the levels of cortisol in the body, which in turn is well-known for its toxic effects on the hippocampal cells (Lupien, et al., 1998), which are critical for the normal memory (Newcomer, et al., 1999; Weiner, et al., 1997). Thus, a stress-induced hypercortisolemia can further aggravate Alzheimer's disease; however, a regular practice of meditation can, through stress reduction and a reduction of serum cortisol levels, provide benefit to patients with Alzheimer's disease. Currently, very limited studies have been conducted with Alzheimer's patients relating the effect of Yoga with preventing cognitive and memory decline. Further research is needed in this area.

Peripheral Nervous System Disorders

Peripheral neuropathy describes damage to the peripheral nervous system, the vast communications network that transmits information between the brain and spinal cord (the central nervous system) and every other part of the body. More than 100 types of peripheral neuropathy have been identified, each with its own characteristic set of symptoms, pattern of development, and prognosis. Impaired function and symptoms depend on the type of nerves (motor, sensory, or autonomic) that are damaged. Peripheral neuropathy may be either inherited or acquired, and causes of acquired peripheral neuropathy include physical injury (trauma) to a nerve, tumors, toxins, autoimmune responses, nutritional deficiencies, alcoholism, and vascular and metabolic disorders. Yoga has also shown benefit in peripheral nervous system disorders. In a study of twenty patients with diabetic neuropathy, forty days of Yoga sessions resulted in improved nerve conduction compared to the control group. Furthermore, a better glycemic control was also achieved by the individuals practicing Yoga (Malhotra, et al., 2002). In a study of forty-two individuals with carpal tunnel syndrome (CTS), eight weeks of Haṭha Yoga sessions showed significant improvements in grip strength and pain reduction in contrast to the control group. The study established that a Yoga-based regimen was more effective than wrist splinting and no supplementary treatment in relieving some symptoms of carpal tunnel syndrome (Garfinkel, et al., 1998).

Fibromyalgia

Fibromyalgia is a condition of heightened generalized sensitization to sensory input presenting as a complex of symptoms including pain, sleep dysfunction, and fatigue. The pathophysiology of the disorder could include dysfunction of the central nervous system's pain modulatory systems, dysfunction of the neuroendocrine system, and autonomic dysfunction/dysautonomia (Lawson, 2008). In a sample of fifty-three female participants with fibromyalgia syndrome (FMS), an eight-week Yoga awareness program consisting of gentle poses, meditation, breathing exercises, coping methods, and group discussions showed that Yoga was helpful in treating a wide range of fibromyalgia symptoms that included improvements in pain, fatigue, stiffness, sleep problems, depression, memory, anxiety, tenderness, balance, vigor, and strength. In addition, participants also exhibited psychological changes in coping with pain through greater utilization of adaptive pain strategies such as problem solving, acceptance, relaxation, activity engagement, and decreased use of maladaptive strategies like confrontation, self-isolation, disengagement, and catastrophizing (Carson, et al., 2010).

Yogic techniques can be used scientifically as a valid adjunct therapeutic method for sustained benefits to patients with FMS. Statistically significant improvements in fibromyalgia manifestations were demonstrated with a meditation-based Stress Reduction Cognitive Behavioral Treatment (SR-CBT) program in a study involving seventy-nine FMS patients. After ten weeks of intervention, symptoms improved in 67 percent of the participants when compared to 40 percent in controls. These represent improvements in global well-being, pain, sleep, fatigue, tiredness upon awakening, and overall functional status among fibromyalgia patients. Furthermore, psychological status also improved by 32 percent among the subjects (Goldenberg, et al., 1994). The effects of Yoga in addition to Tui Na (Chinese massage therapy) was also studied in forty FMS women, which demonstrated improvements in pain perception (Da Silva, Lorenzi-Filho, and Lage, 2007).

Parkinson's Disease

Parkinson's disease (PD) is the second most common neurodegenerative disorder after Alzheimer's disease and affects approximately 7 million people globally and 1 million people in the United States. PD is more common in the elderly with the mean age of onset around sixty years. The prevalence rises from 1 percent in those over sixty years of age to 4 percent of the population over eighty (de Lau and Breteler, 2006). It is characterized by slowness of movement, muscle rigidity, postural instability, and tremors. There have been isolated case reports about the beneficial effects of Yoga on PD (Hall, Verheyden, and Asburn, et al., 2011; Moriello, et al., 2013). A randomized controlled study revealed that a 60-minute Yoga session twice a week improved motor function in individuals with PD (Colgrove, et al., 2012). Claire Henchcliffe, M.D., director of the Parkinson's Disease and Movement Disorders Institute at the New York Presbyterian Hospital–Weill

Cornell Medical Center, conducted a ten-week study in which Parkinson's patients took hour-long Yoga sessions twice a week. She found a gentle Yoga practice increased energy, balance, and coordination. Moreover, Peggy van Hulsteyn has documented various postures and exercises that can benefit individuals suffering with symptoms of PD (Van Hulsteyn, 2013).

DISCUSSION ABOUT YOGA RESEARCH

Yoga is emerging as a widely practiced complementary and integrative therapy. This chapter brings to light the value of Yoga as a noninvasive method in the management of various disorders that improves the overall quality of life. Its efficacy in various neurological disorders has been described in this chapter; however, these studies have certain shortcomings. As with any emerging treatment modality, establishing the most effective method is difficult. In commencing this chapter, the first problem recognized was the broad classification of Yoga. Many studies used the term *Yoga* liberally without specifically identifying the type of Yoga under investigation. There are four classes of Yoga with numerous subtypes under each. Among the various articles described, only a few provided detailed descriptions of the Yoga programs enlisted.

Although studies on certain neurological disorders have shown improvements with Yoga, it is important to recognize that behavioral modification and alterations that are found with a "Yoga lifestyle" may have accounted for the improved outcomes. Socialization, placebo, and self-efficacy effects may have influenced the results. One study has already shown that psychological benefits of an aerobic exercise intervention in a group of healthy young adults could be increased simply by informing subjects that the exercise program was specifically designed to improve psychological well-being (Desharnais, et al., 1993). The issues of placebo effect and self-efficacy, both of which may have a significant impact (Crow, et al., 1999), are difficult to adequately control in nonblind behavioral interventions. Additionally, the absence of statistically significant effects on the mood and cognitive measures needs to be interpreted cautiously because there is a possibility that enhanced mood contributed to these improvements in quality of life and fatigue. This issue is still open to further investigation. Moreover, the mechanism of action of the improvements seen in various studies remains unclear.

Studies measuring the benefits of Yoga-based therapeutic exercise programs should be done with larger sample size and control subjects to offer better statistical support. An important observation made in this chapter is that many of the studies were conducted in India where the philosophy and practice of Yoga originated. The samples reviewed mostly focused on one geographical region where Yoga is particularly ingrained in the culture. Generalizing these findings to other parts of the world and to different populations remains difficult. Only a very small number of studies have actually addressed variables of interest specific to minorities in the United States (Blacks, Hispanics, and Asians). These populations are distinct in their respective vulnerabilities to physical inactivity and specific disorders (Egede and Poston, 2004). Future studies should assess the therapeutic value of Yoga in U.S. minority populations as well.

Studies are also needed to ascertain whether a single course of Yoga intervention with occasional reinforcement can be effective for long-term relief. Since health problems such as carpal tunnel syndrome (CTS) are the leading cause of lost earnings in the workplace, continued evaluations of outcomes are needed to assess long-term effects of Yoga on CTS symptoms, lost time from work, and patient satisfaction. Another aspect, which remains to be determined, is the optimal intensity and duration required to maximize the effectiveness of Yoga programs. Since most of the studies focused only on the short-term health benefits of Yoga with very few including follow-up data, a more comprehensive understanding is still needed in the maintenance aspect of Yoga to achieve long-term effects. It is necessary to have well-designed studies with larger sample sizes to determine the validity of Yoga as an effective therapy for neurological disorders. Despite the many shortcomings in the literature, the potential of Yoga in treating neurological disorders remains vast. Yoga as a prophylaxis can be used as an important tool for health promotion and disease prevention with minimal cost.

CONCLUSION

Yoga has been widely used for health promotion and disease prevention and as a possible treatment modality for neurological disorders. Yoga has also been used as an adjunctive treatment modality for carpal tunnel syndrome, multiple sclerosis, epilepsy, poststroke paresis, and neuropathy of type-2 diabetes. Ongoing research is underway for treatment of fibromyalgia, headache, migraine, Parkinson's disease, chronic back pain, and many other disorders. Additional research on the safety and efficacy of CAM therapies, including research on potential negative interactions between CAM therapies and conventional treatments such as medications, will bring forth the true value of Yoga in neurological disorders and other disciplines of medicine.

REFERENCES

Bastille, J. V., and K. M. Gill-Body. "A Yoga-Based Exercise Program for People with Chronic Post-stroke Hemiparesis." *Physical Therapy* 84.1 (2004): 33–48. Print.

Benson, H., et al. "Decreased Blood Pressure in Pharmacologically Treated Hypertensive Patients Who Regularly Elicited the Relaxation Response." *Lancet* 1.7852 (1974): 289–291. Print.

Berg, K. O., et al. "Measuring Balance in the Elderly: Preliminary Development of an Instrument." *Physiotherapy Canada* 41.6 (1989): 304–311. Print.

Carson, J. W., et al. "A Pilot Randomized Controlled Trial of the Yoga of Awareness Program in the Management of Fibromyalgia. *Pain* 151.2 (2010): 530–539. Print.

Castillo–Richmond, A., et al. "Effects of Stress Reduction on Carotid Atherosclerosis in Hypertensive African Americans." *Stroke* 31.3 (2000): 568–573. Print.

Centers for Disease Control and Prevention. "Stroke." 2012. Web. 18 Jan. 2014. http://www.cdc.gov/stroke/.

Colgrove, Y. S., et al. "Effect of Yoga on Motor Function in People with Parkinson's Disease: A Randomized, Controlled Pilot Study." *Journal of Yoga and Physical Therapy* 2.2 (2012): 112. Print.

Cramer, H., et al. "A Systematic Review and Meta–Analysis of Yoga for Low Back Pain." *Clinical Journal of Pain* 29.5 (2013): 450–460. Print.

Creel, G. L., K. E. Light, and M. T. Thigpen. "Concurrent and Construct Validity of Scores on the Timed Movement Battery." *Physical Therapy* 81.2 (2001): 789–798. Print.

Crow, R., et al. "The Role of Expectancies in the Placebo Effect and Their Use in the Delivery of Health Care: A Systematic Review." *Health Technology Assessment* 3.3 (1999): 1–48. Print.

Da Silva, G. D., G. Lorenzi-Filho, and L. V. Lage. "Effects of Yoga and the Addition of Tui Na in Patients with Fibromyalgia." *Journal of Alternative and Complementary Medicine* 13.10 (2007): 1107–1114. Print.

de Lau L. M., and Breteler, M. M. "Epidemiology of Parkinson's Disease." *Lancet Neurology* 5.6 (2006): 525–535. Print.

Dean, C. M., C. L. Richards, and F. Malouin. "Task-Related Circuit Training Improves Performance of Locomotor Tasks in Chronic Stroke: A Randomized, Controlled Pilot Trial." *Archives of Physical Medicine and Rehabilitation* 81.4 (2000): 409–417. Print.

Desharnais, R., et al. "Aerobic Exercise and the Placebo Effect: A Controlled Study." *Psychosomatic Medicine* 55.2 (1993): 149–154. Print.

Duncan, P. W., et al. "The Stroke Impact Scale Version 2.0: Evaluation of Reliability, Validity, and Sensitivity to Change." *Stroke* 30.10 (1999): 2131–2140. Print.

Egede, L. E., and M. E. Poston. "Racial/Ethnic Differences in Leisure-Time Physical Activity Levels Among Individuals with Diabetes." *Diabetes Care* 27.10 (2004): 2493–2494. Print.

Garfinkel, M. S., et al. "Yoga–Based Intervention for Carpal Tunnel Syndrome: A Randomized Trial." *JAMA* 280.18 (1998): 1601–1603. Print.

Garland, S. J., T. J. Stevenson, and T. Ivanova. "Postural Responses to Unilateral Arm Perturbation in Young, Elderly, and Hemiplegic Subjects." *Archives of Physical Medicine and Rehabilitation* 78.10 (1997): 1072–1077. Print.

Garrett, R., M. A. Immink, and S. Hillier. "Becoming Connected: The Lived Experience of Yoga Participation After Stroke." *Disability Rehabilitation* 33.25–26 (2011): 2404–2415. Print.

Goldenberg, D. L., et al. "A Controlled Study of a Stress-Reduction, Cognitive-Behavioral Treatment Program in Fibromyalgia." *Journal of Musculoskeletal Pain* 2.2 (1994): 53–66. Print.

Hall, E., G. Verheyden, and A. Ashburn. "Effect of a Yoga Programme on an Individual with Parkinson's Disease: A Single-Subject Design." *Disability and Rehabilitation* 33.15–16 (2011): 1483–1489. Print.

Harper, D. M. "Review: Yoga Reduces Low Back Pain and Back-Specific Disability." *Annals of Internal Medicine* 159.8 (2013): JC13. Print.

Holtzman, S., and R. T. Beggs. "Yoga for Chronic Low Back Pain: A Meta-Analysis of Randomized Controlled Trials." *Pain Research and Management* 18.5 (2013): 267–272. Print.

Jain, S. C., et al. "A Study of Response Pattern of Non-Insulin Dependent Diabetics to Yoga Therapy." *Diabetes Research and Clinical Practice* 19.1 (1993): 69–74. Print.

Kabat-Zinn, J., et al. "Effectiveness of a Meditation-Based Stress Reduction Program in the Treatment of Anxiety Disorders." *American Journal of Psychiatry* 149.7 (1992): 936–943. Print.

Lawson, K. "Treatment Options and Patient Perspectives in the Management of Fibromyalgia: Future Trends." *Neuropsychiatric Disease Treatment* 4.6 (2008): 1059–1071. Print.

Lundgren, T., et al. "Acceptance and Commitment Therapy and Yoga for Drug Refractory Epilepsy: A Randomized Controlled Trial." *Epilepsy Behaviour* 13.1 (2008): 102–108. Print.

Lupien, S. J., et al. "Cortisol Levels During Human Aging Predict Hippocampal Atrophy and Memory Deficits." *Nature Neuroscience* 1 (1998): 69–73. Print.

Lynton, H., B. Kligler, and S. Shiflett. "Yoga in Stroke Rehabilitation: A Systematic Review and Results of a Pilot Study." *Top Stroke Rehabilitation* 14.4 (2007): 1–8. Print.

Malhotra, V., et al. "Effect of Yoga Asanas on Nerve Conduction in Type 2 Diabetes." *Indian Journal of Physiology and Pharmacology* 46.3 (2002): 298–306. Print.

Mishra, S. K. *An Overview of Ayurveda and Yoga: Think Horses Not Zebra*. Redwood City, CA: Stanford University Press, 1999. Print.

——. Ayurveda for Depression and Mental Health in "Many Paths to Healing to Depression." In *Natural Healing for Depression; Solutions from the World's Great Health Traditions and Practitioners*, Eds. J. Strohecker and N. Strohecker, New York: Penguin, 1999. Retrieved from Healthy.net. Web. 18 Jan 2014. http://www.healthy.net/Health/Article/Many_Paths_to_Healing_to_Depression/1088/4.

Mishra, S. K., and S. P. Vinjamury. "Neurological Disorders in Ayurveda." *International Journal of Integrative Medicine* 3.1 (2001): 13–16. Print.

Mishra, S. K., et al. "The Therapeutic Value of Yoga in Neurological Disorders." *Annals of Indian Academy of Neurology* 15.4 (2012): 247–254. Print.

Moriello, G., et al. "Incorporating Yoga into an Intense Physical Therapy Program in Someone with Parkinson's Disease: A Case Report." *Journal of Bodywork and Movement Therapies* 17.4 (2013): 408–417. Print.

Newcomer, J. W., et al. "Decreased Memory Performance in Healthy Humans Induced by Stress-Level Cortisol Treatment." *Archives of General Psychiatry* 56.6 (1999): 527–533. Print.

Oken, B. S., et al. "Randomized Controlled Trial of Yoga and Exercise in Multiple Sclerosis." *Neurology* 62.11 (2004): 2058–2064. Print.

Ornish, D., et al. "Intensive Lifestyle Changes for Reversal of Coronary Heart Disease." *JAMA* 281.15 (1998): 2001–2007. Print.

Panjwani, U., et al. "Effect of Sahaja Yoga Meditation on Auditory Evoked Potentials (AEP) and Visual Contrast Sensitivity (VCS) in Epileptics." *Applied Psychophysiology and Biofeedback* 25.1 (2000): 1–12. Print.

Rajesh, B., et al. "A Pilot Study of a Yoga Meditation Protocol for Patients with Medically Refractory Epilepsy." *Journal of Alternative Complementary Medicine* 12.4 (2006): 367–371. Print.

Seyfer, E., and L. Bell. *Gentle Yoga: A Guide to Low-Impact Exercise.* Cedar Rapids: Celestial Arts, 1990. Print.

Shumway-Cook, A., and M. H. Woollacott. *Motor Control: Theory and Practical Applications.* Philadelphia: Lippincott Williams & Wilkins, 2001. Print.

Sirven, J. I., et al. "Complementary/Alternative Medicine for Epilepsy in Arizona." *Neurology* 61.4 (2003): 576–577. Print.

Van Hulsteyn, P. *Yoga and Parkinson's Disease: A Journey to Health and Healing.* New York: Demos Medical Publishing, 2013. Print.

Velikonja, O., et al. "Influence of Sports Climbing and Yoga on Spasticity, Cognitive Function, Mood and Fatigue in Patients with Multiple Sclerosis." *Clinical Neurology and Neurosurgery* 112.7 (2010): 597–601. Print.

Weiner, M. F., et al. "Cortisol Secretion and Alzheimer's Disease Progression." *Biological Psychiatry* 42.11 (1997): 1030–1038. Print.

Winterholler, M., F. Erbguth, and B. Neundtrfer. "The Use of Alternative Medicine by Multiple Sclerosis Patients—Patient Characteristics and Patterns of Use." *Fortschritte der Neurologie-Psychiatrie* 65.12 (1997): 555–561. Print.

Orthopedics and Yoga Therapy

Ray Long, M.D., F.R.C.S.C.

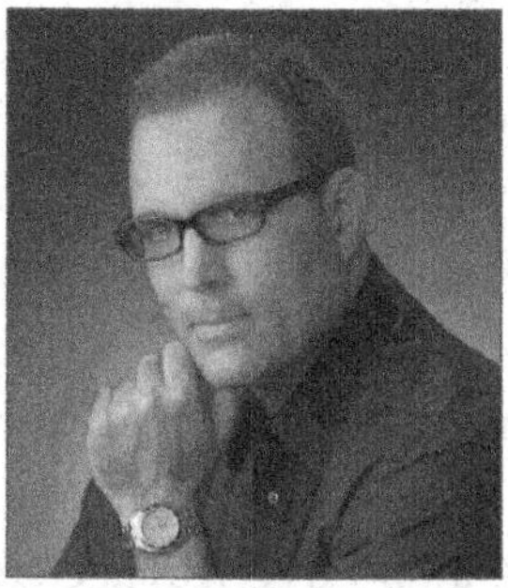

Ray Long is a board-certified orthopedic surgeon specializing in sports medicine and shoulder and elbow reconstruction. Dr. Long graduated from the University of Michigan Medical School and completed his orthopedic residency at the University of Montreal. He then went on to complete fellowships in lower extremity arthroscopy and arthroplasty, shoulder and elbow surgery, and sports medicine.

Dr. Long studied Yoga at the Ramamani Iyengar Memorial Yoga Institute in Pune, India, under the guidance of B. K. S. Iyengar. He has practiced and taught Yoga for over thirty years and is the author of the bestselling *Scientific Keys* and *Yoga Mat Companion* book series combining modern Western science and Yoga. Dr. Long conducts seminars throughout the world on the subjects of anatomy, biomechanics, and therapeutics in Yoga.

INTRODUCTION

A number of years ago, I took a course at the University of Michigan Medical School called "History and Medicine." I was the only participant in the course, which is unfortunate for others because it was one of the most influential experiences of my training. I spent the first week of the course in the archives of the medical library reading journal articles that were at least fifty years old. I randomly perused the preeminent publications of the day, including the *New England Journal of Medicine*, the *Lancet*, and the *Journal of the American Medical Association*. The course director then asked me for my impressions. I could not believe the treatments and therapies utilized and advocated by the leading journals of that period. The logical conclusion, however, indicates that others in the future will likely make similar observations about our current practices (Prasad, et al., 2013). This was my first introduction to the concept of a paradigm shift.

Indeed, I have witnessed such shifts in medicine and, in particular, in the field of orthopedics. Diagnostic tools, such as the MRI, allow visualization of the body in ways we could only dream of forty years ago. Minimally invasive techniques, such as arthroscopy, which were in their infancy during my training, are now the standard of care. Use of the body's own healing and growth factors, such as platelet-rich plasma and cartilage grown from stem cells, is now part of the expanding field of regenerative medicine (using the body to heal the body). Coincident is the growing interest and acceptance of complementary medicine for the treatment of conditions ranging from low back pain (Tilbrook, et al., 2011) to osteoarthritis (Ebnezar, et al., 2011, 2012).

In addition, there has been an explosion of interest in practicing Yoga, both for its healing potential and its ability to enhance quality of life. With the increasing number of practitioners of this powerful healing art, we also have learned about injuries, particularly musculoskeletal ones, that can occur from the practice, underscoring the admonition that anything with healing potential requires caution. Consequently, growing interest has focused on the application of modern Western science to the practice of Yoga, both to enhance its benefits and to minimize the risks of injury.

With this in mind, this chapter explores the intersection of the current paradigms of orthopedics and Yoga. I begin with fundamental concepts of joint structure and function, muscle physiology, and proprioception, as understood in orthopedics and applied to Haṭha Yoga. Next, I discuss the application of the concepts to the treatment of several conditions by presenting actual cases from my experience in both workshops and the clinic. I conclude with considerations for future applications of Yoga as therapeutic in orthopedics.

CONTRIBUTIONS OF ORTHOPEDICS TO YOGA

Joint Mechanics and Physiology

As a general consideration, mobility and stability of the joints are determined by three factors. First is the shape of the bone at the joint—for example, a ball and socket joint versus a hinge joint. Next are the soft tissue stabilizers, such as the ligaments, capsule, labrum, or meniscus. Finally, there are the muscular stabilizers that surround a given articulation. A related subject is the concept of joint congruency. This references the fit of opposing joint surfaces. High joint congruence means that more surface area is in contact; low joint congruence indicates less contact area (Herzog and Frederico, 2006).

A related concept is "joint reaction force," which, in essence, is a combination of all of the factors that can produce pressure within a given articulation, such as the hip or knee. These elements include body weight, the contractile force of the muscles that surround the joint, or even someone "assisting" a practitioner to accomplish a pose. When the articulations are taken to extreme positions, the joint reaction forces tend to be concentrated over a much smaller area, creating the possibility of injury. To understand this, imagine one pound of force spread over 10cm^2 of surface area versus one pound spread over 1cm^2. The force spread over the smaller region is more likely to cause injury. When practicing Yoga, it is best to spread the joint reaction forces over a greater area by maintaining maximum congruency of the joint surfaces. Figure 1 illustrates the bony capsuloligamentous and muscular stabilizers of the shoulder joint.

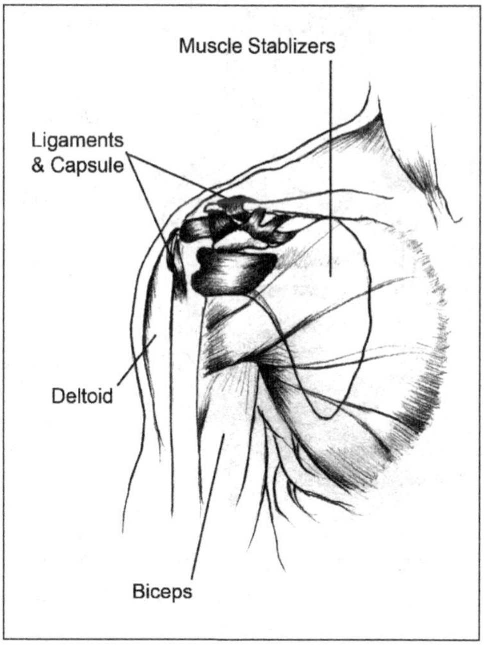

Figure 1: Stabilizers of the Shoulder Joint

The next concept relating to the joints is that of joint "coupling," such as in the hip joint. As the femur flexes in the acetabulum, the pelvis simultaneously tilts forward. Related to this is joint "rhythm." For example, as the pelvis tilts forward, the lumbar spine extends. These are examples of lumbopelvic rhythm (Hasebe, et al., 2013; Murray, et al., 2002; Kuo, Tully, and Galea, 2013). An example from Yoga would be integrating forward flexion of the pelvis in a forward-bending pose like uttānāsana to maintain a proper ratio of forward tilt of the pelvis with lumbar flexion.

One of the main points for Yoga practitioners to take away from orthopedics is that joint surfaces are smooth, curved structures. They adapt best to slow gradual changes, especially in situations where the articulation is near the end of its "physiological" range of motion (as with some Yoga poses). Accordingly, in my practice and teaching, I advocate for deliberately slowing the motion when approaching the endpoint of a pose. Similarly, I utilize gentle engagement of the periarticular muscles to maintain maximum joint surface congruency.

Synovial Joints

Synovial joints—such as the hip, knee, shoulder, and elbow—are surrounded by a capsule, which is lined by a synovial membrane (synovium) that faces the joint cavity. The synovium contains two primary cell types. The first are fibroblast cells, and they secrete synovial fluid that lubricates the joint surfaces, reduces friction during movement, and acts as a shock absorber through fluid pressurization. The fluid also carries oxygen and nutrients to the articular cartilage and removes carbon dioxide. The other cell type lining the synovium is a macrophage cell, which removes debris or other unwanted material from the joint space. Activities that maintain joint range of motion aid in circulating the synovial fluid and bringing unwanted material into contact with the macrophages. Conversely, pathological conditions, such as osteoarthritis, are associated with inflammation and thickening of the synovium (and capsule), reduction in range of motion of the joint, and concomitant diminished circulation of synovial fluid (Scanzello and Goldring, 2012; Sokolove and Lepus, 2013).

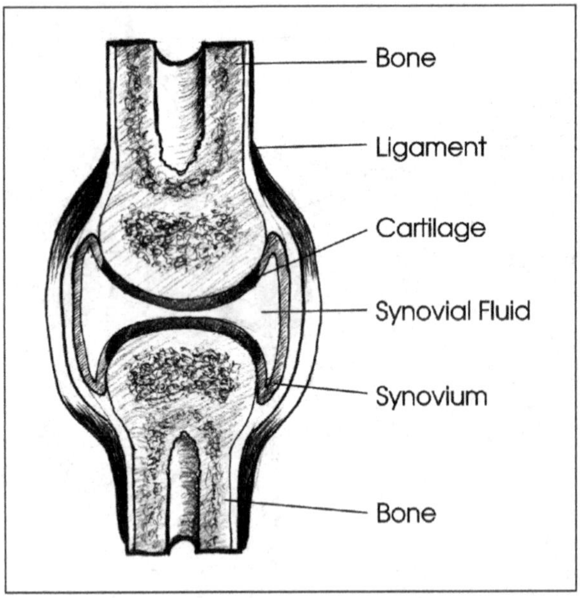

Figure 2: Synovial Joint Capsule

Muscle Physiology

Knowledge relating to the physiology of muscle contraction and stretching is now increasingly integrated into the practice of Haṭha Yoga and is also an area of interest in sports medicine. A number of articles, both basic science and clinical, have been published on the subject. The basic science literature elucidates the structures that contract and lengthen during stretching; these include the contractile elements of the muscle (sarcomeres) and the fascial elements that surround muscles and tendons. In addition, many factors contribute to the way a muscle lengthens, including neurological input, viscoelastic properties (meaning that the stress/strain relationship is dependent on the load and the rate at which the load is applied—a function of the internal friction within the muscle), creep (a type of deformation that has been postulated for fascial elements), psychological factors (such as muscle memory and tolerance), and extramuscular links to synergists (examples would be myofascial connections between muscles of the anterior compartment of the lower leg, which affect muscle length and force transmission; another example would be seen with the hamstrings—virtually all compartments of muscles demonstrate this phenomenon). Individual muscle architecture or shape also plays a role (Taylor, et al., 1990; Kato, et al., 1985).

A basic understanding of the neurological control mechanisms of muscle contraction and stretching is useful for both Yoga practice and therapeutics. One such mechanism is reciprocal inhibition. This process involves relaxation of the muscle on one side of a joint (the antagonist) when the muscle on the other side of the joint (the agonist) contracts. For example, when the brain signals the quadriceps muscle to contract and extend the knee, it also inhibits the hamstrings from contracting (via an inhibitory interneuron in the spinal cord) (Crone, 1993). This inhibitory process occurs on the unconscious level. It can be accessed in Yoga by consciously engaging the quadriceps in a forward bend like uttānāsana. This extends the knee (and stabilizes the joint) and allows the hamstrings to stretch. I use reciprocal inhibition frequently during my Yoga practice, and, when working with therapeutics, by analyzing the muscles that create the form of the pose (as with the example of uttānāsana) and consciously engaging those muscles. This process can become quite refined as one becomes aware of cues for engaging the synergist muscles as well. The result is a refinement in joint stability and form of the pose as well as deep mindfulness in the practice.

Another technique from rehabilitative and sports medicine that I frequently use in my personal practice and in therapeutics is proprioceptive neuromuscular facilitation (PNF). This involves taking a target muscle out to length, holding it there, and then gently contracting it for several seconds. Upon releasing the contraction, the muscle can be taken out to greater length. The exact underlying mechanism of this process is debated, but it is believed to involve proprioceptors within the muscle tendon unit, in particular the Golgi tendon organ (Hindle, et al., 2012). A feedback mechanism appears to be evoked that results in relaxation of the muscle targeted for stretching.

As with reciprocal inhibition, I use the general form of the āsanas to determine which muscles are stretching and which are contracting. Then, I devise a PNF stretch for a given muscle. For example, in a low lunge like ardha-añjaneyāsana (kneeling crescent pose), I might begin to stretch the quadriceps muscle by reaching for the back leg and bending the knee, bringing the heel in the direction of the buttock. After backing off a few degrees from the full length of the stretch, I'd gently press the foot of the back leg into my hand, holding it for several seconds, gradually engaging the quadricep to about 20 percent of maximum contractile force. Finally, I'd relax the quadricep and then gradually draw the foot back toward the buttock, which will almost always take it out to a length that was deeper than the original length. Depending on the muscle group I am targeting and the level of conditioning of the individual, I typically begin with one to two repetitions, of a PNF stretch; as conditioning improves, PNF stretches can be repeated a few times to ensure a new maximum length is established neurologically and into muscle memory. Additionally, I should personally note that I prefer a short warm-up with sun salutations prior to working with any PNF, whether it's my body being self-treated or that of a patient. Data suggests that short duration (6–10 seconds) submaximals (no more than 20 percent of maximum contractile force) are effective guidelines for utilizing PNF in stretching and range-of-motion training (Feland and Marin, 2004).

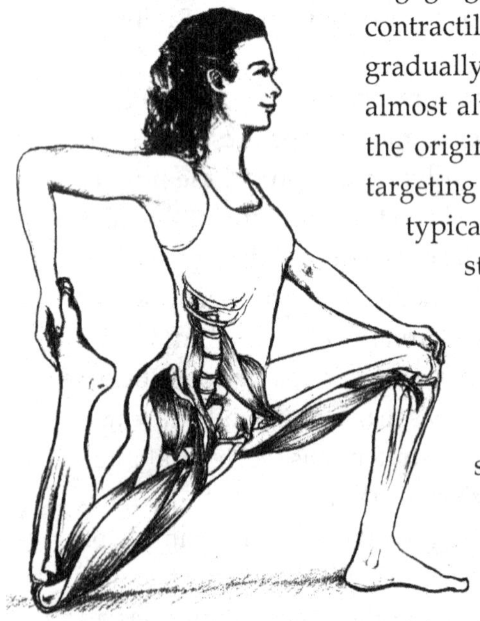

Figure 3: PNF for the Quadriceps in Ardha Añjaneyāsana (Kneeling Crescent)

While these techniques access complex neurophysiological mechanisms (many of which remain undefined and function unconsciously), they are actually quite simple to integrate into āsana practice. In a sense, this parallels the healing benefits of Yoga itself; we perform the practice and the benefits come.

Proprioception

Proprioception refers to the sense of the relative position of neighboring body parts, such as the femoral head within the acetabulum (hip socket), and the muscular force utilized in the movement of those parts. This is distinct from exteroception, which is the perception of the outside world (like the feeling of the feet on the ground), and interoception, which is the perception of the inside of the body (pain, hunger, etc.).

Joint position is detected by specialized nerve endings, known as "proprioceptors," located within the muscles, ligaments, joint capsule, and the periosteum (on the surface of the bones) (Proske, 2006; Fortier and Basset, 2012; Proske and Gandevia, 2012). These receptors communicate information about the joints to the brain via the sensory columns of the spinal cord. Conscious sense of joint position is transmitted to the cerebrum of the brain; unconscious proprioception is communicated to the cerebellum. Many of these receptors, including the muscle spindle and Golgi tendon organ, also play a role in the various stretch reflexes. Figure 4 illustrates this pathway in a cross section of the spinal cord.

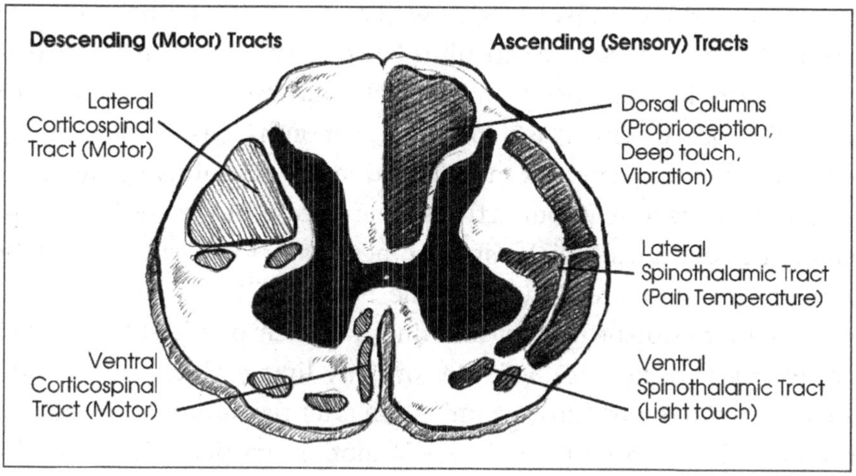

Figure 4: Cross Section of the Spinal Cord

Proprioception has been shown to diminish in pathological conditions, such as knee osteoarthritis (Smith, King, and Hing, 2012; Duman, et al., 2012; Van der Esch, et al., 2012) and generalized ligamentous laxity (joint hypermobility) (Wolf, Cameron, and Owens, 2012; Smith, et al., 2013). Derangements in proprioception can also account for the reduced performance seen in some athletes who participate in events immediately following stretching sessions (Micheo, Baerga, and Miranda, 2012). I suspect diminished proprioception might also play a role in joint pain seen in activities requiring frequent deep stretching, including ballet (Duthon, et al., 2013) and Yoga. Conversely, elite athletes have been shown to possess enhanced proprioceptive acuity (Han, et al., 2013). Various training techniques can be used to improve proprioception and diminish injury risk for various activities, including athletics (Hrysomallis, 2011). An example would be balance training with Yoga āsanas; tree pose and half moon pose are examples of Yoga poses that might assist in this.

CASE STUDIES

Adhesive Capsulitis (Frozen Shoulder)

Idiopathic adhesive capsulitis is a disorder of the shoulder characterized by pain and loss of motion with no identifiable cause. This condition occurs more frequently in women in the fifth-to-seventh decade of life, with an incidence of approximately 3 to 5 percent among the general population. It can be associated with diabetes and thyroid disorders, as well as a variety of other conditions, or it can occur in isolation. Adhesive capsulitis has three phases. The first is the painful or freezing phase that lasts between six weeks and nine months. Next comes the frozen or "stiff" phase, which lasts four to nine months. Last is the thawing phase, which lasts for five to twenty-six months. Adhesive capsulitis frequently resolves with conservative treatment, but arthroscopic release of the shoulder capsule (or manipulation under anesthesia) might be necessary for particularly debilitating cases (Griggs, Ahn, and Green, 2000; Levine, et al., 2007).

Patients with this disorder typically find that their pain resolves and shoulder function returns to normal for activities of daily living, although this can take as long as two years to occur. Close examination after resolution of the active disease often reveals a deficit in patients' range of motion, particularly external rotation and forward elevation of the shoulder.

This residual deficit in shoulder range of motion does not interfere with activities of daily living; however, it can become apparent when taking the shoulder into some of the positions of Yoga, particularly downward dog pose. This manifests as discomfort in the affected shoulder and can be seen as a decrease in forward flexion when compared to the unaffected shoulder.

I have seen two such cases in clinical practice and several others during workshops. Each case had an established history of frozen shoulder that resolved with conservative management (including physical therapy and home stretching). Other shoulder pathologies—including glenohumeral arthritis, rotator cuff injury, or acromioclavicular arthritis—were ruled out with physical exam and radiological studies. An average of approximately 15 degrees of deficit in forward flexion (elevation) and external rotation was noted upon examination.

For stretching, we utilized a combination of seated gomukhāsana (cow face pose) and garuḍāsana (eagle pose), using short duration PNF and passive stretches. For gomukhāsana, I focused on one shoulder at a time, working with a belt in the other hand to facilitate drawing the target shoulder up or down. The lower side shoulder was in internal rotation behind the back, thereby lengthening the external rotators, including the infraspinatus and teres minor muscles. To add PNF to this stretch, I had the practitioner gently press the back of the hand into the back for 8–10 seconds (using minimal force). This contracts the external rotators when they are out to length, creating a facilitated stretch. Then, the practitioner relaxed the pressure into the back and drew the target shoulder upward (with the belt). I repeat the same sequence for the upper side arm, this time pressing the hand into the upper back to engage the subscapularis muscle (an internal rotator). Following the PNF portion of the stretch, the upper arm is gently drawn down the back. For garuḍāsana, we integrated PNF by gently pressing the upper side elbow into the lower side forearm (essentially, squeezing the elbows together for 8–10 seconds) and then drawing the upper side elbow across the contralateral chest. Figure 5 illustrates these stretches.

In each case, the practitioners were able to regain equal, or nearly equal, range of motion of the shoulders in as little as two stretching sessions. Repeat examination in downward dog pose revealed significant improvement to the previous imbalance and little or no remaining discomfort. Long-term retention of these gains in range of motion probably requires regular stretching sessions.

Working with gomukhāsana and garuḍāsana in this manner is an example of combining knowledge from joint biomechanics and stretching (in this case, use of PNF) to assist in resolving residual limitations in range of motion, which are often present after resolution of other clinical symptoms in idiopathic adhesive capsulitis. Accordingly, these poses might be of benefit for improving range of motion in selected patients with deficits following clinical resolution of idiopathic adhesive capsulitis. Note that other pathologies of the shoulder—such as glenohumeral arthritis and rotator cuff injury—should be ruled out by an appropriately trained healthcare practitioner prior to working with this technique. Particular care and attention should be given to slow, gentle, and methodical stretching. No stretches should be forced. If practitioners experience pain in any stretch, they should carefully release the pose. Figure 5 illustrates the muscles stretching in this technique for gomukhāsana and garuḍāsana, respectively.

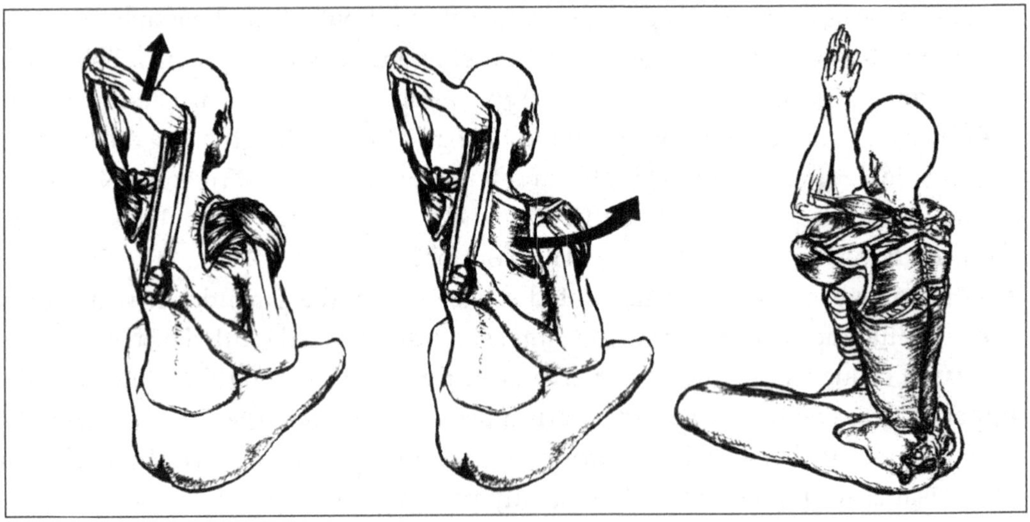

Figure 5: Gomukhāsana and Garuḍāsana PNFs

Piriformis Syndrome

Piriformis syndrome is characterized by buttock and/or hip pain that can radiate into the leg as a form of sciatica. This syndrome is thought to result from a spasm of the piriformis that causes irritation of the sciatic nerve as it passes across (or through) the muscle. Figure 6 illustrates the relationship of the piriformis muscle

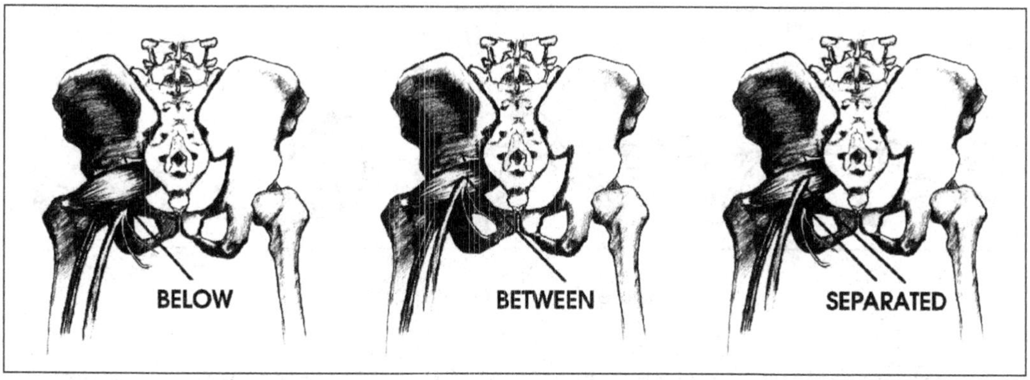

Figure 6: The Relationship of the Piriformis to the Sciatic Nerve

to the sciatic nerve. Spasm in the piriformis can be precipitated by an athletic injury or other trauma (Boyajian-O'Neill, et al., 2008). Tightness or asymmetries in the piriformis muscle can create rotational pelvic imbalances. This, in turn, can lead to imbalances further up the spinal column through the process of "joint rhythm."

Piriformis syndrome is diagnosed through a careful history and physical examination as well as radiological studies. The physical exam includes the FAIR test (flexion, adduction, internal rotation of the hip). The mainstay of treatment involves stretching the piriformis and its neighboring external hip rotators; surgery to release the muscle is reserved for recalcitrant cases.

I personally suffered from piriformis syndrome for a number of years and finally treated it with Yoga. I have also worked with one patient in my clinic and several others in workshops who had been diagnosed with piriformis syndrome. All had buttock and/or sciatic-type pain. In each case, other causes of sciatica were ruled out through physical exam and radiological studies and the FAIR test was positive. There was also no evidence of hip injury or other pathology.

In each case, we worked with a balanced Yoga practice that encompassed a warm-up, standing poses, forward bends, backbends, and hip openers, including reverse pigeon pose. Each of us had significant relief of the sciatic pain from piriformis syndrome through Yoga. In my case, when I do not practice, the pain returns (especially when sitting for long periods). Thus, Yoga āsanas, such as reverse pigeon pose (variations of which are also utilized in conventional physical therapy), appear to be useful as an adjunct in the management of select cases of confirmed piriformis syndrome.

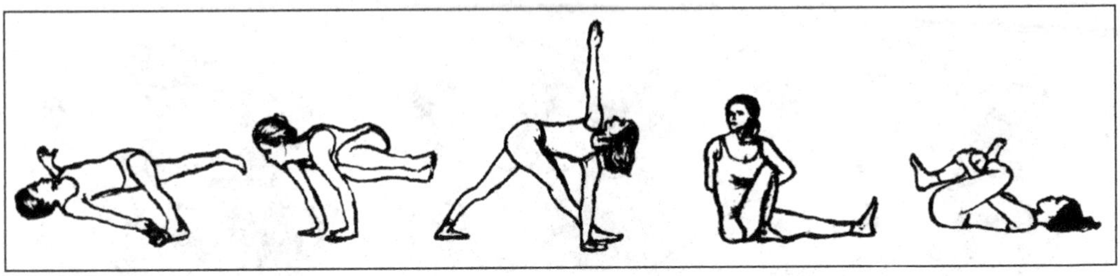

Figure 7: Piriformis Stretches

Analyzing why this pose stretches the piriformis illustrates how an understanding of biomechanics is valuable in Yoga. For example, the actions of the piriformis muscle vary according to the position of the hip joint. When the hip is in a neutral position, the piriformis acts to externally rotate (turn outward), flex, and abduct the joint. When the hip is flexed beyond about 60 degrees, the piriformis becomes an internal rotator and extensor (and remains an abductor). Muscles stretch when we move a joint in the opposite direction of the action of the muscle. In reverse pigeon pose, the hip is flexed and externally rotated, thus stretching the muscle, which extends and internally rotates the hip in this position. Figure 7 (above) illustrates various poses that stretch this muscle. Parāvṛtta-trikoṇāsana (revolved triangle pose), sūcī randhrāsana (eye of the needle pose), and the rotating version of supta padāṅguṣṭhāsana (reclined hand to foot pose) lengthen the muscle by adducting and flexing the hip. Similarly, pārśva-bakāsana (side crow pose) and marīcyāsana III (sage pose III) adduct and flex the hip joint, thereby stretching the muscle, which is an extensor and abductor when the hip is flexing. Figure 8 (left) illustrates a commonly used stretch for the piriformis muscle using reverse pigeon pose.

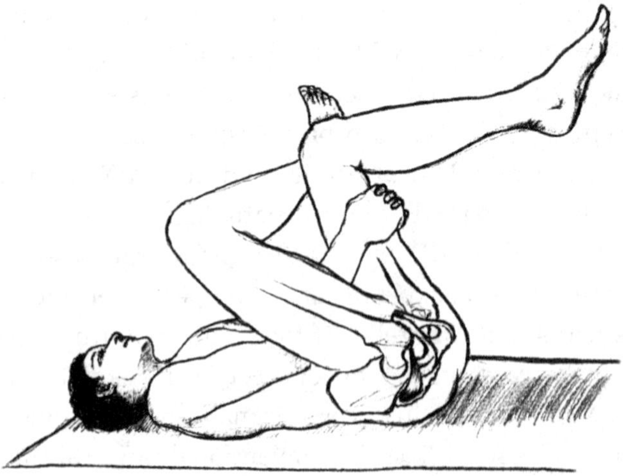

Figure 8: Reverse Pidgeon Pose

Hip Pain in Yoga

One of the most intriguing problems I have encountered recently is hip pain in Yoga absent an underlying condition, such as arthritis or femoral acetabular impingement. I have seen this more frequently in women, but also in men. In two cases from a recent workshop, the practitioners frequently had generalized hip soreness following Yoga practice, especially a hip-opening-type session. Neither had any history of hip injury, surgery, arthritis, or other symptomatic pathology. On examination, there was no evidence of generalized ligamentous laxity or symptomatic labral pathology, and the impingement test was negative (hip flexion to 90 degrees, internal rotation, and adduction).

This is similar to the hyperflexibility scenario seen with ballet dancers , and it led me to theorize that the cause might be similar to the joint pain seen in persons with generalized ligamentous laxity (benign joint hypermobility syndrome). These patients have diminished proprioception about the joints and benefit from muscular strengthening and proprioceptive training.

Accordingly, we worked with co-activation of the muscles of the hip during the workshop. Specifically, we interposed vīrabhadrāsana II (warrior II pose) on each side between the various hip opening poses, such as baddha-koṇāsana (bound angle pose), eka pada raja kapotāsana (pigeon pose), and padmāsana (lotus pose). During the warrior II, we used brief simultaneous engagement of the hip adductors and abductors in an intermediate version of the pose (the hip and knee flexing less than 90 degrees). We held this pose for 20–30 seconds, using the cue to visualize pressing the inside of knee into an immoveable object while simultaneously pressing the outside of the knee into a similar object (the knee remains centered and does not move). For each practitioner, the hip pain was significantly diminished or completely gone when integrating this technique. Furthermore, the practitioners later confirmed that applying this technique in their practice and teaching had a similar result.

This leads me to postulate that some of the hip pain experienced by Yoga practitioners might be related to reduced or inadequate proprioception in the hip joint after stretching the muscles surrounding the joint. This reduction in proprioception could lead to microinstability in the joint, with abnormal contact pressure (joint reaction forces) leading to pain. If so, this would be similar to pain from joint instability elsewhere in the body. In fact, microinstability of the hip is an emerging concept in orthopedics. Furthermore, considering that among asymptomatic volunteers, labral tears were identified in 69 percent of hip joints, I could reasonably expect to find a labral tear in these practitioners (Register, et al., 2012). If the pain, however, was related to diminished proprioception, then the labral tear would be an incidental finding. Thus, the possibility of integrating proprioception-type training (using the Yoga poses themselves) is worth considering as the pathophysiology of hip pain from Yoga (and other activities) becomes better defined.

POTENTIAL FOR THE FUTURE FOR YOGA AND ORTHOPEDICS

Studies have demonstrated that knee osteoarthritis is associated with decreased quadriceps strength (Hafez, et al., 2013) and proprioception, with a possible role for both deficiencies in the pathogenesis of the disease. We know that maintaining range of motion of synovial joints, such as the knee and hip, is beneficial for both circulation of the synovial fluid and clearance of debris (via macrophages) from the joint space. Judiciously applied forces across the joint surfaces have been shown to increase cartilage volume and decrease defects in certain studies (Urquhart, et al., 2011; Racunica, et al., 2007). Thus, it might be possible to develop Yoga-training regimens that strengthen the periarticular muscles of the hip and knee, increase proprioception, enhance synovial fluid circulation, and apply healthy joint reaction forces—with a view to working with the body to prevent arthritis of these joints.

In conclusion, knowledge of the musculoskeletal system will continue to expand in orthopedics. This knowledge can be utilized for safer and more effective practice and teaching of Haṭha Yoga. Similarly, as science progresses, we can anticipate that the healing benefits of Yoga will become better defined and more integrated into mainstream medicine, especially for certain orthopedic conditions.

REFERENCES

Boyajian-O'Neill, L. A., et al. "Diagnosis and Management of Piriformis Syndrome: An Osteopathic Approach." *Journal of the American Osteopathic Association* 108.11 (2008): 657–664. Web.

Crone, C. "Reciprocal Inhibition in Man." *Danish Medical Bulletin* 40.5 (1993): 571–581. Web.

Dewberry, M. J., et al. "Pelvic and Femoral Contributions to Bilateral Hip Flexion by Subjects Suspended from a Bar." *Clinical Biomechanics* 18.6 (2003): 494–499. Web.

Duman, I., et al. "Assessment of the Impact of Proprioceptive Exercises on Balance and Proprioception in Patients with Advanced Knee Osteoarthritis." *Rheumatology International* 32.12 (2012): 3793–3798. Web.

Duthon, V. B., et al. "Correlation of Clinical and Magnetic Resonance Imaging Findings in Hips of Elite Female Ballet Dancers." *Arthroscopy* 29.3 (2013): 411–419. Web.

Ebnezar, J., et al. "Effect of an Integrated Approach of Yoga Therapy on Quality of Life in Osteoarthritis of the Knee Joint: A Randomized Control Study." *International Journal of Yoga* 4.2 (2011): 55–63. Web.

Ebnezar, J., et al. "Effects of an Integrated Approach of Hatha Yoga Therapy on Functional Disability, Pain, and Flexibility in Osteoarthritis of the Knee Joint: A Randomized Controlled Study." *Journal of Alternative and Complementary Medicine* 18.5 (2012): 463–472. Web.

Esola, M. A., et al. "Analysis of Lumbar Spine and Hip Motion During Forward Bending in Subjects with and Without a History of Low Back Pain." *Spine* 21.1 (1996): 71–78. Web.

Feland, J. B., and H. N. Marin. "Effect of Submaximal Contraction Intensity in Contract-Relax Proprioceptive Neuromuscular Facilitation Stretching." *British Journal of Sports Medicine* 38.4 (2004): E18. Web.

Fortier, S., and F. A. Basset. "The Effects of Exercise on Limb Proprioceptive Signals." *Journal of Electromyography and Kinesiology* 22.6 (2012): 795–802. Web.

Griggs, S. M., A. Ahn, and A. Green. "Idiopathic Adhesive Capsulitis. A Prospective Functional Outcome Study of Nonoperative Treatment." *The Journal of Bone and Joint Surgery* 82-A.10 (2000): 1398–1407. Web.

Hafez, A. R., et al. "Treatment of Knee Osteoarthritis in Relation to Hamstring and Quadriceps Strength." *Journal of Physical Therapy Science* 25.11 (2013): 1401–1405. Web.

Han, J., et al. "Level of Competitive Success Achieved by Elite Athletes and Multi-Joint Proprioceptive Ability." *Journal of Science and Medicine in Sport,* n. pag. [Epub ahead of print]. 12 Dec. 2013. Web. pii: S1440–2440(13)00514–8. http://www.ncbi.nlm.nih.gov/pubmed/24380847.

Hasebe, K., et al. "Spino-Pelvic-Rhythm with Forward Trunk Bending in Normal Subjects Without Low Back Pain." *European Journal of Orthopaedic Surgery and Traumatology* 24.2 (2013): n. pag. Web.

Herzog, W., and S. Frederico. "Considerations on Joint and Articular Cartilage Mechanics." *Biomechanics and Modeling in Mechanobiology* 5.2 (2006): 64–81. Web.

Hindle, K. B., et al. "Proprioceptive Neuromuscular Facilitation (PNF): Its Mechanisms and Effects on Range of Motion and Muscular Function." *Journal of Human Kinetics* 31 (2012): 105–113. Web.

Hrysomallis, C. "Balance Ability and Athletic Performance." *Sports Medicine* 41.3 (2011): 221–232. Web.

Kato, E., et al. "Acute Effect of Muscle Stretching on the Steadiness of Sustained Submaximal Contractions of the Plantar Flexor Muscles." *Journal of Applied Physiology* 110.2 (1985): 407–415. Web.

Kuo, Y. L., E. A. Tully, and M. P. Galea. "Lumbofemoral Rhythm During Active Hip Flexion in Standing in Healthy Older Adults." *Manual Therapy* 15.1 2010: 88–92. Web.

Levine, W. N., et al. "Nonoperative Management of Idiopathic Adhesive Capsulitis." *Journal of Shoulder and Elbow Surgery* 16.5 (2007): 569–573. Web.

Micheo, W., L. Baerga, and G. Miranda. "Basic Principles Regarding Strength, Flexibility, and Stability Exercises." *PM&R* 4.11 (2012): 805–811. Web.

Murray, R., et al. "Pelvifemoral Rhythm During Unilateral Hip Flexion in Standing." *Clinical Biomechanics* 17.2 (2002): 147–151. Web.

Prasad, V., et al. "A Decade of Reversal: An Analysis of 146 Contradicted Medical Practices." *Mayo Clinic Proceedings* 88.8 (2013): 790–798. Web.

Proske, U. "Kinesthesia: The Role of Muscle Receptors." *Muscle Nerve.* 34.5 (2006): 545–558. Web.

Proske, U., and S .C. Gandevia. "The Proprioceptive Senses: Their Roles in Signaling Body Shape, Body Position and Movement, and Muscle Force." *Physiological Reviews* 92.4 (2012): 1651–1697. Web.

Racunica, T. L., et al. "Effect of Physical Activity on Articular Knee Joint Structures in Community-Based Adults." *Arthritis and Rheumatology* 57.7 (2007): 1261–1268. Web.

Register, B., et al. "Prevalence of Abnormal Hip Findings in Asymptomatic Participants: A Prospective, Blinded Study." *American Journal of Sports Medicine* 40.12 (2012): 2720–2724. Web.

Scanzello, C. R., and S. R. Goldring. "The Role of Synovitis in Osteoarthritis Pathogenesis." *Bone* 51.2 (2012): 249–257. Web.

Smith, T. O., J. J. King, and C. B. Hing. "The Effectiveness of Proprioceptive-Based Exercise for Osteoarthritis of the Knee: A Systematic Review and Meta-Analysis." *Rheumatology International* 32.11 (2012): 3339–3351. Web.

Smith, T. O., et al. "Do People with Benign Joint Hypermobility Syndrome (BJHS) Have Reduced Joint Proprioception? A Systematic Review and Meta-Analysis." *Rheumatology International* 33.11 (2013): 2709–2716. Web.

Sokolove, J., and C. M. Lepus. "Role of Inflammation in the Pathogenesis of Osteoarthritis: Latest Findings and Interpretations." *Therapeutic Advances in Musculoskeletal Disease* 5.2 (2013): 77–94. Web.

Taylor, D. C., et al. "Viscoelastic Properties of Muscle-Tendon Units. The Biomechanical Effects of Stretching." *American Journal of Sports Medicine* 18.3 (1990): 300–309. Web.

Tilbrook, H. E., et al. "Yoga for Chronic Low Back Pain: A Randomized Trial." *Annals of Internal Medicine* 155.9 (2011): 569–578. Web.

Urquhart, D. M., et al. "What Is the Effect of Physical Activity on the Knee Joint? A Systematic Review." *Medicine and Science in Sports and Exercise* 43.3 (2011): 432–442. Web.

van der Esch, M., et al. "The Association Between Reduced Knee Joint Proprioception and Medial Meniscal Abnormalities Using MRI in Knee Osteoarthritis: Results from the Amsterdam Osteoarthritis Cohort." *Osteoarthritis Cartilage* 21.5 (2013): 676–681. Web.

Wolf, J. M., K. L. Cameron, and B. D. Owens. "Impact of Joint Laxity and Hypermobility on the Musculoskeletal System." *Journal of the American Academy of Orthopedic Surgeons* 19.8 (2011): 463–471. Web.

Psychiatry and Yoga Therapy

Elizabeth Visceglia, M.D., RYT-500

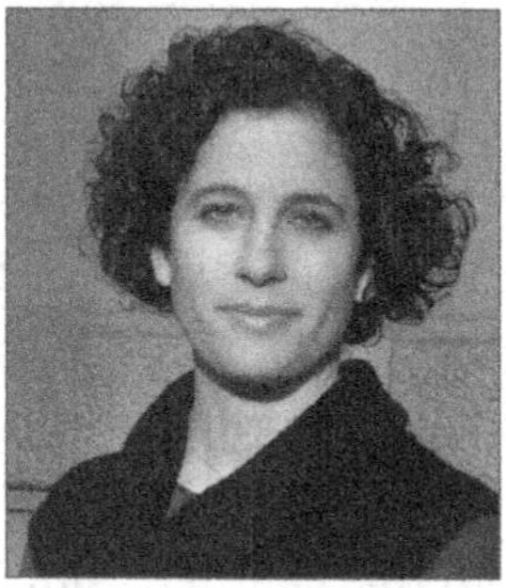

Elizabeth Visceglia, board certified in psychiatry, is a twenty-year student of Yoga. She met her teacher, Guruji Prakash Shankar Vyas, a kriyā yogī, nearly fifteen years ago when she was living in Varanasi, India, and she continues to study and practice with him. Her first published study found that Yoga has a profoundly positive impact on people with schizophrenia, their symptoms, and their quality of life, and she continues to do research on Yoga and schizophrenia. Dr. Visceglia also supervises Yoga Therapists working in the mental health field. A former AIDS educator in Kenya and a graduate of Mount Sinai School of Medicine, Dr. Visceglia has a private practice in Brooklyn, New York, where she lives with her family.

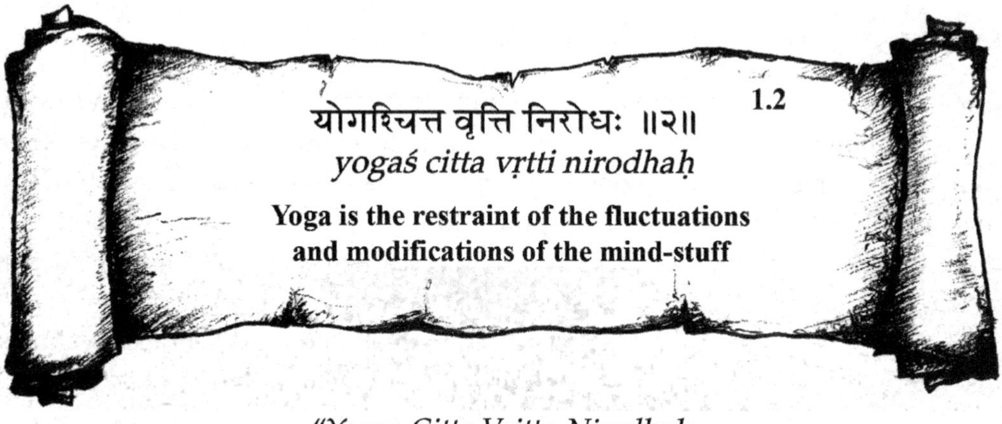
1.2
योगश्चित्त वृत्ति निरोधः ॥२॥
yogaś citta vṛtti nirodhaḥ
Yoga is the restraint of the fluctuations and modifications of the mind-stuff

"Yogas Citta Vritta Nirodhah
(The restraint of the modifications of the mind-stuff is Yoga.)"

—Patañjali's Second Yoga Sūtra

INTRODUCTION

While psychiatry and Yoga might seem at odds at first glance, their goals are remarkably similar: the transformation of mind. Whether the mind has lost touch with shared reality and spins into psychosis, whether it has sunk into a deep and seemingly unremitting depression, or whether it is simply overactive and responds to every stimuli it encounters creating a sense of psychic instability for the individual, attempts to restrain the mind from these tendencies can take many forms. In psychiatry, there is a focus on psychopharmacology and on an intellectual or experiential understanding of the difficulties from which one suffers in the hope that this may lead to transformation. As the tradition of Yoga clearly states and modern evidence-based medicine is now confirming, therapeutic Yoga has a wide range of applications to many of these same psychiatric problems by activating a cascade of physiologic and emotional changes and by utilizing the healing power of breath, movement, and the awareness of mind and body.

I explore two different sorts of psychiatric difficulties in this chapter—one psychotic disorder and one mood disorder—to begin to elucidate ways Yoga has been found to be therapeutic for a wide spectrum of suffering. I examine up-to-date evidence of Yoga's effectiveness, explore potential mechanisms that might explain this effectiveness, and consider ways to integrate some of the principles and practices of Yoga into mental health care.

PSYCHOTIC DISORDER: SCHIZOPHRENIA

Jim is a fifty-seven-year-old man (names and identifying details have been changed to protect patients' privacy throughout this chapter) with a long history of schizophrenia, multiple hospitalizations, childhood physical and sexual abuse, and a history of polysubstance abuse. In response to auditory hallucinations, he had lit himself and his apartment on fire several years ago and was transferred from prison to a state hospital when he was found "not guilty by reason of insanity."

Having spent over two years in the state hospital, Jim was frustrated, alienated, and angry; he would have regular outbursts on the ward, saying how meaningless his life was and how enraged he felt at the state for keeping him locked up. He called it the state's "system of social control." These explosive periods of anger often required additional medication sometimes against his will. He repeatedly stated that he preferred being in jail where "at least you knew when you were getting out," and he was depressed, isolated, intimidating, and hard to reach. In addition, he had a variety of medical problems including HIV, hepatitis C, and hypertension.

Jim began taking therapeutic Yoga classes twice a week, initially in a group setting and eventually individually. He engaged in simple stretches and movements coordinated with breath as well as prāṇāyāma (breathing exercises) that emphasized long, smooth exhalations. We encouraged Jim to notice his body and thoughts without judging them and included āsanas (Yoga postures) of all categories: standing poses, balancing poses, twists, forward bends, backward bends, inversions, and Yoga nidrā (relaxation). After several months, the changes were apparent to everyone who knew him. He stopped requiring extra medication for agitation and became motivated enough to start painting again, something he had not done for many years. He began to spend his free time creating beautiful, seasonal murals, which were hung on his ward and throughout the hospital. He also began to articulate that "everyone is responsible for his own mind," and he started practicing Yoga outside class as well. He received a higher level of privilege, and the hospital staff noticed that he was less hostile, more motivated, and better related.

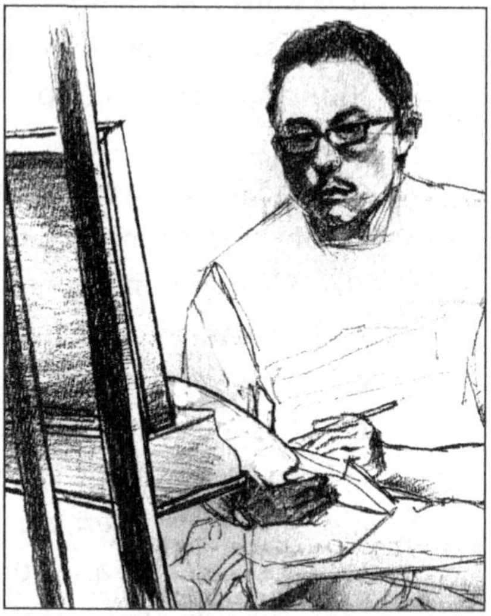

By engaging in the sensations and grounding the experience of the body, Jim and many like him are able to become present to a calm refuge in their own minds that otherwise eludes them. Antonio Damasio writes about the ways "the body provides a ground reference for the mind" (Damasio, 1994). In a most simplistic way, moving the body gently and calmly can affect the chaos of the thoughts so eventually the person mirrors the smooth, orderly movements of the body.

People with schizophrenia have been found to have a heightened baseline level of physiological arousal, in which the body is chronically agitated even under normal conditions (Zahn, Carpenter, and McGlashan, 1981). Simultaneously, the parasympathetic nervous system, the body's means of calming itself, has been found to be underactive (Toichi, et al., 1997). This hyper-responsivity to stress can lead to overactivation of the hypothalamic-pituitary-adrenal axis (HPA). The HPA then produces higher levels of the stress hormones, cortisol and epinephrine, which increase the body's state of alert and lead to increased blood pressure, increased respiratory and heart rates, and other physiologic and emotional changes. When these hormones are chronically released, as is often the case in schizophrenia, they strain the entire body and mind and can lead to chronic mental and physical distress. Additionally, high levels of cortisol can interfere with some cell functions leading to dopamine dysregulation (Mizoguchi, et al., 2008), long considered a hallmark of schizophrenia, and augmented cortisol release has itself been found to exacerbate psychotic symptoms in schizophrenia (Walker, Mittal, and Tessner, 2008).

There is an accumulating body of evidence that schizophrenia may be linked to chronic inflammatory-related changes in the brain (Fan, Goff, and Henderson, 2007). This autoimmune reaction unleashes a cascade of proinflammatory cytokines and several of these cytokines are associated with changes in the glia, which are cells that support and protect neurons in the brain and nervous system, and can effect myelination, create blood brain barrier leakage, and disturb cerebral vasculature (Falcone, Carlton, and Franco, 2009). These inflammatory changes are also linked to several metabolic disturbances common in schizophrenia including type 2 diabetes (Fan, Goff, and Henderson, 2007), which "atypical" antipsychotics worsen even further (Jufe, 2008). The practice of Yoga, however, has been found to produce increased levels of melatonin, a powerful anti-inflammatory, antioxidant, and free-radical scavenger (Bushell and Theise, 2009). This melatonin may counteract the effects of the inflammatory cascade of schizophrenia.

Furthermore, it seems that Yoga's emphasis on long exhalation and conscious slow breathing reactivates the parasympathetic nervous system. The beneficial effects of yogic breathing are wide-ranging. Particular yogic breathing exercises, such as ujjāyi and bhastrikā, seem to affect the autonomic nervous system and may help reregulate the schizophrenic's dysfunctional autonomic nervous system (Sageman, 2004). Alternate nostril breathing has been found to lower both systolic and diastolic blood pressure (Raghuraj & Telles, 2008), and yogic breathing exercises such as sudarśana kriyās have been found helpful in women with schizophrenia (Sageman, 2004). Lengthened exhalation in the form of prāṇāyāma or mantra has also been found to produce favorable psychological and physiologic effects (Bernardi, et al., 2001).

Physiologically, yogic breathing helps to stimulate the vagus nerve and strengthens the body's means of relaxing itself. Yet, to date, the precise mechanism remains unclear. Lengthened exhalation and breathing with increased airway resistance (as in ujjāyi prāṇāyāma in Yoga) have been hypothesized to effect physiologic change through vagal nerve stimulation (Brown and Gerbarg, 2005). It seems that ujjāyi breathing "stimulates vagal nerve afferents to the brain . . . [which] induces a parasympathetic reduction in heart rate and most likely a withdrawal of sympathetic input to the heart" (Brown and Gerbarg, 2002). Dr. Kevin Tracey has also concluded that there is a vagal/cholinergic anti-inflammatory system whereby vagal activation seems to dampen inflammation. He concludes that meditation and related practices likely induce their benefits through such vagal stimulation (Tracey, 2002). Activating the vagus nerve can lead to other neuroendocrine changes, including increased acetyl choline release in the liver, spleen, heart, and gastrointestinal tract, all of which can further inhibit the release of proinflammatory cytokines from tissue macrophages (Olivo, 2009). These cascades of changes stimulated in Yoga Therapy may begin to bring remedy and relief to nervous system disequilibrium in those with schizophrenia.

Clients participating in Yoga Therapy frequently notice the transformative capacity of the breath. Jim mentioned how in the past he never noticed that he held his breath when he was stressed. When asked how Yoga has been helpful, he stated, "Now at least I remember to breathe." Jim and others have had remarkable effects from a very simple intervention, one that consists of simple movements coordinated with breath. Duraiswamy, et al. (2007) found statistically significant improvements in negative symptoms of schizophrenia on the Positive and Negative Syndrome Scale (PANSS) and in perceived quality of life through regular Yoga practice versus a control group who performed the same amount of calisthenics. In a pilot study I authored and taught Yoga for at Bronx State Psychiatric Hospital, we found similar results: statistically significant improvements in all subscales of the PANSS except for thought disturbance and improvements in perceived physical and psychological health on the World Health Organization Quality of Life Scale (Visceglia and Lewis, 2011). This intervention led to no unwanted effects of any sort, was low cost, and was even found to be effective with several of the more "treatment resistant" patients in the hospital.

Strikingly, even the same group Yoga practice seems to affect individuals differently and in most constructive ways. One woman with schizophrenia who had severe paranoia and lived at a shelter removed her heavy jacket, boots, and sunglasses for the first time ever in a Yoga class; simultaneously, another with ongoing somatic preoccupations stopped discussing the fishes living in her belly and began to articulate the stiffness she felt in her body as a side effect of her medications and her grief at her life situation immediately after we all practiced Yoga together. Another man living in a state hospital refused to publicly admit he was having auditory hallucinations but freely shared information about "this little voice I'm hearing" in Yoga class. From my experiences, therapeutic Yoga practice has both the generalized positive effects discussed above as well as particular individual effects that are often subtler and more difficult to predict at the outset of treatment.

MOOD DISORDER: MAJOR DEPRESSIVE DISORDER

Lindsey was a twenty-eight-year-old female, seen as an outpatient, but with a history of inpatient hospitalizations for severe depression. She had several suicide attempts, posttraumatic stress disorder due to a history of childhood sexual abuse, difficulties sleeping and trusting other people, and had a strong somatic component to her illness. Lindsay had trouble forming a therapeutic alliance and was emotionally fragile on presentation.

Early on, it was clear that staying present during her therapy appointments was very challenging for her. She commonly arrived to sessions near to tears and cried throughout the sessions. For her, it was a way to isolate herself from the therapy and from me. Because talking seemed almost beyond her in these early months and her symptoms seemed very overwhelming, we started using prāṇāyāma when she arrived each week. Typical prāṇāyāma practices included:

1. Simple diaphragmatic breathing with a lengthened exhalation of at least four seconds
2. Following her breath with her awareness while she held her hand to her belly and felt it rise during inhalation and fall during exhalation
3. Ujjāyi breathing
4. Nāḍī śodhana (alternate nostril breathing—done either mentally or physically with the hand)
5. A balancing breathing exercise

These were all very effective in helping her calm down enough to participate during the session. Had she presented with a less agitated depression (with no history of mania), more stimulating breathing exercises such as kapālabhāti (breath of joy) would likely have been effective in reenergizing her. I have used kapālabhāti successfully with depressed clients with prominent psychomotor retardation and anergia/lethargy.

As Lindsey began to trust our work together, slowly we added basic standing poses with awareness of her breath and body. This helped her stay present no matter what physical and emotional experiences she encountered. Doing things as simple as feeling her feet supporting her body beneath her, inhaling as she moved to stand on tiptoes, and exhaling back to flat feet helped Lindsey breathe through and accept the discomforts of her moment-to-moment experience without retreating into pure emotional display. She reported, "It has always been hard for me to stay present when I am upset; my mind likes to go a million other places, but somehow breathing helps me just be here." Over time, we tapered her off the antidepressant she came to me on, and she became interpersonally engaged enough to form a therapeutic alliance and partake in the challenging work of therapy. During her treatment, we continued to begin our time together with prāṇāyāma, a "check-in" of how she felt physically, and simple āsana; we also used these tools during the session whenever excessive emotionality began to interfere with her treatment or one of us felt it might be helpful. We both agreed that the integration of Yoga into our work together made her treatment more successful.

The evidence for the effectiveness of Yoga as a treatment for depression is impressive. Yoga seems to have a positive effect on mood in psychiatric inpatients as evaluated by the Profile of Mood States (Lavey, et al., 2005), and several recent studies point to its effectiveness in outpatient mood as well. A particular sequence of breathing exercises known as Sudarśana Kriyā Yoga (SKY) has been found to alleviate anxiety, depression, and stress (Brown and Gerbarg, 2005). In another study, SKY led to remission of depression on the Beck Depression Inventory and Hamilton Rating Scale of Depression at a rate of 67 percent, with the tricyclic antidepressant Imipramine, achieving 73 percent remission and electroconvulsive therapy (ECT) at 95 percent (Janakiramaiah, et al., 2000). Young adults with depression who participated in two 1-hour Iyengar Yoga āsana classes weekly for five weeks were found to have significant improvements in the Beck Depression Inventory, State-Trait Anxiety Inventory, and Profile of Mood States and normalized cortisol levels (Wooley, et al., 2004). Similar results were found in a comparable study where women who perceived themselves as emotionally distressed participated in a three-month Yoga program and subsequently reported both pain relief and improved mood compared to women in a control group (Michalsen, et al., 2005). A recent review article found that, while further investigation is required, the overall evidence suggests that Yoga is a beneficial intervention for depression (Pilkington, et al., 2005).

Yoga's physiologic effects on depression may be understood on a variety of levels. First, there is a significant body of evidence indicating that physical exercise can effectively treat mild to moderate depression (Stammes and Spijker, 2009) and Yoga itself shares the same benefits of any exercise program. This is likely due to that fact that it was developed specifically as a tool for mental and physical healing. Several of these proposed mechanisms are similar to those that may be at work in the case of schizophrenia as well. Elevated cortisol levels in depression are one of biological psychiatry's most consistent findings (Tafet, et al., 2001) and are widely believed to be due to persistently elevated HPA activity that occurs with chronic stress (Kahn, 1998). This elevated cortisol then leads to hyperactive uptake of serotonin and may be a biochemical link between psychosocial stress and depression (Post, 1993). Participating in just one Yoga class has been found to decrease cortisol levels (Brainard, et al., 1997), which suggests one mechanism through which Yoga may be effective in depression.

Furthermore, depression is associated with low levels of melatonin secretion as compared to controls (Claustrat, et al., 1984). As discussed, Yoga tends to elevate melatonin levels and melatonin goes on to stimulate the vagus (Bushell and Theise, 2009), thus reenergizing the parasympathetic nervous system, which is the body's rest and relaxation system, and countering the effects of the overstimulated HPA axis. Depression is also associated with lowered gamma-aminobutyric acid (GABA) levels in the cortex (Sanacora, et al., 1999) and treatment with selective serotonin reuptake inhibitors has been found to be one way to increase GABA concentrations (Sanacora, et al., 2002). Similarly, Yoga āsana has been found to increase GABA levels by up to 27 percent with no change in lev-

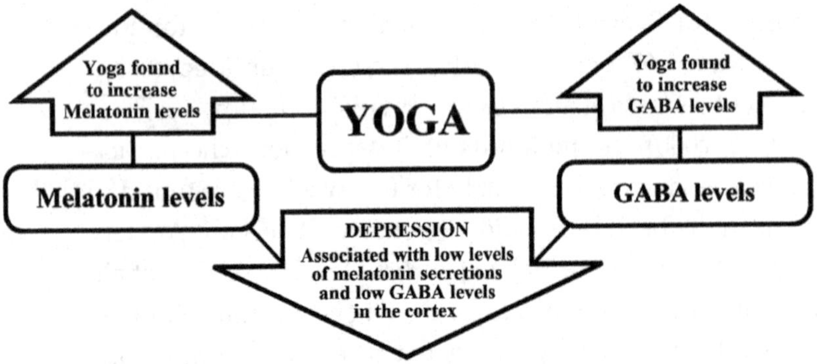

els for controls (Streeter, et al., 2007), another potential mechanism for Yoga's effectiveness.

Particularly with depression, Yoga lends itself to a variety of types of interventions. Just participating in a regular Yoga class seems to have a positive effect on mood. In addition, certain practices from Yoga can be effectively interwoven in a therapeutic session, particularly when there is a desire to better understand and integrate somatic phenomena or when just talking starts to feel repetitive or stuck. I can hardly think of a single patient I have worked with who did not have intermittent anxiety or insomnia. As a result, I teach virtually all my patients about the calming benefits of slow diaphragmatic breathing, repeatedly counting breaths to 10 or down from 10 to 0, mental alternate nostril breathing, and other simple prāṇāyāma. They are able to notice the results right away and very often this eventually empowers them enough to give up the medication they had grown accustomed to using to effect these same emotional and physical changes. One patient of mine had used sleep medications for over nine years and, within months of learning diaphragmatic breathing techniques, she had given up the medications completely. Another had a nearly lifelong history of untreated chronic depression, and by using activating breathing exercises and a meditation technique that focused on his ongoing experience of his physical body, his depression resolved without the use of any medications. Deep and careful inquiry into the realities of the body is where Freud began with his hysterical patients—individuals suffering from physical symptoms without organic cause. Accordingly, it seems quite fitting to utilize an ancient discipline to access the experiences of the body and their powerful effects on the mind to restore function and balance.

INTEGRATION AND INTERVENTIONS

As is clear from these examples, therapeutic Yoga practice effects changes in the brain and body on a multitude of levels. It is a low-cost intervention with no significant dangers or side effects when utilized by a knowledgeable practitioner. In fact, there are many well-documented physical health benefits in addition to mental health benefits. Yoga has been found to be effective in the treatment of post-traumatic stress disorder (PTSD) (van der Kolk, 2006), anxiety (Kirkwood, et al., 2005), depression (Pilkington, et al., 2005), obsessive-compulsive disorder (OCD) (Shannahoff-Khalsa, et al., 1999) and a variety of other psychiatric difficulties.

To begin to utilize some of the tremendous healing benefits of Yoga, it is not necessary to know how to twist the body into acrobatic positions. Benefits can come from a seemingly simple breath-oriented practice. When working with a client, first encourage her/him to begin the process of noticing her/his own mind and body without judgment. Suggest that he/she witness the sensations in his/her body and the rhythms of his/her own breath, as well as any qualities his/her breath contains in that moment. Gently encourage him/her to begin to lengthen the exhalation longer than the inhalation and as long as comfortably possible while noticing any effects this may have. Help the client breathe three-dimensionally: moving the breath in the front, back, and both sides of the body. As greater ease develops in the breath, focus on deep, slow, smooth abdominal breathing that utilizes the diaphragm to its full capacity. The hands may be placed on the lower belly to help sense the abdomen's expansion during inhalation and the release during exhalation. Practice watching the breath in the mind's eye as it moves through nostrils, throat, chest, and abdomen, and then returns back up this path and out the nostrils.

Profound changes can be accomplished easily and accurately with these sorts of breathing exercises, particularly when combined with Yoga nidrā (yogic sleep, a form of guided meditation). Numerous variations of effective breathing exercises exist too. For example, invite the client to inhale and count silently "one" to herself, then exhale and count silently "one," then inhale "two" and exhale "two," then "three," up to ten or whatever number you have chosen. If he/she makes a mistake, falls asleep, or finds that "thinking" is happening, start over at one. If he/she would like, when he/she gets to ten he/she can count back the same way to zero. Another simple and effective exercise is to imagine that all breathing is happening in alternating nostrils beginning in the left nostril (more beneficial for the parasympathetic system). Start with an exhale and count down from some number, say thirty-five, to zero. Again, if you lose track, start over from the beginning. Mental alternate nostril breathing is also very effective, typically starting and finishing with the left nostril, and this can also be done with breath counting if desired.

These breathing exercises all have a calming effect on the nervous system, which makes them widely applicable for anxiety, insomnia, many kinds of depression, and a variety of other difficulties. For someone with a severe depression for example, more activating breathing exercises like kapālabhāti (breath of fire) would be included. These stimulating techniques are best taught by an experienced practitioner who has learned from a reputable teacher.

Depending on your training, you and your client might choose to add light stretches to the breathing over time and explore movements or positions he/she feels drawn to do. When he/she begins to feel comfortable with a slow and strain-free breath, consider a simple walking meditation in which he/she inhales for two steps and exhales for three steps. Over time you can lengthen the inhalation and exhalation, and eventually the inhalation and exhalation may become equal in length. Or simply let the breath be as it is and count the number of steps in each inhale and exhale, allowing the steps to vary as they may. Whatever the body may or may not be doing, allow the focus to remain with the breath. As the mind wanders, gently refocus it on the experience of the breath moving in and out of the body at that moment.

Personally, in my training from Prakash Shankar Vyas, a Kriyā Yogi from Varanasi, India, I was taught that the entire system of Yoga practice is what makes it effective. Living an ethical life and practicing every category of āsana, prāṇāyāma, and meditation are necessary components of a complete system for mental wellness. With this in mind, blending Western "talk therapy" with insights from the rich philosophical tradition of Yoga can strengthen our tools for mental healing. Educating clients about Yogic concepts such as nondualism, equanimity, nonharming, attention to the present moment, and restraint from judgment can contextualize and deepen important psychotherapeutic insights. These philosophical concepts can be reinforced by the wisdom that emerges from ongoing attention to the breath, the body, and the mind, just as they were by Yogis thousands of years ago.

CONCLUSION

For Yoga Therapy to be effective, the first step is our own commitment to its insights and practices. The more we practice, the more real our understanding becomes of Yoga Therapy's transformative powers and the better we are able to communicate the techniques and their benefits to clients. While the possibility that something as ordinary as breathing can unleash our bodies' innate capacity to heal goes against many of the conventional beliefs of psychiatry, we must seriously consider the other simple tools we have all witnessed transforming patients: conversation, empathy, and human connection. Adding the insights of Yoga to these modest psychiatric tools has the potential to enhance the work we are already doing, evolve mental health care, and transform mental wellness.

REFERENCES

Bernardi, L., et al. "Effect of Rosary Prayer and Yoga Mantras on Autonomic Cardiovascular Rhythms: A Comparative Study." *British Medical Journal* 22.323 (2001): 1446–1449. Print.

Brainard, G., et al. "Plasma Cortisol Reduction in Healthy Volunteers Following a Single Yoga Session of Yoga Practices." *Yoga Research Society Newsletter.* Philadelphia, PA: Neurology, Jefferson Medical College, No. 18, 1997. Print.

Brown, R. P., and P. L. Gerbarg. "Sudarshan Kriya Yogic Breathing in the Treatment of Stress, Anxiety, and Depression." *Journal of Alternative and Complementary Medicine* 11.2 (2005): 383–384. Print.

——. "Yogic Breathing and Meditation: When the Thalamus Quiets the Cortex and Rouses the Limbic System." Paper presented at the "Science of Breath" International Symposium on Sudarshan Kriya Pranayama and Consciousness, New Delhi, India. March 2–3, 2002. Print.

Bushell, W. C., and N. D. Theise. "Toward a Unified Field of Study: Longevity, Regeneration, and Protection of Health Through Meditation and Related Practices." *Annals of the New York Academy of Sciences* 1172 (2009): 5–19. Print.

Claustrat, B., at al. "A Chronobiological Study of Melatonin, a Biochemical Marker in Major Depression." *Biological Psychiatry* 19.8 (1984): 1215–1228. Print.

Damasio, A. *Descartes' Error.* New York: Penguin, 1994. Print.

Duraiswamy, G., et al. "Yoga Therapy as Add-On Treatment in the Management of Patients with Schizophrenia: A Randomized Controlled Trial." *Acta Psychiatrica Scandinavica* 116.3 (2007): 226–232. Print.

Fan, X., D. C. Goff, and D. C. Henderson. "Inflammation and Schizophrenia." *Expert Review of Neurotherapeutics* 7.7 (2007): 789–796. Print.

Falcone, T., E. Carlton, and K. Franco. "Inflammation, Psychosis and the Brain."*Psychiatric Times* July 10, 2009. Web. www.psychiatrictimes.com/schizophrenia/inflammation-psychosis-and-brain.

Janakiramaiah, N., et al. "Antidepressant Efficacy of Sudarshan Kriya Yoga (SKY) in Melancholia: A Randomized Comparison with ECT and Imipramine." *Journal of Affective Disorders* 57.1–3 (2000): 255–259. Print.

Jufe, G. S. "Metabolic Syndrome Induced by Antipsychotic Drugs: The Problem of Obesity." *Vertex* 19.83 (2008): 338–347. Print.

Kahn, A. *Neurochemistry of Schizophrenia and Depression.* Clovis, CA: A. J. Publishing, 1998. Print.

Kirkwood, G., et al. "Yoga for Anxiety: A Systematic Review of the Research Evidence." *British Journal of Sports Medicine* (2005) 39: 884–891.

Lavey, R., et al. "The Effects of Yoga on Mood in Psychiatric Inpatients." *Psychiatric Rehabilitation Journal* 28.4 (2005): 399–402. Print.

Michalsen, A., et al. "Rapid Stress Reduction and Anxiolysis Among Distressed Women as a Consequence of a Three-Month Intensive Yoga Program." *Medical Science Monitor* 11.12 (2005): 555–561. Print.

Mizoguchi, K., et al. "Persistent Depressive State After Chronic Stress in Rats Is Accompanied by

HPA Axis Dysregulation and Reduced Prefrontal Dopaminergic Neurotransmission." *Pharmacology and Biochemistry of Behavior* 91.1 (2008): 170–175. Print.

Olivo, E. L. "Protection Throughout the Lifespan: The Psychoneuroimmunologic Impact of Indo-Tibetan Medicine and Yoga Practices." *Annals of the New York Academy of Sciences* 1172 (Sept. 2009): 163–171. DOI:10.1111/j. Web.

Pilkington, K., et al. "Yoga for Depression: The Research Evidence." *Journal of Affective Disorders* 89.1–3 (2005): 13–24. Print.

Post, J. M. "Transduction of Psychosocial Stress into the Neurobiology of Recurrent Affective Disorders." *American Journal of Psychiatry* 149.8 (1993): 999–1010. Print.

Raghuraj, P., and S. Telles. "Immediate Effect of Specific Nostril Manipulating Yoga Breathing Practices on Autonomic Respiratory Variables." *Applied Psychophysiology and Biofeedback* 33.2 (2008): 66–75. Print.

Sageman, S. "Breaking Through the Despair: Spiritually Oriented Group Therapy as a Means of Healing Women with Severe Mental Illness." *Journal of the American Academy of Psychoanalytic Dynamic Psychiatry* 32.1 (2004): 125–141. Print.

Sanacora, G., et al. "Reduced Cortical Gamma-Aminobutyric Acid Levels in Depressed Patients Determined by Proton Magnetic Resonance Spectroscopy." *Archives of General Psychiatry* 56.11 (1999): 1043–1047. Print.

Sanacora, G., et al. "Increased Occipital Cortex GABA Concentrations in Depressed People After Therapy with Selective Serotonin Reuptake Inhibitors." *American Journal of Psychiatry* 159.4 (2002): 663–665. Print.

Shannahoff-Khalsa, D. S., et al. "Randomized Controlled Trial of Yogic Meditation Techniques for Patients with Obsessive-Compulsive Disorder." *CNS Spectrums*, 4.12 (1999): 34–47. Print.

Stammes, R., and J. Spijker. "Physical Training to Treat Depression." *Tijdschrift voor Psychiatricie* 51.11 (2009): 821–830. Print.

Streeter, C. C., et al. "Yoga Asana Sessions Increase Brain GABA Levels: A Pilot Study." *Journal of Alternative and Complementary Medicine* 13.14 (2007): 419–426. Print.

Tafet, G. E., et al. "Correlation Between Cortisol Level and Serotonin Uptake in Patients with Chronic Stress and Depression." *Cognitive, Affective and Behavioral Neuroscience* 1.4 (2001): 388–393. Print.

Tracey, K. J. "The Inflammatory Reflex." *Nature* 420.6917 (2002): 853–859. Print.

Toichi, M., et al. "The Influence of Psychotic States on the Autonomic Nervous System in Schizophrenia." *International Journal of Psychophysiology* 31.2 (1997): 147–154. Print.

Visceglia, E., and S. Lewis. "Yoga Therapy as an Adjunctive Treatment for Schizophrenia: A Randomized, Controlled Pilot Study." *Journal of Alternative and Complementary Medicine* 17.7 (2011): 601–607. Print.

Walker, E., V. Mittal, and K. Tessner. "Stress and the Hypothalamic Pituitary Adrenal Axis in the Developmental Course of Schizophrenia." *Annual Review of Clinical Psychology* 4 (2008): 189–216. Print.

Wooley, A., et al. "A Yoga Intervention for Young Adults with Elevated Symptoms of Depression." *Alternative Therapies in Health and Medicine* 10.2 (2004): 60–63. Print.

Zahn, T. P., W. T. Carpenter, and T. H. McGlashan. "Autonomic Nervous System Activity in Schizophrenia." *Archives of General Psychiatry* 38.3 (1981): 251–266. Print.

YOGA THERAPY AND SPORTS SCIENCE

LeRoy R. Perry, D.C.

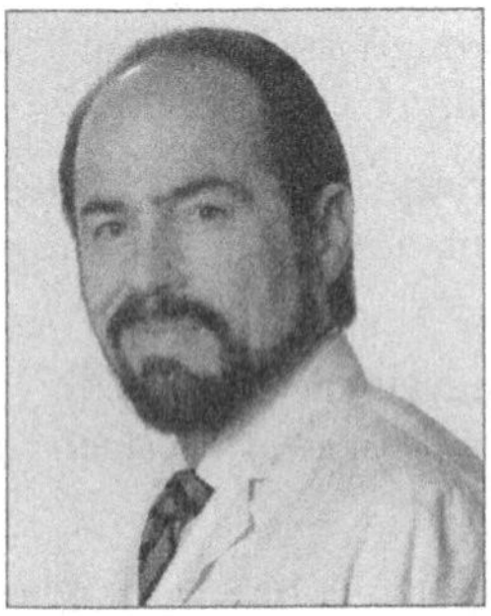

LeRoy R. Perry Jr. is a chiropractic orthopedist, pedorthist, Ayurvedic wellness counselor, inventor, and innovator in sports science. Dr. Perry, the founder and president of the prestigious International Sportscience Institute (ISI) in Los Angeles, was the first chiropractor to serve as an official Olympic team doctor—and did so five times. He was also the first chiropractor to officially work the World Series as the doctor for the Los Angeles Dodgers in 1977, and he has treated athletes from more than forty-five countries. During the 1988 Olympics in Seoul, South Korea, NBC featured a report on Dr. Perry and his work. With cofounder Wilt Chamberlain, Dr. Perry created the Foundation for Athletic Research and Education, an organization that teaches athletes how to enhance performance through proper diet, exercise, and biomechanics. Dr. Perry has been the chiropractor for many famous Yoga teachers including Yogi Bhajan, Bikram Choudhury, Ana Forrest, and Dr. Larry Payne, and he donates his time as chairman of the Sports Science and Medical Advisory Board for America's schools. He was honored in 1991 by the Soviet team during the closing ceremonies of the Track and Field World Championships in Tokyo when he was asked to carry the Soviet flag. This was the last time the flag was ever carried in an athletic event. For more on Dr. Perry's work, please visit www.DrLeRoyPerry.com.

INTRODUCTION

The practice of sports medicine is the application of science to sports. In the real world of health-related sports professionals, we call the scientific practice *sports science* because the word *medicine* is usually related to drugs and/or surgery. Sports science describes the physics of the body and the application of motion, i.e., the kinetics of the body, while sports medicine falls under the larger umbrella of sports science. A sports scientist is someone who practices anything from biomechanics of movement to physical rehabilitation, athletic training, peak performance training, coaching, computer analysis, joint manipulation, decompression of the spine, and/or Yoga Therapy. The intention of any therapist, be it from sports science or Yoga Therapy, is not to see how much they can treat people, it is to teach people to be able to perform correct movements on their own.

Personally, I've found that in the heart or psychology of athletes, you have to reinforce their goal within them. That is how passion and desire for achievement are created and stimulated in an athlete. In Yoga, it is called saṁkalpa (intention, purpose, or determination). When a Yoga teacher works with a Yoga student and that person has a unique ability to do special types of movements or has an inclination to be able to progress in certain practices, the Yoga teacher recognizes and embraces those movements, qualities, and abilities and trains the student accordingly. In sports science, this is called a patient-centered or athlete-centered approach. Instead of forcing the athlete or Yoga practitioner to adapt to the training regimen, the training is adapted to best fit the athlete's special skills and sport-specific individual goals.

THE SPORTS SCIENCE TRIAD OF HEALTH

The basis for how I train athletes has its foundation in the sports science triad of health. The sports science triad of health is made up of three parts: 1) The athlete's structure and function, 2) The athlete's biochemical physiology—the nutrition, acid/alkaline balance, and water intake of the athlete's body, and 3) The athlete's psychological, mental, and/or metaphysical state since the mind is the foundation and source of an athlete's health and success. Included in the third part are meditation, concentration,

The Athlete's Triad of Health

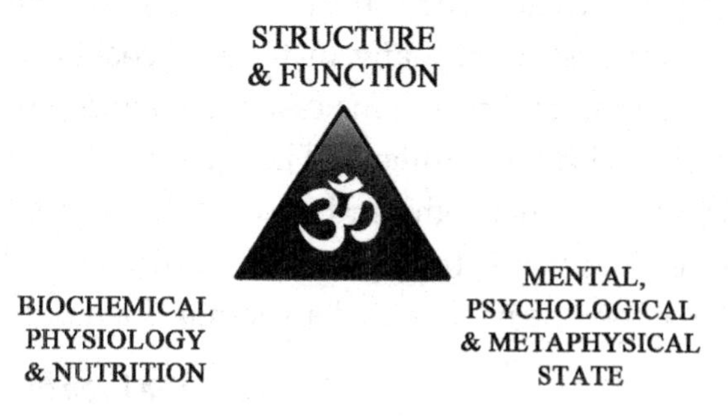

prayer, and the athlete's ability to stop, visualize, and meditate before and during competition.

In sports science and Yoga Therapy, a person should not be treated only from a limited structural point of view of the body. We must look beyond the physical form. Ayurveda, Yoga's sister science, believes that you are what you metabolize and absorb, not just what you eat. Additionally, an athlete's water intake also biochemically affects the levels of alkalinity in his/her body (think of alkalinity as being cool, blue, and soothing and acidity as hot, red, irritating, inflamed, and damaging). We similarly need to understand the mental aspects of the person: where they want to go with their dreams, hopes, and ambitions. In Yoga, we call this bhāva (mood or mental state). Regardless of which concept of the triad we are training—structure, nutrition, or mental state—our goal is to create homoeostasis through a comprehensive plan that addresses all aspects of the person and reinforces the development of top-level training techniques, the ultimate enhancement of human potential.

YOGA THERAPY AND SPORTS TRAINING

Just as different monks and scribes sometimes added and/or eliminated information in the early evolution of the Holy Bible, as Yoga has evolved, different masters and gurus found that not every posture or practice was good for each person. They made modifications to the tradition when necessary and started adding their input on the postures and practices that they thought would be beneficial to Yoga practitioners in their own personal methodology. This flexibility in its delivery is the essence of Yoga Therapy and one of the key features that links it with sports science and distinguishes it from regular Yoga. Yoga Therapy is a practice tailored to the needs and aspirations of the individual. The job of the Yoga Therapist, like a good coach, is to help each student/patient/athlete find and reinforce this path.

Interestingly, many of today's coaches and trainers don't know where their stretching and programs came from and have unknowingly embraced yogic principles with their athletes. They just don't call it Yoga. They call it isometric kinetic training or neuromuscular rehabilitation or foundational training or something else. So, what is the fundamental difference between these disciplines that do not have the title of *Yoga* and an actual Yoga practice? What is missing?

Well, the breath, of course!

It all starts with the breath. You have to breathe! In Yoga, breathing practices are called prāṇāyāma, which are revitalization techniques every athlete and non-athlete should learn. The breath impacts agility, balance, and coordination . . . everything! It creates present moment awareness and helps to calm stress. If you don't breathe well, then you don't physiologically assimilate oxygen; if there is no oxygen, the mitochondria are not going to work efficiently at the cellular level and you have no endurance; if you have no endurance, you have no hope for success in athletic performance. This is the importance of breathing and why Yoga (and embracing all of its aspects beyond just its physicality) is so powerful and necessary in sports training and athletics. When one starts to breathe properly by bringing the air in and letting the air flow out, he/she is re-oxygenating the body, increasing healing potential, and tapping into his/her ability to get into a blissful state.

One of the biggest problems I see with athletes is that they really don't know how to breathe. They are exercising and training, and, yet, they simply don't know how or when to take a deep breath. No one has really taught them or coached them about breathing, and this is where Yoga Therapy can be so beneficial. Additionally, if the muscles are too tight in the upper body and chest, the person often can't breathe efficiently, which will decrease muscular output by overutilizing secondary respiratory muscles as part of a normal breathing pattern. As an example of this, distance runners commonly need to be coached to let the jaw relax so they can let the air in and breathe better. Jim Bush, a five-time national champion track and field coach at UCLA, shared with me that this is one of the first things he teaches his athletes: to relax the jaw. Ultimately, Yoga therapeutically applied to sports training influences athletes to relax and helps them get air into their bodies, giving them the vital energy they need to function and excel.

COMPRESSION VERSUS DECOMPRESSION

What is the chief component that creates a bad back or a bad neck in Yoga and in sports? The answer is compression. Compression is the body's number-one enemy. Compression equals trauma. There are two types of compression: 1) macro-trauma usually related to significant impact like getting hit by a truck or falling off a bike and breaking an arm, and 2) micro-trauma, which is from daily accumulative impact and bad habits that create mechanical stress, such as running, lifting, and/or throwing incorrectly or doing Yoga exercises without good form.

In sports science, reversing compressive load pathomechanics (disease-producing movements) can be the difference maker between a winning performance and a debilitating injury. Pathomechanics, improper biomechanics, can cause a breakdown of joints, damage bones, create inflammation, intensify pain, and create compression. The forces of gravity create further compression, and impact also increases compressive forces—and sports have a lot of impact! As Yoga Therapy relates to sports, it is of the utmost importance that we understand the forces of compression and teach people proper techniques to decompress their spines/bodies, relieving pressure physically, emotionally, and/or mentally.

FINDING NIRVANA AND "THE ZONE"—THE COMPETITIVE UNIVERSE WITHIN

Perhaps one of Yoga Therapy's greatest boons to sports science is how it teaches athletes to calmly self-initiate the internal yogic trance state. In Yoga, this is known as samādhi (total absorption), in Buddhism as nirvāṇa (enlightenment), and, athletically, it is thought of as the competitive universe within "The Zone." Athletes can train and reinforce this meditative ability when they work out, when they study, when they are running, when they are jumping and throwing, when they prepare for competition, and when they are on the field of play actually competing.

When athletes are working out, they commonly go inside themselves and are in that blissful nirvanic state. Most of them simply don't know what that is called because they come from a Western culture, and no one puts it in that terminology. In sports science, we change the yogic nomenclature so that people can relate to it and can train themselves to access it within. Lots of times, especially at the beginning, we're coaching them to find "The Zone," a defined mind-set, a deep concentration that a coach might describe to an athlete that they need to get into to perform better.

Once an athlete is in "The Zone," over time he/she can learn how to replicate that experience and understand its rhythm and flow of body, breathe, movement, and time. In athletic training, this process is known as deprogramming and reprogramming the athlete. Deprogramming is teaching the athlete what they are doing wrong, like instructing a baseball player to bring his shoulder down, keep his shoulder over his hip, and tighten up his swinging motion. It teaches the athlete to not waste energy or lack attention. Reprogramming is reinforcing and teaching the athlete what they are doing right, like a baseball player shifting his weight during the swing from the back foot to the front foot, creating velocity from the rotation of his hips, and following his swing all the way through. It teaches the athlete how to harness energy and power while maximizing focus. In Yoga, deprogramming would be using commands/instructions like "don't arch back so much" and "don't poke your chin," while reprogramming would be using commands/instructions like "drop your front ribs toward your back ribs to initiate the core" and "bring your chin slightly in toward your neck." It is merely teaching people to develop proper habits: evolving from bad habits that don't serve our purpose or performance toward good habits that help us achieve, do our best, enhance our performance, and improve the quality and longevity of our lives. It is this competitive Universal Intelligence, which athletes can learn to apply to every aspect of their lives, that makes them winners.

Now, not everybody is the same, so intellectually people are not going to relate to instructions in the exact same way. A good sports scientist, whether a doctor, coach, trainer, or Yoga Therapist/teacher, should realize this and figure out how to communicate with that specific person. He/she takes responsibility to teach people to recognize and be aware of their unfulfilling habits and replace and reinforce them with good habits that can be trained and maintained. It is essentially the same with teaching athletes to find their state of samādhi, their nirvanic state, "The Zone." We reprogram/educate the athlete to understand how his/her mind and body are interlinked and dependent upon each other in re-creating a new habit, a feeling, and the ease of the position or skill. When the action begins on the field, the athlete's preparation then has the opportunity to take over, and his/her intuition and innate ability does the rest.

EVOLVING AN ATHLETE'S TRAINING

After an athlete has been deprogrammed, he/she must be reprogrammed with a goal. The athlete and coach also have to have a methodology in place of achieving that goal in a way that is safe and doesn't risk him/her getting hurt. My East German sports science friends called it the rule of 10 percent. For example, if an athlete is going to do ten bicep curls when training, we would tell him/her to only increase the weight 10 percent every three days. Let us say the athlete eventually goes up to 20 percent, but he/she gets stiff and sore with the increase. Well, then we would back off 10 percent for three days then resume the activity. If he/she tries that and is still too tight and sore, then we back the athlete off 20 percent, which in this case would be to the original weight. He/she goes back and tries lifting it again for three days. If he/she can do it, great. He/she then goes back up 10 percent and so on. The one caveat is that if he/she has to back off as much as 30 percent below the beginning weight, he/she must stop all activity and reset the plan, possibly with supervision by coaches and trainers.

In sports science, we are very aware that the human body can adapt to almost any stimuli, any challenge. We must therefore constantly change the workload required to achieve greater physiological demands upon the body. Workload is defined as the actual load or weight/mass, distance traveled, times spent and speed at which the effort was performed (WK=MDTS), so as you increase the workload you must safely increase the difficulty of the athlete's training and be ready to grade him/her up to the next level, especially if he/she is doing too many repetitions or too long a hold in a certain exercise or āsana. The mantra of sports science protocols and how to practice Yoga and apply Yoga Therapy are the same. Our goal is always balance and coordination first, strength second. As one's practice and skills improve so will his/her ability to deal with new challenges.

CREATING CORE

The term *core spinal stability* is the proper term for the enhancement of human performance. Typically, when people talk about core stability it is in reference to strengthening the abdomen. This is not core stability in movement and athletics! That is only one-third of the equation in how to really understand the biomechanics of the core. To enhance human performance in sports, you need to strengthen the spine in 360 degrees around the spine. This is what we refer to as core spinal stability.

Taking it a step further, to strengthen athletes, we must think of the core as the entire body, not just the abdomen. If you think of the spine as a bow and arrow, you can think of the string as the erector muscles. When the erectors are too tight, the bow bows more. When the bow bows, the front of the abdomen is getting pushed out and the lumbar spine and facet joints get compressed. Yet, if the erectors are elongated, the pelvis can fall and find a normal and neutral pelvic tilt, which must be able to be controlled.

The most important part to understanding core spinal stability is knowing how to strengthen what part of the body and when. If an athlete has dominant chest muscles, am I going to spend time with him doing bench presses? No way! I'm going to have him strengthen/work his upper back. That is how we create true core spinal stability. In sports science, our goal is to achieve balance to figure out ways to stretch the tight muscles, strengthen the weak muscles, and enhance proper balance with coordination. Core spinal stability creates the foundation of balance/strength and the stability we all need to stay injury free and perform to our highest throughout our lives. The quality of your life depends upon your core spinal stability.

THE ATHLETE'S WILL

In Cuba back in the 1970s, I was invited to lecture at the 1st International Congress of Applied Sciences. At the time, some Eastern Bloc countries were doing calf biopsies of 5-year-old athletes studying the fast-twitch vs. slow-twitch muscle fibers, which would presently be viewed as a highly objectionable practice. They would take these young athletes with "x" amount of fast-twitch muscle fibers and turn them into sprinters, jumpers, or gymnasts and, if the child had more slow-twitch powerful muscle fibers, he/she would most likely be ushered into a heavier sport, which would require pushing/pulling and lifting. I was asked what I thought about the methods that some of the countries were using to train athletes. I said I believed in free will and giving every athlete the opportunity to maximize his/her potential physically, mentally, and emotionally.

You see, you can have an athlete with impeccable genetics, great physiology, lots of fast-twitch muscle fibers, keen visualization ability, and superior practical training that finely tunes his/her body. But, what happens to the young athlete who receives a biopsy at five years old and then is forced to become a sprinter? Maybe that young athlete wants to become a violinist or participate in a different sport. You've directly taken the athlete's will, his/her desire, out of the equation.

Yet, people need will to become a successful, accomplished athlete. You can influence an athlete to achieve great physiological feats if they are given options to think about an embrace. It must come from within. You cannot take the average person and teach him/her about winning. The desire has to be kindled in an athlete's will in competition. You need that subjective part of the person; otherwise the athlete will never find his/her meditative self . . . and that is the place from which champions are created. People who haven't been there might not be able to understand. But when you know, you know. There is a certain swagger and a certain attitude with champion athletes and people who excel in their jobs and their lives. Yoga works to develop that kind of willpower and personal volition through focus, concentration, and an oriented intention. These attributes are all vitally important to develop in top-level athletes and spending the time to work on these skills and developing the will to win may be the difference between a champion and a nonqualifier.

THE USE OF VISUALIZATION IN SPORTS SCIENCE

In the former Soviet Union, now Russia, there is a special place called Bele Noći Sanitarium in the Baltic where back in the 1970s the Supreme Soviet and the KGB would go for indoctrination two weeks every year with their entire families. I was lucky enough to be invited to and spend time at Bele Noći Sanitarium as a journalist and doctor. I did eight hours of filming a TV program for them, which was later aired on Soviet TV. The Sanitarium had special chamber rooms where light, sound, and temperature were all controlled. Inside this highly regulated space, people would learn how to do visualization exercises much like the techniques that are routinely taught in Yoga. The Soviets would sit their athletes down and repeatedly show them videos with perfect technique, perfect form, and perfect motion to program the athletes so all they knew was *perfect*. Ultimately, it was all about getting them into a deeper state of consciousness, a meditative state like "The Zone."

Olympic champion high jumper, Dwight Stone, and gold medalist sprinter, Carl Lewis, were both patients of mine and would commonly visualize the races and the movements in their mind. Dwight would stand as if he was looking at a video of himself running, visualizing where every step would go, where he was going to plant, how high he was going to jump, how he was going to approach the bar, and how he would go over the bar, all with perfect visualization.

Working with many of the best Olympic athletes in the world, it was always clear to me that if an athlete could achieve peace and stillness within himself/herself and find a deep meditative state like in Yoga, he/she would be able to build some inner consciousness and create a balance within. One of my athletes and close friends, Mac Wilkins, a two-time Olympic gold medalist in the discus, is a perfect example of such an athlete. Today, he teaches other athletes to understand and initiate that state of balance to influence the mental, emotional, and character aspects of athletic competition that are needed to not only be successful but to achieve greatness. I truly believe there is a genius within all of us. Tapping into Universal Intelligence to me is the ultimate achievement and accomplishment of experiencing Nirvana.

AYURVEDA AND SOMATOTYPING FOR ATHLETES

Ayurvedic medicine is one of the fastest growing areas of sports science today. In classical Sanskrit literature, Ayurveda is made up of *Ayur* (life) and *Veda* (wisdom, knowledge, or science) and together means the "science of life." Traditionally, Ayurveda is one of the oldest forms of medicine in the East and observes health as the balance of the three main doṣas (constitutions) called vāta, pitta, and kapha. Each individual is primarily one doṣa and most people are a combination of two or more doṣas that contribute to his/her overall makeup. To maintain health and prevent potential disease, different practices and therapies are provided to bring equilibrium back to the doṣas.

Surprisingly, the doṣa principles of balance in Ayurveda are similar to those found in the study of morphology and somatotyping in the West. Somatotyping is the study of body types and shapes. There are three basic body shapes: endomorph, mesomorph, and ectomorph. People with different somatotypes tend to be good at different sports. For example, a high jumper or swimmer has stronger ectomorphic traits, a boxer or triathlete has stronger mesomorphic traits, and a weight lifter, wrestler, or a shot putter has stronger endomorphic traits but all with a significant mixture of mesomorphic traits.

Additional details combining doṣas and somatotyping can be found in the following table and can used to better understand the nature and constitution of athletes.

DOṢAS AND SOMATOTYPING FOR UNDERSTANDING THE NATURE AND CONSTITUTION OF ATHLETES

DOṢA	BODY TYPE	PSYCHIC CENTERS AND ELEMENTS	PHYSICAL CHARACTERISTICS	PERSONALITY TRAITS
Vāta	Ectomorph	Heart and throat; 4th & 5th cakras; Ether and air	Thin and lean, flat chest, delicate build, young appearance, tall, lightly muscled, narrow shoulders and hips, little fat and muscles, long arms and legs, thin face, high forehead, large brain, stooping posture	Self-conscious, preference for privacy, introverted, inhibited, socially anxious, artistic, mentally intense, emotionally restrained
Pitta	Mesomorph	Dantien and solar plexus; 2nd & 3rd cakras; Fire and water	Hard and firm muscular physique, strong arms and legs, overly mature appearance, wide shoulders and narrow hips, rectangular shape, thick skin, upright posture, very little body fat, warrior and gladiator class	Adventurous, desire for power and dominance, courageous, indifference to thoughts of others, assertive, bold, zest for physical activity, competitive, love for risk
Kapha	Endomorph	Root and dantien; 1st & 2nd cakras; Water and earth	Heaviness, underdeveloped muscles, round shape, large frame, wide hips, overweight, overdeveloped digestive system, high percentage of body fat, slim wrists, narrow shoulders, prominent abdomen	Love of food especially sugar, carbohydrates, and starches, tolerance, evenness of emotions, loves comfort, sociable, constant cravings, good humored, relaxed, need for affection

THE APPROACH AND ASSESSMENT

Sports science is an art dependent on science. How do we treat people in sports science using yogic principles? Well, first you have to know what you want to treat and how you want to treat it. The thinking process of a sports scientist is thus very much the same as a forensic detective. We are trained to study the academic, but, as famous German sprinting coach Bert Sumser said during a 1975 lecture at the University of Mainz, "Study the academic, learn everything there is to know about the academic and science, then throw the books away, and do what works." In essence, he was telling us to think outside the box. In order to do that, there has to be some type of diagnostic, intellectual process going on in the teacher's/therapist's mind to know what is applicable to that particular person.

The initial exam I do is a complete orthopedic, neurological, and biomechanical exam, including gait analysis and all range-of-motion tests from head to toe and all circumference measurements. Then I do a complete muscle examination with some slight sports science modifications. For example, normally the adductors are tested with the legs straight. In sports science, we do it straight, 45 degrees, 90, and 130, or as close to the chest as possible and with bent knees as close to the abdomen as possible. We test the muscle in four different components of movement, and we do comparable testing throughout the body. In sports science, we check how the body performs through a wide range of motions and situations like one would experience when in the field of play. From that muscle examination and prior exams, I can specifically determine the points of instability in the athlete. As part of the treatment, I observe how a person's body compensates, especially through his/her sport-specific actions, and determine ways I can help him/her add the yogic principles of stirrha (steadiness in balance and coordination) and sukha (ease and flexibility) to his/her training.

THE EVOLUTION OF YOGA THERAPY AND SPORTS SCIENCE

A sports scientist is a student of athletics, biomechanics, physics, engineering, biology, and/or the clinical sciences. As such, a sports scientist is empowered to think differently. He/she looks at the obvious with an understanding that he/she does not know it all, but rather that we are students of performance studying the reflection of those bodies that we are honored enough to take care of, to improve, and to learn from. Each athlete we learn from improves our understanding and inspires us to help others in accomplishing greater deeds and greater triumphs.

Sports science is based upon science, but it is also based on the intuition of the practitioner. We must learn to study the academic and we must apply it to ourselves. As we become more at one with our intuitive selves and we feel and experience the process, we can tap into Universal Intelligence and make better decisions. Therefore, the thought process of a Yoga Therapist and sports scientist are one and the same. We strive to achieve excellence in all things.

Often coaches interested in stretching and flexibility have heard of Yoga, but they have rarely participated in it, and their preconceived idea may or may not be correct. If I were speaking to a trainer or a coach, I would ask him/her to just stay open to the idea and try taking and experiencing a Yoga class for himself/herself. It has been my experience in life that, until we become subjective of our thoughts, concerns, and fears about something we are exposed to for the first time, we may not be accurate. For example, reincarnation was initially something I did not believe in. Through the years, I had many discussions on the topic with actress, Shirley MacLaine, a close friend of mine and patient for over thirty-five years. Finally, I became more open to the idea when I began studying Ayurveda and Ayurvedic medicine. I have now learned to challenge all ideas while keeping an open mind, and I think coaches and athletes who do the same in reference to Yoga Therapy will gain a lot of value from the practice. Through meditation, prayer, and Yoga, Universal Intelligence is obtainable by all. The more you open up your mind, the more creative and intuitive you become.

I believe all sports scientists, doctors, coaches, and trainers need to learn about Yoga and participate for themselves. Similarly, Yoga Therapists must learn about the sport of the athletes they wish to work with. THERE IS NO FREE LUNCH! Both sides need to do the work! Do not expect an athlete, sports scientist, coach, or trainer to embrace Yoga if the Yoga Therapist knows nothing about the needs of the athlete and his/her particular sport. PARTICIPATE! Find a coach in the sport of interest and ask questions. Build a relationship and feel and experience the athletic activity. Think of working with a gladiator in an arena. You do not train a gladiator by handing him a bushel of flowers; you give a gladiator a sword and shield. The first time I visited the Coliseum in Rome, I understood and felt this principle innately. Like a gladiator, an athlete must learn to fight to survive—and this is the truth. In sports competition, the goal is to win and anything less is unacceptable. Yoga Therapists must understand this warrior mentality in sports to be successful in teaching athletes and coaches. Only then will the Yoga Therapist understand the athlete's needs and how to apply the yogic sciences appropriately.

Yoga Therapy adapted to the needs of the athlete can assist athletes in achieving his/her personal and competitive goals and potential.

In the end, Yoga Therapy is the perfect complement to sports training because it is extremely safe and effective for enhancing athletic performance while minimizing stress. For Yogāsanas, people are trained to work on a mat. For sports, you have to get that philosophy of agility, balance, and coordination off the mat and onto two feet. Coordination during movement is important to experience for both the athlete and the Yoga practitioner. Together the practices of Yoga and sports science support each other like players on the same team because they are both applied sciences where experience is the key to understanding and unlocking performance obstacles. Performance is important; however, competing to the highest level of personal achievement without injury is the crowning achievement.

The one thing I know for sure is that the human body is adaptable to everything—altitude, weather, temperature, environment, and activity. In order to enhance human performance in sports science, there is an underlining goal. The goal is to constantly teach the athlete how to achieve balance. If the athlete understands how to develop and maintain balance, then he/she is going to have skills to better prevent injuries and stay in the game, performing to his/her maximum potential. At its essence, preventive care is simply balance, so teaching people balance is teaching them prevention. I'm not just referring to the person's postural balance; I'm talking about his/her triad of health: structural, biochemistry/diet, and mental attitude. If we can teach people the principles of homeostasis and balance and they learn how to apply them to everything they do in their lives, then everyone wins, there will be less injuries, athletes will perform better, and people will have longer and healthier lives with improved quality.

Joe Weider, the "Father of Fitness" and my personal workout partner for over twenty-five years, said, "Never quit, only those who quit lose." Through his mentorship and many others' wisdom and influence, I have learned to never quit, to never give up, and it has made me a better doctor, a better sports scientist, and a better person. The best sports science advice I can share with anyone, whether they are athletes, Yoga practitioners, or patients, is simply, "Look deeply into your heart and follow your dreams."

REFERENCES

LIFE.

The Psychology of Yoga Therapy

Ira Israel, L.M.F.T., L.P.C.C.

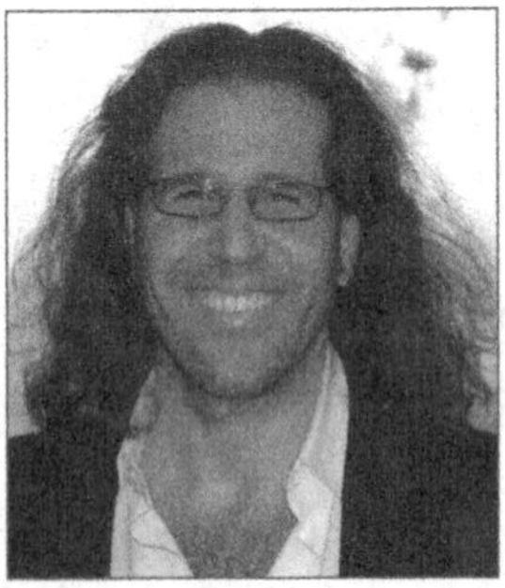

Psychotherapist **Ira Israel** is a licensed marriage and family therapist, a licensed professional clinical counselor, a certified Yoga Therapist, and an E-RYT500 Yoga instructor. He has a bachelor of arts degree in sociology from the University of Pennsylvania, a master of arts degree in psychology from Antioch University, a master of arts degree in religious studies from the University of California at Santa Barbara, and a master of arts degree in philosophy from the University of Connecticut. Mr. Israel is on the teaching faculty at Esalen Institute and Omega Institute and is the author of three mindfulness and Yoga DVDs: *Mindfulness for Urban Depression, Mindfulness Meditations for Anxiety,* and *Yoga for Depression and Anxiety.*

INTRODUCTION

As reported in Patricia Cabral, Hilary Meyer, and Dr. Donna Ames's study on the "Effectiveness of Yoga Therapy as a Complementary Treatment for Major Psychiatric Disorders: A Meta-Analysis," Yoga is an efficacious conjoint therapy for treating and regulating mood disorders such as depression, anxiety, and posttraumatic stress disorder (PTSD) (Cabral, Meyer, and Ames, 2011). As a licensed psychotherapist and certified Yoga Therapist, I have found that the qualities of self-discipline, self-inquiry, and the delayed gratification that a commitment to a consistent Haṭha Yoga practice engenders bode favorably for treating and regulating mood disorders. Additionally, I have observed that the underlying philosophical tenets of Hinduism and Buddhism—such as ahiṁsa (nonviolence) and metta (loving-kindness)—resonate particularly well with creative people who are challenged by existential questions, which often manifest in the form of depression, from living in a highly competitive, consumer-based society that puts pressure on them to be constantly motivated and productive.

Until recently, there have been relatively few psychotherapists who have used Yoga as a conjoint therapy to help patients self-regulate their moods and overcome depression, anxiety, and PTSD. Historically, Yoga consisted of religious and spiritual practices done by ascetics and renunciants in monasteries and ashrams. Only relatively recently has the emphasis of Yoga shifted toward the physical āsana practice and in doing so has become more popular with laypeople. Although Yoga Therapy is only now beginning to be employed to treat psychological disorders, the Western field of psychotherapy is quite open for exploration and the initial results, as clearly documented in studies such as the one mentioned above by Cabral, Meyer, and Ames.

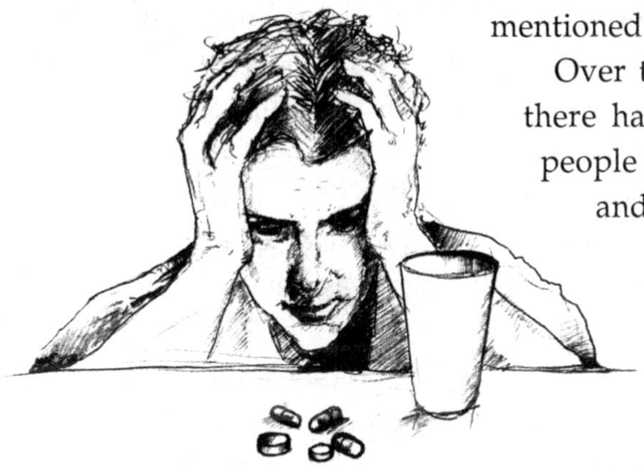

Over the last thirty years in America and Europe, there has been a tremendous rise in the number of people who receive prescriptions for anti-anxiety and antidepressant medications. Over 100 million prescriptions are given in America every year for antidepressant medication (Mojtabai and Olfson, 2011) and over 10 percent of Americans, or 30-plus million people, over the age of twelve years old take antidepressant medication on a daily basis (Pratt, Brody, and Gu, 2011). Current research demonstrates that a variety of Yoga sequences and breathing practices have been found to be helpful with treating and/or co-managing mood disorders. Yet, I am personally unaware of any evidence-based studies unequivocally proving that prescriptions of specific āsanas (postures or poses) or specific āsana sequences are valid and reliable for treating specific mood disorders. Some correlations, though, seem intuitive: for example, inversions stimulate the flow of blood to the brain; the flow of blood to the brain stimulates activity; stimulated brains may result in improved moods. In terms of empirical evidence, I would argue that it is the Yoga practice and commitment to that practice and lifestyle that has positive effects on moods, not placing the physical body in particular poses (even though maybe at some later date studies may conclude that moving or stretching the body in certain ways positively affects moods).

HOW YOGA WORKS REGARDING COGNITION

According to Patañjali, the person who codified the origins of the modern Yoga practice, one of the outcomes of practicing Yoga is "the cessation of movements in the consciousness" (Iyengar, 1993). Recent trends in psychology, including Aaron Beck's Cognitive Therapy and Albert Ellis's Rational Emotive Behavioral Therapy, have proposed that thoughts precede emotions. More precisely, negative thinking and negative mental states result in negative emotions. Thus, if one can learn to observe and regulate one's cognitive processes, then one will have a modicum of control over one's emotional states. Put in the most simplistic terms possible, a glass can either be observed as half-empty or half-full depending on the observer's perspective.

In scientific terms, physical exercises like those found in most Haṭha Yoga practices raise endorphins and dopamine levels (Kay, 2013). Studies have shown that, although antidepressants prove more helpful in the very short term, exercise trumps antidepressants in the long run for mood regulation as a long-term treatment and has no side effects (Gill, Womack, and Safranek, 2010).

In addition, there is a meditative quality about the way Haṭha Yoga is typically practiced. While it can be argued that āsana-based Haṭha Yoga was developed to help ascetics prepare for seated meditation by warming up the spine and loosening up the hips, the majority of styles of Haṭha Yoga that are practiced today in the West link expansive movements to deep, fluid inhalations and contracting movements to deep, fluid exhalations. Oceanic, wave-like guttural breathing called ujjāyi breathing is also an integral part. Linking breath to movement is known as Vinyāsa Flow Yoga and functions similarly to a moving meditation, taking the practitioner out of the shallow breathing that corresponds with being in fight-or-flight mode and placing a primacy on long, deep, relaxing breaths. Vinyāsa Flow Yoga is more akin to the exercise one would find in ballet, Chi Gong, and Tai Chi rather than running sprints or lifting weights. Because of the dance-like nature of linking one's breathing and movements, it is easy to see how Yoga could be referred to as a moving meditation. Recent books such as Rick Hanson's *The Buddha's Brain* refer to the recent scientific research on meditation that has been overwhelmingly positive (Trafton, 2011). So whether we use Yoga to prepare our bodies for seated meditation, or we use it as a moving meditation unto itself, both ultimately result in decreased stress, more positive moods, and an enhanced ability to accept and regulate negative moods.

MINDFULNESS MEDITATION IN PRACTICE

Recently there has been a tremendous rise in interest in mindfulness practices in general and mindfulness meditation in particular in the fields of psychology and Yoga Therapy. An important distinction, though, needs to be made between Yoga and mindfulness regarding the worldview and the intention of the practitioner. According to the viewpoint of Advaita Vedānta, which was taught by Swami Shankara in the eighth century and made popular in Western culture in the 1960s by the Beatles, the primary purpose of meditation is to allow the practitioner to transcend his/her ego and everything perceived through his/her senses (maya) in order to taste, realize, and experience his/her inner divinity, oneness, and perfection. Thus, if one is looking for the psychological causes or culprit for *malaise* in terms of Hinduism, it is the thinking mind. The thinking mind busies itself creating stories about the no longer existent past and projects imaginations about the not yet existent future. At its essence, the human mind was designed to act as a protective, defensive mechanism to try to stave off traumas. However, just as meditators are fond of saying, "The mind has a mind of its own," most people do not realize why they are acting and reacting to certain stimuli in a particular manner. Since one uncompromising quality of the mind is that it cannot be instructed to shut itself off, in the Hindu lineage an "anchor" or focus of thought is used to trick the mind into taking a break. This anchor can be the breath, a mantra, visualizations, or sensations—anything that subtly lulls the overactive mind into relaxing for a brief respite.

Buddhists, on the other hand, believe that there is no Self and no God or divinity; there is nothing to transcend and nothing to transcend to. Instead, the mind is akin to a muscle, and we must exercise it through meditation so that it grows stronger, and, in doing so, we will gain insights into how the mind is operating. As in the Hindu lineage, the anchor or focal point of Buddhist mindfulness meditations can be the breath, a mantra, visualizations, or sensations; or, the focus of the mind can be the mind itself, and the thoughts, emotions, and/or sensations rising to one's awareness. However, the *intention* of the meditations is very different in the two traditions. This is an important distinction because it helps patients in Yoga Therapy examine the assumptions they have about their own minds, their worldviews, their own psychological compositions, their emotional experience, and their own empowerment.

In America, Yoga has been separated from its Hindu origins and mindfulness separated from its Buddhist origins; I am not advocating any religious dogma when I talk about Yoga or mindfulness. Personally, I believe that discerning the intention and worldview of the practitioner greatly eases practicing Yoga and/or meditation for him or her. Is the intention to transcend the ego to temporarily release the mental chatter or noise in the head? Or is the intention to train the mind to concentrate on desired phenomena for longer and longer periods of time? Due to the fact that most people find meditation to be extremely challenging, anything a Yoga Therapist can do to facilitate a patient's meditation practice is helpful. Regardless of the intention, the results of both types of meditations are similar: greater peace of mind, equanimity, calmness, tranquility, and ease.

In one popular type of mindfulness meditation, meditators are instructed to openly monitor their thoughts and feelings nonjudgmentally. Monitoring one's thoughts creates a distance between whatever one considers to be his/her essential Self—whatever part of us that observes the thoughts—and the thoughts and emotions that arise to consciousness. This slight perceived distance between the watcher and the thoughts implies that we are not limited to gaining our personal identities through our thoughts, as Descartes unfortunately proposed in his *cogito ergo sum:* "I think therefore I am." Open-monitoring meditation allows one to get a sense of being greater than the limited mental soundtrack that rolls through our heads. Cultivating the ability to be nonreactive, particularly to negative thoughts that arise, is extremely important when trying to regulate one's moods. If one can recognize the negative thoughts that trigger negative emotions and one has cultivated nonreactivity by being able to nonjudgmentally observe his/her thoughts and refrain from reacting, then one can make pro-active decisions regarding how to appropriately act or react.

Open monitoring of thoughts teaches people that they have a choice regarding whether they should listen to their thoughts or choose to just let them pass. Emotionally deregulated people tend to be highly reactive. They listen to their thoughts and instantaneously react in visceral and often irrational manners. Little incidents occur and they catastrophize them, adding meanings onto events and phenomena that are not necessarily accurate or beneficial. For instance, I have had adult patients who hear mere suggestions that were intended by their parents to be helpful as criticism. A parent aims to be helpful when he/she suggests something benign such as "Why don't you add a little pepper to that recipe?" or "Why don't you move the car up a little before you try to parallel park?" But the son or daughter assimilates such a suggestion as "I can never do anything right!" or "I'll never be good enough!" Both Yoga as a moving meditation and meditation itself teach us how to cultivate nonreactivity; they teach us how to avoid adding extra meaning to thoughts and reactions that arise. For example, if one cannot touch the floor in trikoṇāsana (triangle pose), it does not mean that one is a bad person or that one's practice is deteriorating. One quickly learns that everyone's physical practice will be different every day, so being able to attain a position or stretch really does not mean anything. Thus, when teaching, I often remind students of one of Shakespeare's famous lines from *Hamlet* Act II Scene ii: "There is nothing either good or bad, but thinking makes it so." Both Yoga and meditation were designed to take the practitioner *beyond* his/her ephemeral thoughts, *beyond* thinking, *beyond* mind chatter to help the practitioner *dis-identify* with his/her mental soundtrack and all of the judgments that lie therein. Because labeling phenomena as "good" or "bad" is a function of our minds, "good" and "bad" does not arise outside human cognition. Yoga stills the natural fluctuations of our agitated minds so that we can have a better understanding of what is transpiring and our mind's relationship with what is occurring.

Another popular style of mindfulness meditation is known as *labeling thoughts*. In the meditation, the meditator not only observes the thoughts, he/she labels what types of thoughts they are. The thoughts are either about something in the past, present, or future, and they either have a negative, neutral, or positive charge. For example:

1. Thinking about something in the past and the thought is neutral, neither positive nor negative—"I went to the zoo last week."—is **REMEMBERING**.
2. Thinking about the past and the thought has a positive charge—"The chopped salad I ate last Friday was amazing!"—is **REMINISCING**.
3. Thinking about the past and the thought has a negative charge—"I can't believe he broke up with me via text message!"—is **REGRETTING**.
4. Thinking about something in the present and the thought is neutral, neither positive nor negative—"I wonder if it's going to rain tomorrow."—is **WONDERING**.

5. Thinking about the present and the thought has a positive charge—
"Boy, I would really like to have a vegan hot fudge sundae right now."
—is **DESIRING**.

6. Thinking about the present and the thought has a negative charge—
"I cannot believe that girl on the next mat chose that nail color!"—is **JUDGING**.

7. Thinking about something in the future and the thought is neutral, neither positive nor negative—"I'm going to email my ex when I get home."
—is **PLANNING**.

8. Thinking about the future and the thought has a positive charge—"I hope he has enough money so we can honeymoon at the Four Seasons in Kauai."
—is **FANTASIZING**.

9. Thinking about the future and the thought has a negative charge—
"If that brown spot isn't melanoma now, then it certainly will be some day!"
—is **FEARING**.

Labeling thoughts often demonstrates to the practitioner how limited the mind is and the redundancy of one's thoughts. The point of the technique is to raise one's consciousness around how the mind operates and to eventually empower the practitioner to realize that, although the mind has a negativity bias, choices are available and it is not always necessary or beneficial to act or react to the thoughts arising to consciousness.

DISCIPLINE AND DELAYED GRATIFICATION

In their landmark study, "Delay of Gratification in Children," Walter Mischel, Yuichi Shoda, and Monica Rodriquez demonstrated that children who were able to delay gratification at age four or five became adolescents whose parents rated them as more academically and socially competent, verbally fluent, rational, attentive, and able to deal well with frustration and stress (Mischel, Shoda, and Peake, 1988). Emotionally deregulated people often have poor impulse control. Being able to delay gratification and control impulses for immediate gratification is something that Yoga teaches all practitioners. Of course, all Yoga sequences have poses that each individual will enjoy and poses that each individual will find challenging; cultivating discipline to continue through the challenging poses to complete a sequence and arrive in the restfulness of śavāsana (corpse pose) is something that every Yoga student learns.

There is also a second type of delayed gratification experienced by Yoga practitioners: learning the poses incrementally. Practitioners who are not naturally hyper-flexible and/or who are not former gymnasts and ballerinas notice that the suppleness of their limbs increases over time. Although touching one's toes is not necessary for practicing Yoga, as the body becomes more limber, Yoga practitioners often take pride in overcoming perceived shortcomings such as stretching farther than previously possible or stretching more easily than previously experienced.

Similarly, carving out 60 or 90 minutes from our day also demonstrates delayed gratification in the form of discipline as one does not eat, check email, or attend to any other matters during that time. Regarding discipline, most practitioners also make specific commitments to practice Yoga a certain number of times per week. I believe that it is in these subtle attributes of practicing Yoga on a regular basis—namely, delayed gratification and discipline—that will ultimately be found to be the links between the scientific research and the psychological and emotional benefits of Yoga.

CONCLUSION

The majority of the physical Haṭha Yoga that is practiced in the West helps to regulate and treat mood disorders on the physical level similar to the manner in which exercise helps regulate and treat mood disorders by raising endorphins and dopamine levels. Secondly, it helps practitioners disidentify with their thought processes and gain respites from thinking in general and negative self-talk. Practicing Yoga addresses mood disorders on the mental level by stilling, quieting, and focusing the mind. On the emotional level, Yoga Therapy helps regulate and treat mood disorders by allowing the practitioner to cultivate nonreactivity to his/her thoughts; similar to practicing mindfulness meditation, equanimity and equipoise are developed as the practitioner grows to realize the distance between one's essential Self—one's "core" or "higher power"—and one's temporary and fleeting mental and emotional states. The instruction that I use when teaching both Yoga and meditation is, "You are not your thoughts; you are not just the thoughts rolling through your head."

The benefits of Yoga Therapy as a conjoint therapy to treat mood disorders are evident and constantly evolving in Western medicine. Patañjali's second Yoga sūtra, "Yoga is the cessation of the movements of consciousness" (Iyengar), helps many clients cultivate nonreactivity to the negative thoughts that engender negative moods. Additionally, because of the underlying philosophy, Yoga Therapy is particularly effective for treating creative people who often suffer from existential despair. Although Yoga has been secularized in North America, the spiritual component and the myths and stories, such as that of the *Bhagavad Gītā,* assist many people in gaining a more interesting understanding of what their dharma (vocation) is and what they are doing with their lives.

To explain these concepts further, we must remember that Yoga and meditation are practices. They are means, not ends. As writer Gertrude Stein famously said, "There's no there *there,*" meaning that there is nothing to achieve, no perfect pose, no place to get to, no bonus karma points for being able to put your ankles behind your neck or for holding a pose for an extended period of time. Yoga teaches us to release our expectations and just show up and "be" with and "be" in our bodies. What we learn through practicing Yoga is to disregard our egos, which primarily manifest psychologically as negative voices in our heads echoing, "There's something wrong with you. Everyone else is better at this than you are. You'll never be good at this. Why are you wasting your time? You should just give up and stop making a fool of yourself."

Essentially, our minds are built to make judgments, and these judgments are primarily based on fears; fears are primarily based on either ignorance and/or are reactions to past traumas. Judgments and prejudices inhibit us from showing up authentically and limit us from being truly present in the present moment. What Yoga and meditation teach us is present-time awareness of our bodies and our breaths—to be mindful of our *prāṇa,* or essential life source.

A central tenet of Yoga is *ahiṁsa,* or nonviolence and nonharming. One quickly learns through the practice of Yoga to regard overly judgmental forms of critical thinking as being harmful in many ways. Practicing Yoga teaches us that ahiṁsa must start with the way we treat our own bodies. This is why and how Yoga can help practitioners build self-esteem, confidence, and self-love and further helps him/her to overcome the negative self-talk that has been conditioned into us early in our lives.

Whenever I conclude teaching a Yoga class, after the final supine resting pose, *śavāsana,* I have the students gently return to a comfortable seated position, and I instruct them to move their hands into a prayer pose at the level of the hearts. From there, I suggest that they take any benefits cultivated during the Yoga practice off the mat and into the world by:

1. Raising their thumbs in prayer to their foreheads, silently asking for clarity of consciousness
2. Lowering their thumbs in prayer to their lips, silently asking for clarity of communication
3. Lowering their thumbs in prayer back to their hearts silently, asking for clarity of sentiments, clarity of emotions

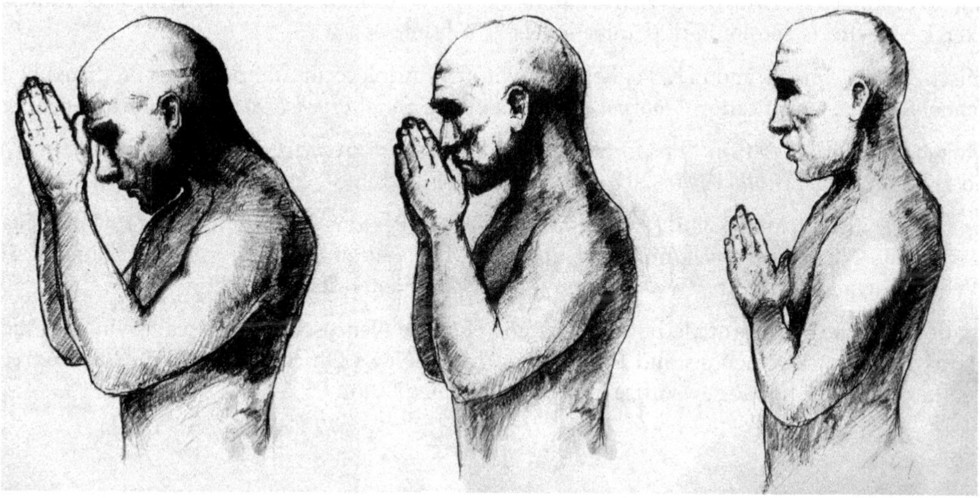

The psychological benefits of Yoga as a conjoint therapy to help regulate and treat mood disorders have been barely tapped in North America. As Yoga becomes more popular and more studies are conducted, I am confident that Yoga will move from being a conjoint therapy to being a therapy unto itself in the various fields of mental health. The yogic lifestyle and the belief system that buttress the physical practice of Haṭha Yoga are great tools that we can employ to treat our culture's epidemics of depression and anxiety and learn how to live more fulfilling and peaceful lives.

REFERENCES

Cabral, P., H. B. Meyer, and D. Ames. "Effectiveness of Yoga Therapy as a Complimentary Treatment for Major Psychiatric Disorders: A Meta-Analysis." *Primary Care Companion for CNS Disorders* 13.4 (2011). Web. Retrieved February 11, 2014. http://www.ncbi.nlm.nih.gov/pmc/articles/PMC3219516/.

Hanson, R. *Buddha's Brain: The Practical Neuroscience of Happiness, Love, and Wisdom.* Oakland, CA: New Harbinger, 2009.

Iyengar, B. K. S. *Light on the Yoga Sutras of Patanjali.* London: Thorsons, 1993; Harper Collins, 2002. Print.

Gill, A., R. Womack, and S. Safranek. "Clinical Inquiries: Does Exercise Alleviate Symptoms of Depression?" *Journal of Family Practice* 59.9 (2010): 530–531. Web. Retrieved from U.S. National Library of Medicine February 11, 2014. http://www.ncbi.nlm.nih.gov/pubmed/20824231.

Kay, S. (Demand Media). "Exercise and Its Effects on Serotonin & Dopamine Levels." Healthy Living, azcentral.com. 2013. Web. Retrieved 13 February 2014. http://healthyliving.azcentral.com/exercise-its-effects-serotonin-dopamine-levels-2758.html.

Mischel, W., Y. Shoda, and P. K. Peake. "The Nature of Adolescent Competencies Predicted by Preschool Delay of Gratification." *Journal of Personality and Social Psychology* 54.4 (1988): 687–696. Print.

Mojtabai, R., and M. Olfson. "Proportion of Antidepressants Prescribed Without a Psychiatric Diagnosis Is Growing." *Health Affairs* 30.8 (2011): 1434–1442. Print.

Pratt, L., D. Brody, and Q. Gu. "Antidepressant Use in Persons Aged 12 and Over: United States, 2005–2008." NCHS data brief, no. 76. Hyattsville, MD: National Center for Health Statistics, 2011. Web. PDF available at http://www.cdc.gov/nchs/data/databriefs/db76.htm.

Trafton, A. "The Benefits of Meditation: MIT and Harvard Neuroscientists Explain Why the Practice Helps Tune Out Distractions and Relieve Pain." MIT News Office. 5 May 2011. Web. Retreived February 11, 2014. http://newsoffice.mit.edu/2011/meditation-0505.

YOGA THERAPY AND CANCER

Jnani Chapman, R.N., B.S.N., C.M.T., C.Y.T., E-RYT 500

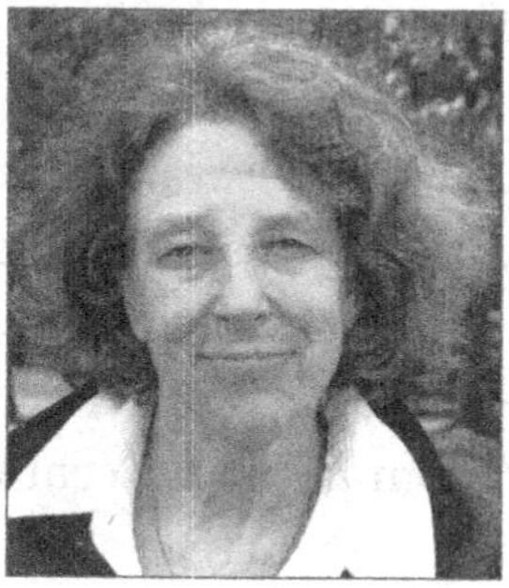

Jnani Chapman is founder and director of YCat Yoga Therapy in Cancer and Chronic Illness, a three-level certification training for Yoga teachers and health professionals. She is an integrative medicine specialist providing Yoga Therapy, acupressure, and massage at St. Mary's Medical Center in the oncology and elder services departments in San Francisco, California. Jnani is a twenty-nine-year staff member of the Commonweal and Smith Center cancer help programs, and she teaches Yoga for Dean Ornish, M.D.'s prostate cancer, postresearch participants in Sausalito, California. She was a stress-management specialist for Dr. Dean Ornish's heart disease reversal research and clinical programs from 1986–1999. Executive director of the International Association of Yoga Therapists from 1994–1998, Jnani was also a founding clinician at the UCSF Osher Center for Integrative Medicine, and she created the Yoga programs for the UCSF Comprehensive Cancer Center from 1997–2009. She is a consultant on Yoga research studies nationally and internationally and balances her work life with kayaks and sailing on San Francisco Bay.

YCAT YOGA THERAPY ORIGINS

Since the mid-1990s, I have been training other Yoga teachers and many health professionals to use Yoga Therapy with people who have been diagnosed with cancer, heart disease, and other chronic illnesses. I also work with people through the end of life and train others to support people through the dying process. The professional Yoga training work began as ten-day workshops: I taught everything I believed essential to know from a nursing and medical perspective in using Yoga during cancer treatment and in cardiac rehabilitation. This work has evolved into a three-level training, YCat Yoga Therapy, whose skilled 300-hour graduates are serving people in medical settings around the United States and several other countries (Chapman, 2013). YCat is specifically designed from a physiological nursing perspective, and YCat teachers are expected to communicate the physiological mechanisms that underlie the practices they teach as health educators. YCat Yoga Therapy is appropriate for people who are at any point along a life continuum in dealing with illness, disease, and the normal aging process.

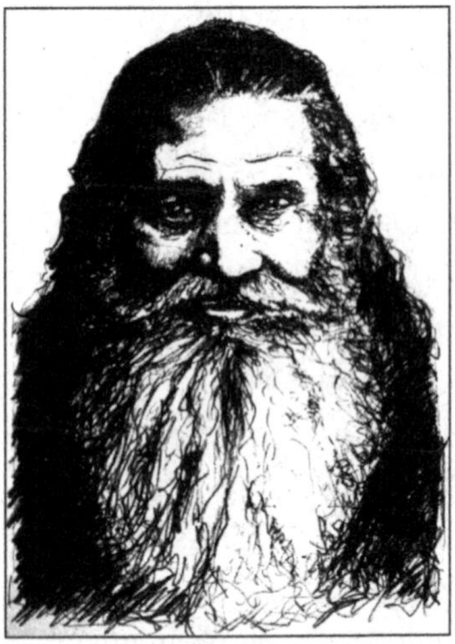

Swami Satchidananda

YCat Yoga Therapy developed from Integral Yoga, founded by Swami Satchidananda. Swami Satchidananda's teachings center on the inner spiritual "self" inherent in all beings and in life. The structure he created for an Integral Yoga class invokes that connection to the "inner self." It moves from an initial centering practice into physical activity with active stretches, postures, and movement sequences; then, for the remaining 40 percent of time, students move attention inward through Yoga nidrā (relaxation), prāṇāyāma (breathing), and dhyāna (meditation) before a centering reminder of inner essence closes each class (Chapman, 2013; Satchidananda, 2006).

Lineages of teaching in Yoga vary greatly in determining what aspects of Yoga get highlighted in thought and practice. Many traditions focus all effort on meditation, others on movement, and others on sound vibration and chanting. Originally, lineages derived through familial handing down to the next generation of an oral tradition of stories, parables, and tales from ancient scriptures. Swami Satchidananda's adage: "Truth Is One, Paths Are Many" (Satchidananda, 2008) was his way of giving permission for the many paths that can be followed to lead to an experience of oneness of the "All in All and the All in Everything" that Yoga says is our own true nature and our native home (Chapman, 2013).

With Swami Satchitananda's encouragement and blessing, a traditional hour-long Integral Yoga beginner class was prescribed as a daily commitment to the research participants in Dean Ornish, M.D.'s program for reversing heart disease from 1986–1990 (Ornish, 1992). I was one of the research Yoga teachers, and I continued teaching in Ornish's weeklong clinical lifestyle retreats through 1999. We also delivered his program at the Medical Center at the University of California, San Francisco, where I worked as an integrative medicine specialist, Yoga Therapist, and nurse educator from 1987 until 2009. Today, the Ornish program for reversing heart disease is a covered Medicare benefit that provides 72 hours of a comprehensive lifestyle intervention at sites whose staff has trained to deliver his program. Ornish has also completed groundbreaking work using Yoga and lifestyle change in early stage prostate cancer.

Swami Satchidananda and his teachings inspired a generation of thinkers, creators, and leaders, like Dean Ornish, M.D., in coronary artery disease and early stage prostate cancer and Michael Lerner, Ph.D., in public health and cancer support. Ornish's and Lerner's visions continue to change outcomes for people in medical crises and will become the new norms for healing in our world. Their work has inspired a generation of Yoga teachers like Elizabeth Lakshmi Kanter and Pat Devi Fitzsimmons at Inova Hospital system in the greater Washington, D.C., area and Tali Ben-Shariff at University of Pennsylvania Medicine's Abramson Cancer Center in Philadelphia. These YCat Yoga Therapists and many others are providing health education, stress management, and motivation for lifestyle changes through Yoga in ways that reduce distressing side effects and help people feel better. May the stories herein shine a light on YCat Yoga Therapy, its purposes and practices, and its service to healing along the continuum of cancer diagnosis and treatment.

YCAT YOGA THERAPY BASICS: AN ACTIVE LISTENING PRESENCE

The trajectory of people who can benefit from Yoga Therapy in illness includes people who may be receiving many types of medical treatments simultaneously, including tests and procedures, various classes of pharmaceuticals, and surgeries and radiation therapy. This includes people who may be in rehabilitation and recovery after medical interventions that are hoping to prevent relapses and recurrences. It may also include people who are finished with medical interventions because all of the standard treatments and experimental research avenues have been exhausted or because something inside them said, "No more," and they decided to follow that voice. Either way, these are people who may be nearing the end of the continuum of life.

The underlying and principle goal in YCat Yoga Therapy is to create an environment to maximize the possibility of connection to essence. A cancer diagnosis often comes with an immediate experience of shock and trauma (Serra et al., 2012). The body moves into a high-tension, high-stress "alarm" mode known as the stress response. The YCat Yoga Therapist leaves personal fears and feelings aside in order to create a container of support to receive the lived experience of the person's fears and feelings. Because YCat Yoga Therapists are meeting people in vulnerable states and circumstances, they must be using Yoga in their own personal lives as a way of life and as a transformational discipline. YCat Yoga Therapists draw from their personal experiences to come to know "Self at essence," which creates the opportunity for the client to also experience this "Self at essence." It has been my continued witnessing over two decades of teaching the YCat curriculum that, when someone has had an experience of "Self at essence," this connection holds stronger than a well-positioned anchor, no matter how brutal the storm. Once that connection is established, healing is a profound byproduct—whether someone is healing into life or into death.

Being present to the feelings and needs of another person is the foundation of any yogic relationship. Have you had those moments with friends or strangers when suddenly everything seems clear and open, a new insight, a new behavior inserts itself naturally and harmoniously as if it had always been there? Those moments of inspiration come from when people are actively listening and receiving the entire situation. In Yoga Therapy, one of the greatest services we can give our clients is this active listening presence, especially when they are dealing with cancer or chronic illness. When we are actively listening, the mind and its chatter is on hold in some way. It is not actively concocting a response or busy with planning what to say next. The mind is in "receive mode." As it receives each word, each phrase from another, it underlines and highlights the particulars of what it is hearing and opens up possibilities. When our minds are busy preparing what we are going to say, we are not really listening. When we are not really listening, we are not really receiving the communication. This is the "react" mode, not the "receive" mode. When we do not receive a communication, it leaves the delivery person stuck with the whole package.

Offering complete attention to another human being can be very healing in and of itself. It comes before any movement and breathing practices are initiated, just as in Patañjali's *Yoga Sūtras,* the ethical precepts of Yoga—the *yamas* and *niyamas*—come before the āsanas (movements) and prāṇāyāma (breath control) (Satchidananda, 1990, p. 124–127; 152–153; 158). People are often preoccupied in their minds, thinking of their own responses and experiences; setting that mental activity aside, however, helps the other person allow their experience and receives that person as if a guest is being invited in to one's home. There is safety in this dynamic of neither pushing away nor pulling. Being open to receiving provides the opportunity for whatever needs to express itself in the moment.

"The only place we can ever be
is where we are at each moment."

—ROCCA (*ROCCA, 2011*)

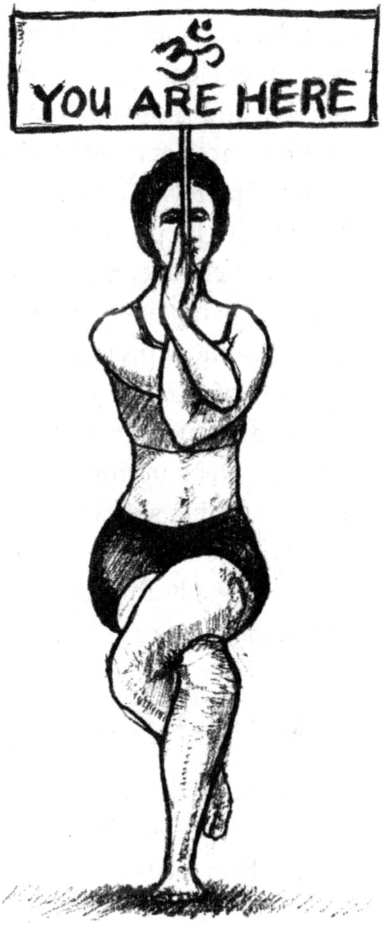

Whenever we are in a new place, we need to find our bearings; we hunt for the wall chart that says, "You are here!" We see the arrow pointing to the spot we are standing on, and, by knowing where we are, we can navigate forward. This is the service that active listening provides to people. In speaking, they can hear themselves without our adding or subtracting; this permission to speak, to say, to share, to talk allows the speaker to find his/her bearings in the "here and now" and to move forward.

A diagnosis of cancer can mean being inundated by advice from well-meaning friends and family: see this doctor, read this book, try these supplements, see this practitioner. The diagnosis, itself, is enough to put most receivers into a state of shock, anxiety, and stress (Carlson, et al., 2004; Serra, et al., 2012). Well-meaning advice can unwittingly add insult to injury, trauma to trauma. Instead, when people are raw and vulnerable, allow them to express themselves, their fears, and their feelings. Receive their fears and feelings for them. We human beings need to be received and validated by one another. Another common experience of the newly diagnosed is that the well-meaning people in their lives disappear. When people are uncomfortable about what to say or how to approach difficult subjects, it is often easier to avoid the situation completely. This unfortunately leaves people feeling further isolated and alone. Pulling back to avoid communicating is as innocently egregious as offering well-intentioned, but stress-inducing statements like, "Don't feel that way; you are going to be alright." The simple act of being present to another human being, giving the gift of our attention, is often all that is needed in any moment. In this way, Yoga Therapists can become role models to family and friends who can emulate how to hold this receptive space for their loved ones.

When our communications are not received, we can all become like stuck records unable to release a trapped thought, emotion, or feeling. When someone truly hears us and truly receives us, we can move to the next note and sing the next song. Healing is possible when fears and feelings are validated by being listened to and received. The old wounds we carry even prior to diagnosis from the circumstances of childhood and life are often softened and muted; sometimes they heal completely. For feelings are not right or wrong, they just *are*—to the extent that we can be present to our feelings and accept them, those feelings are free to move and change. But when we resist the feelings that are cycling through us, by labeling them "bad" and trying to push them away or by stuffing them or trying to change them prematurely, we are actually solidifying them in place and creating more of a problem. The basic yogic premise of bringing awareness to things as they are includes working toward accepting them as they are, along with two essential steps in things moving, shifting, and changing. Through the practice of active listening shifts will evolve naturally, allowing things to move toward more peace and acceptance, more joy and integration, more harmony and balance—even alongside the realities of cancer treatments, side effects, progression, and end of life.

YCAT YOGA THERAPY: THE WOUNDED HEALER MODEL

The model of the wounded healer is crucial for YCat Yoga Therapists. This concept is eloquently described by Rachel Remen, M.D., the medical director of Commonweal, which hosts a weeklong cancer help retreat center in California founded by Michael Lerner, Ph.D., in 1985. Dr. Remen, the author of two books, *Kitchen Table*

Wisdom and *My Grandfather's Blessings* (Remen, 1996, 2000), says that the wounded healer model suggests that it is my personal wounds that allow me to see, to recognize, and to be present for other people and their personal wounds. In this model, there is a "level playing field": I am not standing above as an expert; rather, I stand beside as an equal—another human being who has known suffering and who has wounds. The degree to which we can be present to our own inadequacies and insufficiencies becomes a part of the container that allows therapists to be present for the fears and feelings in our clients. Our awareness of our own limits can protect our clients from doing something harmful to themselves in practice and in life. Moreover, anyone who has or has had cancer or other life-threatening illnesses can immediately sense condescension and ingratiation in others around them. Alarms go off like big blips on a radar screen. It is a healthy thing that these perceptive qualities develop over time in survivors; it shifts their experience from being "specimen-ized" to being empowered. Long-term survivors have generally learned how to navigate rough seas and know when the winds are clear and the waters are safe for deep sharing. Only in these pools will they reveal what is most true for them. Being present to ourselves and listening to our own needs, our own fears, and our own feelings is an essential step in being able to be there in truly healing ways for others through the gifts of our presence and attention.

THE WITNESS PRACTICE: CHECKING IN WITH SELF

Awareness is the first step to change. Yet, this practice is not trying to change anything. In fact, practitioners are encouraged to let things be exactly as they are without trying to change anything. The practice of being a witness cultivates a level of awareness and develops a level of acceptance over time that carries into observing what happens when waiting for test results or after receiving test results as well as many other potential challenges during cancer treatment. Over time, this awareness of self will cue the person into enacting practices to maintain or restore balance as needed moment to moment.

Early in any session, the YCat Yoga Therapist will verbally guide student practitioners through an awareness meditation designed to allow a nonjudgmental observation of aspects of the individual self that are present in that actual moment. This practice typically begins by looking at, noticing, and paying attention to sensations and feelings that are in the physical body. These observations may include habituated and recurrent patterns or recent developments. The guiding process in a witness practice suggests a consistent flow of awareness and does not let the awareness rest in any one place to examine that area in depth. The guidance moves from place to place in an ordered way though the physical aspects of being, and then guides with transitional sentences from the physical level to the emotional level, then to the thinking level, and on to the energetic level. Is there fatigue or tiredness, restlessness, activity, or a sense of hyperactivity? They are not cued, yet each person can notice things at each level of being and acknowledge whatever is present for them in that moment (McCall, 2007).

Awareness notices what needs to change, so this first step can be painful. It is uncomfortable to see our issues and problems. We may have been distracting ourselves to avoid seeing things as they are. Our habit patterns may not serve our lives or our health, and reinforcing those patterns also habituates us in ways that can prevent change. Sometimes our resistance is based on past conditioning and old habits patterns. However, it does not serve to challenge anybody's resistance (Chapman, 2013). The value in Yoga Therapy comes when the principles and practices connect with one's direct experience. We let the focus rest with aspects of Yoga philosophy that resonate as true. How the mind and the senses perceive and receive Yoga concepts and ideas and bring them into daily experiential awareness matters. If it rings true, it has use and value. Otherwise, we let it go.

"Accept what is and know that things change."

—T. K. V. DESIKACHAR (*DESIKACHAR, 1996*)

Acceptance may be the only real power that any of us have. People may always have things that are hard for them to accept about themselves and things that they really want to change. This is the nature of being human. When we find a way of accepting what is, as it is, that acceptance provides the ground of being that can allow freedom of movement. Resistance creates persistence, which keeps things stuck and limits our capacity to shift, to change, and to grow. Many times the Yoga practices can get under our resistance to enable us to accept our quirks, our shortcomings, and the unique things about ourselves that make us who we are. This acceptance of ourselves opens us into new, healthier ways of being.

GUIDED IMAGERY: THE MIND AND IMAGINATION

Mary Lynn Tucker is a nurse practitioner who lives in Virginia near Roanoke. Mary Lynn is a YCat graduate and a long-time YCat faculty member. She chooses Yoga Therapy practices with clients based on lengthy intakes that discern individual client's needs and goals. She worked privately with a friend and Yoga student, Justine, who was using Yoga to modulate the severe pain associated with the end stages of her colon cancer. In imagery sessions, Justine would describe images as they came to her mind and into her sensory experience. Frequently, these images were of heat and sunlight and their movement was wavelike. These images were comfortable and familiar in Justine's external environment and collecting them internally reduced her pain symptoms from distressing to manageable. It also allowed her to get sleep. She was highly conscious and coherent and "not on any pain meds at all" for the last days of her life. After receiving her stage-3 colon cancer diagnosis, Justine had three active years of Yoga and physical exercise that included gardening and hiking. Mary Lynn attributes Justine's graceful departure from life to "her beautiful attitude . . . a will and spirit that believed in the ability to manifest one's true desires."

Working with imagery is working with the creative faculties of the mind. Over time, an ability to project forward intent and desire develops like a photograph. An invisible imprint forms that allows the imagination to construct physical dimensions into the image. In talking about Justine, Mary Lynn says there was a "quality of contentment inherent in her that accepted her life, yet, simultaneously, she engaged a direct action of her mind and will through her imagery practice." Justine was at peace with her circumstances and simultaneously able to exert emotional and mental effort though her self-directed imagery practice, bringing her great peace. Mary Lynn's role was in reflecting Justine's own images back to her. This is not prescriptive imagery: "Go here, do this." This imagery process is a living, moving thing generated by the client. Mary Lynn likens it to witnessing a dream while being aware that you are dreaming it. She says, "In imagery you go in there and you can make it come out the way you want it to come out." Guiding a person by reflecting their own images of deep meaning back to them is often an experience of empowerment and mastery as well as an experience of awe and mystery.

Investigators at New York Beth Israel Medical Center evaluated the impact of guided imagery on patients undergoing radiation therapy for breast cancer. They saw statistically significant improvements from baselines in objective measures, including blood pressure, respiration rate, and pulse rate showing a decrease in sympathetic response. A validated health subjective questionnaire was collected with patient reports at the end of radiation therapy and indicated overall satisfaction with 86 percent describing the intervention as helpful and 100 percent saying they would recommend it (Serra, et al., 2012).

Another one of Mary Lynn's clients, Alison, uses the behavioral Yoga principle of pratipakṣa bhāvana in action. Swami Satchidananda translates *pratipakṣa bhāvana* as "cultivate the opposite" or "act as if" (Satchidananda, 1990, p. 127), which is another form of self-guided imagery. Alison was struggling financially because she had to accept full-time disability. To counter her sense of lacking resources, she engaged in practicing pratipakṣa bhāvana. Whenever she was feeling trapped financially and strapped for money, she would immediately extend herself and her possessions out to others in sweeping gestures of generosity. She told Mary Lynn, "It always works wonders. When I give, it's like someone has turned on the waterspout of the universe and blessings are all around me."

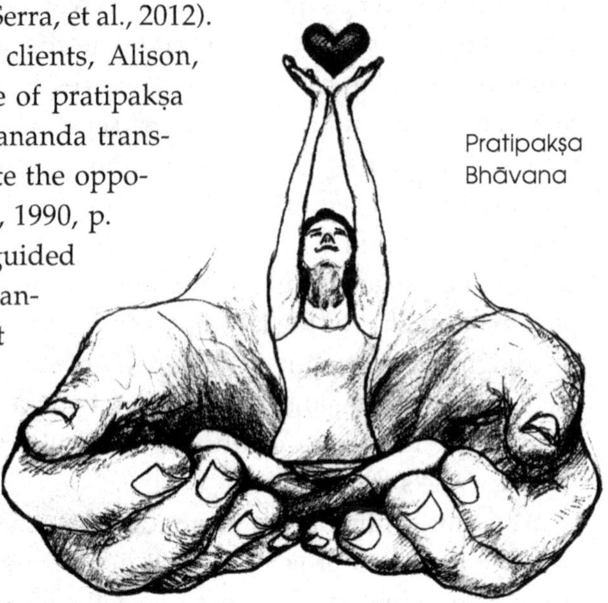

Pratipakṣa Bhāvana

By opening her coffers and spreading good will, far and wide, that good comes bouncing right back to Alison in ways that affirm hope and keep her spirits alive.

YOGA THERAPY AND CREATIVITY: A DOOR TO HEALING

Creativity is innate. It is native to each of us. Larry LeShan, Ph.D., is a psychotherapist and prolific author who has worked with cancer survivors in New York City for many decades. His book, *Cancer as a Turning Point*, is a classic in the mind-body genre (LeShan, 1990). LeShan encourages patients to "find their own song." He may ask someone, "When in life did any creative spark get stifled?" or "How can you let that creativity back into daily life?" LeShan sees people who extend their lives and some who go into long remissions by reconnecting to their creativity. Finding one's own, and possibly unique, ways of expressing creativity helps the creative juices to flow from deep within and grooves channels for profound healing to occur. Yoga Therapists may listen to stories of stifled creativity in helping clients to reconnect to their creativity. Opportunities that allow expression to our innate creative nature are multiplied when we give people, including ourselves, permission and encouragement. It is empowering to everyone.

In 1996, I represented Commonweal at a symposium on healing at T.K.V. Desikachar's teaching center in Chennai, India. The event was sponsored by the photography magazine, *Aperture,* which was founded in the 1950s by three photographers: Ansel Adams, Dorothy Lang, and Minor White. The *Aperture* mission statement is to bring light to the dark places on the planet through the photographic medium. *Aperture's* former executive director, Michael Hoffman, brought together healers from both ancient and recent traditions of medicine. The intention was to creatively capture the act of healing from each tradition in photographs. Auspicious healers from Tibetan medicine, Oriental medicine, Yoga as medicine, Ayurveda, and anthroposophical medicine were present, in addition to others. While at the symposium, I met Tibetan physician Dr. Tenzin Choedrak, who survived incarceration and torture by the Chinese for twenty-two years in a Tibetan prison and thereafter was a senior personal physician to His Holiness the Dalai Llama. Cinematographer Franz Reichle documented the infinite compassion of Tenzin Choedrak's practice in his film *The Knowledge of Healing* (Reichle, 1997). The filmmakers shared Tenzin's story with me. They told me how when Tenzin arrived in Dharamasala after his release, the Dalai Llama asked how he had survived the tortures that had taken the lives of so many younger monks. Tenzin replied that he never allowed himself to hate his captors, only to feel sorry for their ignorance, and that he continuously repeated the mantra sacred to Buddhists: *oṁ māṇi padme hūṁ*. The Dalai Lama translates this mantra as "praise to the jewel in the lotus." He encourages reflection on its meaning during chanting: That enlightenment (the jewel) comes from within (the lotus), that wisdom and altruism purify the mind, body, and speech to transform an experience of duality into realization of nonduality or essence—which from a Buddhist perspective is "emptiness" (Gyatso, 2014).

For some people, chanting can be a useful tool to reawaken creativity. In chanting, sound is vibrationally moving through people. Making sounds is like turning on a generator. A person can feel the sound as it resonates through the body and can hear it as it moves out into space. Allowing sound to move in and through oneself is a way of being vibrationally engaged in the moment. Initially, some may be self-conscious when chanting. Freely opening into this creative expression for all to see *and* hear can be scary for many people. However, there is a safety in numbers when groups chant together that can help lessen any self-consciousness that might stifle creative expression. Encouraging new chanters to listen to the middle of the room where all the voices meet can reduce some of this self-consciousness. As sounds build into an experience of vibration and creativity is channeled, many parts of us that have been wanting expression, perhaps after years of having been silenced, can be given voice and released (Chapman, 2013).

THE THERAPEUTIC RELATIONSHIP

A therapeutic relationship is not a relationship of friends, although there may be some aspect of friendship. It is not a relationship of family, although there may be some familial aspects in it. Typically, a therapeutic relationship has a beginning, a middle, and an end. The end of a therapeutic relationship can come because someone is unable to come to class anymore, because they can't afford the expense, because they move away, and sometimes because they die. The qualities present in a therapeutic relationship will include safety, comfort, trust, caring, confidentiality, empathy, an ability to listen, respect, compassion, honoring, honesty, attention, nonjudgment, acceptance, boundaries, being able to relate, observation skills, communication skills, confidence in teachings, sensitivity to needs, giving and receiving feedback, eye contact, mirroring, patience, flexibility, intuition, spontaneity, nonattachment to outcome, nonattachment to perceptions, rapport, regard, faith, humor, truthfulness, ability to assess, sacred space, healing environment, openness, and love (Chapman, 2013).

Safety is the essential ingredient in therapeutic Yoga interactions. Safety means that anything that needs to come up for the student is welcome. If you need to cry for the whole class, you are welcome. I will not badger you by asking what is wrong. I will give plenty of opportunity for you to share if you choose to, both before and after class or by phone later. Your autonomy and your integrity are intact here. This establishes the kind of safety vital for Yoga Therapy in healing. Our therapeutic relationship means that I am here for you; I am here to serve you.

When pressed for space, some medical institutions have placed Yoga classes in waiting rooms and other public areas. However, being in the public eye can leave people feeling unsafe and they may not communicate this or be able to communicate this. Adding a group ritual to envelop the space can sometimes build safety in these situations, but sharing may remain superficial, and "I'm fine today" may be all anyone is willing to say to a group or even the therapist. No worries; the practices will still benefit the students. Giving advanced warnings like "The plant manager may come in today to check the heating system," or "We may be interrupted by intercom voices today" can relieve some of the surprise factor that can unsettle a sense of safety for the group. If continuing interruptions by the overhead speaker persist, I may say out loud, "Well, you can say all you want, but nobody will walk in here who doesn't belong. This is our space and we claim it for peace." In therapeutic relationships, humor can also be very important. The ability to make light of ourselves, our actions and behaviors, our thoughts and habit patterns can encourage new sprouts to grow in thinking and behaving.

Like most YCat Yoga Therapists working in medical settings, Sharen Lock describes her work at Moffitt Cancer Center in Tampa, Florida as "inspiring and enriching." Since 2010, Sharen has worked twenty hours a week creating a safe space for people in hospital beds, in the blood and bone marrow transplant units, in the infusion center, in private sessions, and in group courses and classes. She describes the work as "planting seeds for healing." She says, "By encouraging practice in chairs, nobody is excluded; all our marketing shows pictures of people doing very simple Yoga practices. We want to demystify Yoga and show that everyone is welcome regardless of age or level of physical health."

Initially, Sharen found that the concept "less is more" was challenging for her as an approach to Yoga. "I wanted the classes to progress," she remembers, "yet I came to see over and over that the nonphysical components of Yoga, and the breath in particular, are even more powerful than the physical components. Also, I realized how important it is to be comfortable with silence. It can be more powerful than trying to find the right words to say." Additionally, she found that guiding an imagery practice was not comfortable for her. "I avoided it until I saw that imagery created safe, healing places and the images generated gave people peace. I decided not to analyze it or judge it, and just went with it. As a result, many people have told me that the imagery is their favorite part of our Yoga practice."

Another challenge for Sharen was seeing how people were hard on themselves and judgmental. "Validating what people say, because their feelings and emotions are real, helps build safety and trust in group classes. Facing trauma triggers our old wounds and losses, and I commonly see this play out in front of me. I witness a lot of anger, fear, pain, and suffering, but I also witness great courage, authenticity, and grace. I am deeply honored and grateful that when people open up to share their feelings, I get to watch these issues resolve." She identifies her biggest challenge as working with clients who were former athletes or people who had a strong physical Yoga practice: "They want to get back to what they used to do and they fight the fact that this is no longer a reality. They are hard on themselves, as if they feel they are not doing real Yoga anymore. Nevertheless, every interaction teaches me something, even if the session does not flow smoothly. There is less attachment to the end result for me, and I hope for more acceptance for them in the present moment. This work really is 'service.'" Lastly, Sharen adds, "When I work with someone around the same age as me, it makes me intensely aware of my own life and its fragility. This is a daily reminder to live in the present moment and not hold back waiting for life to happen."

YOGA THERAPY AND COMMUNITY: SAṄGHA AND VERBAL CHECK-IN

Check-in is the community's time for sharing. It is an opportunity to hear from each member present. A check-in typically begins each session in a YCat course class. The teacher's responses to what comes into the room, through the spoken word of each participant, is crucial: "I hear you, I respect you, I appreciate your concerns, and validate you in your sharing." These are all appropriate and supportive responses. The teacher may share pieces of Yoga philosophy in response or may tell a short story to highlight something relevant and/or important. When unsolicited external confirmation comes back in a student's response, the teacher can affirm that choice of statements and story. A spontaneous interject in response to each person's sharing can move the whole group in deep ways (Chapman, 2013).

In a 12-week Yoga in breast cancer treatment and recovery course, a patient named Jasmine shared that she had stayed in bed all week and couldn't get out of her pajamas. She said she had been so depressed that she knew, "I had to come to class tonight." The moment she spoke the words, the feeling for everyone in the room became dark and heavy. It required an immediate response to avoid losing her or the class. So, I shared something personal from my past about a time when loss was upon me and it colored my world black. I shared the coping mechanisms I used to protect myself and the Yoga practices that helped move me through grief, anger, and sadness. I shared how time also helped. And, then, I said to Jasmine, "The fact that it was worth it for you to get dressed to come to class tonight, Jasmine, after a week of doldrums, tells me just how much this class means to you. I am so grateful that you made the effort, and I pray that your efforts are rewarded deeply. I am so glad that you are here. Thank you for recognizing this class as a place of safety. Can we talk after class?" After class, in privacy, I provided her with a professional referral. But, in that moment of checking in, Jasmine was seen, validated in her feelings, and acknowledged for her importance to the group; the group held together and its sense of safety in sharing was reinforced.

Recognizing what you are sharing and how you are sharing your own personal story can maintain and deepen a therapeutic relationship: This is therapeutic use of self (Chapman, 2013). The story I told Jasmine was not about me, even though the story was about me. Telling this story was all about being of service to another. The need to express that particular story came from a perspective of service and not self-aggrandizement. What stories we choose to share and how we share those stories within a therapeutic relationship requires great intention and care. What comes back is a good indicator of how our stories are received. And, if a particular sharing does have an unintended response and comes to be a mistake, there is inevitably something that can be done to heal the situation: an apology. Apology is another means of engendering trust. Revealing one's own imperfections and learning another's edges can be just as therapeutic as exhibiting expertise. I remember once on the last night of an Integral Yoga New Year's retreat, Swami Satchidananda gave us a clear message about mistakes. He said, "May you all make a lot of mistakes this year," and he laughed as jaws dropped in response to what he'd said. Then, he went on to say, "Mistakes are good; that is how we learn. Never feel bad for making a mistake; just don't make the same mistakes over and over again." He gave the analogy of the director on a movie set saying, "Make a mistake, take it again and again. Take 1, take 3, take 20 . . . " (Satchidananda, 1988). Realistically, even a physician calls what he/she does his/her "practice." Mistakes are an important aspect of our learning and form the basis for growth in Yoga. For persistence in practice will eventually make our actions perfect.

THE BREATH AND PRĀṆĀYĀMA

Swami Satchidananda says that the breath is the bridge between the physical world and the invisible world (Satchidananda, 1993). Once the mechanics of a breathing practice have been mastered a person can include imagery with the breathing to deepen its effect. Sandra Gilbert is an Integral Yoga Teacher, a YCat graduate, and a long time YCat staff and faculty member. Sandra's parents both died of cancer. Working with her mother at the end of her life motivated Sandra to steep her consciousness in YCat Yoga concepts and ideas. She encourages her students to take time for mental assimilation and somatic integration. Sandra knows that the body has its own innate wisdom; she guides students to a tactile, kinesthetic body awareness that honors its evolutionary roots. She says, "Cooperating with communications from the body creates an environment for healing to take place. Listening to and providing the body with what it needs makes the most sense for healing," and adds that, "Pushing the body and forcing it to accommodate the mind and its habituated drives and desires can be detrimental to healing."

Sandra's YCat Breath Awareness Practice

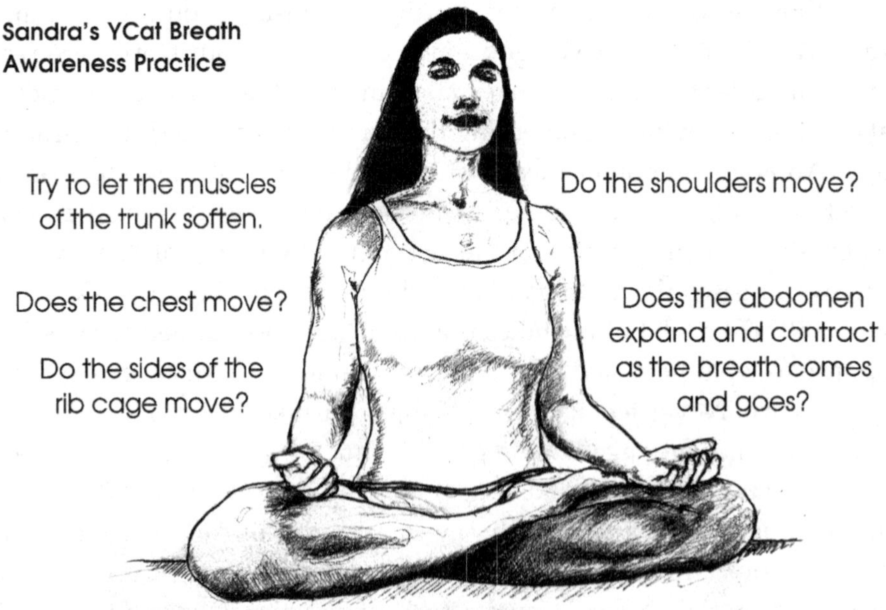
Try to let the muscles of the trunk soften.
Does the chest move?
Do the sides of the rib cage move?
Do the shoulders move?
Does the abdomen expand and contract as the breath comes and goes?

Before moving back to Nashville, TN, Sandra enacted the YCat curriculum in New York City in cardiac and pulmonary rehab at Mount Sinai Medical Center in the infusion center and with breast cancer patients and at Beth Israel Hospital. She also taught for Orthodox Jewish women with cancer through Chai Lifeline. Here is Sandra's YCat Breath Awareness Practice:

> Watch the natural breath. Hold back any attempt to control it. Let the breath come and go, come and go. It was already doing that before you started to think about it. As you let it come and let it go, please notice what areas of the body are involved automatically with breathing. Does the abdomen expand and contract as the breath comes and goes? Do the sides of the rib cage move? What about the shoulders? What about the chest? Try to let the muscles of the trunk soften so that they can move easily and effortlessly on the ebb and flow of the breath. This practice can extend for 5 or 6 minutes while timing the inhale and exhale to an even in and even out count. For example, a 2 count in and 2 count out, or a 3 count in and 3 count out, and so on (Chapman, 2013).

Once the body stays relaxed with "even in and even out breath," a person is ready to begin consciously controlling the breath by developing the ability to move a full volume of air in and out with ease and without force or strain. The trunk muscles move passively as air comes and goes in a series of complete breath cycles. Over time, a person will be able to extend the exhalation to *twice* as much time spent on the out breath verses the in breath (Chapman, 2013). The "extended exhalation breath" needs to feel easy and comfortable. It can build to include an abdominal muscle contraction with each exhalation as long as that easy, comfortable pattern remains. Research supports this breathing style for a variety of physical, psychological, and emotional issues, which can be found in detail in Dr. Elizabeth Visceglia's chapter "Psychiatry and Yoga Therapy" in this text. The extended exhalation breath can be practiced for 3 to 6 minutes throughout the day as a transition between activities or it can be used as a focus for meditation. Here is the YCat extended exhalation breath practice:

> Allow the breath to flow out slowly and evenly for 3, 4, or 5 seconds. Then, quicken the inhalation to let the same amount of breath come in, in half that time. Work toward a twice-as-long exhalation, comfortably, letting the practice build with time. Do not extend the exhalation for any longer than twice the inhalation: It is a 2:1 ratio. The inhalation will become more efficient by taking the same

amount of air in over less time. Let time for the exhale be determined by how effortlessly it can be sustained. This will help it become easier to extend the exhalation. Pay attention to how all parts of the body feel during the extended exhalation practice. If the body tenses or feels tight this is a signal that one is trying too hard. Accept the pattern that feels natural and let the practice be rhythmic and steady. Let the body relax in a comfortable position while practicing this technique. When there is an easeful 2:1 exhalation to inhalation, begin extending the length of time of the practice. As the practice develops, people find that the lung capacity naturally deepens with time. Initially, doing two seconds in and four seconds out will grow to three seconds in with five or six seconds out, and eventually, to longer durations that maintain the 2:1, exhale:inhale ratio.

When significant anxiety is present, the YCat curriculum suggests to move away from teaching any controlled breathing. Instead, guide the anxious person into a Yoga nidrā deep relaxation state and then direct the person's awareness toward how the breath has naturally deepened. This is cuing an acceptance and nonresistance to things as they are and encourages passive observation through statements like, "Notice the freedom in the movement of the breath." Eventually, the discovery of a deeply relaxed breath will allow a person to move toward being able to control the breath at will, and then he/she can use it as a tool to replace the anxious state of being. Anxiety and tension will give way to relaxation and will become cued into his/her being with repeated practice.

YCAT YOGA THERAPY IN ĀSANA: MOVEMENT, POSTURE, AND POSITIONING

Therapeutically modified Yoga classes for people in cancer treatment can start from any position including a hospital bed, but, typically in the community, YCat Yoga Therapists start students in a seated position in chairs. This provides a chance to observe students to ensure that they are doing what feels right for their bodies and are not doing what they think they are supposed to do based on what they've seen in books or based on wanting to please me as the teacher. There are more chair poses and floor poses in YCat adaptive āsana than standing poses because standing poses require full-body energy and can therefore be much more tiring for people in cancer treatment. Fatigue is the number-one side effect of cancer and its treatment, making it imperative to progress slowly to allow students to build stamina and endurance gradually. It is important to not overtire a body that is working for healing much harder internally than a body that is fit and healthy (Carlson, et al., 2004).

Stephanie Sohl, Ph.D., is a YCat Yoga Therapist working in integrative medicine research at Vanderbilt University in Nashville, TN. Stephanie has learned to not demonstrate in classes at her personal flexibility capacity when providing movement and breathing sequences to people in the chemotherapy infusion suite. She says, "Demonstrating at the capacity I suspect a person will be able to master allows that student an experience of success that will encourage them in continuing the practices. This gives people permission to feel where they are comfortable and they are less likely to try to go further to a position that may not be safe." Stephanie continues, "When newbies come to class they initially want to do more of the advanced stretches that they see the old timers accomplish easily. I allow this and simply observe when there is likely no harm involved. As I continue to demonstrate adaptations to the poses that can provide similar benefits, I inevitably notice that the newer students find their own grooves of right effort with no strain."

Research studies show that adaptive Yoga can help people feel better physically and emotionally at almost any point during their cancer recovery. Some of these studies have come out of the work of Suzanne Danhauer, Ph.D., at Wake Forest's Medical Center in Winston Salem, NC (Carlson, et al., 2007; Danhauer, et al., 2008; Kiecolt-Glaser et al., 2014). Lynn Felder, a YCat Yoga Therapist, has been the Yoga teacher on most of Danhauer's studies. Herself a survivor of stage-4 ovarian cancer, Lynn credits Yoga with her "spontaneous remission," which occurred in conjunction with traditional surgery and chemotherapies. She has since retired from her job in the news industry and now reaches many people who are using Yoga during their cancer treatment through her research, open classes, and private sessions.

"The best lessons that I got from my cancer experience were in learning to slow down, to honor my body, and to allow it to heal," Lynn says. "I had a hard time accepting that my body was different because of the cancer and the treatment. The body was weaker, stiffer. The fatigue was unbelievable. Where I had run, biked, hiked, and danced, now I got winded just walking around the block. Thanks to Yoga, I realized that I could create conditions in which healing could occur: I listened to my body and let it rest. I stopped trying to make it do stuff. When—and only when—I had the strength, I walked and I went to Yoga āsana practice. Yoga lays out the welcome mat to health." Lynn says Yoga gave her ways to "reduce stress on the mind and body and plant the seeds of possibility." Her personal journey with cancer and Yoga educates and inspires students, clients, and research participants. "I invite people to switch their focus from what their mind tells them about their bodies to what their bodies are telling them."

Swami Satchidananda frequently said, "It's all from God and it's all for good" (Chapman, 2013).When things feel bad, it is hard for the mind to consider that it could be for good. It is human nature to avoid the painful and to seek the pleasurable in life. Whatever arises for us in any moment is coming up for healing, and how we hold it in attitude makes a difference in our potential for healing. Any present moment may contain memories of events or feelings that are in process on the way to healing. Meeting these memories and feelings with unconditional love and acceptance may enable healing to take place instantly in that present moment. In this way, while many patients are grateful to the medical procedures that help save their lives in cancer treatment, they are equally as grateful to the Yoga practices they find along the way that help make life worth living.

CASE REPORT: *LIVING ON THE EDGE WITH METASTATIC BREAST CANCER*

Stephanie Sugars was thirty-five years old when her initial breast cancer diagnosis came in 1991. When it recurred in 1992, after she dutifully followed all medical advice, she "felt betrayed." In the years since, Stephanie has become a strong survivor; she has lasted in pursuit of life and health in spite of living a stage-4 metastatic cancer reality. A few years ago Stephanie was obsessed in wanting to know the exact processes involved in how people die: "What organs shut down? And how?" She was on a mission and using the full force of her life of advocacy, justice, and human rights work to interview and converse with anyone she could engage in discussing end-of-life scenarios. She went to grief workshops and death cafes (deathcafe.com) and attended the end of life conversations held at the New School at Commonweal, which are available on their website. I shared stories with her of deaths that I have attended. Stories of people who died alert, conscious, and without distress; stories of people who died after several or many days of being unconscious, but arousable; and stories of people who fought death even as life was shaking them off like a dog shakes off rain. Finally, I told Stephanie that each death was unique, like a snowflake or a fingerprint.

Stephanie's life has been a balancing act. She has an active, vibrant life, full with life's joys and sorrows, and, simultaneously, she's living with death. It reminds me of the character played by Bill Murray in the film adaptation of the W. Somerset Maugham story by the same name, who learns that the difficult path is like walking on "the razor's edge" (Byrum, 1984). The ever going ebb and flow of opposites always dance together dynamically for her. Each up, each down, each gain, each loss has smoothed a honed stone, a solid self that holds it all inside her and gives it all way, wherever she can possibly extend. Now, staring down death, she intends to see it, to know it, and to face it.

During this same period of Stephanie's query into death, another twenty-plus-year cancer survivor living with a rare cancer and decades of multiple surgeries that continue, multiple physical disabilities, and multiple indignities asked me, "To balance this disease and life, one has to do their *inner work.* Do you agree?" She is the expert, however, and does her own inner work. She continued, "Of course, there is no guarantee of life and living, but it is so much easier to survive when I do not have an adversarial relationship to my body or cancer." I ask about the pain that she began experiencing almost a year ago, after the last surgery. The last time we had seen each other, the pain was obvious and obviously debilitating: She was talking about places that are lines drawn across the sand and informing me that, when life takes her across that line, she will choose to say, "Enough." Now, I hear a different tune. "It is just pain," she said. "I am not taking anything. I am not fighting it or trying anymore to change it. I am living with it." If you ask specifically how she went from there to here, she will mention something vague, something she calls "inner work."

Similarly, Stephanie's inner work began in childhood with the awareness of being different. She was born with a rare genetic disorder called Peutz-Jeghers syndrome (PJS) and the atmosphere was always full of fear around her. She was not allowed to run and tumble with other children. Her skin was pale and adults compared her arms and legs to sticks. PJS is also known as juvenile polyposis and dramatically increases the likelihood of future cancer in those diagnosed. Stephanie was preverbal for her first PJS surgery and had a "near death" experience. She knew from inside herself the feeling of "being dead," and she associated this place with "pre being born" (Sugars, 2013). She describes the feeling as "so familiar, a feeling of remembering on a deep level, something so at home, at ease." To this day, Stephanie can recall the curious warm interest that came to her about embodiment. It came as a "wanting to know."

Stephanie describes her early adult life as "counterculture." Because of her multiple PJS surgeries and removal of body parts, Stephanie decided "to make an experiment" of her "own body and psyche" to find ways to survive outside medical realms. She needed to be able to identify herself as more than her disease. Erich Schiffman became her guide in Yoga as Stephanie was determined to bring vigor to her chronically anemic body. She studied Coyote Medicine with Lewis Mehl-Madrona and did trance work and soul journeying. She found family and a sense of belonging by participating in the well-being of others. She chose activism, advocacy, and service as her offerings. These were her gifts to the macrocosm. While life was taking things away, she was giving back to life.

A few months ago Stephanie was asked to be one of the "midwives" in the dying process of a dear friend. The friend was another woman with metastatic breast cancer; her cancer had spread to her bones and to her brain. Stephanie had been fearful of brain metastases, not wanting them in her own brain. She has watched lives become traumatized by cancers in the brain. Whether a primary tumor or a metastasis, tumors in the brain can be incredibly challenging. Depending upon what areas of the brain are affected, a person's ability to move, to speak, and to reason can be impacted. Stephanie's brain has been such a vital organ; it has enabled Stephanie to search databases and websites, to read voraciously to cull information, and to disseminate it to people in need. Being of service to others is a prime value that gives meaning to Stephanie's life. She will readily admit to her attachment to her "mind and to ideas," which made the thought of losing them distressing.

Thankfully, Stephanie's fear shifted through her service to her friend. She recalls, "It gave me a lot of relief, in fact." Her friend had lost her independence and needed to rely on family to drive her and to reorient her when confusion was present. Stephanie would lie with her. Sometimes they would both nap; sometimes they would "just stare into each other's eyes." After the friend's death, Stephanie shared in the duties of preparing her friend's dead body. She experienced "a light in the room" and reported that "a deep feeling of reverence" came over her and it took her fear away. She adds, "I realized from this experience that death does not have to be medicalized. Now I will be satisfied with a good enough death."

Stephanie calls herself a "statistical outlier," and this is a factual truth that acknowledges how few women with metastatic breast cancer make it to twenty-three years of living with cancer. She researches options and chooses what treatment options she will accept and which ones she will forego. In 1996, Stephanie was a resident of a clinic in Germany dedicated to anthroposophical medicine. While there, she began receiving injections and infusions of a medicine called Iscador, which is an extract of mistletoe, and continues these treatments to date.

Over and over, Stephanie has risen above all the losses and challenges that life has sent her way. She has learned how to listen to her body, how to protect it in movement, and how to let it be still. My prayer for Stephanie is that she be satisfied with a life that is good enough to live.

CONCLUSION

Many of my Yoga colleagues who work primarily with Yoga Therapy as āsana and other forms of structural Yoga have shown profoundly beneficial effects with Yoga's influence on anatomical structure and function in the human body. Studies from exercise science and physiology have shown that balancing activity with rest and movement with stillness have an important place in prevention and rehabilitation (Boyle, et al., 2012). Extensive research evidence shows that exercise reduces mortality and recurrences in cancer. Exercise, in fact, has some of the strongest correlations seen so far in integrative medicine research for reducing mortality and morbidity in cancer treatment (Boyle, et al., 2012; Ibrahim, et al., 2011; Kushi, et al., 2012; Liu, et al., 2011; Moore, et al., 2010; Moorman, et al., 2010; Meyerhardt, et al., 2006; Ornish, et al., 2005; Speck, et al., 2010; Schmitz, et al., 2010; Steindorf, et al., 2013; Wolin, et al., 2011; Wu, et al., 2013). Yoga Therapists can provide clients with educational and motivational rationales for being regular with exercise and explain the similarities and differences between Yoga āsana and exercise.

Moreover, Yoga Therapists working in the treatment of cancer can help clients become reacquainted with their bodies, establish healthier relationships with the body, explore movement and stillness in the body, and also assist them in finding a deeper connection within themselves to what is transcendental. Thus, the movements in Yoga Therapy are not ends in themselves, but doors into this deeper connection to self, at essence. When someone has had a direct connection to what Swami Satchidananda refers to as the "peace within," this experience provides a context for holding all of life's ups and downs. It enables a deep resilience and a resonant potency that engenders trust and healing. May all beings access this healing resonance and direct its power for healing to and through one's self and on to heal our communities and the planet we share.

REFERENCES

Boyle, T., et al. "Physical Activity and Risks of Proximal and Distal Colon Cancers: A Systematic Review and Meta-Analysis." *Journal of the National Cancer Institute* 104.20 (2012): 1548–1561. Print.

Byrum, John, Dir. *The Razor's Edge.* Author. W. Somerset Maugham (1944). Perf. Bill Murray, Theresa Russell, Denholm Elliot, Catherine Hicks, James Keach. Columbia, 1984. Film.

Carlson, J. W., et al. "Yoga for Women with Metastatic Breast Cancer: Results of a Pilot Study." *Journal of Pain and Symptom Management* 33.3 (2007): 331–341. Print.

Carlson L. E., et al. "High Levels of Untreated Distress and Fatigue in Cancer Patients." *British Journal of Cancer* 90.12 (2004): 2297–2304. Print.

Chapman, J. *YCat Yoga Therapy: Yoga for People with Cancer & Chronic Illness Manual.* Buckingham, VA: Integral Yoga Academy Press, 2013, Rev. Ed. Print.

Danhauer, S., et al. "Restorative Yoga for Women with Ovarian or Breast Cancer: Findings from a Pilot Study." *Journal of the Society for Integrative Oncology* 6.2 (2008): 47–58. Print.

Desikachar, T. *Using Yoga in Healing.* Aperture Symposium. Chennai, India. Overheard, 1996. Print.

Desikachar, T. K. V. (2005). Health, healing and beyond: Yoga and the living tradition of Krishnamacharya, (cover jacket text). Aperture, US.[Reference unclear. Specifically, the word "Overheard." Did Desikachar make a comment at symposium that was overheard by someone? A more correct designation would be "Personal conversation" But editor finds nothing online for this symposium OR "Using Yoga in Healing." See reference below this, found on web. Is this the one intended? If not, please provide more detailed source info for 1996 source.]

Gyatso, T., 14th Dalai Lama of Tibet. "On the Meaning of: Om Mani Padme Hum." Tran. Ngawang Tashi (Tsawa). From a lecture at the Kalmuck Mongolian Buddhist Center, NJ. Web. Retrieved 1 March 2014. http://www.sacred-texts.com/bud/tib/omph.htm.

Ibrahim, E. M., et al. "Physical Activity and Survival After Breast Cancer Diagnosis: Meta-Analysis of Published Studies." *Medical Oncology* 28.3 (2011): 753–765. Print.

Kiecolt-Glasser, J., et al. (2014). "Yoga's Impact on Inflammation, Mood, and Fatigue in Breast Cancer Survivors: A Randomized Controlled Trial." *Journal of Clinical Oncology.* Published online before print 27 January 2014. Print. http://jco.ascopubs.org/content/early/2014/01/21/JCO.2013.51.8860.

Kushi, L. H., et al. "American Cancer Society Guidelines on Nutrition and Physical Activity for Cancer Prevention: Reducing the Risk of Cancer with Healthy Food Choices and Physical Activity." *CA: A Cancer Journal for Clinicians* 62.1 (2012): 30–67. Print.

Lerner, M. *Choices in Healing.* Cambridge: MIT Press, 1994. Print.

LeShan, L. *Cancer as a Turning Point.* New York: Penguin, 1990. Print.

——. *How to Meditate.* New York: Little, Brown & Co, 1974. Print.

Liu, Y., et al. "Does Physical Activity Reduce the Risk of Prostate Cancer? A Systematic Review and Meta-Analysis." *European Urology* 60.5 (2011): 1029–1044. Print.

McCall, T. *Yoga as Medicine.* New York: Bantam, 2007. Print.

Meyerhardt, J., et al. "Impact of Physical Activity on Cancer Recurrence and Survival in Patients with Stage III Colon Cancer: Findings from CALGB 89803." *Journal of Clinical Oncology* 24.22 (2006): 3535–3541.

Moore, S. C., et al. "Physical Activity, Sedentary Behaviors, and the Prevention of Endometrial Cancer." *British Journal of Cancer* 103.7 (2010): 933–938. Print.

Moorman, P. G., et al."Recreational Physical Activity and Ovarian Cancer Risk and Survival." *Annals of Epidemiology* 21.3 (2011): 178–187. Print.

Ornish, D. *Dr. Dean Ornish's Program for Reversing Heart Disease.* New York: Balentine, 1992. Print.

Ornish, D., et al. "Intensive Lifestyle Changes May Affect the Progression of Prostate Cancer." *Journal of Urology* 174.3 (2005): 1065–70. Print.

Ornish, D. *The Spectrum.* New York: Ballantine, 2008. Print.

Reichle, F., Dir. *The Knowledge of Healing.* Perf. The 14th Dalai Lama and Dr. Tenzin Choedrak. Icarus, 1997. Film.

Remen, R. *Kitchen Table Wisdom.* New York: Riverhead Books, 1996. Print.

——. *My Grandfather's Blessings.* New York: Riverhead Books, 2000. Print.

Reynolds, M. Comp. words and music. "Magic Penny." Northern Music Corporation, 1958. CD.

Rocca, P. "A Question of Existence and Time." *The Stupid Way Blog.* 21 November 2011. Web. http://thestupidway.blogspot.com/2011/11/time–and–existence–are–as–important–for.html.

Satchidananda, S. *The Yoga Sutras of Patanjali.* Buckingham, VA: Integral Yoga Publications, 1990. Print.

——. *The Breath of Life: Integral Yoga Pranayama.* Buckingham, VA: Integral Yoga Publications, 1993. Print.

——.*Healing from Disaster.* Buckingham, VA: Integral Yoga Publications, 2006. Print.

——. *To Know Yourself.* Buckingham, VA: Integral Yoga Publications, 2008. Print.

Schmitz, K. H., et al. "American College of Sports Medicine Roundtable on Exercise Guidelines for Cancer Survivors." *Medicine and Science in Sports and Exercise* 42.7 (2010): 1409–1426. Print.

Serra, D., et al. "Outcomes of Guided Imagery in Patients Receiving Radiation Therapy for Breast Cancer.: *Clinical Journal of Oncology Nursing* 16.6 (2012): 617–623. Print.

Speck, R. M., et al. "An Update of Controlled Physical Activity Trials in Cancer Survivors: A Systematic Review and Meta-Analysis." *Journal of Cancer Survivorship* 4.2 (2010): 87–100. Print.

Steindorf, K., et al. "Physical Activity and Risk of Breast Cancer Overall and by Hormone Receptor Status: The European Prospective Investigation into Cancer and Nutrition." *International Journal of Cancer* 132.7 (2013): 1667–1678. Print.

Sugars, S. "I Wish I'd Known Earlier . . . Palliative Care Is Not a Mandate Not to Treat." Center for Advancing Health. Web. 13 August 2013. Web. Retreived March 4, 2014. http://www.cfah.org/blog/2013/i-wish-id-known-earlier-palliative-care-is-not-a-mandate-not-to-treat.

——. Peuts-Jeghers listserv. Association of Cancer Online Resources. Acorg.org. 2013. Retreived March 4, 2014. Web. http://listserv.acor.org/scripts/wa-ACOR.exe?A0=PJS.

Stortz, M. "Yoga Therapy for Cancer Survivors." *Coping with Cancer.* May/June 2013. Web. Retreived March 4, 2014. http://copingmag.com/cwc/index.php/search/articles/yoga_therapy_for_cancer_survivors .

Wolin, K., et al. "Physical Activity and Risk of Colon Adenoma: A Meta-Analysis." *British Journal of Cancer* 104.5 (2011): 882–885. Print.

Wu, Y., et al. "Physical Activity and Risk of Breast Cancer: A Meta-Analysis of Prospective Studies." *Breast Cancer Research* 137.3 (2013): 869–882.

Yoga Therapy and Nursing

Felicia Tomasko, R.N., E-RYT500

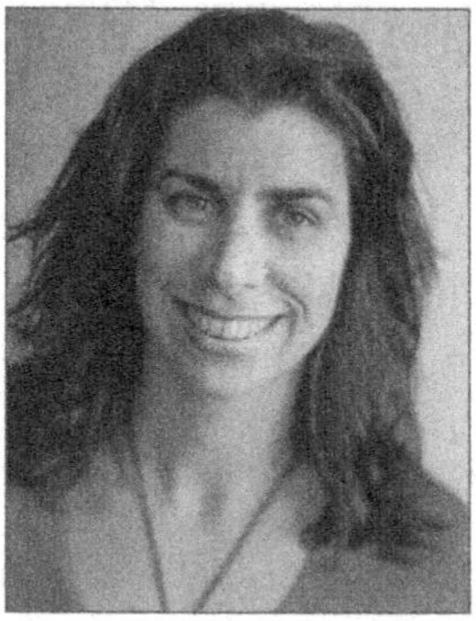

Felicia Tomasko combines her training and experience as a Yoga Therapist, Ayurvedic practitioner, writer, and registered nurse in her writing, private practice, and teaching. Her work as the president and editor-in-chief at the Bliss Network, producing *LA YOGA Ayurveda and Health* magazine and *Find Bliss* magazine, focuses on educating people on the importance of the interconnected traditions of Yoga, Ayurveda, and Yoga Therapy. She maintains a private practice in Yoga Therapy and Ayurveda. Additionally, she teaches Yoga Therapy integrated with Ayurveda and modern Western biomedicine in teacher-training programs around the world, including in the Yoga Therapy RX program at Loyola Marymount University. Felicia is the past president of the California Association of Ayurvedic Medicine, has served multiple terms on the board of directors of the National Ayurvedic Medical Association, and has represented Traditional World Medicines on the board of the Academic Consortium for Complementary and Alternative Health Care (ACCAHC).

INTRODUCTION

The fields of Yoga Therapy and nursing are complementary in many ways. The American Nurses Association says, "Nursing is the protection, promotion, and optimization of health and abilities, prevention of illness and injury, alleviation of suffering through the diagnosis and treatment of human response, and advocacy in the care of individuals, families, communities, and populations" (ANA, 2014). Similarly, in Ayurveda, the oldest known therapy in the yogic traditions, nursing has a long history and the role of nurses is embedded in the source texts. The *Caraka Saṁhitā*, considered to be the most ancient of the Ayurvedic textbooks, says that nurses are a vital part of the health promotional team and should be "endowed with good conduct, cleanliness, character, devotion, dexterity and sympathy and who are conversant with the art of nursing and good in administering therapies" (Sharma and Dash, 2002). *Caraka* goes on to describe some of the holistic duties of these nursing attendants, including cooking soup, porridge, and other dishes, bathing, massaging, lifting, seating of patients, and grinding of drugs. "These attendants should all be willing workers." In keeping with the holistic nature of healing understood in Ayurveda and Yoga Therapy, as well as the comprehensive view of this person's role, *Caraka* also insists that nurses should be versed with vocal and instrumental music, literature to recite to patients, ancient lore, short stories, sacred texts, mythology and the *Purāṇas,* and they should be able to understand desires, be obedient (good team players), and have knowledge of the context of time and place (Sharma and Dash, 2002).

When reading this definition, it reminds me in many ways of my own training as a nurse. While my formal education did not include music or literature, there was an emphasis on understanding the cultural and demographic context of the patient at hand (context of time and place) as well as sensitivity to his/her tradition (prayer, mythology, religion). Bathing, lifting, moving, massaging, preparation of medicines, and proper body mechanics were all part of my training as well as the training of a modern nurse. The connection of philosophy and practice as described through the literature of Ayurveda, Yoga Therapy, and modern Western medical practice signifies the universality of this type of holistic caregiving. Personally, I feel that nursing is a discipline like Yoga Therapy that is concerned with the wellness of the mind, body, and spirit of the individual, the family, and the community. At their core, Yoga Therapy and nursing together maintain an emphasis on caring, compassion, the whole person, and an understanding of spirituality that is unique to their fields within health care.

THE EVOLUTION OF NURSING

In the Western healthcare system, the professional field of nursing famously originates with Florence Nightingale. Born in Italy in the 1820s, Nightingale advocated for increased training, status upgrades, and increased respect for nurses. Her work in the Crimean War beginning in 1854 instituted what were seen at the time as radical reforms, including wholesome food and clean sheets for recuperating soldiers (A&E Networks, 2014). She established the Nightingale Training School for Nurses at St. Thomas' Hospital in London in 1860, further revolutionizing the training of nurses. The profession today still refers to her legacy and a version of the oath that many nurses still take upon graduation is dubbed the Florence Nightingale Pledge, first composed in 1893 by Mrs. Lystra E. Gretter and a committee at the Farrand Training School for Nurses in Detroit, Michigan (ANA, 2014).

At the present time, nursing is an area of current growth and development in health care. As they have always been, nurses are on the front line with patients and often have more contact with patients than their doctors. Moreover, nursing research and the application of other effective modalities within nursing is also a growing specialization within the field. In a 2014 continuing education for nurses article in *Advance Healthcare Network for Nurses,* Joan Lorenz, R.N., PMHCNS-BC, said, "I felt like a real pioneer when I began my master's thesis research on Haṭha Yoga at Yale University School of Nursing in 1978" (Lorenz, 2014). In the course of her time researching the physical benefits of Yoga practice for people whose medication regimens had the side effect of stiffness and rigidity, Joan discovered that there was no nursing research at that time in the United States related to Yoga (or research done by any other U.S.-based healthcare professions) as research related to Yoga was only published in medical journals in India. This has changed dramatically since 1978 in all of the healthcare professions, including nursing, with a growing body of published evidence-based research confirming the positive influence of Yoga Therapy. A 2012 article in *Holistic Nursing Practice* by Nkechi Rose Okonta, M.S.N., R.N., reviewed a variety of studies to investigate the evidence specifically related to Yoga Therapy and reducing blood pressure in people with hypertension (Okonta, 2012). Okonta found in her comprehensive review that Yoga is an effective methodology for reducing high blood pressure because of its ability to positively impact the body's general adaptation syndrome. She states that "Yoga Therapy is a multifunctional exercise modality with numerous benefits. Not only does Yoga reduce high BP [blood pressure] but it has also been demonstrated to effectively reduce blood glucose level, cholesterol level, and body weight" (Okonta, 2012).

While research throughout the medical community investigating the therapeutic benefits of Yoga has been increasing, this proliferation is specifically seen within the nursing literature. Nurses are evaluating the therapeutic benefit of Yoga practices and techniques and are publishing their own research. Advance practice nurses Juyoung Park, Ruth McCaffrey, Dorothy Dunn, and Rhonda Goodman found in a pilot study that chair Yoga reduced pain and depressive mood and improved health, well-being, and physical function in older adults with osteoarthritis (Park, et al., 2011). A review of Yoga-related articles published in nursing journals conducted by advance-practice nurses Alyson Ross and Sue Thomas found that Yoga outperformed generic exercise techniques when considering the regulation of the hypothalamic-pituitary-adrenal (HPA axis) and the sympathetic nervous system (Ross and Thomas, 2010). Yoga Therapy and nursing research is increasing related to the activity of the HPA axis, which is involved in a variety of physiological activities, including regulation of the body's stress response, blood pressure, and the endocrine system as a whole. A school-based Haṭha Yoga intervention in a group of prehypertensive seventh graders found that the Haṭha Yoga practices demonstrated the potential to reduce resting blood pressure. As nurses are important team members, not only in healthcare or hospital environments, but also in educational settings, the demonstrated efficacy of simple Haṭha Yoga programs for prevention can be significant (Sieverdes, et al., 2014). While beyond the research studies, the nursing literature includes recommendations for the use of Yoga as part of a holistic program.

NURSING DIAGNOSES AND PRACTICE

One of the ways in which the nursing profession today identifies how to work with individuals and groups is through the classification and system of nursing diagnosis. The development of the current system of nursing diagnosis began in 1973, instigated at the First National Conference on the Classification of Nursing Diagnoses (NANDA, 2014). These are significantly different from the types of diagnoses that physicians use to identify diseases and the disease process and are more akin to the holistic assessments and evaluations that would typically be performed by a Yoga Therapist. According to NANDA International, the organization that sets up the criteria for nursing diagnoses, "Nursing diagnoses define the knowledge of professional nursing" (NANDA, 2014). NANDA continues, "The diagnostic process in nursing differs from the diagnostic process in medicine in that, in a majority of situations, the person or persons who are the focus of nursing care should be intimately involved as partners with nurses in the assessment and diagnostic process. This is because the focus of nursing care is the whole person or persons' achievement of well-being and self-actualization" (NANDA, 2014).

NANDA International identifies 216 diagnoses that address patient systems rather than the medical diagnoses that label pathologies. "To achieve positive changes in behaviors that affect health, people and nurses together identify the most accurate diagnoses that have potential to guide nursing care for the achievement of positive health outcomes. Nursing interventions for diagnoses of human responses offer additional ways, besides treating medical programs, that the health of people can be promoted, protected, and restored" (NANDA, 2014).

According to NANDA International, these diagnoses are divided into thirteen holistic domains or categories and forty-seven classes or subcategories and include:

1. Health promotion—health awareness and health management
2. Nutrition—ingestion, digestion, absorption, metabolism, and hydration
3. Elimination/exchange—urinary system, gastrointestinal system, integumentary system, and pulmonary system
4. Activity/rest—sleep/rest, activity/exercise, energy balance, cardio-pulmonary responses, and self-care
5. Perception/cognition—attention, orientation, sensation/perception, cognition, and communication
6. Self-perception—self-concept, self-esteem, and body image
7. Role relationship—caregiving roles, family relationships, and role performance
8. Sexuality—sexual identity, sexual function, and reproduction
9. Coping/stress tolerance—posttrauma responses, coping responses, and neurobehavioral stress
10. Life principles—values, beliefs, and value/belief/action congruence
11. Safety/protection—infection, physical injury, violence, environmental hazards, defensive processes, and thermoregulation
12. Comfort—physical comfort, environmental comfort, and social comfort
13. Growth/development—growth and development

When we consider these various groupings of diagnostic criteria in nursing, we see an emphasis on the whole person in health and healing, just as there is in Yoga Therapy. Importantly, Heather Herdman, Ph.D., R.N., the executive director of NANDA International states that it is vital to "look past the diagnosis to the patient" (Comment and Herdman, 2014); therefore, nursing diagnoses must take the patient into account. Through this process of diagnosis, the field of nursing addresses the spiritual-psychosocial-sexual nature of the individual as well as his/her physiological and psychological aspects while emphasizing prevention, self-image, minimizing the stress response, and empowering patients' belief systems. The nature of the nursing diagnoses and the emphasis on whole-person care means that the nurse as a healer is a natural point of integration. "Nursing diagnosis, as a classification system for nursing phenomena, can serve as a mechanism to enhance visibility of this healing role of the nurse" (Daniels and McCabe, 1994). In an effort to refine these domains, categories, and the diagnoses themselves, NANDA International continually purviews and reviews these concepts to assist nurses in making more accurate and effective diagnoses in order to help patients. The emphasis on holistic evaluation, the experience of the patient, viewing the human response, and the importance on not only wellness but also on self-actualization reveal the commonality between the core philosophy and teaching of nursing and the field of Yoga Therapy.

HOLISTIC NURSING

The field of nursing as a whole recognizes holistically minded distinctions in the process of patient care. The American Holistic Nurses Association (AHNA) is an organization within the field of nursing that specifically focuses on the holistic aspects of the profession from a more targeted point of view and one that embraces Yoga and Yoga Therapy. Founded in 1998, AHNA has 4,500 members (as of 2014) and is "the only full-service professional organization representing the nation's holistic nurses" and is "at the forefront of policy relating to holistic nursing and integrative health care" (AHNA, 2014).

AHNA states, "Holistic nursing is defined as all nursing practice that has healing the whole person as its goal" (AHNA, 1998). The commitment of AHNA has led to the field of holistic nursing becoming recognized as an official nursing specialty in 2006, with its own scope and standards of practice (AHNA, 2014). This recognition is by the American Nurses Association (ANA), the professional organization that represents the United States' 3.1 million registered nurses (AHNA, 2014). Holistic nurses, according to the AHNA, "Integrate complementary and alternative modalities (CAM) into clinical practice to treat the whole person and view healing as a partnership between a person seeking treatment and their practitioner" (AHNA, 2014).

More than simply acknowledging Yoga, the practice of Yoga is encouraged in the literature of AHNA for practitioners in their own self-care and is offered at the annual AHNA conferences each year. Under the auspices of the category Mind-Body Medicine (AHNA, 2014), the use of Yoga as a therapeutic modality is also encouraged by the AHNA and can be the key to treatment in many patients' cases. Ultimately, the integration of techniques of Yoga Therapy into nursing is "to help nurses optimize the 'art' of nursing through remaining calm and centered while assisting patients . . . [and] to provide easy gentle exercises and meditation techniques that can be taught to patients" for maintenance of their health and well-being and to reduce stress (AHNA, 2014).

YOGA THERAPY IN NURSING PRACTICE

One of the important tasks of a nurse is to assist in taking care of the patient's mental, emotional, and spiritual well-being. Many of the therapeutic benefits of Yoga are found beyond the practice of āsana in the form of prāṇāyāma (breathing) and meditative techniques used for healing. In my own experience working in hospital settings, I found numerous opportunities to incorporate the techniques of Yoga into practice and great healing benefits followed. For instance, taking a patient through a few moments of deep breathing before giving an injection or starting an IV can have the effect of calming the patient's nervous system and reduce the negative experience or pain of the procedure. This simple and basic Yoga Therapy technique has become a standard recommendation for people to reduce pain before receiving shots or injections, especially in children. Information for parents disseminated by the Centers for Disease Control and Prevention suggests that parents take deep breaths with their child to "blow out" or reduce the pain (CDC, 2014). Another study investigating wound healing found that people who received instructional relaxation and guided imagery and listened to relaxation CDs three days before and seven days after surgery experienced reduced stress and improved wound healing responses (Broadbent, et al., 2012). As the healthcare provider with the most patient contact before and after surgery, nurses can either teach guided imagery or provide therapeutic reinforcement of the use of the technique before or after surgery. In addition, every time vital signs are checked, which is frequent in preoperative and postoperative patients, provides a meaningful opportunity to take a few moments to remind a person to repeat their own use of healing imagery or relaxation techniques.

The six *ṣaṭkarmas,* or cleansing kriyā practices described in the *Haṭha Yoga Pradīpikā,* are also important techniques in Yoga Therapy that can be utilized by nurses. Specifically, the use of neti, or as it is commonly referred to in Western medicine, nasal irrigation, is one that has become a part of the nursing profession in many settings. Studies confirm the traditional usages of neti (nasal irrigation), which include improving the symptoms of sinusitis. Neti even leads to reduced usage of sinus medication in affected patients (Heatley, et al., 2001). The use of nasal saline washes is documented to be well tolerated and beneficial for the majority of people with chronic rhinosinusitis (Harvey, et al., 2007). Its use is even taught to nurses and detailed in nursing textbooks; one example of which can be found in the widely used text *Lippincott's Nursing Procedures* (Lippincott, Williams, and Wilkins, 2013). This example of a traditional Yoga Therapy practice that is already part of the nursing lexicon provides evidence for the complementary, connected, and integrated nature of the two fields.

Adding to the use of the techniques listed above, researchers Sears, Bolton, and Bell evaluated a preoperative program employing a holistic approach before and after surgery utilizing guided imagery, an eye pillow, the use of aromatherapy, and a written healing plan personalized for the individual. Their research found that this combination effectively reduced both the pain and the anxiety associated with surgery. The authors' conclusion included a recommendation for the incorporation of this method in healthcare settings and mentions the role of nurses in the implementation of this holistic approach. "Nurses are in a prime position to deliver these interventions, given their frequent direct contact with patients" (Sears, Bolton, and Bell, 2013).

YOGA THERAPY APPLIED TO NURSES

In addition to using Yoga Therapy with patients and in hospital settings, nurses themselves are encouraged to incorporate Yoga into their own lives and routines for its ability to reduce stress in clinical environments. Mukunda Stiles, one of my own personal mentors in Yoga Therapy, repeatedly instructed us that any part of a Yoga Therapist's ability to teach his/her students comes from the strength of his/her own practice. According to the American Holistic Nurses Association, "The practice of holistic nursing requires nurses to integrate self-care, self-responsibility, spirituality, and reflection in their lives. This may lead the nurse to greater awareness of the interconnectedness with self, others, nature, and spirit. This awareness may further enhance the nurse's understanding of all individuals and their relationships to the human and global community, and permits nurses to use this awareness to facilitate the healing process" (AHNA, 2014). It will often increase nurses' effectiveness and thereby improve their relationships with patients.

While vacations, sick leave, or drugs and medication may be short-term fixes, Ingrid Kollak, Ph.D., R.N., encourages nurses to "find a level of self-care that both reduces your vulnerability and enhances your resilience." The suggested self-care regimen includes the various components of the practice of Yoga. As stated in her book, *Yoga for Nurses*, Yoga is effective because it helps to "break the vicious circle of stress to help calm your mind and become focused" (Kollak, 2008). "Short breaks for Yoga exercises (asana) can fit into the work routine and provide quick help" (Kollak, 2008). A 2013 paper in *Workplace Health & Safety* confirmed Dr. Kollak's support for the benefits of Yoga. The "high rates of stress and burnout among nurses and other health care providers" need a solution. "A growing body of evidence supports the physical and psychosocial benefits of Yoga and suggests the potential for Yoga to support self-care and reduce stress among health care providers" (Alexander, 2013).

CONCLUSION

According to the American Holistic Nurses Association, a holistic nurse is an instrument of healing and a facilitator in the healing process. This same definition could easily apply to Yoga Therapists and their role in the discovery of how to achieve balance in mind, body, and spirit for patients. As the field of holistic nursing continues to grow and develop alongside the expansion of Yoga Therapy into medical settings, and, as current trends continue, the connection between the two disciplines and practices will continue to become even more integrated over time. In the decades since Yoga and Yoga Therapy have proliferated in the Western world, the interest by nursing and nurses in the therapeutic benefits and application of Yoga are also increasing.

The components of the profession that drew me to nursing as a practitioner were the same ones that fueled my passion for Yoga Therapy: the roles of advocate, coach, teacher, spiritual support, caregiving, facilitator, and the person whose mission it is to see the whole person in the healing process. The role of the nurse as described in the Ayurvedic source texts, including the *Charaka Samhita,* mirror Florence Nightingale's vision for this essential part of the healthcare delivery team.

While people like advanced practice nurse Joan Lorenz saw themselves as pioneers in the field decades ago, they have been joined by a growing cadre of nurses integrating Yoga as a complementary therapy. These nurses are studying Yoga Therapy, working in tandem with Yoga Therapists, completing research into Yoga Therapy, and looking for ways in which to incorporate techniques from Yoga Therapy into everyday nursing-care plans and the advocacy of holistic patient care. The practices of Yoga, naturally used to address nursing diagnoses, can be effective complementary modalities at all levels of practice and in multiple settings to further nurses' mission in caring for individuals, community, and society.

REFERENCES

A&E Networks. "Florence Nightingale." The Biography.com website. n.d. Web. Accessed 26 Jan. 2014. Accessed http://www.biography.com/people/florence-nightingale-9423539.

Alexander, G. "Self-Care and Yoga-Academic-Practice Collaboration for Occupational Health." *Workplace Health & Safety* 61.2 (2013): 510–513. Print.

American Holistic Nurses Association (AHNA). "Description of Holistic Nursing." 1998. Web. Accessed 1 Jan. 2014. http://www.ahna.org/About-Us/What-is-Holistic-Nursing.

——. ("Holistic Nursing Speciality Status." 2014. Web. Accessed 30 Jan. 2014. http://www.ahna.org/About-Us/ANA-Specialty-Recognition.

——. "Mission Statement." 2014. Web. Accessed 15 Jan. 2014. http://www.ahna.org/About-Us/Mission-Statement.

——. "What is Holistic Nursing?"2014. Web. Accessed 30 Jan. 2014. http://www.ahna.org/About-Us/What-is-Holistic-Nursing.

——. "Descriptions of Healing Modalities." 2014. Web. Accessed 30 Jan. 2014. http://www.ahna.org/Home/For-Consumers/Holistic-Modalities.

American Nurses Association (ANA). "About ANA." 2014. Web. Accessed 30 Jan. 2014. http://www.nursingworld.org/FunctionalMenuCategories/AboutANA.

——. "What Is Nursing?" 2014. NursingWorld.com. Web. Accessed 1 February 2014. www.nursingworld.org.

——. "Florence Nightingale Pledge." 2014. Web. Accessed 27 Jan. 2014. http://nursingworld.org/FunctionalMenuCategories/AboutANA/WhereWeComeFrom/FlorenceNightingalePledge.aspx.

Broadbent, E., et al. "A Brief Relaxation Intervention Reduces Stress and Improves Surgical Wound Healing." *Brain, Behavior, and Immunity* 26.2 (2012): 212–217. Print.

Centers for Disease Control and Prevention (CDC). "Tips for a Less Stressful Shot Visit." 2014. Web. http://www.cdc.gov/vaccines/parents/downloads/tips-factsheet.pdf.

Comment, T., and H. Herdman. "What Is Nursing Diagnosis and Why Should I Care?" 2014. Web. Accessed 15 Feb. 2014. http://www.nanda.org/What-is-Nursing-Diagnosis-And-Why-Should-I-Care_b_2.html.

Daniels, G. J., and P. McCabe. "Nursing Diagnosis and Natural Therapies. A Symbiotic Relationship." *Journal of Holistic Nursing* 12.2 (1994): 184–192. Print

Harvey, R., et al. "Nasal Saline Irrigations for the Symptoms of Chronic Rhinosinusitis." *Cochrane Database of Systematic Reviews.* 18 Jan. 2007 (3): CD006394. Web. Abstract available at http://www.ncbi.nlm.nih.gov/pubmed/17636843.

Heatley, D. G., et al. "Nasal Irrigation for the Alleviation of Sinonasal Symptoms." *Otolaryngology and Head and Neck Surgery* 125.1 (2001): 44–48. Print.

Kollak, I. *Yoga for Nurses.* New York: Springer, 2008.

Lippincott, Williams, and Wilkins. *Lippincott's Nursing Procedures,* Sixth Edition. Netherlands: Wolters Kluwer Publishers, 2013, pp. 819–822. Print.

Lorenz, J. M. "Understanding Yoga: Research Shows Yoga's Benefits for Low Back Pain, Cancer, Diabetes, Osteoarthritis, High Blood Pressure, and More." Advance Healthcare Network for Nurses. 2014. Web. Accessed 10 Jan. 2014. http://nursing.advanceweb.com/Continuing-Education/CE-Articles/Understanding-Yoga.aspx.

North American Nursing Diagnosis Association (NANDA). *International Nursing Diagnoses: Definitions and Classification 2012–2014,* Ninth Edition. New York: Wiley-Blackwell, 2011 , p. 72. Print.

——. "International Diagnosis Development." 2014. Web. Accessed 1 March 2014. http://www.nanda.org/nanda-international-diagnosis-development.html.

——. "International History." 2014. Web. Accessed 1 February 2014. http://www.nanda.org/nanda-international-history.html.

Okonta, N. R. "Does Yoga Therapy Reduce Blood Pressure in Patients with Hypertension?: An Integrative Review." *Holistic Nursing Practice* 26.3 (2012): 137–141. Print.

Park, J., et al. "Managing Osteoarthritis: Comparisons of Chair Yoga, Reiki, and Education (Pilot Study)." *Holistic Nursing Practice* 26.6 (2011): 316–326. Print.

Ross, A., and S. Thomas. "The Health Benefits of Yoga and Exercise: A Review of Comparison Studies." *The Journal of Alternative and Complementary Medicine* 16.1 (2010): 3–12. Print.

Sharma, R. K., and B. Dash, trans. *Caraka Samhita* (*Text with English Translation & Critical Exposition Based on Cakrapani Datta's Ayurveda Dipika*). Varanasi, India: Chowkhamba Sanskrit Series Office, 2002, pp. 289–290. Print.

Sears, S. R., S. Bolton, and K. L. Bell. "Evaluation of 'Steps to Surgical Success' (STEPS): A Holistic Preoperative Medicine Program to Manage Pain and Anxiety Related to Surgery." *Holistic Nursing Practice* 27.6 (2013): 349–357. Print.

Sieverdes, J. C., et al. "Effects of Hatha Yoga on Blood Pressure, Salivary Amylase, and Cortisol Among Normotensive and Prehypertensive Youth." Published online ahead of print 12 Mar. 2014. *The Journal of Alternative and Complementary Medicine.* Web. http://online.liebertpub.com/doi/abs/10.1089/acm.2013.0139.

YOGA THERAPY AND NUTRITION

David R. Allen, M.D.

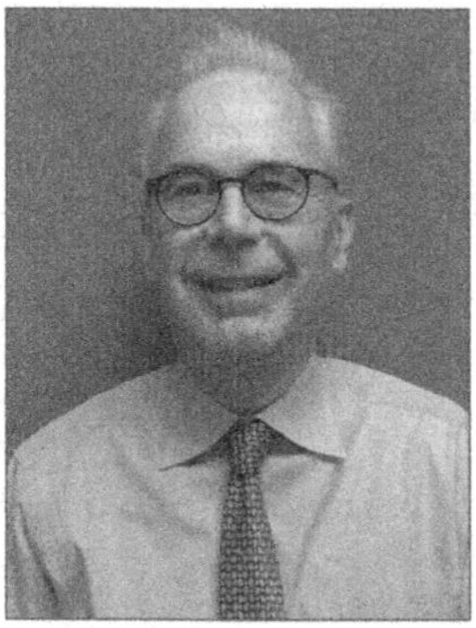

David Allen is a graduate of the University of California at Berkeley and the University of California at Los Angeles Medical School. His advanced training includes studies in internal medicine, traditional acupuncture, and classical homeopathy. He is a lecturer and codirector at Loyola Marymount University's Yoga Therapy Rx program. Dr. Allen also lectures at the Esalen Institute and has a private practice in integrative medicine in Los Angeles, CA.

INTRODUCTION

Diet is one of the most important aspects of being and staying healthy. Every day we are learning how our food choices are related to the development of chronic diseases. Heart disease, cancer, obesity, and diabetes have been shown to be directly related to what we eat (Willett and Stampfer, 2013). Food is information for our DNA. How we bathe our genes has a direct effect on how they express themselves. It has been shown that genes can express themselves differently depending on the environment to which they are exposed (Kaput and Rodriquez, 2004). Therefore, to a great extent, we hold the fate of our health in our diet and lifestyle choices. If we expose our genes to sugar, junk, and fast food, the phenotype, or how we appear and what is expressed in our body and mind, is one of disease. With millions of Americans being overweight, sedentary, and living on junk food, we are facing a crisis of illness of unprecedented proportions. How, then, do we decide what is the best diet to promote optimum health in Yoga Therapy? If you go into the diet section of your local bookstore or peruse online, you will see the vast selection of different diet books, and it can be incredibly confusing. Each book tells you that if you just eat one way and follow that plan you can achieve health, perfect weight—and maybe even eternal life! These diets can be vegan, low fat, low carbohydrate, Mediterranean, Atkins, gluten-free, macrobiotic, ayurvedic, allergy-free, elimination-oriented, rotation-based, designed for your blood or body type, and/or raw, just to name a few! In this chapter, we will explore these options and offer some answers to the questions of how to live a long, healthy life.

DR. ALLEN'S KEY OBSERVANCES TO A HEALTHY DIET

In the *Yoga Sūtras,* Patañjali outlines five *niyamas,* or observances, in the second limb of classical Aṣṭāṅga Yoga that lead the Yoga practitioner to a healthy lifestyle. The five observances according to Patañjali are satya (truthfulness), saṁtoṣa (contentment), tapas (austerity), svadhyāya (self-study), and īśvara praṇidhāna (devotion). In a similar way, below are ten key observances that can lead one to a healthy yogic diet when diligently followed:

1. Eat local organic foods in season, avoiding foods with pesticides, chemicals, synthetic fertilizers, and GMOs.
2. Minimize sugar, junk food, refined carbohydrates, white flour, and foods with a high glycemic index.
3. Eat regular meals and track caloric intake to restrict calories in a proper way.
4. Drink your solids and chew your liquids.
5. Use nutritional supplements appropriately.
6. Eat less as you grow older and prevent dementia and disease through diet.
7. Keep the body hydrated and drink plenty of water.
8. Practice detoxifications regularly.
9. Have your own food allergies tested to maximize your body's efficiency.
10. Try to eat in a calm relaxed manner, avoiding television and upsetting situations while ingesting and digesting.

HOW HEALTHY IS YOUR DIET?

As humans, we often feel that we are eating better than we really are. Take this simple test to see how healthy you are eating. Be honest with yourself because you can always improve on what you are currently doing:

1. Do you have several servings of vegetables each day?
2. Do you have several varieties of vegetables every day?
3. Do you eat several pieces of organic nontropical fruit each day?
4. Do you eat dried peas and beans (legumes, lentils, chickpeas, kidney beans, green peas, etc.) every day?
5. When you consume meat is it grass fed?
6. Do you avoid soda and/or soft drinks?
7. Do you avoid high mercury fish like tuna, swordfish, etc.?
8. Do you avoid sweets such as ice cream, cookies, and cakes?

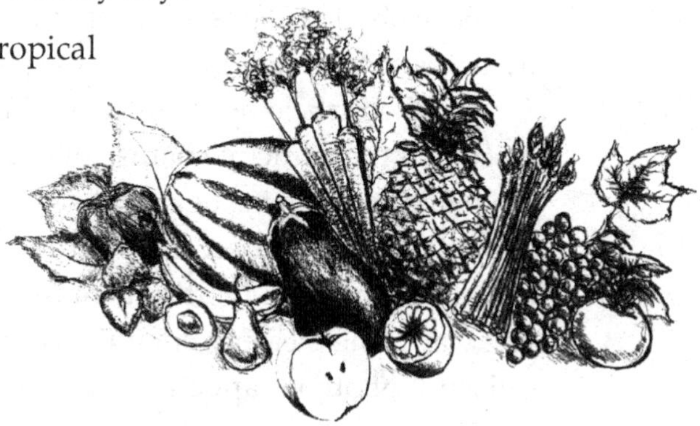

If you answered no to two or more of these questions then your diet could use improvement. Pay attention to the yogic tips you'll find in this chapter to improve your eating habits and your health.

GLYCEMIC INDEX

For thousands of years in India and throughout the world, our ancestors were drawn to sweet foods in an environment that was low in carbohydrates, high in fat, and moderate in protein. Our taste buds were developed to crave and prefer sweet-tasting foods that were generally safe foods in nature, whereas bitter foods in nature often caused harm. If we think of the Native Americans of the southwest United States, they were lean, tough, and lived for thousands of years in harmony with their environment. Their genetic makeup, when put in that specific geographic area, produced healthy human beings. Fast-forward to the present, and the same group now suffers from epidemics of diabetes, hypertension, and heart disease because their diet no longer fits their genetic structure.

For many of us, both yogis and nonyogis alike, our modern diet no longer fits what our genetics were designed to consume. Most of the chronic degenerative diseases today are caused by our lifestyle choices. Our health is literally in our hands. In September 2013, *Scientific American* published an entire issue on food. It raised the question as to whether it was the total calories that we consumed or the types of calories (protein, carbohydrates, or fat) that mattered the most (Taub, 2013). For years the relationship between carbohydrate consumption and obesity and diabetes has been observed. It is clear that the modern diet, high in sugar and refined carbohydrates, contributes greatly to the poor health of the American public.

Another article by Paul Kenny in the same issue of *Scientific American* in 2013 discussed the addictive nature of overweight behavior (Kenny, 2013). Many modern foods are high in sugar and activate our reward circuits in a powerful way. An addictive cycle gets set up where you "can't have just one," similar to the Lay's brand potato chip advertisement from a few years ago. The more you eat, the more you want. The pleasure circuits overwhelm leptin, the hormone secreted by our fat cells to shut off our appetite, and we keep eating.

The glycemic index is a number that indicates how quickly a particular food raises the blood sugar levels in the body. The higher the number, the quicker the sugar rises in the blood. It can be tricky because not all high glycemic foods taste sweet. Even foods like potatoes and whole grains can be broken down easily and move into the bloodstream quickly. When high glycemic foods enter the bloodstream, the body produces large amounts of insulin. Insulin causes the glucose to be used as fuel or to be stored as fat. Over time, the glucose that isn't burned in the muscles can lead to obesity and insulin resistance. Insulin resistance promotes fat storage in the abdominal area where fat becomes much more dangerous. Abdominal fat is metabolically active and increases deadly inflammation in the body. High levels of insulin can also cause reactive hypoglycemia, where the blood sugar drops. This can lead to shakiness and fatigue. For example, just look at a high school class after they eat lunch. Half of the class is asleep and the other half is bouncing off the walls!

Glycemic Index

Level	*Glycemic Index*	*Glycemic Load per serving*
HIGH	70 or more	20
MEDIUM	50–69	11 to 19
LOW	49 or less	10 or less

Glycemic Load of Certain Foods

FRUITS	*Glycemic Index*	*Carbs (grams per serving)*	*Glycemic Load per serving*
Apple, 1 average	38	16	6
Banana,1 whole, ripe	51	26.5	14
Orange, 1 whole	42	12	5
Raisins, 1/2 cup	64	44	28
Watermelon	72	6	4
Strawberries	40	152	3.6
VEGETABLE	*Glycemic Index*	*Carbs (grams per serving)*	*Glycemic Load per serving*
Broccoli, 1/2 cup steamed	6	2	1
Carrots, 1 cup raw	47	6	3
Corn on cob, 1 ear	53	29	15
Grean Beans, 1/2 cup	28	5	1
Baked potato, white	85	30.5	26
Spinach, 1/2 cup steamed	6	3.5	1
Sweet Potato	61	28	17
Tomatoes, 1 cup raw	61	28	17
GRAINS	*Glycemic Index*	*Carbs (grams per serving)*	*Glycemic Load per serving*
Bagel	72	89	33
Corn Tortilla	70	24	7.7
Pumpernickel bread 1slice	41	26	4.5
White bread, 1 slice	70	25	8.4
Wheat Bread	70	28	7.7
French Bread, 1 slice	95	64	29.5
Whole wheat pita	57	64	17
Bran muffin 1 medium	60	113	30
Corn Bread 1 slice	110	60	30.8
Oatmeal 1 cup	58	234	12.8
Oatmeal, instant 1 cup	65	234	13.7
Corn Flakes 1 cup	92	28	21.1
Kellog's Special K 1cup	69	31	14.5
Grape Nuts 1/2 cup	75	58	31.5
Cheerios	74	30	13.3
Coco Pops	77		20.2
Popcorn 1 cup	55	8	2.8
Rice White, 1 cup cooked	64	36	23
Rice brown, 1 cup cooked	55	33	18
Barley	25		10.6
Buckwheat	54		16
Quinoa	53		13
LEGUMES	*Glycemic Index*	*Carbs (grams per serving)*	*Glycemic Load per serving*
Baked beans 1 cup	48	253	18.2
Chickpeas, boiled 1 cup	31	240	13.3
Kidney Beans 1 cup	27	256	7
Lentils 1 cup	29	198	7
Soy Beans 1 cup	20	172	1.4
Pinto Beans 1 cup	39	171	11.7
Chana Dal	8 to 11	3.9	2.4
BEVERAGES	*Glycemic Index*	*Carbs (grams per serving)*	*Glycemic Load per serving*
Apple Juice 8 oz	40	30	12
Pepsi 8 oz	58	25	15
Tomato Juice, 1/2 cup	38	10	4

Additionally, there are foods that have a higher glycemic index, but have a low impact when eaten in normal portion sizes. For instance, carrots have a high index; however, they are okay if eaten in small portions. If you have diabetes, are overweight, or have low blood sugar then you should avoid any food that has a glycemic index of over 45. You can help your health by limiting high glycemic foods like potatoes and bananas, grains, sugar, and fruit juice. Many dietitians suggest emphasizing beans, vegetables, seeds, nuts, and healthy animal protein. On page 223 is a chart of the glycemic load of various foods to ease and assist in choosing the right foods with a low glycemic index.

DETOXIFICATION

We are inundated with toxins and heavy metals in our modern world. A recent study showed that the average child born in the United States had more than 287 different chemicals in the umbilical cord blood at birth (Environmental Working Group, 2005). The average adult has 1,000 times more lead in his/her bones than the Inca Indians had 500 years ago. Since the industrial revolution began, we have poured millions of tons of waste into the environment. These toxins cause, or contribute to, many modern illnesses. There is no way to maintain health in today's world without a consistent detoxification program.

What do we really mean by detoxification and what is the healthiest way to go about it? All food, and, in fact, everything that we ingest goes from the intestine through the liver. The liver is where many of these toxins accumulate. Most toxins are fat-soluble and are stored in the fat cells. This is one of the reasons that the "yo-yo diet syndrome" of repeated weight loss and gains can be so destructive to your health. With weight loss also comes exposure to all of the toxins stored in the fat cells.

The first step then is to promote liver health and help detoxify the liver. The liver detoxifies in two steps, which change the toxins from a fat- to a water-soluble product that can be eliminated through the gut or the kidneys. The first step, or phase, is to address the cytochrome p450 system. This system takes the toxins and makes an intermediate product of the toxin that then goes through phase two, the final step in the liver's detoxification. Both phases require certain nutrients for this detoxification process to occur smoothly and for the liver to be healthy such as N-acetyl cysteine, glutathione, vitamin C, and B vitamins, as well as many others. The body also requires a certain amount of protein each day to stay in a positive balance. If we have less protein than what we need, the body may break down muscle to try to maintain that balance. Many detoxification programs fall short in the required nutrients and protein to leave the body in a healthy state after the program is over. This is why many detox programs can leave a person weak and depleted.

So, what is the best way to go about detoxifying? The program I generally recommend is as follows:

1. Do a three-day detoxification four times a year at the change of the seasons. Use hypoallergenic protein powder three to four times a day and drink plenty of water. The USDA's recommendation for water can vary depending on your activity level and the climate you are living in. This protein powder must contain all of the nutrients for the liver as well 50 to 60 grams of hypoallergenic protein. During this three-day period, you may want to have one or two colonic therapies to help clean out the colon.

2. One day per week from dinner to dinner (or pick a whole day if you wish), regularly use the protein powder three to four times a day without any other food. If you do this one day per week, it will prepare you for the 3-day intensive cleansing program. This also allows a more gradual detoxification and minimizes any uncomfortable symptoms that may occur.

3. Use a far-infrared sauna. This type of sauna gives you the benefits of a regular sauna, but at a temperature that allows a longer time in the heat. Follow each sauna with several charcoal capsules so that the toxins will be eliminated from the intestine and will not be reabsorbed.

4. Use a loofah scrub each day when you shower. Moderately and vigorously scrub your skin until you feel a slight tingling or glow. Remember the skin is an organ of elimination, so by doing this you help get rid of toxins.

CALORIC RESTRICTION

One of the only proven ways to increase longevity and health is through caloric restriction. It has been shown in animals and in primates that a lower caloric diet, as long as it is high in micronutrients, can increase life span as well as decrease the development of chronic degenerative diseases and cancers (Roth, Ingram, and

Lane, 2001). Caloric restriction can activate the SIRT 1 gene. In the scientific study of genetics, when this gene is turned on there is an increase in DNA repair and the suppression of bad or disruptive genes. The SIRT 1 gene can also cause the breakdown of fat cells and promote weight loss. This gene also seems to contribute to the longevity effect. So far, calorie restriction and resveratrol, a substance found in red wine, are the main things that can activate these genes.

Most of these studies suggest a reduction of 30 to 40 percent of your daily calories (Everitt and Le Couteur, 2007). If you were consuming 2,000 Kcal per day you would have to drop it down to 1,200 Kcal. An alternative is to fast completely one day and then eat normally the next. This can be challenging for most of us, and compliance, except for the most dedicated, is usually poor or short-lived. So how do we get the benefit of caloric restriction and still live in the modern world? Unfortunately, you would have to drink a lot of red wine to achieve the positive effect, which is impractical. The following are ways to get the greatest benefits out of caloric restriction:

1. Decrease your total caloric intake by 30 to 40 percent. Measure your total calories for a few days, average them, and then again, decrease the total by 30 to 40 percent.

2. Decrease your caloric intake 20 percent and increase your exercise to burn up 10 to 20 percent of your calories. By increasing your exercise and burning calories you can get the same result without such a severe reduction of calories consumed.

3. Alternate fasting and eating. Fast or decrease your calories by 40 percent one day and eat normally the next.

4. Fast for twelve hours each day from 6 or 7 p.m. to 6 or 7 a.m., decrease your caloric intake by 10 to 15 percent, and increase your exercise to burn 10 to 15 percent of your calories. This is the most practical, easiest, and preferred method for most of us.

Lowering your intake of carbohydrates and unhealthy fats is the best way to achieve the goal of 10 to 15 percent reduction of calories. Carbohydrate is 4 Kcal per gram, protein is 4 Kcal per gram, and fat is 9 Kcal per gram. The fat and sugar in fast foods and soft drinks account for a high percentage of calories in the standard American diet (SAD). Ancient man ate 75 percent of his calories from fat, 20 percent from protein, and 5 percent from carbohydrates. The modern recommended diet is 60 to 70 percent carbohydrates, 15 to 30 percent protein and 15 to 30 percent fat (HHS and USDA, 2005). Following a lower carbohydrate diet like our ancestors did, consuming healthy fats, and adding vigorous exercise can help us achieve the benefits of a reduced calorie diet. This will go a long way to help us live longer and healthier both as yogis and nonyogis alike.

ORGANIC OR REGULAR FOODS?

There is controversy as to whether the higher cost of organic foods warrants the possible health benefits. Organic means that the foods are grown without pesticides, chemicals, and synthetic fertilizers. Organic beef and chicken are raised without pesticides or antibiotics while organic milk and eggs are from animals that are raised organically. There are new studies that show organic foods have lower levels of pesticides and other chemicals (USDA, 2002). These pesticides and chemicals can accumulate over time and have significant effects on our health. Other studies show that in some cases organic foods are higher in certain minerals and vitamins (USDA, 2002).

The Environmental Working Group is an organization that is a good source of information about healthy food and household and personal products. They publish the dirty and clean fruits and vegetables lists. The following foods highest in pesticides are known as the "dirty dozen" and should always be organic:

Grapes	Cucumbers	Potatoes
Spinach	Peaches	Celery
Cherry tomatoes	Apples	Bell peppers / hot peppers
Strawberries	Kale	Nectarines

The cleanest or the least contaminated foods known as the "clean 15" are:

Avocados	Onions	Eggplant
Pineapples	Sweet corn / corn	Grapefruit
Kiwi	Cantaloupe	Mushrooms
Cabbage	Sweet peas	Papayas
Mangoes	Asparagus	Sweet potatoes

Additionally, there is a lot of current debate on the use of genetically modified foods (GMOs). Current research says they are safe. As a doctor, I feel they should be avoided. From the yogic perspective, GMOs have never been used in human history. We don't really know the long-term health effects, so, until we do, they should be avoided.

FOOD AND GLUTEN ALLERGIES AND SENSITIVITIES

For thousands of years, human beings ate food on a seasonal basis. Ancestral man did not eat the same foods every day. Modern humans, on the other hand, eat too many of their calories from too few foods (Allen, 2014). Nowadays, we can have tropical fruits and vegetables in the coldest climates in the winter. Because of the constant repetition of foods to which we expose our bodies, we can develop food allergies and sensitivities from a lack of variation within our diets. Realistically speaking, grains were only introduced into the diet of humans around 12,000 years ago. The diet of humans for millions of years was devoid of grains. This is one of the reasons grains, especially wheat, cause so many problems for people today.

Food allergies and food intolerances contribute to many physical and mental disorders. Recurrent ear infections in children, abdominal pain, nasal allergies, skin rashes, attention deficit disorder, autistic spectrum, depression, dementia, autoimmune disease, and fatigue are common problems caused by foods (Patten and Williams, 2007). When many of my patients eliminate gluten and dairy from their diets, more than 50 percent of their presenting symptoms are often eliminated! The most common allergic foods are unfortunately the foods we consume the most. They include wheat, soy, citrus, peanuts, milk, cheese, gluten, and corn.

So how do we test for and treat food allergies? Well, there are many blood tests for food allergies. We can test antibodies to foods or test for lymphocyte activation by foods. There are skin tests, prick testing, and intradermal, as well as sublingual testing. All of these tests can be helpful, but none are perfect, even though they can give us useful information as to what foods may be causing our health problems. The simplest way to test for food allergies is called elimination-provocation. We take a food, say wheat, and we eliminate it from the diet for three to four weeks. We keep a food diary, or a journal of what we eat, and track our symptoms. If our symptoms improve or are eliminated, we then reintroduce the food and see if the symptoms reappear. Once we eliminate a food our sensitivity to its effect can diminish. It can stay diminished if we avoid it daily or decrease its frequent use—much like we refine our practice of āsanas over time in Yoga Therapy. We can also initiate a rotational diet, which consists of eating each family of food once every four to five days. For example, if we eat wheat on Monday, we eat it again on Friday. By keeping a food diary we can begin to detect a la Sherlock Holmes which foods cause our symptoms.

Gluten is becoming more and more of a substance of concern in the modern diet. We now think of gluten as being related to a wide spectrum of disorders. There can be wheat allergy, celiac disease, or basic gluten sensitivity. All of them can have digestive symptoms like abdominal pain and diarrhea, but 50 percent of those with gluten spectrum disorder have no abdominal symptoms whatsoever. Gluten sensitivity can cause abdominal pain, eczema, headaches, fatigue, depression, joint pain, and numbness of extremities (Sapone, et al., 2012; Volta and DeGiorgio, 2010). The typical blood tests for celiac disease often miss gluten sensitivity. There are, however, more sensitive tests, like the gluten tests from Cyrex Laboratories, that are often positive when the traditional tests are negative. Future research will likely highlight gluten's deleterious effect on the gut and intestinal system, thus limiting gluten intake in wheat-based and/or processed foods helps to promote healthy digestion and longevity while decreasing inflammation and disease.

HOW TO HAVE A HEALTHY BRAIN AND PREVENT DEMENTIA

When I was a medical student, the diet of choice to prevent illness was a low-fat diet. When you lower fat in the diet you have to increase the amount of carbohydrates. This increase of carbohydrates, especially refined carbohydrates, may be contributing to some of the health problems we face today. For example, brain disease is starting at an earlier age and now affects people under fifty-five years old, and approximately 15 percent of people over seventy years old are now affected by dementia (Mayers, 2012).

How does our diet contribute to dementia? As previously mentioned, a diet high in carbohydrates can contribute to insulin resistance and elevated blood sugar levels. When our blood sugar is high it attaches to proteins and forms an AGE (advanced glycosolated end-product). One dangerous form of AGE is formed when a glucose molecule attaches to an LDL ("bad" cholesterol) protein. When glucose attaches to an LDL protein, the AGE it forms increases damage to the blood vessels in the heart and in the brain. Other proteins that have combined with glucose can be a source of free radicals. These dangerous free radicals can then oxidize LDL cholesterol, causing the double threat of glycosolated LDL and oxidized LDL, which together can be dangerous and deadly to the brain by increasing inflammation and free radical production.

Fructose can be dangerous to the brain as well. Not necessarily the fructose found in fruit, but the high fructose corn syrup found in soft drinks and many other products. The intake of fructose has increased 1000 percent in the last few decades (Bray, 2004). When you increase the fructose in your diet you increase dangerous abdominal fat, increase insulin resistance, and increase the incidence of hypertension, all risk factors for dementia. Diabetes also carries with it an increased risk of dementia. Fructose is 10 times as likely as glucose to increase AGEs (McPherson, Shilton, and Walton, 1988), which can trigger inflammation in the brain. Moreover, the sugar substitute, aspartame, is toxic to the brain. Avoid it at all costs!

I once asked a world-renowned neurologist, who is an expert in preventing dementia, what he ate every day. This was his brain health program:

- Breakfast: Eggs, vegetables, tea
- Lunch: Large salad, with a variety of vegetables
- Dinner: Animal protein and vegetables
- Supplements: CoQ10, Multiple vitamin/mineral, resveratrol, green tea extract, essential fatty acids, alpha lipoic acid, coconut oil, and glucoraphain.

According to *The Lancet*, the world's leading general medical journal and specialty journals *Oncology*, *Neurology*, and *Infectious Diseases*, nearly 50 percent of Alzheimer's cases can be prevented with lifestyle modifications (Barnes and Yaffe, 2011). The five most important modifications in that regard are controlling diabetes, controlling blood pressure, managing obesity, managing depression, and exercising.

SUPPLEMENTATION

Nutritional supplements are always a complement to a healthy diet. Diet is the foundation and supplements are required based on the specific needs of the person. There is some controversy as to whether supplements are necessary or if they just create expensive urine. There are several studies that show the quality of our current food supply is deficient. By the time the food gets from the field, to the central warehouse, to the market, and finally to your dinner table, it can lose up to 40 to 60 percent of its nutritive value (Thomas, 2007). We also live in a stressful world, exposed to numerous toxins, which facilitate irregular eating patterns and poor food choices. All of these situations require increased nutrient intake.

There is also biochemical individuality. The Recommended Daily Allowance (RDA) is only the minimum required to prevent illness. It does not represent the amount needed for optimal health for each individual. Biochemical individuality means that we all require different amounts of nutrients based on our uniqueness as human beings. For example, there is an enzyme called MTHFR, which activates folic acid. This activated folate has many uses like serotonin production, detoxification, creating red and white blood cells, and making DNA. If you have a mutation on this enzyme, you will have difficulty activating folate and will be prone to depression, immune dysfunction, and low energy. If you have this mutation, you would need an increased intake of the active form of folate, 5-methly folate. In fact, taking regular folic acid could actually be harmful to your immune system. Another example is vitamin D. Vitamin D deficiency is epidemic in the United States and many people do not even know their vitamin D levels are low. I have tested hundreds of patients and found fewer than 5 percent have sufficient levels. Low vitamin D levels can lead to osteoporosis, immune dysfunction, and dementia.

There are also people with certain medical conditions that require medication and further supplementation. Patients taking a statin drug for high cholesterol often need to supplement with CoQ10, vitamin E, and omega-3 essential fatty acids. The statin drug inhibits the production of these nutrients and can lead to severe muscle inflammation if not properly supplemented and balanced. CoQ10 at high doses has also been shown to slow the progression of Parkinson's disease (Shults, et al., 2002).

Lastly, I recommend that everyone take at least a good multivitamin-mineral supplement. If you have a specific medical condition, you may need certain other nutrients. Please consult with a nutritionally oriented doctor to be evaluated.

AYURVEDIC DIET: THE ORIGINAL FOOD PLAN FOR YOUR BODY TYPE

A chapter on Yoga Therapy and nutrition would be incomplete without at least a brief discussion of the Ayurvedic diet. Ayurveda is a system that has been in existence for thousands of years. It focuses on mind-body balance and the balance of the three doṣas, or body types: vāta, pitta, and kapha. According to Ayurveda, everyone is a combination of earth, air, water, fire, and space. This is similar to the five elements in Chinese Medicine, which substitutes metal for space. These elements combine in different ways to form the three body types listed above, which are covered in great detail in this book in Mukunda and Chinnamasta Stiles's chapter "Structural Yoga Therapy and Ayurvedic Yoga Therapy" and Dr. Vasant Lad's chapter "Ayurveda and Yoga: Complementary Therapeutics." In Ayurveda, there are six different tastes, and each taste has an effect on our body energy and can be used to put us in or out of balance. Every person has a combination of the elements and body types, but usually one type will be predominant. This balance seems to be genetic, and, therefore, it doesn't change throughout our life. Each of these types can be in or out of balance, and when they are in balance a person is in optimum health.

Vāta

People who are tall, slender, sensitive to cold, creative, can have anxiety and worry, and be excitable, but also can tire quickly and burn out. They are the ectomorphs and often have dry skin and hair. Vāta individuals can catch cold easily and can also have insomnia. Diseases most common to vāta are heart disease, inflammatory arthritis, skin disease, lung conditions, asthma, and nervous disorders. Nutritionally, vātas need cooked, warm, and nourishing foods; foods that are easy to digest.

Pitta

The Pitta body types are mesomorphs—strong, well built, confident, aggressive, demanding or pushy, and perfectionists. They can be competitive and passionate. They are the achievers and business executives. They can suffer from anger, dislike hot weather, and have premature gray hair or hair loss. Typically, they have strong digestion and can eat anything. Under stress they can suffer from boils, skin rashes, stomach ulcers, gastritis, and heartburn. Nutritionally, pittas need cooling foods and green vegetables while minimizing salt and fats.

Kapha

These are the endomorphs, who are physically strong and sturdy, and usually the largest of the body types. They have a slow and steady energy and are often described as loyal and good in relationships. When out of balance, they can get obese and have poor circulation and poor digestion. They dislike cold, damp weather and can suffer from colds, headaches, and allergies. Nutritionally, kaphas need to be warmed and stimulated. They are best avoiding salt, oily foods, and refined sugars while using all types of spices.

CONCLUSION

Just as in Patañjali's *Yoga Sūtras,* Yoga Therapy has many facets. A healthy diet is just one aspect of a successful Yoga practice that is at the foundation of health and healing. It is important to realize that food is information for the body and brain and is one of the basic ways we inform our DNA. Just like we inform our bodies of position and breath when practicing āsana and meditation, nutrition gives us an opportunity to become aware of how food can affect our consciousness and practice.

REFERENCES

Allen, D. Personal observation from over 1000 patient questionnaires in my medical practice. 2014.

Barnes, D. E, and K. Yaffe. "The Projected Effect of Risk Factor Reduction on Alzheimer's Disease Prevalence." *The Lancet* (*Neurology*) 10.9 (2011): 819–828. doi: 10.1016/S1474–4422(11)70072–2. Epub 19 July 2011. Print/Web.

Bray, G. "Consumption of High-Fructose Corn Syrup in Beverages May Play a Role in the Epidemic of Obesity." *American Journal of Clinical Nutrition* 79.4 (2004): 537–543. Print.

Environmental Working Group. "Body Burden: The Pollution in Newborns—Benchmark Investigation of Industrial Chemicals Pollutants, and Pesticides in Umbilical Cord Blood." 14 July 2005. Web. Retreived February 27, 2014. http://www.ewg.org/research/body-burden-pollution-newborns.

Everitt, A.V., and D. G. Le Couteur. "Life Extension by Calorie Restriction in Humans." *Annals of the New York Academy of Sciences* 1114 (2007): 428–433. Print.

Kaput, J., and R. L. Rodriquez. "Nutritional Genomics: The Next Frontier in the Postgenomic Era." *Physiological Genomics* 16.2 (2004): 166–177. Print.

Kenny, P. J. "Is Obesity an Addiction?" (aka "The Food Addiction"). *Scientific American* 309.3. 20 August 2013. Web. http://www.scientificamerican.com/article/is-obesity-an-addiction/?page=5.

Mayers, P. C. "Changing Patterns of Neurological Mortality in 10 Major Developed Countries." *Public Health* 127.4 (2012): 357–568. 17 April 2013. Web. doi: 10.1016/j.puhe.2012.12.018.

McPherson J. D., B. H. Shilton, and D. J. Walton. "Role of Fructose in Glycation and Cross-Linking of Proteins." *Biochemistry* 27.6 (1988): 1901–1907. Print.

Patten, S. B., and J. V. Williams. "Self–Reported Allergies and Their Relationship to Several Axis 1 Disorders in a Community." *International Journal of Psychiatry in Medicine* 37.1 (2007): 11–22. Print.

Roth, G. S., D. K. Ingram, and M. A. Lane. "Caloric Restriction in Primates and Relevance to Humans." *Annals of the New York Academy of Sciences* 928 (2001): 305–315. Print.

Sapone, A., et al. "Spectrum of Gluten-Related Disorders: Consensus on New Nomenclature and Classification." *BMC Medicine* 10 (2012): 13. BioMed Central.com. doi:10.1186/1741-7015-10-13. Web. http://www.biomedcentral.com/1741-7015/10/13.

Shults, C. W., et al. "Effects of Coenzyme Q_{10} in Early Parkinson Disease: Evidence of Slowing of the Functional Decline." *Archives of Neurology* 59.10 (2002): 1541–1550. Print.

Taub, G. "Which One Will Make You Fat?" *Scientific American* 309.3 (2013): 60–69. Print.

Thomas, D. "The Mineral Depletion of Foods Available to Us as a Nation (1940–2002): A Review of the 6th Edition of McCance and Widdowson." *Nutrition and Health* 19.1-2 (2007): 21–55. Print.

U.S. Department of Health and Human Services (HHS) and U.S. Department of Agriculture (USDA). Dietary Guidelines for Americans, 2005. 6th Edition, Washington, DC: U.S. Government Printing Office, January 2005. Web. http://www.health.gov/dietaryguidelines/dga2005/document/.

U.S. Department of Agriculture (USDA). (2002). Consumer Brochure: The National Organic Program. "Organic Food Standards and Labels: The Facts." 2002. Accessed 15 Jan. 2014. Web. http://www.ams.usda .gov/AMSv1.0/nop.

Volta, U., and R. DeGiorgio. "Gluten Sensitivity." *The Lancet* (*Neurology*), 9.3 (2010): 233–235. Print.

Willett, W. C., and M. J. Stampfer. "Current Evidence on Healthy Eating." *Annual Review of Public Health* 34 (2013): 77–95. Web. 13 Jan. 2013. doi: 10.1146/annurev–publhealth–031811–124646.

Willett, W. C. (1994) "Diet and Health: What Should We Eat?" *Science* 264 (1994): 532–537. Print.

Yoga Therapy for the Cardiovascular System

Art Brownstein, M.D., M.P.H., D.Y.Ed., F.A.C.P.M.

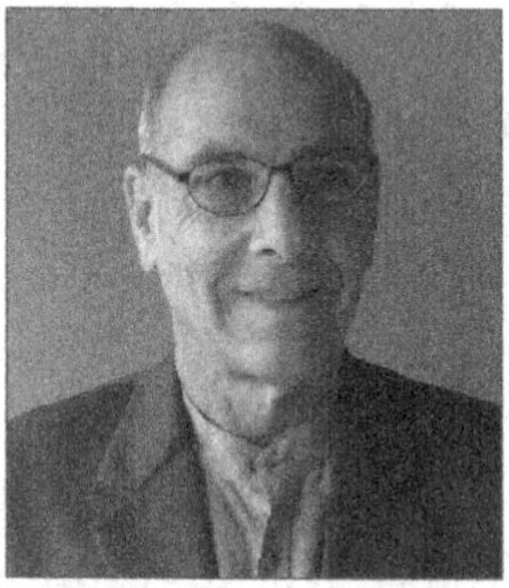

Art Brownstein is a former assistant clinical professor of medicine in the John A. Burns School of Medicine at the University of Hawaii at Manoa and a former staff physician in Dr. Dean Ornish's renowned program for reversing heart disease. He is a diplomate of the American Board of Preventive Medicine, a founding diplomate of the American Board of Holistic Medicine, and the only American physician ever to receive a diploma in Yogic education from the government of India. A recipient of the prestigious Air Medal by the U.S. Air Force, Dr. Brownstein is the author of two books, *Healing Back Pain Naturally* and *Extraordinary Healing: The Amazing Power of Your Body's Secret Healing System.*

INTRODUCTION

The cardiovascular system, which includes the heart and blood vessels, is responsible for delivering blood and life-sustaining oxygen and nutrients to every cell and tissue and is one of the most important systems in the entire body. The heart, the central organ of the cardiovascular system, weighs only about ten ounces, yet pumps about twelve tons of blood a day. It beats, on average, seventy-two times a minute, and when properly cared for, can sustain a steady rhythmic pace for approximately one hundred years.

Diseases of the cardiovascular system, while potentially deadly, are highly responsive to Yoga Therapy. This is not just because of the tremendous prevalence of these types of diseases in modern society (e.g., high blood pressure and heart disease), but primarily because of their underlying causes and mechanisms. While previously these illnesses were thought to be of genetic origin, many researchers now consider them "diseases of modern civilization" since they have been strongly linked to our high-stress, modern lifestyles. Even though Western medicine has developed sophisticated technological and pharmaceutical solutions for the management of cardiovascular illnesses (and intervening during their acute flare-ups), studies show that drugs and surgery do little to address the underlying causes of these diseases.

In reality, thoughtful evaluation of the current epidemic of cardiovascular diseases will reveal that Yoga Therapy is far superior to any other modern remedy for the treatment and prevention of these diseases. And while the scientific evidence to support this claim is based on research that is relatively new, the techniques and methods that have established the efficacy of Yoga Therapy for cardiovascular diseases are rooted in the ancient wisdom that was described by Patañjali more than 1,500 years ago.

According to data from the Centers for Disease Control and Prevention (CDC), heart disease is currently the number-one killer in the Western world, resulting in about 600,000 deaths annually (CDC, 2013). There are also 78 million Americans presently suffering from high blood pressure (CDC, 2013). As of this writing, more than 30 million suffer with diabetes, which not only directly affects the blood vessels but also increases the risk of heart disease and stroke (CDC, 2013). From both an individual and public health perspective, using Yoga to help heal the cardiovascular system has the potential to do an enormous amount of good. The successful use of Yoga in treating, curing, and preventing cardiovascular disease, as demonstrated by the monumental clinical research of Dr. Dean Ornish (in addition to studies conducted by others) serves to dramatically raise public awareness about the effectiveness of Yoga Therapy. It also helps to further the global acceptance of Yoga, debunking the superficial image of Yoga as merely a system of stretching, but, rather, endorsing the fact that Yoga is a genuinely authentic, deep, and powerful system of healing.

Yet, ironically, because of the potential serious nature of cardiovascular diseases, including the very real possibility of sudden death through a heart attack, or a devastating lifelong paralysis via stroke, in addition to other potentially life-threatening consequences seen during acute flare-ups of these diseases, many Yoga Therapists may be tempted to shy away from treating patients with cardiovascular disease, especially those who may lack training in professional health care.

However, as Dr. Dean Ornish has so eloquently shown during his nearly four decades of pioneering clinical research, even severe, advanced heart disease can be reversed and healed without drugs or surgery through the thoughtful and intelligent application of Yoga Therapy when used in the context of other related beneficial lifestyle changes. For these reasons, Yoga Therapists everywhere should not hesitate to step up to the challenge of applying their knowledge, skills, heart, and training in Yoga Therapy to help people who are suffering from the devastating effects of cardiovascular illnesses and, in so doing, demonstrate to the world that the science of Yoga, while based on ancient wisdom, is more relevant and more urgently needed today than ever before.

HISTORY

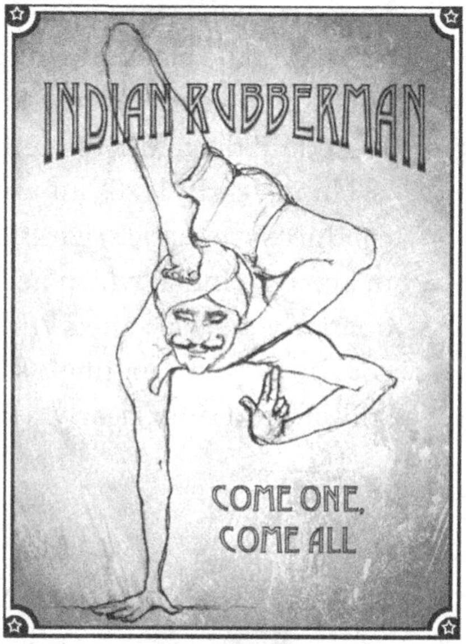

In the ancient land of India, during the relatively recent period of European colonization, most dramatically witnessed from the early 1500s until the mid-1900s, not much credence was given by the West to the practice of Yoga. At best, Yoga was viewed as a novelty, considered to be nothing more than a circus sideshow act, dominated by Indian "rubber men" who could stretch their muscles and attain great flexibility, as they wrapped their legs around the back of their heads while performing all sorts of bizarre body positions like contortionists. Prior to the twentieth century, in the eyes of the West, Yoga held little practical merit other than perhaps being a system of stretching that could improve physical flexibility.

Toward the latter part of this period, however, sporadic reports began to slowly filter into the West about certain accomplished yogic practitioners who could slow down their hearts voluntarily. Other yogic practitioners claimed they could even stop their hearts while remaining buried underground for up to a week at a time (and in some extreme cases, even longer), without oxygen, food, or water. Occasionally, these yogic burial demonstrations were attended by Indian physicians who claimed they were authentic. Slowly, a growing number of scientists in India began to believe that certain advanced practitioners of Yoga could exert control voluntarily over their cardiovascular system, including the lowering of blood pressure at will, slowing the resting heart rate, and decreasing respiratory rate (Raghavendra, et al., 2013).

Naturally, Western physicians and scientists scoffed at the idea that a human being could accomplish such feats (as many still remain skeptical to this day). While numerous challenges were issued to Western scientists during this period to come to India to witness firsthand these yogic demonstrations, most fell on deaf ears. No Western doctor would risk his career or reputation to travel halfway around the world to be a part of such a charade.

The hidden secrets of Yoga, a science estimated to be between five and ten thousand years old, with all its methods and techniques, its emphasis on breath control, deep relaxation, meditation, and physical postures, its ability to influence the autonomic nervous system and the brain, as well as its ability to slow down heart rate and modulate blood pressure, while exerting an overall, positive, health-enhancing effect on the entire cardiovascular system in general, would remain hidden to the West until the mid-twentieth century.

In the early 1920s an unknown Indian yogi, Swami Kuvalayananda, began to conduct systematic scientific studies in Yoga at the Kaivalyadhama Yoga Institute in Lonavla, India, which he founded in 1924. He began publishing his findings in a quarterly journal called *Yoga Mimamsa*, the first journal of its kind devoted to discovering and promoting a scientific understanding of Yoga (Note: *Yoga Mimamsa* is still in print after nearly a century of continuous publication). Swami Kuvalayananda went on to found the first hospital of its kind to treat diseases using only yogic methods (the SADT Gupta Yogic Hospital in Lonavla), which is still operational to this day. Many people interested in Yoga research from India and other parts of the world began to visit Kaivalyadhama Institute in Lonavla. Although he passed in 1966, even today in India, among Yoga researchers and scholars, Swami Kuvalayananda is widely acknowledged as the most important figure of his time to help usher Yoga into the modern scientific age.

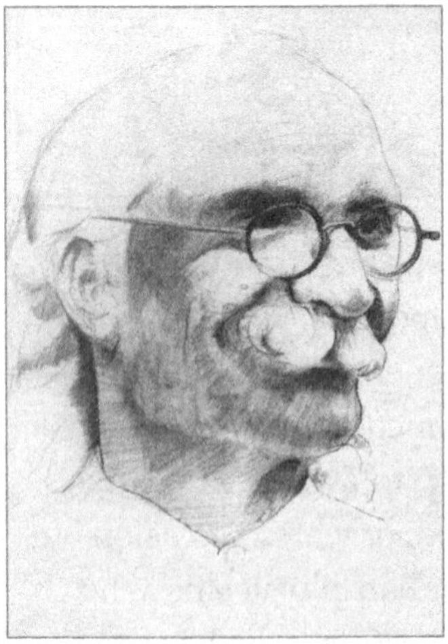

Swami Kuvalayananda

In 1935 a French cardiologist, Dr. Thérèse Brosse, the first known Western scientist to bring EKG equipment to India to study Yoga, conducted experiments that were later published in which she claimed that certain advanced Yoga practitioners could slow their hearts at will and, in some cases, for brief periods, stop their hearts altogether (Wenger, Bagchi, and Anand, 1961). While the methodologies of her studies were later challenged by other scientists, she is generally given credit for being the first Western scientist to suggest that, through the practice of Yoga, one could develop a certain mastery and influence over the cardiovascular system through voluntary means.

In the 1950s, American psychologist Basu Bagchi of the University of Michigan Medical Center and Professor M.A. Wenger of UCLA came to the Kaivalyadhama Yoga Institute to study and work with Swami Kuvalayananda. In a collaborative effort with Professor B. K. Anand, then Chairman of the Department of Physiology at the All India Institute of Medicine in New Delhi (the largest medical school in Asia), they utilized more extensive electrophysiological monitoring technologies than Dr. Brosse to analyze Yoga practices for the cardiovascular system. In the early 1960s they published their findings in several scientific journals, including *Circulation* (Wenger, Bagchi, and Anand, 1961). This latter publication is regarded as the first peer-reviewed scientific article appearing in the West that links the practice of Yoga to its potential beneficial influence on the cardiovascular system.

From the late 1960s onward, studies on the physiological effects of Yoga and the cardiovascular system began to appear in other peer-reviewed scientific Western journals. In 1969, Dr. K. K. Datey, an Indian cardiologist, published his work on Yoga Therapy using śavāsana (corpse pose) for hypertensive patients (Datey, et al., 1969). His work was supported by a series of published studies conducted by Dr. Chandra Patel, an Indian physician from England, who also demonstrated that the practice of śavāsana could lower blood pressure (Patel and North, 1973, 1975). Other studies have since verified these earlier studies, including the work of Dr. A. H. Brownstein and Dr. Mark Dembert, U.S. Air Force and Navy aviation medicine specialists who studied the lowering of blood pressure through Yoga Therapy in military aviators (Brownstein and Dembert, 1989).

In the late 1960s, Dr. Herbert Benson, a renowned cardiologist at Harvard, working with Dr. Keith Wallace, a postdoctoral student from UCLA (and a TM student of the late Maharishi Mahesh Yogi), became the first person in the world to prove that meditation can lower blood pressure (Benson, 1974). At the same time, he helped elucidate the mechanisms on how meditation influenced the autonomic nervous system through what he called the relaxation response, which is the physiological counterpoint to the fight-or-flight response seen during times of stress.

These changes can be measured through such parameters as heart rate and blood pressure, oxygen consumption, metabolic rate, and pupil diameter in the eyes, which are increased by stress and decreased during periods of relaxation. Dr. Benson demonstrated that the regular participation in Yoga practices that elicit the relaxation response is the key to counteracting the harmful effects of stress that lie at the root of most cardiovascular illnesses (Benson, 1975).

In 1970, Elmer and Alyce Green, pioneering scientists in the field of biofeedback and the autonomic nervous system invited Swami Rama to the Menninger Institute in Topeka, Kansas, to study his yogic abilities. They conducted a series of experiments in which Swami Rama could demonstrate his ability to voluntarily induce cardiac atrial fibrillation for seventeen seconds and to increase the blood flow to one side of his right hand while decreasing the blood flow on the opposite side, resulting in a 10 degrees Fahrenheit temperature change between the two sides of his hand. Prior to this time, such voluntary control of the autonomic nervous system was considered impossible.

YOGA AND HEART DISEASE: THE WORK OF DR. DEAN ORNISH

After more than a decade of research, in 1988 Dr. Dean Ornish, Clinical Professor of Medicine at the University of San Francisco School of Medicine, founder of the Preventive Medicine Research Institute in Sausalito, California, and student of the late Swami Satchidananda, became the first person in the world to prove that heart disease could be reversed without drugs or surgery. His methods relied primarily on Yoga and a low-fat, plant-based diet, which was considered the traditional diet of yogis in India.

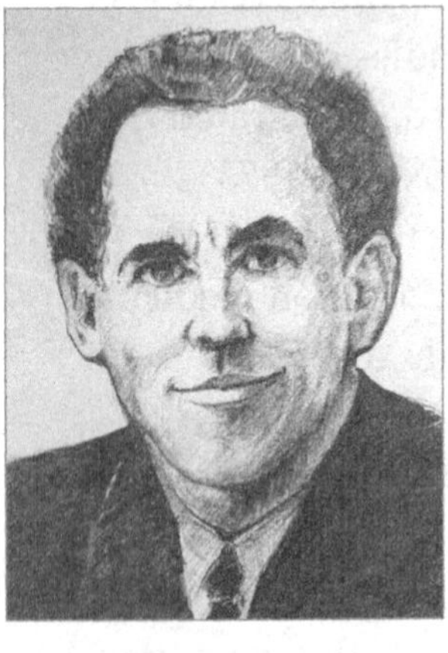

Dr. Dean Ornish

Dr. Ornish has authored numerous scientific articles and books to date, has appeared on the *Oprah Show* many times, has helped cure heart disease of thousands of patients, including those of celebrities, politicians, and corporate CEOs and executives. He served as President Clinton's personal heart consultant and was appointed by him to the White House Commission on Complementary and Alternative Medicine Policy. President Obama appointed him to the Presidential White House Advisory Group on Prevention, Health Promotion, and Integrative and Public Health.

After nearly four decades of research in applying Yoga to help heart patients reverse their heart disease, regain their health, and discover the joy of living, Dr. Ornish's program has finally been approved by Medicare, the gold standard for mainstream medicine in America. Thanks to Dr. Ornish, Yoga Therapy has now entered the heart of conventional mainstream Western medicine, opening the door for the wider field of Yoga to become recognized as the incredibly powerful, health-restoring, spiritually transformative discipline and science that it is.

WHAT TYPE OF PATIENT WITH CARDIOVASCULAR DISEASE IS ELIGIBLE FOR YOGA THERAPY?

Anyone who has been diagnosed with underlying cardiovascular disease, or anyone who has had a major life-threatening cardiovascular event, including heart attack, arrhythmia, or stroke, is eligible for Yoga Therapy. This may include anyone who has undergone one or more invasive procedures for a cardiovascular problem, including open heart surgery, angioplasty (with or without stent placement), one or more radiofrequency ablation procedures, a pacemaker or internal defibrillator implantation, or any one of a number of related procedures. It may also include anyone who has a strong family history of cardiovascular disease or who is at risk for contracting one or another form of it and is interested and motivated to prevent it.

The only cautionary exception to the above-mentioned categories is the case when someone's health is extremely fragile or has an imminent life-threatening cardiovascular diagnosis that has not been properly stabilized and may require urgent surgical intervention or some other life-prolonging procedure. For such a patient, it is important to refer that patient back to their cardiologist or primary-care physician and let him/her get stabilized first, before beginning a Yoga Therapy program. When in doubt about a patient's stamina and health status, it always better to error on the side of caution, and to not take unnecessary risks. For this reason, a medical clearance letter from a patient's primary-care doctor or cardiologist will minimize the possibility of your being confronted with such a difficult situation even though you may have to turn away someone who is genuinely interested in Yoga Therapy, but too medically unstable to participate. Before anyone can participate in Dr. Ornish's program, a medical clearance letter as mentioned above is a standard prerequisite.

When working with this group of patients, even in the absence of cardiovascular fragility, it is recommended for the Yoga Therapist to be trained in CPR and to know emergency protocols, including when to call 911. When administering Yoga Therapy in a supervised hospital or clinic program, where trained staff, including nurses and doctors, are usually available, proper contingency planning in advance, combined with good communication and teamwork will help prepare for any untoward possibility.

MEDICAL HISTORY/INTAKE

The following information should be elicited prior to implementing Yoga Therapy for a patient with a history of cardiovascular disease.

- List of known medications, including all prescription, over-the-counter medications, herbs, and supplements, and an awareness of their potential side effects
- Allergies
- Tests or studies conducted to date on the cardiovascular problem (blood tests, EKG results, x-ray reports, etc.)
- Referring physician's diagnosis
- Medical Clearance letter from patient's cardiologist and/or primary care physician giving permission for patient to participate in Yoga Therapy for his/her cardiovascular condition. (This must include current contact information for cardiologist or referring doctor.)
- Medical history including a list of prior illnesses and hospitalizations in addition to any concomitant illnesses, conditions, injuries, or other underlying problems/medical conditions that might limit a patient's participation in Yoga Therapy. For example, patients with heart disease may also have severe arthritic conditions such as those of the knees, hips, or spine, which may require modification of certain poses and/or additional props to accommodate these conditions.
- Prior experience with Yoga, in addition to any expectations, fears, and other potential psychological or physical barriers to the introduction and practice of Yoga for therapeutic purposes

METHODS

The general principle to follow with Yoga Therapy, as it is with Yoga, is to remember that Yoga Therapy is for the individual, not the other way around. In other words, in Yoga Therapy for patients with cardiovascular illness, certain Yoga āsanas and other practices may need to be modified for the benefit of the patient. This also means that while definite preplanned routines and sequences of Yoga practices can be introduced to and prescribed for each patient, it is important to exhibit sensitive pacing and flexibility in the introduction of these practices. As a general rule, in the beginning, to avoid overwhelming the new practitioner, it is better to introduce fewer poses than more. The saying, "Slow but steady wins the race," applies here.

Despite dealing with potentially life-threatening conditions, it is also important for the Yoga Therapist to keep a lighthearted spirit to make Yoga Therapy enjoyable, so that each participant will be more inclined to develop a regular daily Yoga practice of his/her own. If you try to move too fast or introduce too many things at once, the yogic practices that you are trying to implement for therapeutic purposes could backfire and result in an injury, or a worsening of the underlying condition, or the patient may develop an aversion to Yoga that will result in its nonutilization. If this is the case, all your training and efforts will have been in vain, and you will not get the results you are looking for. Rather, you will likely feel frustrated. What I am trying to say can possibly be best stated in the following sayings borrowed from the annals of conventional medical practice:

"The secret of the care of the patient
is in caring for the patient."

—FRANCIS W. PEABODY M.D. (*OGLESBY 1991*)

"It is much more important to know
what sort of a patient has a disease
than what sort of a disease a patient has."

—WILLIAM OSLER (*SILVERMAN 2003*)

All of this is really no different from how any sincere, dedicated Yoga instructor introduces the practice of Yoga to a new student. The only difference is that in the case of Yoga Therapy for the cardiovascular system, the new student just happens to have certain health issues related to this system. If the Yoga Therapy is introduced properly, over time, the Yoga Therapy will evolve into a successful daily Yoga practice, which is the goal. If this occurs, there will be a good chance that the cardiovascular health issues will disappear altogether or, at the very least, diminish significantly.

While, to date, strict guidelines or protocols outside Dr. Ornish's program have not been scientifically established for the application of Yoga Therapy for diseases of cardiovascular origin (with the possible exception of those that rely primarily on the practice of meditation, such as those founded by Dr. Herbert Benson, Jon Kabat-Zinn, and others), and because there is no hard and fast rule to a particular order and/or sequence of methods, practices, or techniques that are first introduced to the patient with cardiovascular disease, it is a wise principle in general to start the patient out with the gentlest, simplest, and easiest technique available. For most people, this will be śavāsana, even though it may need to be modified with pillows and bolsters to accommodate those with orthopedic limitations so that they may be more comfortable during the practice.

YOGA RELAXATION (ŚAVĀSANA)

Most clinical programs that utilize Yoga Therapy for patients with cardiovascular disease prefer to start with śavāsana for a number of reasons. First, it requires the least amount of physical effort of all the āsanas and related yogic practices. Second, it is simple and easy on the body and in general does not cause strain to the heart, lungs, joints, or muscles. Third, in this respect, it utilizes the least amount of energy. For these reasons, it is generally considered one of the safest, if not *the* safest, of all yogic practices for those with cardiovascular disease.

People with severely weakened hearts and damaged cardiovascular systems will be comforted to know that they can perform this practice without too much physical difficulty. This will give them a sense of accomplishment and help instill confidence at a time when their confidence has most likely significantly waned, especially if they have just suffered a heart attack or have gone through major open-heart surgery. Knowing that they can learn something new will help them build self-esteem and self-confidence. These qualities, when combined with the direct benefits of the Yoga practice itself, will further cement their relationship with Yoga in a beneficial way. The more they can adhere to a regular Yoga practice, the more their health will improve.

This was what Dr. Ornish was able to confirm through his research in which his older, sicker patients showed greater improvement than the younger, healthier patients, not only subjectively, but as measured by quantitative angiography and cardiac PET scans (Ornish, et al., 1990). At first, this confounded researchers, as these findings went totally against conventional wisdom. However, deeper inquiry into the matter discovered that, because they had the most to lose as well as the most to gain, the older, sicker patients were more motivated to follow the program than the others. The improvements in subjective health and measured physiological parameters were directly linked to the regularity of adhering to their daily Yoga practices. As patients' health improved, they saw the intrinsic value of regularly performing their Yoga practices. The more Yoga they did, the better they felt. The better they felt, the more they wanted to do their Yoga. It became a win-win, self-perpetuating cycle.

While the traditional preferred method for śavāsana is in a supine position, with the patient on his/her back, shoulders relaxed, feet about shoulder-width

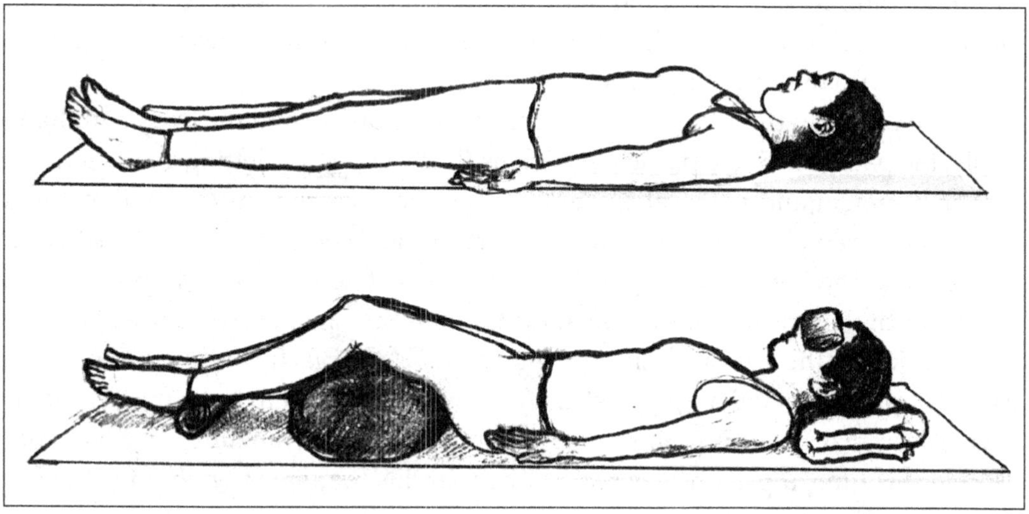

Śavāsana (top) and Śavāsana with Props (bottom)

apart, hands along the side of the body, palms facing up, śavāsana can also be performed in prone position (caturaṅgadaṇḍāsana; crocodile pose) or laterally on either side. It can be modified through body positioning or the use of props and pillows so that the patient is comfortable. If the patient is uncomfortable, the physical discomfort will be a source of distraction for the mental component of the practice.

It must be remembered that, as simple as it appears to the outside observer, the practice of śavāsana is more than just a pose. If taught correctly, it is a profound mind-body practice that, not only increases personal awareness of the body, but also reveals to the patient how physical tension is created and sustained by mental tension. It also helps introduce the patient to elementary breath awareness, preparing them for the practice of prāṇāyāma, which will follow.

While śavāsana lacks the conventional upright spine and seated posture associated with most forms of traditional meditation, for those with significant physical disabilities, including those of the spine or lower extremities, including the knees, as well as the cardiovascular system, śavāsana can also serve as an effective platform for meditation. Along with a resting posture that will minimize strain on the heart and lungs, it is relatively easy for the Yoga Therapist to introduce simple breathing practices as well as complementary meditation techniques such as guided imagery/visualization during the latter stages of śavāsana. These will also aid in helping to calm the mind and, if the imagery is relevant to the heart and blood vessels, can serve to help further deepen and focus the patient's energies and awareness into their healing process.

In śavāsana, with the mind fully focused on the breath and the body simultaneously, the patient actively participates in his/her progressive letting go of fear, control, and mental and physical tension. As he/she does this, he/she will come to experience deep abiding peace and comfort in the region of the heart that could best be described, even if only momentarily, as a state of pure saṁtoṣa (contentment). With the practice of śavāsana, for the first time in a person's life, they may come to know the true meaning of the word *relaxation*. In my own experience as both a physician and a Yoga instructor introducing Yoga to beginning students, I have seen that, for many, this alone will not only be therapeutic but revelatory. During this time, a person may feel at one with his/her spirit or soul for the first time in his/her life.

If this be the case (and I can assure you it happens more commonly than not), you can be sure that the patient has caught and experienced the true meaning and spirit of Yoga. Even if nothing further is accomplished, your role as a Yoga Therapist in facilitating this experience can be viewed as nothing less than a stunning clinical and spiritual success.

The duration of time for a śavāsana practice when used in the context of Yoga Therapy for those with cardiovascular disease is not the same as those encountered in normal health clubs and spa Yoga venues, where classes last for one hour, or one and a half hours at most, and where śavāsana is limited to 5 to 10 minutes maximum. While regular āsana routines in Yoga Therapy can vary according to the needs of the patient, the very first time a patient with cardiovascular disease is introduced to śavāsana, the patient should not feel rushed but should be given adequate time to relax and experience the true therapeutic depth and power of the practice. A minimum of 20 to 30 minutes is recommended and possibly longer. In other words, in Yoga Therapy for cardiovascular diseases, the very first time a patient is introduced to Yoga, the practice of śavāsana will occupy the lion's share of the first Yoga session.

As it is in many traditional schools of Yoga in India, in Yoga Therapy, an āsana routine not only begins with śavāsana but also ends with śavāsana. It is only after the patient begins to improve and has the stamina to tolerate a more rigorous posture (āsana) routine with more variety, that the śavāsana that is given at the beginning of an āsana sequence can be shortened to 5 to 10 minutes, whereas another, longer version of śavāsana is routinely given at the end of the practice sequence. This second and final practice of śavāsana should last for at least 20 to 30 minutes.

Because of the relatively few instances in which it is contraindicated, and because śavāsana is considered to be the safest and most effective way to introduce patients suffering from cardiovascular illness to Yoga, Dr. Dean Ornish has adopted it in his groundbreaking work on reversing heart disease. He not only begins each Yoga session with śavāsana but ends each session with it as well. (Note: In Dr. Ornish's original program, research participants who demonstrated reversal of heart disease after one year practiced Yoga twice a day for one and a half hours per session, which meant that their total daily dose of śavāsana was about one hour per day.)

With the mind calm and quiet, and the body relaxed, śavāsana becomes a perfect segue into the practices of prāṇāyāma and meditation, which, for those who are able, can be practiced in peaceful seated positions.

OTHER ĀSANAS

Because the body is a singular unit with all anatomical regions being physiologically interconnected, in reality all poses (āsanas) that can be tolerated without strain or discomfort will have benefits that will ultimately be of value to the heart and blood vessels. That is why many experts who have worked in the field of Yoga Therapy geared toward cardiovascular illness do not distinguish between any one particular āsana as being superior to another. Having said this, because there are so many āsanas to choose from in the entire field of Yoga (by some estimates, 84,000 Yoga poses exist), in this continually evolving, relatively new discipline of Yoga Therapy for patients with cardiovascular diseases, a few underlying principles can help guide us in selecting the best āsanas and āsana sequences for each patient.

As it is for the basic underlying principles in Yoga, these same principles apply in Yoga Therapy for patients with cardiovascular system illnesses: No forcing or straining, relaxed breath, focused yet calm, serene mind with an engaged, optimistic attitude intent on a healing outcome. Practicing the prescribed āsanas (poses) with an indifferent, apathetic, or even hopeless attitude will not yield positive, concrete results. At the same time, an overzealous participant who is in a hurry to heal is at risk of injury or exacerbation of an underlying cardiovascular condition. A balance between a patient, sober, measured effort and hopeful, eager, enthusiasm must be struck. Also, a certain degree of flexibility and patience on the part of the Yoga Therapist must be applied in remembering that certain poses may need to be modified to best meet the individual health requirements of each patient.

While Dr. Ornish has described the āsana sequence he successfully used in his program for reversing heart disease in his first bestselling book, *Dr. Dean Ornish's Program for Reversing Heart Disease* (1990), during the decade since, his āsana sequence has been somewhat scaled back and simplified to make it more inclusive to a wider range of people suffering from various types of cardiovascular disease.

EXTEND THE SPINE/EXPAND THE CHEST

In my work with patients with heart disease and diseases of the blood vessels, there is an interesting relationship between the spine and heart that, when properly understood, can become a guiding principle in āsana selection and routines for patients in this category. While the finding is based on clinical observations alone and needs to be more thoroughly researched, in general, poses that extend the spine, and consequently expand the chest, appear to benefit the patient with heart disease and diseases of the blood vessels, provided they can be easily tolerated and that no forcing or straining occurs in their execution.

The beneficial mechanism that occurs with spinal extension appears to be simply mechanical, but there are biochemical benefits that also may be involved. Because the chest is expanded when the spine is extended, with an expanded chest, there is more space created in the region of the heart. The lungs are also able to open and expand to a greater degree with poses (āsanas) that help to extend the spine. Postures (āsanas) that help extend the spine and expand the chest appear to increase both blood flow and oxygenation to the heart and lungs as well as all the organs in the body that are consequently served by the circulatory system.

Some of the evidence for the benefits to the cardiovascular system seen in these types of poses can be appreciated when studying what happens in the reverse scenario. For example, it is well known that many heart attacks occur when a person is bending forward, to, let's say, tie a shoelace. The forward bent position (known as spinal flexion) compresses the chest, forcing the abdomen and diaphragm against it, which decreases the space for the heart, as well as the lungs, restricting their movement, diminishing blood flow as well as oxygenation to both the heart and lungs. The entire circulatory system becomes impaired, as does the other organs in the body that are dependent on adequate blood flow. The diaphragm, which helps to regulate breathing, is further impaired in such a flexion position. Among other things, all of these changes can severely compromise bloodflow to the heart muscle, precipitating a heart attack in a heart that is already in a compromised condition of health. In patients with enlarged abdomens due to obesity, these adverse effects are even more pronounced.

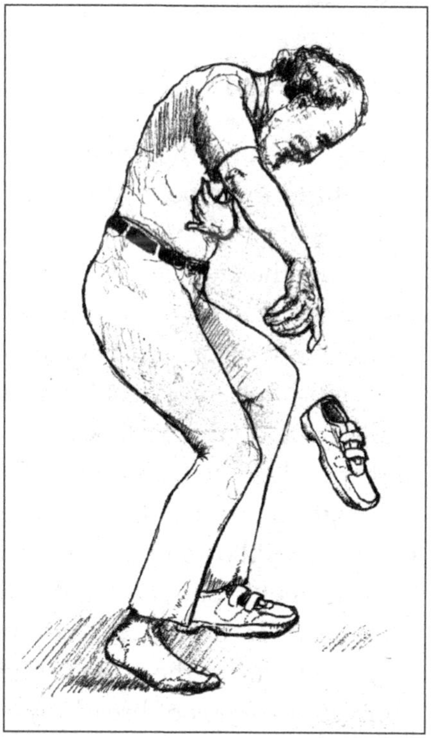

People with kyphotic (bent forward in the upper spine) curves in their spine (think of the Hunchback of Notre Dame) are known to be prone to breathing problems related to reduced lung volumes and diminished ability to oxygenate the heart and blood. The bent forward position compresses the lungs and reduces their ability to expand and fill up with oxygen. Many of these patients go on to have shortened life spans and may develop heart conditions in their later years. Spinal extension helps to correct kyphosis and reverse the factors that serve to compress the heart and lungs and circulation.

In the decade that I worked with Dr. Dean Ornish, a large percentage of the patients I saw had undergone previous spine surgery prior to their developing heart disease. So, although it has not been studied as thoroughly as it needs to be, there appears to be a clear link between spinal posture and cardiovascular disease. Perhaps this is why the health of the spine has always been such a central principle in the field of Yoga.

SUPINE POSES

After śavāsana, although it is not a hard and fast rule, it is convenient for patients to continue on to poses done in the supine position (see illustrations opposite). It is an easy transition because they are already lying on their backs. Simple poses that bring the knees toward the chest, one knee at a time, as tolerated, with gentle breathing, and no forcing or straining, followed by simple leg raises and then hamstring stretches can help to loosen and warm the muscles in the lower extremities, hips, and lower spine, while improving circulation. Gentle spinal twisting while lying on the back, knees bent and slowly brought to one side of the body and then the other can follow. Each pose can be maintained for 30 seconds or so, although for some patients, 15 seconds or less may be all they can tolerate in the beginning. Pillows or bolsters can be incorporated to help support the knees if needed. As the patient demonstrates he/she can tolerate it, over time, each pose can be extended to 1 to 2 minutes or more, provided they are comfortable. Be sure not to hurry the patient during or between any of these movements. Maintaining awareness of breath throughout is essential to a successful supine āsana routine. Remember to allow adequate time for rest and recovery of breath and heart rate in between each pose.

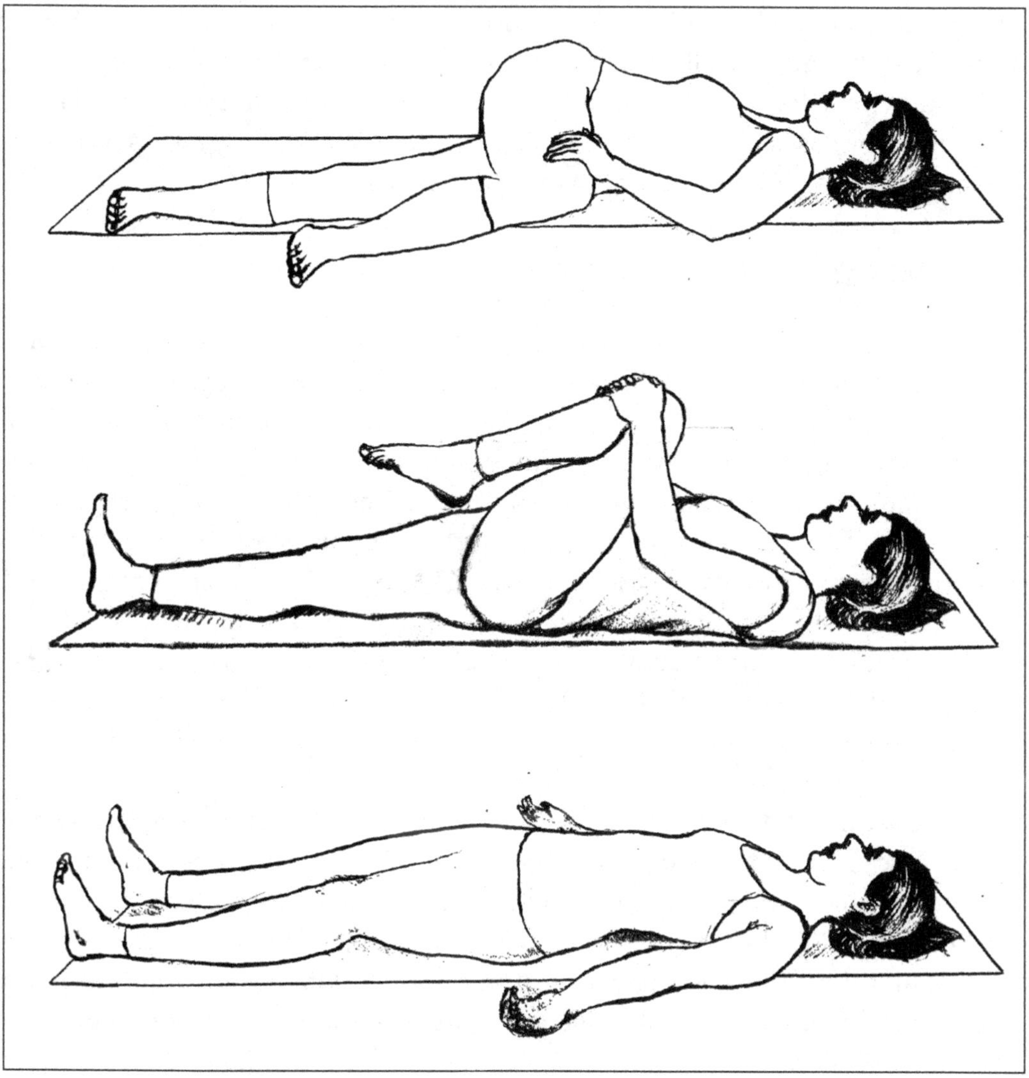

Supine Routine

INVERTED POSES

While generally contraindicated for those with high blood pressure and certain forms of heart disease, Dr. Ornish has used a very gentle modified inverted pose whereby patients, still lying on their backs, can place both feet and legs up on a chair or against the wall. There should be no forcing or straining and the patient should feel comfortable during this practice. Inverted poses aid the return of blood from the feet, reduce swelling in the lower extremities, and act as a gentle overall aid to the circulatory system. But it is important not to overdo them, especially in the beginning, as they can raise blood pressure if done in excess, especially in patients with fragile or weak cardiovascular systems.

ABDOMINAL POSTURES/ĀSANAS

From laying on the back, patients can be gently transitioned to a series of abdominal poses, as tolerated. Because of the intense abdominal pressure generated by these poses, in addition to the pressure that is exerted on the chest and heart, this series requires a very cautious, conservative approach in the beginning, especially among those patients who have recently undergone major open heart surgery, have suffered a recent heart attack, have high blood pressure, or have any other underlying cardiovascular condition that contributes to a weakened, fragile heart. Breath awareness is critical to this series of āsanas (poses). In this respect, it is important not to hold the breath, in spite of the abdominal pressure sometimes impairing the ability to breathe freely. It is also important to remind patients not to eat for three hours prior to a Yoga Therapy session, especially when abdominal poses are introduced.

Once on the abdomen, patients can lay with their feet slightly apart. Hands and arms can be folded underneath the head—which can then be turned to one side or the other. The position is sometimes called makarāsana (crocodile pose), but it can be modified to suit the needs of the patient. Pillows or props can be used at any time to make a patient feel more comfortable. With the eyes gently closed, mind focused on breath, this is the preferred resting position in between abdominal āsanas.

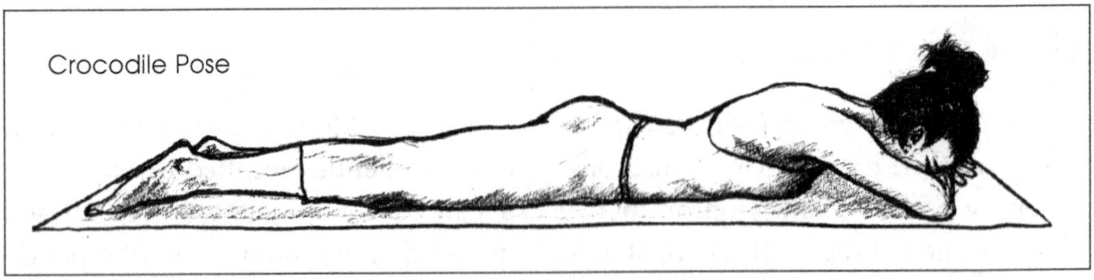

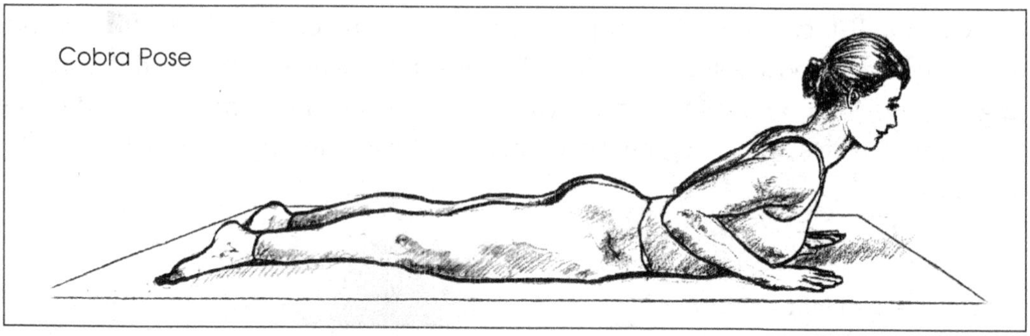

Gentle bhujaṅgāsana (cobra pose) without forcing or straining, and without breath-holding, can be performed one to three times, holding anywhere from 5–10 seconds, building up to 30 seconds and beyond, each time, slowly increasing the amount of time in the pose slowly but steadily as tolerated over several weeks to months. Cobra pose helps extend and strengthen the spine while opening the chest, creating more space for the heart and lungs. This improves blood flow and oxygen to the heart and blood vessels. It also helps to tone the abdomen and core further stabilizing the spine and contributing to improved posture.

After cobra pose, ardha salabhāsana (half-locust pose) can be performed a maximum of one to three times, as tolerated, following the same timing as cobra pose. Full locust pose should be postponed until the patient has been performing half locust for at least three to six months without any discomfort in the chest region. In fact, many Yoga Therapists who work with cardiovascular patients consider full locust optional at best, and probably not worth the risk of agitating the heart, due to the intense pressure felt in the abdomen and chest with this pose. For these reasons, half locust, practiced sincerely, is generally considered safer and of more of a reliable benefit in the long run for patients with cardiovascular illness.

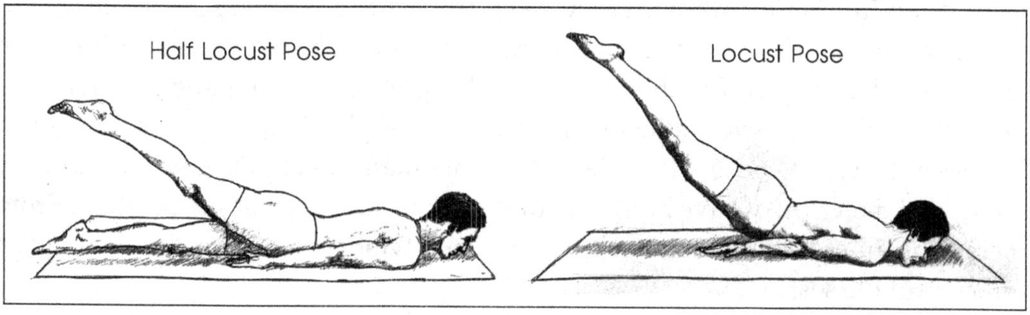

Once half-locust pose is completed, patients can remain in caturaṅgadaṇḍ-āsana (crocodile pose—still on their abdomens) for a brief rest/relaxation/breathing respite. After 5 minutes or more in crocodile pose, this signals the end of the abdominal series for a beginning course of Yoga Therapy for cardiovascular patients.

Fish Pose with Props

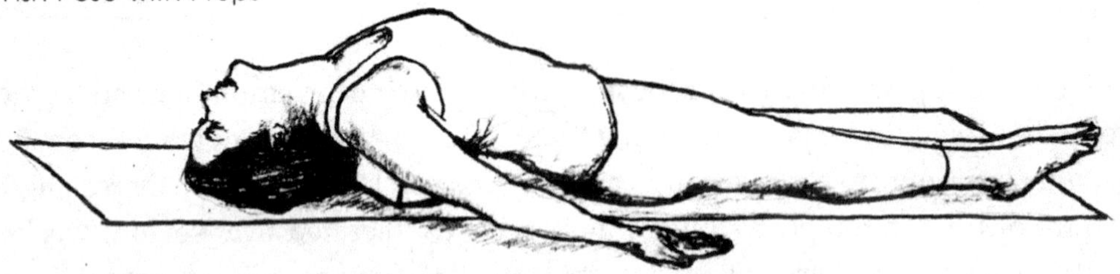

From the abdominal position, the patient can gently turn back onto his/her back. A pillow can be positioned lengthwise and placed underneath the spine to help support the patient in matyāsana (fish pose). Alternatively, a bolster or folded blanket can be used for support in arching the spine in this position. Make sure the neck, while arched backward, is not strained in any way. This is an excellent pose for extending the spine, opening the chest, and expanding the space for the heart and lungs. People experiencing chest pain will often find almost instantaneous relief in this position, especially when it is supported by slow, deep, gentle breathing. It is relatively safe and easy to perform, requiring very little energy output, thus reducing the possibility of straining the heart in any way. Remember to have the patient keep his/her shoulders relaxed as he/she focuses on his/her breathing. Try to see if the patient can feel his/her chest and heart widening and opening in this pose. Continue to have the patient breath in and out as he/she comfortably maintains this position. If the patient is not comfortable, make whatever adjustments are necessary to help him/her remain in this very beneficial pose. Have the patient maintain this final pose for a minute or so, and then slowly have him/her come back to a resting supine position. From here, it is an easy transition back to śavāsana, which should be the final āsana practice of the session.

ŚAVĀSANA AT CLOSE OF ĀSANA SEQUENCE

Make sure you give a generous dose of śavāsana (20 to 30 minutes) at the end of the āsana practice routine to not only give the patient adequate time to experience deep relaxation but to ground him/her in the rhythm of this amount of time required for śavāsana to work its proven therapeutic magic. I say *magic* because I have seen impossible conditions of the heart and blood vessels get significantly better with the regular practice of this technique, especially when done in conjunction with other lifestyle changes as recommended by Dr. Ornish. Plus, early studies with Yoga and blood pressure, as reported by Dr. Datey and Dr. Chandra Patel, relied almost exclusively on śavāsana to document Yoga's ability to lower blood pressure.

In today's hurry-up world of stress and high-speed living (e.g., "life in the fast lane"), there is a tendency to look for shortcuts while cutting corners to save time. Even in the world of Western Yoga, this exists, and, unfortunately, when it occurs, śavāsana is usually the first āsana practice to get cut from the routine. This is a critical mistake I have consistently witnessed in health clubs, spas, and Yoga studios across the United States for the past thirty years, a mistake I must confess I have also made while teaching Yoga in such venues. Unfortunately, this is a bad habit that should not get transferred to the field of Yoga Therapy, especially when attempting to introduce Yoga to patients with cardiovascular disease because, ultimately, the entire effort of integrating Yoga into Western medicine will become seriously diluted when śavāsana is short changed. Śavāsana is the most underrated, and yet one of the most powerful practices in the entire field of Yoga Therapy that can be safely and effectively administered to even the most seriously ill patient with cardiovascular disease. As such, it should be respected and given its full measure of time to work so that it can be properly used for the powerful therapeutic practice that it is.

STANDING POSES

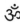

Standing poses are to be approached very cautiously and are generally avoided in the beginning sessions of Yoga Therapy for heart patients for several reasons. First, poor balance is a common issue especially for the senior population and age groups in which heart disease and blood vessel diseases are most prevalent. Those who have suffered from strokes will often find standing poses very difficult, at least to start out on. Second, many heart patients and patients with high blood pressure are often on multiple drug regimens of upward of ten to twenty different powerful medications. Many of these drugs interfere with normal adaptive changes in blood pressure that allows for adequate blood flow to the brain when these patients are standing. They can often experience light-headedness and dizziness, due to the effects of the medication, which can cause a dangerous drop in blood pressure. This phenomenon is known as orthostatic hypotension. Falls with resultant head trauma, including skull fractures and concussions, are not uncommon in this group.

This isn't to say that standing poses are to be avoided altogether in all patients with cardiovascular disease. In fact, as they progress with the other āsanas, and develop their stamina and flexibility, standing poses can be gently introduced and, in the long run, will be of significant benefit in reducing the amount of falls due to improving balance and stability. Standing poses can improve balance, as well as leg strength. But in the beginning, it is safer to not introduce them for at least three to six months or so.

SITTING POSES

Most traditional schools of Yoga in India emphasize the importance of sitting with a straight spine in one or more of a number of seated āsanas, including lotus pose, specifically for the practices of prāṇāyāma and meditation. But for most Americans, especially those with cardiovascular disease who may never have practiced Yoga before, in the beginning of their practice, they will find it intolerable to sit on the floor in even a modified form of one or more of the traditional Yoga seated poses. A chair will most likely be more comfortable as they learn to develop breath awareness and quiet their mind through the practices of prāṇāyāma and meditation.

BREATHING/PRĀṆĀYĀMA

Generally, for people with cardiovascular diseases, yogic breathing can be introduced at any time. Matra Majmundar, an occupational therapist and colleague at Stanford Medical Center who worked on the heart transplant service, taught prāṇāyāma techniques to patients in the ICU who had recently returned from the operating room for heart transplant surgery. They were just waking up from their anesthesia, still intubated with breathing tubes in place, still connected to ventilators, as she helped allay their anxiety by gently guiding them through a series of prāṇāyāma breathing practices that helped calm and relax their minds. Sedative and anti-anxiety drug use, normally administered postoperatively to these patients, was significantly reduced through her work.

For most patients, as it is for Yoga students and practitioners in general, prāṇāyāma is usually practiced in one of the more traditional Yoga seated poses. However, for many patients with cardiovascular disease, especially Westerners who may have arthritic joints, bad knees, hips, or spines, etc., a chair is often required, at least in the beginning. Some patients may even need to start out practicing breathing in some other modified supine or reclining position such as śavāsana (corpse pose). The simpler, gentler prāṇāyāma practices, such as ujjāyi (breathing with sound) or anuloma viloma (alternate nostril breathing) or one or more of their variations, are preferred over some of the more vigorous forms of prāṇāyāma, such as kapālabhāti (high-frequency diaphragmatic breathing, with forced exhalation and passive inhalation), at least in the beginning (Kuvalayananda, 1931).

Prāṇāyāma helps to calm and quiet the mind, reduce anxiety, and soothe the nervous system, while setting the stage for meditation. In fact, for some, prāṇāyāma itself can serve as a form of meditation. Either way, prāṇāyāma, although mediated through the breath, works on the higher centers of the brain to slow down and calm the mind and nervous system. This has a calming, soothing effect on the cardiovascular system, including the heart and blood vessels. Prāṇāyāma has the ability to help reduce heart rate, lower blood pressure, and reduce oxygen consumption of the heart and body (Upadhyay, 2008).

As the breath is known to be the link between the body and the mind, prāṇāyāma has traditionally been valued for its powerful influence on the nervous system. So powerful is its influence that Swami Kuvalayanda and his colleagues at Kaivalayadhama used to call prāṇāyāma the quintessential practice for "nerve culture." (Kuvalayananda, 1931). In other words, we can educate and modify our nervous systems through our breath. It is not surprising to know that this is how many great yogis, such as Swami Rama and others, were able to exert such tremendous control over their hearts and blood vessels.

When practiced properly, prāṇāyāma neutralizes stress and the fight-or-flight response by activating the relaxation response, which slows the heart rate, lowers blood pressure, decreases oxygen consumption, and decreases sympathetic nervous system activity, all of which decrease the workload and strain on the heart and the blood vessels. Prāṇāyāma should be taught in a way that encourages the patient's breath to be smooth and relaxed.

A patient may start with two to three rounds of ujjāyi (breathing with sound) or anuloma viloma (alternate nostril breathing) and may slowly increase to up to ten rounds of each per session. By slowing the breath, making it smoother and deeper, with each inhalation and exhalation, the patient should notice a pleasant calming quality with the practice. While 15 to 20 minutes or 30 minutes a day may be devoted to prāṇāyāma, the benefits of prāṇāyāma will accrue with regularity of practice.

MEDITATION

Meditation, or dhyāna, according to Patañjali, is the seventh stage of yogic practice that leads to samādhi, the highest stage of conscious evolution in the yogic path. Meditation encompasses many different methods and techniques, which have, as their common goal, a very focused, profound sense of mental quietude that leads to total absorption of consciousness in the present moment. A meditative state is one that reflects an expanded awareness, deep peace and serene contentment, as well as an elevation of consciousness. It is intensely therapeutic and healing, and exerts an extremely calming influence on the nervous system and cardiovascular system. Dr. Dean Ornish has used meditation for many years as an integral part of the stress management component in his program for reversing heart disease.

Maharishi Mahesh Yogi, with his famous students, The Beatles, introduced and popularized meditation in the West. His particular style, known as TM, or Transcendental Meditation, is based on an ancient yogic technique whereby a specific mantra, which is a word or phrase charged with a spiritual meaning and vibrational quality, is repeated a set number of times. The traditional number is 108. This results in a deep calming and quieting of the mind and a relaxation of the heart and blood vessels. Studies more than forty years ago at Harvard with Dr. Herbert Benson, who used a variation of the Maharishi's technique, scientifically proved that meditation could lower blood pressure. It was through this work that Dr. Benson discovered the relaxation response, the neurophysiological antithesis of the fight-or-flight reaction, which has been found to significantly reduce stress while helping to restore and maintain superior health of the heart and blood vessels.

When introducing meditation to patients with cardiovascular disease, there may be some confusion as to the meaning of the word, what it implies, and how to practice it. For many Westerners, meditation can be a very foreign and threatening concept. A good Yoga Therapist working with patients with cardiovascular disease will take the time to give an introduction to the subject of meditation in general, will answer all questions and allay all fears, and will carefully explain and demonstrate the techniques of the various methods that he/she will introduce to the patient. He/she will then gently introduce the subject on a practical level with, perhaps, some simple prāṇāyāma or oṁ chanting. A number of different methods of meditation may be introduced over time, including meditating on a sound, a mantra, or some other method, including the integration of creative guided imagery or visualization if the therapist has training in these techniques. Even deep, thoughtful prayer can be considered a form of meditation.

Over time, patients will be encouraged to choose one or more preferred techniques for their own individual meditation practice. And while it may take a while to find a favorite meditation technique, and because our tastes may change over time, so might our preferred meditation technique change. Traditionally, with the body supple and relaxed after āsanas, and the mind calm, focused, and serene after prāṇāyāma, meditation can be practiced for up to 30 minutes at a time or more. As with all practices in Yoga, the key to success with meditation is regularity of practice.

A WORD ON A YOGIC DIET FOR THE CARDIOVASCULAR SYSTEM

While many people believe that diet is a totally separate subject from Yoga or Yoga Therapy, they are very much mistaken. Many diseases of the Western world, such as heart disease, high blood pressure, diabetes, and cancer, which Albert Schweitzer correctly identified as "diseases of modern civilization," have been directly linked to not only stress but to our faulty diets (Schweitzer, 2009). The rising epidemic of obesity, which predisposes us to the clogged arteries seen in coronary artery disease (which sets the stage for fatal heart attacks), has also been strongly linked to diabetes as well as hypertension. Obesity is an example of how out of balance our diets and eating habits have become.

The Sanskrit word *mitahara,* described in ancient yogic texts, such as Gorakshanatha's *Haṭha Yoga Pradīpikā,* as well as in the *Upaniṣads,* describes dietary guidelines for those interested in attaining success in Yoga. The underlying premise of mitahara is one of moderation in food intake, while emphasis has traditionally been on a primarily plant-based, low-fat diet as superior to all others for this purpose. The average American diet at present is anything but this. If you study the recommended diet of Dr. Dean Ornish, which he has found so integral to his reversing heart disease program, you will find precise dietary guidelines that were advised by the ancient Yoga masters, which you can pass on to your patients.

> *"Take half stomachful of wholesome food. Fill a quarter with pure water. Leave the rest free. This is Mitahara. Mitahara plays a vital part in keeping up perfect health. Almost all diseases are due to irregularity of meals, overeating and unwholesome food."*
>
> —SWAMI SIVANANDA

BHAKTI YOGA/KARMA YOGA

Bringing the spirit of Yoga into everyday life and creating a healthy yogic lifestyle is the ultimate goal of Yoga. It is also the goal of Yoga Therapy for people suffering with cardiovascular disease. Although the point of embarkation, as well as the motivation for stepping onto the yogic path, may initially seem to differ, in reality, the spiritual path of Yoga and the healing path of Yoga Therapy are ultimately one and the same. The saying, "All roads lead to Rome," applies to both aspects of Yoga.

As Dr. Ornish has repeatedly reminded us, Yoga Therapy for the cardiovascular system is not just about opening arteries, improving blood flow to the heart, lowering blood pressure, and normalizing blood sugar, even though as he proved through his meticulous research, it can do all of these things. Beyond these physiological improvements, applying the principles of Yoga in the spirit of living more from our hearts, in the spirit of love, is the ultimate goal of Yoga Therapy for those suffering with cardiovascular disease. This concept is the same goal that Patañjali wrote about centuries ago in his *Yoga Sūtras.* In Sūtra 1.23, he says, "Īśvara praṇidhānad Va" and describes that one of the ways to attain samādhi is through surrender to the divine, which exists within us all.

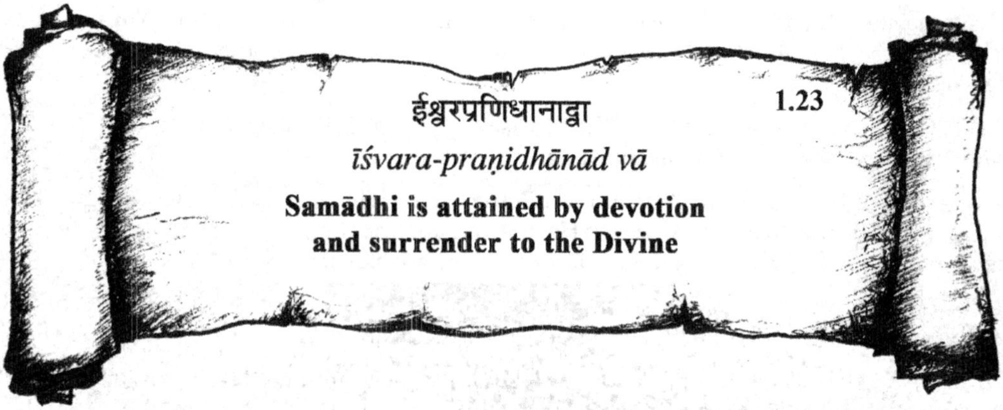
ईश्वरप्रणिधानाद्वा
1.23
īśvara-praṇidhānād vā
Samādhi is attained by devotion
and surrender to the Divine

"The physical heart is a metaphor for the spiritual heart."

—DR. DEAN ORNISH (Ornish, 1999)

In the fields of Bhakti Yoga and Karma Yoga, which are not confined to a Yoga mat, but, rather, exist with the realm of our everyday lives, becoming a lover of the divine as well as a selfless servant of humanity are the twin qualities ascribed to some of the greatest saints and Yoga masters of the past, as well as to those of us who aspire to such lofty goals in the present and the future. As *Yoga* means union and describes both the goal and process of attaining this goal, the purpose of our lives should be to become one with the Divine Living Source of Love, the greatest healing power in the universe, which exists within us all. This is the promise that Yoga and Yoga Therapy hold for all of humanity. Let us realize this true Spirit of Yoga and serve this Spirit with all our hearts, minds, and souls.

REFERENCES

Benson, H., J. F. Beary, and M. P. Carol. "The Relaxation Response." *Psychiatry* 37.1 (1974): 37–46. Print.

Benson, H. *The Relaxation Response.* New York: Harper Collins, 1975. Print.

Boston Medical Library at the Francis Countway Library of Medicine. Distributed by Harvard University Press, Cambridge, Mass.

Brownstein, A. H., and M. L. Dembert. "Treatment of Essential Hypertension with Yoga Relaxation Therapy in a USAF Aviator: A Case Report." *Aviation, Space, Environmental Medicine* 60.7 (1989): 684–687. Print.

CDC (Centers for Disease Control). "Heart Disease." 9 Jan. 2013. Web. Retrieved 21 Feb. 2014. http://www.cdc.gov/nchs/fastats/heart.htm.

———. "High Blood Pressure." 2013. Web. Retrieved 21 Feb. 2014. http://www.cdc.gov/bloodpressure/. PDF available from American Heart Association at http://www.heart.org/idc/groups/heart-public/@wcm/@sop/@smd/documents/downloadable/ucm_319587.pdf.

———. "2011 National Diabetes Fact Sheet." 24 Oct. 2013. Web. Retrieved 21 Feb. 2014. http://www.cdc.gov/diabetes/pubs/factsheet11/fastfacts.htm.

Datey, K. K., et al. "Shavasana: A Yogic Exercise in the Management of Hypertension." *Angiology* 20 (1969): 325–333. Print

Kuvalayananda, S. *Pranayama*. Lonavala, India: Kaivalyadhama Press, 1931, 61–76. Web. Ebook download available at http://www.scribd.com/doc/150994782/pranayama-1931-from-kuvalayanand-of-lonavala.

Oglesby P. *The Caring Physician: The Life of Dr. Francis W. Peabody*. Cambridge, MA: Boston Medical Library in the Countway Library of Medicine, 1991. Print.

Ornish, D. *Love and Survival*, New York: Harper Collins, 1999. Print.

Ornish, D., et al. "Can Lifestyle Changes Reverse Coronary Heart Disease?" *Lancet* 336.8708 (1990): 129–133. Print.

Patel, C. "Yoga and Bio-Feedback in the Management of Hypertension." *Lancet* 302.7837 (1973): 1053–1055. Print.

——. "12-Month Follow-Up of Yoga and Bio-Feedback in the Management of Hypertension." *Lancet* 305. 7898 (1975): 62–64. Print.

Patel, C., and W. R. North. "Randomized Controlled Trial of Yoga and Bio-Feedback in the Management of Hypertension." *Lancet* 2.7925 (1975): 93–95. Print.

Raghavendra, B. R., et al. "Voluntary Heart Rate Reduction Following Yoga Using Different Strategies." *International Journal of Yoga* 6.1 (2013): 26–30. Print.

Satchidananda, S. *The Yoga Sutras of Patanjali: Commentary on the Raja Yoga Sutras*. Yogaville: Integral Yoga Publications, 1990. Print.

Schweitzer, A. *Out of My Life and Thought*. Baltimore: Johns Hopkins University Press, 2009. Print.

Silverman, M. (2003). *The Quotable Osler*. Philadelphia: American College of Physicians, 2003. Print.

Upadhyay, D. K. "Effect of Alternate Nostril Breathing Exercise on Cardiorespiratory Functions." *Nepal Medical College Journal* 10.1 (2008): 25–27. Print.

Wenger, M. A., B. Bagchi, and B. K. Anand. "Experiments in India on 'Voluntary' Control of the Heart and Pulse." *Circulation* 24 (1961): 1319–1325. Print.

Yoga Therapy for Rehabilitation Professionals

Matthew J. Taylor, P.T., Ph.D., E-RYT500

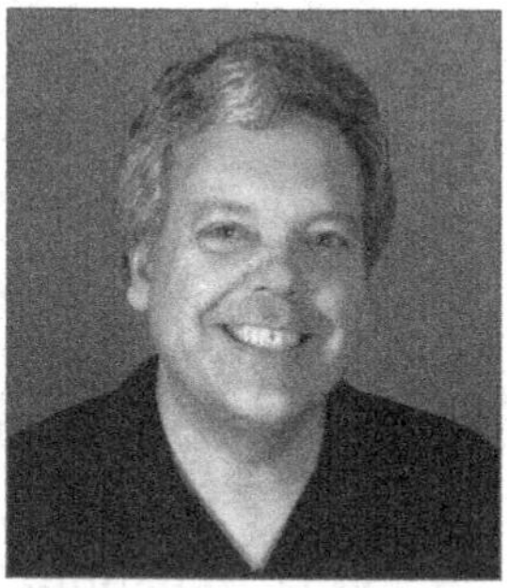

Matthew J. Taylor has over thirty years of clinical experience in orthopedic and sports physical therapy. A leader in advancing rehabilitation toward a gentle, integral, whole person approach, he received his master's degree in physical therapy from Baylor University in 1981 and a Ph.D. from the California Institute of Integral Studies with an emphasis on adult education in transformational learning and change. Dr. Taylor served as a physical therapist and active duty Army Medical Specialist officer in the United States Army from 1980 through 1988 and became a certified, advanced level Yoga Therapist in 1998. Since then, Dr. Taylor has taught hundreds of licensed rehabilitation professionals how to integrate mind-body science into traditional rehabilitation and has published two books. He also served as both the president of the International Association of Yoga Therapists (from 2008–2010) and as the IAYT representative on the board of the Academic Consortium for Complementary and Alternative Health Care.

INTRODUCTION

This chapter is for medical rehabilitation professionals. Chances are that through either personal or clinical experience there is some curiosity about the therapeutic potential of Yoga and how to bridge that experience with traditional paradigms. This chapter brings together many facets of Yoga Therapy in rehabilitation I wish I knew when my interest was first piqued in 1996.

We begin by discussing the increasing popularity of Yoga Therapy and the relationships between Yoga, mind-body science, and modern physical rehabilitation. In particular, the rehabilitation professions are abuzz about finding a whole-person or bio-psychosocial approach to care, and you will learn how such an approach is the heart of Yoga Therapy in a brief history and description of the paradigms shaping Yoga therapeutic principles. Then, the most common examination and intervention principles are described in functional detail. The chapter concludes with a vision for the future of Yoga Therapy and rehabilitation.

THE DEFINITION OF YOGA THERAPY

What is Yoga Therapy? Who can do Yoga Therapy? How is it like traditional rehabilitation? The short answer is that, while Yoga Therapy is rooted in ancient principles, it is quite embryonic in its emergence into Western culture and medicine. Right now [at the time of publication] anyone may claim to be a Yoga Therapist because there are no accepted standards nor is there a definitive scope of practice. Still, Yoga Therapy shares many commonalities with traditional rehabilitation, including practitioners offering to deliver therapeutic relief of ailments and consumers seeking to gain relief from the practitioners. This has been the natural and often unconscious enculturation of Yoga into the Western healthcare model. Unfortunately, the process has also constrained Yoga's full therapeutic potential. In order to embrace the greatest possibility Yoga Therapy offers rehabilitation professionals, let's start by defining Yoga Therapy.

In December 2007, the International Association of Yoga Therapists (IAYT) offered its first definition of Yoga Therapy following eighteen years of discussion and discernment (Taylor, 2007). Each word was carefully chosen to provide an in-depth understanding of Yoga Therapy relative to rehabilitation:

> *"Yoga Therapy is the process of empowering individuals to progress toward improved health and well-being through the application of the philosophy and practice of Yoga."*

Process/Progress Toward: Yoga Therapy is an ongoing process versus an event. The primary complaint is understood to be a single manifestation of imbalance in health rather than an isolated part to be fixed. Hence an extended inquiry and adaptation of behaviors can provide relief even beyond the resolution of the original complaint. In general, Yoga Therapy is better suited for persistent lifestyle-related complaints rather than acute maladies or traumas.

Empowering: A Yoga Therapy practice rejects the disempowering "expert fixes the broken" model of health and rightfully restores the responsibility and power of healing to the individual.

Toward Health and Well-Being: Yoga Therapy is health care, not sick care. It is a wellness model for optimizing the health of not only the individual but the individual's relationships, community, and planet. Yoga Therapy is not a pathology-based model. It focuses on what is working versus what is lost or dysfunctional and optimizes what can be optimized. Yoga Therapy even offers a person in late-stage terminal disease various processes and practices to move toward healing and wholeness.

Application: Yoga Therapy is a practice that requires action and discipline. Passivity, dependence, and detachment have no place in the process.

Philosophy and Practice: Yoga Therapy is more than postures. Yoga Therapy is a holistic life science, a bio-psychosocial model of wellness that covers every aspect of the human experience from pregestation to death. Practice of the methods and technologies of Yoga without the study of the philosophy reduces Yoga Therapy to just another mechanistic model of pathology.

YOGA THERAPY AND THE INTERDEPENDENCE MODEL

The previous definition of Yoga Therapy is neither exhaustive nor complete, but it does serve the purpose of highlighting contrasts to our rehabilitative paradigms. Contrast that definition with the new paradigm in orthopedic physical therapy that suggests the hip may actually influence function in the shoulder. In the guest editorial of the November 2007 *Journal of Orthopedic and Sports Physical Therapy,* editors proclaimed, "Regional Interdependence: A Musculoskeletal Examination Model Whose Time Has Come." Most important, the editorial concludes, "Further investigation of the regional-interdependence concept in a systematic fashion may add clarity to the nature of many musculoskeletal problems and guide subsequent decision making in clinical care. Regional interdependence is a model whose time has come" (Wainer, et al., 2007).

While such an interdependence model is very helpful in managing rehabilitation cases, the historical context has been lost. Over 3,000 years ago, the *Taittirīya Upaniṣad* of the Indian Vedanta describes the five yogic sheaths, or kośas, which are described in detail in this text in Gary Kraftsow and Claire Collins's chapter "The American Viniyoga Institute," Joseph Le Page's chapter "Integrative Yoga Therapy," and Mukunda and Chinnamasta Stiles's chapter "Structural Yoga Therapy and Ayurvedic Yoga Therapy." The kośa model of body integration extolls the value of understanding that, not only is physical regional interdependence important in optimizing health, so too are all of the other aspects of the human experience, including social, emotional, psychological, and spiritual influences. The kośa model bears many similarities to both the regional interdependence model and the bio-psychosocial model used in rehabilitation. Historically, it is then more accurate to say that the new models in rehabilitation resemble the earlier kośa model from India.

So how does this ancient model and its techniques and technologies fit in with traditional rehabilitation and mind-body medicine in the West?

YOGA THERAPY IN A WESTERN MEDICINE CONTEXT

Yoga is classified as part of complementary and alternative medicine (CAM) as defined by the National Center for Complementary and Alternative Medicine (NCCAM). CAM is a group of diverse medical and healthcare systems, practices, services, and products that aren't part of conventional medicine. A recent survey revealed that of those who used Yoga specifically for therapeutic purposes, 21 percent did so because it was recommended by a conventional medical professional, 31 percent did so because conventional therapies were ineffective and 59 percent thought it would be an interesting therapy to explore. Through such means, Yoga has gained popularity in Western culture and is now the most common mind-body therapy in Western complementary medicine (Wolsko, et al., 2004). Yoga Therapy's unique ability to facilitate spiritual, physical, and psychological benefits is appealing as a cost-effective alternative to conventional interventions.

Yoga Therapy is an emerging field with a professional association of over 3,000 members, 40 percent of whom have dual training to include physical therapists, occupational therapists, and speech and language pathologists. The organization, the International Association of Yoga Therapists (IAYT), has sponsored annual research symposiums since 2007 with researchers from around the world to build its evidence base and solidify its rightful place in the Western conversation of health and medicine. IAYT's *International Journal of Yoga Therapy* has been listed on PubMed since 2011.

Reading like the scope of a physical therapist, Yoga Therapy utilizes movement, proprioception/awareness, breath modification, and education principles as tools for rehabilitation. Conceptually, it is important to know that Yoga refers to that enormous body of precepts, attitudes, techniques, and spiritual values that have been developed in India for over 5,000 years. Yoga describes a method of discipline or means of discovering the integral nature of the body and mind (i.e., modern mind-body science), and it is considered a standard practice in Eastern medicine. It is only our parochial perspective that makes Yoga Therapy appear "new" or foreign as a therapy in the West.

GUIDING PHILOSOPHICAL CONCEPTS WITH REHABILITATION IMPLICATIONS

Yoga originally developed with origins from the Hindu, Jain, and Buddhist traditions, but it is not a religion itself. Yoga is a philosophical life science with practical applications. Thus, the practice of Yoga is congruent with all religious traditions and demands no belief in deities or practices that would conflict with an individual's spiritual tradition. The physical postures and motor performance outcomes, which characterize so much of Yoga within Western culture, is solely a by-product of what is more accurately described as a technology for the evolution of the mind or consciousness. Therefore, Yoga Therapy provides an experiential bridge to the emerging mind-body science of current pain and motor theories. The felt sense or awareness by the individual of the mind-body connection is actually the rediscovery of what has been the basis of the practice of Yoga for thousands of years. The basic tenet of all branches of Yoga focuses not just on conceptualization of this connection but also on literally experiencing the unity of the mind and body, as well as developing spiritual, psychological, and physical health.

The eight-limbed path of Yoga outlined by Patañjali in Chapter 2, Sūtra 29 of the *Yoga Sūtras* acts as a practical science for the relationships between thoughts, emotions, memories, intentions, and actions. As seen in the figure on page 268, each limb emphasizes moral and ethical conduct as well as self-discipline (Taylor, 1998). Traditionally, the student begins with the yamas (moral precepts) and niyamas (qualities to nourish). When well grounded in the practice of the first two limbs, the student embarks on the other six limbs in a recursive and inclusive application similar to Covey's "Seven Habits" (Covey, 2004).

2.29

यमनियमासनप्राणायामप्रत्याहारधारणाध्यानसमाधयोऽ
ष्टावङ्गानि॥२९॥

Yamaniyamāsanaprāṇāyāmapratyāhāradhāraṇādhyānasamādh
ayo'ṣṭavaṅgāni

The eight limbs of Yoga are yama (moral precepts/ethical restraints), niyama (qualities to nourish/social adherences), asana (postures/movements), pranayama (breathing exercises/energy expansion), pratyahara (sense withdrawal/decreased reactivity to sensation), dharana (concentration), dhyana (meditation), samadhi (absorption/ecstatic union).

PATANJALI'S EIGHT-LIMBED PATH OF YOGA

LIMB	DESCRIPTION
Yamas	Moral precepts: nonharming, truthfulness, nonstealing, chastity, greedlessness
Niyamas	Qualities to nourish: purity, contentment, austerity (exercise), self-study, devotion to a higher power
Āsana	Postures/movements: A calm, firm steady stance in relation to life
Prāṇāyāma	Breathing exercises: The ability to channel and direct breath and life energy (prana)
Pratyāhāra	Decreased reactivity to sensation: Focusing senses inward; nonreactivity to stimuli
Dhāraṇā	Concentration; unwavering attention, commitment
Dhyāna	Meditation; mindfulness, being attuned to the present moment
Samādhi	Ecstatic union; flow; "in the zone"; spiritual support/connection

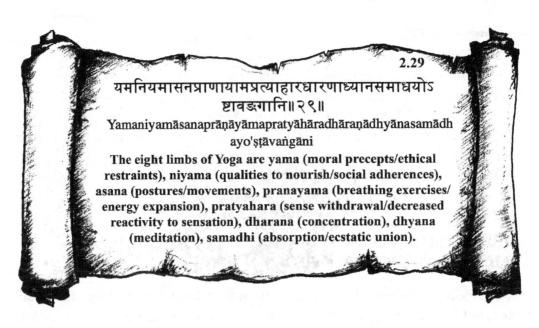

Yoga has developed techniques and technologies for practitioners to question and verify the nature of reality through their direct experience. The techniques and technologies go beyond the Western stereotype of Yoga as complex poses and meditation. An authentic practice of Yoga combines rigorous practice discipline with a wide array of physical and mental exercises rooted in moral and ethical principles that address every aspect of modern life to include consumer patterns, nutritional decisions, and vocational choices. Therefore, utilizing Yoga Therapy allows the patient and therapist to embody a holistic approach to life and health as a wellness and prevention practice designed to generate a lifelong series of healthy lifestyle choices. Since its introduction into Western culture in the late 1880s, there has been a significant shift in emphasis from spiritual outcomes of practice to more physically based outcomes. This shift toward more physical outcomes is the result of the adoption of the West's mechanistic reductionist worldview. Curiously, as Western science advances, it is now coming to reveal that the Yoga model offers a balance of both the Western linear perspective and the Eastern nonlinear perspective of holism as it relates to human health.

THE PRACTICE AND TECHNOLOGIES OF YOGA THERAPY

Yoga Therapy is being used as a treatment in Western culture from major university hospitals to Yoga studios. What is commonly referred to as Yoga in the West is usually Haṭha Yoga, which is comprised of various styles, including, but not limited to, Vinyāsa, Aṣṭāṅga, Bikram, Power, Iyengar, etc. Haṭha focuses on physical postures, deep breathing, and meditation. These practices are what is popular in the media and sold in the gyms. Haṭha's popularity is attributed to its physical familiarity with a typical Western athletic workout. It should be understood not to be the equivalent of Yoga Therapy as Yoga Therapy includes other forms of Yoga, which focus on ethics, mudrā (hand movements/gestures), bhāvana (guided imagery and meditation), jñāna (self-study), and/or diet. All styles of Yoga are believed to lead to the same path of personal fulfillment through self-transformation, yet as described below in the context of health challenges, the tools of Yoga Therapy are far richer and broader than mere Yoga-like postures adapted as therapeutic exercises (Taylor, 2004).

A central feature of Yoga Therapy is that each practice can be modified depending on the participant's abilities and state of health. These characteristics make

Yoga Therapy ideal, accessible, and easy to utilize for all age groups. The only prerequisite for participating in Yoga Therapy is that the participant be breathing. Yoga Therapy stresses the importance of the participant's developing awareness of how what they think, believe, perceive, and have been told influences their physical posture and mobility, the quantity and quality of breathing, and the level of central nervous system vigilance. All of these ultimately affect flexibility, health, and vitality (Taylor, 2004).

Below are descriptions of some of the most frequently used Yoga technologies available to the rehabilitation professional:

1. **Āsanas**, or physical postures, are the third limb of Patañjali's classical eight-limbed system mentioned in the figure on page 268 and have been demonstrated to generate greater cardiovascular fitness, strength, mood modifications, and flexibility (Kolasinski, 2005). Yoga postures teach increased body awareness and optimal biomechanical positioning of the body in space both in static and dynamic movement. Each āsana has a unique focus for enhancing awareness and skill of the effect of thoughts, emotions, memories, and breathing on comfort and stability. The selection of the āsana is far more complex than just a biomechanical assessment to address stability and inflexibility of the musculoskeletal system. Postures for deep relaxation are introduced from the beginning in order to facilitate perception, reflection, and calming of the central nervous system. Maintenance of selected postures allows for the elongation of muscles safely and naturally with gravity assistance and the further discovery of previously unknown postural patterns of holding and tension. The selection and sequencing of āsana includes not only principles that correlate to therapeutic exercise progression but also those that effect breathing patterns, thoughts, emotions, and spiritual insights.

2. To differentiate Yoga Therapy āsana from a traditional rehabilitation use of exercise, consider the following:
   - Follow mindful procedures entering into, holding, and emerging from each āsana.
   - Coordinate and slow down movements while breathing for ease and comfort throughout the āsana.
   - Noting one's breath sensations and other bodily sensations is a commonly

prescribed practice in Yoga Therapy to decrease the agitation and distraction of the thinking mind in the prefrontal cortex of the brain and helps one to become aware of the deeper patterns of fear, attraction, and revulsion found in the limbic system of the brain.

- Every āsana has a counter-āsana. Deliberate, careful movements that make up the experience of āsana explore the polarities of one's experience and are ancient processes that now in modern rehabilitation terminology are known as "pacing, scaling, graded exposure, and desensitization" and address fear avoidance, hyperesthesia (increased sensitivity to stimuli), and kinesiophobia (fear of movement).
- Āsana selection is by an understanding similar to traditional therapeutic progression in terms of load and imposed challenges/perturbations, remembering there are emotional, intellectual, and spiritual responses. The selection of postures is covered in detail by respective lineages.
- Āsanas are adapted with props such as belts, blocks, and blankets in order for the individual to approximate a more complex posture like the way orthotics, assistive devices, and prostheses are employed in traditional rehabilitation.

3. **Prāṇāyāma** is the fourth limb of Yoga. There are over one hundred different combinations of Yoga breathing patterns that may be employed. Each is designed to enhance awareness and experience of this vital bodily function tied, not only to respiration, but also to consciousness and action. Breathing techniques in Yoga Therapy are energy-management tools to curb the effects of increased stress, mood imbalance, and pain. One's patterns of inhalation and exhalation bridge the connection between breathing, the mind, and the emotions (Ekerholt and Bergland, 2008).

   Germane to rehabilitation is the interplay of respiration and the autonomic state of the patient. If a person is stuck in a thoracic, sympathetic/fight-or-flight, chest-breathing pattern, he/she is utilizing accessory respiratory musculature of the cervical spine and thoracic cage to breathe. In that situation, there is a significant load and postural imbalance placed on the body's upper kinetic chain and the lumbopelvic basin at a rate of over 17,000 breaths per day. In Yoga Therapy, alternative breathing patterns through prāṇāyāma decrease these loads and assist in deeper self-reflection and awareness to discover the source of the threat (real or perceived) to the individual that is eliciting the sympathetic response.

This empowers the individual to address the etiology of the response rather than just "tough through" the rehabilitation or overcome the biomechanical limitations of the moment. The development of such introspective reflection yields new understanding for the individual and therapist. The process generates new strategies for action (i.e., movement with intention and diminished fear) (Ekerholt and Bergland, 2008).

4. **Pratyāhāra** (withdrawing of the senses) and **dhāraṇā** (concentration) are important skills that increase attention and awareness. They are the fifth and sixth limbs of Yoga. Practicing these enhances awareness during both rehabilitation and activities of daily living. They silence the hypervigilant/overactive sympathetic mode of the central nervous system via augmentation of the integration of the limbic system with the prefrontal cortex and the resultant interplay with the sensory and motor homunculi. In other words, these practices act on the brain to decrease a person's reactivity to stimuli, increase one's concentration and focus, and create adaptive motor strategies beyond habituated patterns. These concepts are being employed by the military to address PTSD and other symptoms of central nervous system hypervigilance (Pullen, Resources for wounded soldiers). These technologies are more volitional and differ from meditation, the seventh limb, Dhyāna.

5. **Dhyāna** (meditation) is a conscious mental process that induces a set of integrated physiological changes. The practice results in uninterrupted concentration aimed at quieting the mind and body. Daniel Siegel, M.D., of the UCLA Mindfulness Research Center defines the mind as a "process that regulates the flow of energy and information" in his neurophysiology research, "The Mindful Brain" (Siegel, 2007). This intra and interpersonal "attunement" increases awareness, promotes muscle relaxation, encourages the adoption of more efficient postures and patterns of movement, and results in the prevention and reduction of misalignment, cumulative stress, and pain.

   Meditation is active awareness of all the processes of the mind. It includes sensations, images, feelings, and thoughts. It is not the abolition of all thoughts. Meditation may be the quintessential sensorimotor integration practice in Yoga Therapy. Siegel suggests such a practice impacts the therapeutic relationship. He cites the deleterious effects on the patient's ability to breathe well and attain mindfulness if the therapist is stressed, distracted, and lacking in personal integration. The literature indicates that teaching not only meditation but all of the Yoga Therapy techniques, the therapist has a tendency to assume similar introspective, self-reflective qualities that mirror the desired outcomes. Consequently, the state of the mind of the therapist influences the patient's ability to integrate the intervention.

6. **Mudrā** are precise ways of holding the hands, fingers, tongue, and/or body to produce specific effects in the mind and body. Viewed in Yoga Therapy as a delicate interface between the individual and the rest of reality, the fingers and hands are far more than just a robotic tool. When a client suffers from the loss of function of the fingers or hands, mudrā offer a gateway to discovering a subtle reality for the patient locked up inside and provide a practical road back to full interface with his/her world. The incorporation of mudrā generates a natural segue to visual and motor imagery as the perception of these experiences is often most easily described by images and metaphor rather than abstract conceptual language.

7. **Bhāvana** (imagery) and **Yoga nidrā** (deep rest) are Yoga Therapy technologies that provide for hemispheric integration of the mind and body as well as conscious and subconscious integration of memories, emotions, and conceptual limitations of the individual. Closely related to motor imagery in current rehabilitation, these are tools of mental representation of sensation and movement without any body movement and/or in conjunction with movement. Yoga Therapy demands a purposeful use of image, metaphor, imagination, visualization, and sensation to invite whole-brain participation and discovery. The therapist's language facilitates creativity in the experience for the individual while the vocalization of the experience by the individual deepens his/her embodied experience and communicates potential clinical information for decision making by the therapist.

In conclusion, these techniques and technologies of Yoga Therapy may have seemed far removed from traditional rehabilitation, but closer study yields many commonalities between them. An integrative, bio-psychosocial approach to rehabilitation both revisits the very old and also becomes the new evolution of Yoga as it incorporates the insights of modern imagery and research.

YOGA THERAPY PRINCIPLES OF EXAMINATION AND ASSESSMENT IN REHABILITATION

This section examines the key principles of Yoga Therapy for both examination and intervention in rehabilitation. The following principles suggest entry points where one may begin a seamless integration into even the most conservative rehabilitation practices.

Examination Principles

- **Postural Assessment** is foundational and begins from the base(s) of support (BOS) in all standard postures (sitting, standing, gait, supine, and prone). Before the primary complaint is addressed, imbalances in the BOS are identified first by the patient and then, if not recognized or sensed, illuminated by the therapist both through proprioception and visual feedback. A fundamental principle of Yoga is that alignment of structure dictates the flow or communication of prāṇa (one's life force) or what in present-day language would be described as ground reaction forces and Newton's third law of motion. Yoga Therapy's regional interdependence model dictates that to initiate instruction awareness and balance of the BOS are pivotal.

- **Postural Holding Habits** are where the individual discovers postural holding patterns with open-ended questions such as, "Where do you feel the most tension in your body in this position?" and "Which leg is tighter and denser feeling than the other?" etc. The therapist's questions empower the individual to become aware of his/her self. The therapist is helping to identify not only postural but breathing, emotional, and spiritual patterns that reflect the hypervigilant/overactive sympathetic mode of the central nervous system on the part of the individual. These patterns become the touchstone for the home-care programs.

- **Postural Awareness and Accuracy** is where the individual learns to accurately describe observed asymmetries in his/her various postures without first looking or merely repeating what he/she has been told, but by what he/she can sense in the moment. This includes regional areas such as which foot is turned in or out; higher shoulder; shorter rib cage; greater seat pressure right or left; which shoulder is higher off the table; which palm faces more backward; etc. Active participation by the individual during assessment introduces topics such as neuroplasticity, and the individual's awareness has the opportunity to correct itself on the spot. As the individual generates an introspective attitude, he/she senses, then confirms visually and resenses if his/her postural choices were accurate or inaccurate, which assists in restoring sensory and cortical maps.

- **Breath Assessment** includes all the Western parameters of rate, volume, and quality while the therapist studies closely the regional movements associated with the act of respiration. The therapist may ask his/herself or the patient, "Is there movement in the abdomen? How much and in which directions?" And there are similar questions for the upper quarter: "Is there lateral movement of the rib cage that generates upper extremity movement? The sternum, scapula, head, or clavicles? Tone of the tongue, eyes, facial musculature? A thoracic or diaphragmatic recruitment?" As before, the therapist questions the individual to sense and assess his/herself versus telling him/her of the dysfunction. This pattern of recursive observation, sensing, and education weaves throughout the assessments an interlacing with the other principles. The therapist can introduce the importance of respiration patterns, and with over 17,000 repetitions per day, failure to provide an efficient and stable BOS/base(s) of support around breathing will make all other attempts to alter function much more difficult or impossible.

- **Self-Assessment of the Organs of Sensing (Eyes, Ears, Nose, Tongue, and Skin)** is essential for "stabilization of the mind." A preponderance of focus on the thoughts (one of the senses in Yogic theory) generates a lack of awareness of the other sensing fields or an "instability" of the senses. Therefore, in Yoga Therapy individuals are made aware of these fields to initiate moving the mind off the fixation to thinking. If tension is noted around any of the organs of sensing, further questions are asked or expanded should the individual note imbalances in his/her responses. The process moves activation from primarily the prefrontal cortex and limbic systems of the brain to the brain's sensory centers, generating ease and central nervous system acquiescence during the evaluation to facilitate optimal motor learning in the "intervention" phase.

These are only a small percentage of the available tools of assessment for the Yoga Therapist. Many include observation of movement patterns, strength, and flexibility, which are redundant to traditional rehabilitation assessments while others require extensive training and study beyond the scope of this chapter. The boundaries blur between evaluation, assessment, and interventions as well as the roles where the individual becomes a partner in assessment and the therapist takes on the role of learner in addition to the role of expert.

Intervention Principles

Interventions and treatment plans in Yoga Therapy in both the clinic and at home are arrived at through a truly collaborative patient-centered process. Yoga Therapy intervention strategies include, but are not limited to:

- **Manual Therapy/Neuromuscular Reeducation** in Yoga Therapy is not considered a unidirectional intervention from the therapist to the individual. Manual contact in Yoga Therapy is seen as in the language of Siegel, intrapersonal attunement. The state of the therapist's mind and body is an equal concern in determining the effectiveness of the intervention. An imbalance in the therapist affects the quality of the intervention. The therapist self-monitors his/her state, his/her intention, and also that of the patient throughout hands on care. A sense of reverence of touch, intention, and gentleness creates a state of therapeutic presence, allowing for greater sensitivity and decreased overload or unintentional violence.

- **Therapeutic Exercises** focus on the precision of movement facilitated through concentration and specificity of movement. Traditional therapeutic exercises become āsana when they are synchronized with the breath and studied for the relationship between the distal and proximal segments of the extremities and the relationship between the extremities and the spine. The intention of the action in an āsana is held clearly, the mind scans for sensations, emotions, and thoughts that arise and all are performed while maintaining the posture. Thus, āsana is a very detailed process in comparison to counting repetitions or striving to reach some end point of movement in traditional rehabilitation.

- **Directed Therapeutic Activities** are engaged by scanning the patient's entire experience beyond just gross movement to include awareness around the BOS/base(s) of support, thoughts, emotions, and other sensations. If the activity reveals breaches in awareness or new insights, those are explored at that time in real time. For instance, difficulties in a dressing situation like donning a jacket reveal a lack of side bend and rotation to the opposite side. In response, an āsana that incorporates those components is introduced to enhance weight shifting and side bend. The activity of putting on the jacket is then revisited. If the process fails to transfer, a discussion around any perceived fear or hesitancy may yield additional insights. In Yoga Therapy, limitations are teaching points with successive layers of inquiry going beyond biomechanics. Tying one's shoes, reaching for the seat belt, and grooming one's hair take on a playful sense of discovery and many levels of exploration, experimentation, and discovery about one's self. Intention, attention, and action blend together in a myriad of patterns creating fun and cycles of inquiry for both patient and therapist.

- **Home Exercise Programs** are composed of the various Yoga Therapy techniques and technologies chosen to reinforce new learning or invite new awarenesses that the therapist believes will foster additional understanding. For example, an individual with a persistent left temporomandibular joint (TMJ) disorder has a habit of clenching the right hand at rest. An āsana that opens and stretches the right palm and arm may enhance the mind-body connection to a level that the clenching becomes an activity that raises the patient's awareness, allowing for change of the previously unconscious habit. This process informs the next step of interventions.

  Besides the formal home program, the individual is encouraged to regularly return to awareness throughout his/her day, especially when frustrated or during an exacerbation of symptoms. Referred to as "off the mat" Yoga, the individual is expected to return with a full list of experiences to explore and introduce into the session rather than waiting for the therapist to create the agenda.

- **Internal "Passive" Exercises** include the previously listed Yoga Therapy techniques of bhāvana and Yoga nidrā that augment the qualities of nonreactivity and equanimity to stimuli and environments. These modalities require participation by the patient to match their lexicon and life experiences. They can also be incorporated during otherwise passive modalities such as ice, electrical stimulation, and/or ultrasound. Broadening their vocabulary of description of sensation, movement, and activities along the guidelines within motor imagery studies and the use of precise, detailed visioning is encouraged. This "movement" of the mind from frontal cortex to memory with its interplay in the limbic center and self-regulation of the breath develops a resiliency demanding a fully engaged patient. It is this active exploration where the seeds of fear and suffering are discovered and within the light of awareness the seeds wither and make way for integration and healing. In modern rehabilitation, this is an interesting juxtaposition to overcoming and simply pushing through pain, which is often utilized when dealing with fear avoidance, depression, and anxiety.

VISION FOR YOGA THERAPY IN MEDICAL REHABILITATION

The intention of this chapter is to build a bridge between the worlds of Yoga Therapy and medical rehabilitation and to stimulate creative discovery of the possibilities of Yoga Therapy within traditional rehabilitation. Please understand that this summary of Yoga Therapy and traditional rehabilitation is only a rearview mirror look at what has already been . . . and what stretches out ahead is even more exciting! Personally, I see the interface of Yoga Therapy and rehabilitation as the fertile seedbed for real health reform. The study of Yoga Therapy holds the potential for healing to move through our world in ways and rates we only long to see. The time has already arrived, and we are all needed to step forward to allow the best future to emerge.

REFERENCES

Covey, S. R. *The Seven Habits of Highly Effective People.* New York: Free Press, 2004. Print.

Ekerholt, K., and A. Bergland. "Breathing: A Sign of Life and a Unique Area for Reflection and Action." *Physical Therapy* 88.7 (2008): 832–840. Print.

Kolasinski, S. L., et al. "Iyengar Yoga for Treating Symptoms of OA of the Knees: A Pilot Study." *Journal of Alternative & Complementary Medicine* 11.4 (2005): 689–693. Print.

Siegel, D. J. *The Mindful Brain.* New York: W. W. Norton, 2007. Print.

Stankovic, L. "Transforming Trauma: A Qualitative Feasibility Study of Integrative Restoration (iRest) Yoga Nidra on Combat Related Post-Traumatic Stress Disorder." *International Journal of Yoga Therapy* 21: (2011) 23–37.

Taylor, M. J. *Integrating Yoga Therapy into Rehabilitation*. Scottsdale, AZ: Embug Publishing, 1998. Print.

——. "Yoga Therapeutics: An Ancient Practice in a 21st-Century Setting." *Complementary Therapies in Rehabilitation: Evidence for Efficacy in Therapy, Prevention, and Wellness*, 2nd ed. Ed. C. Davis. New York: Slack, 2004. Print.

——. "What Is Yoga Therapy? An IAYT Definition." *Yoga Therapy in Practice* (Dec. 2007): 1–3. Web. PDF available at http://www.matthewjtaylor.com/whatisYRx.pdf.

Wainer, R. S., et al. "Regional Interdependence: A Musculoskeletal Examination Model Whose Time Has Come." *Journal of Orthopaedic and Sports Physical Therapy* 37.11 (2007): 658–660. Print.

Wolsko, P. M., et al. "Use of Mind-Body Medical Therapies: Results of a National Survey." *Journal of General Internal Medicine* 19.1 (2004): 43–50. Print.

TOTAL HIP REPLACEMENT CASE REPORT

This case report on Yoga Therapy postelective total hip replacement was selected for its novelty because the individual's presentation is an extreme of what the reader will encounter with a "routine" hip replacement due to progressive osteoarthritis. Elements of all of the components of the case report will be present in most lower extremity arthoplasties, but, from a teaching perspective, this unique case amplifies what will ordinarily require the Yoga Therapist's keen attention to find. The case is written in conjunction with the foregoing discussion in this chapter.

Initial Presentation

History: Marge (not her real name) presented as a sixty-one-year-old left-handed office worker seven months post right total hip arthroplasty. Rather than the usual history of a slow, gradual increase in pain, loss of motion, and compensatory movement, Marge had been living forty-eight years with a fused hip joint (arthrodesis) as the result of a slipped capital femoral epiphysis at the age of thirteen. She initially, as a teenager, spent several months in a bodycast and then, two months after release from that, suffered a femoral fracture and underwent an intramedullary rod ORIF surgery of the same leg. During the past several years, her right knee and low back had both become increasingly painful and unresponsive to conservative care, forcing her decision to attempt this relatively rare, high-risk restoration of hip motion through a full hip joint prosthesis. She'd completed conventional physical therapy and felt she'd plateaued in comfort and function but thought there must be something more she could do.

Kośa Assessment

- **Anna (Physical):** Significant wasting around the entire right hip, with muscles thin and tight. Ambulated with straight cane, zero degrees of hip extension in terminal stance phase, Trendelenburg and decreased stance time on right. Sit-stand, she weight shifted left and used both arms up and down. She has a half-inch shorter right leg measured radiographically. Operative report states inability to reattach psoas common tendon but did attach thin gluteus medius tendon. Right knee had 12 degree valgus vs. 5 on left and was nontender to palpation. Thigh girth 3 inches suprapatellar was 2.5 inches less than left.
- **Prāṇa (Energetic):** Muscle strength right hip was fair abduction, fair minus hip flexion (unable to initiate hip flexion supine without assist), quadriceps fair plus, hip extension fair plus but limited to zero degrees. Chest/neck breathing pattern with R > L limited diaphragmatic descension with tight, fibrous obturator and pelvic floor musculature on the right. Right rib cage collapsed with 1 inch loss of vertical dimension and restricted lateral and anterior-posterior excursion. Very tight and fibrous scalenes, upper trapezius, and anterior chest muscles bilaterally.
- **Mano (Emotional):** Noted apprehension over the limited improvement to date. Also stress with new move to the Valley, new job, and the need to move her disabled mother to the region against her will. Being worked up medically for tachycardia episodes and unable to get and stay asleep most nights.
- **Vijana (Thinking):** Often distracted, frequently consumed by worry and considerable self-doubt regarding wisdom of the procedure even though back and knee are much better since. Looking toward retirement but didn't want to be disabled during it.

- **Ananda (Spirit):** Questioning "fairness" of her life experience, to include growing up with fused hip, pain of past several years, and now the "hardness" of this rehab experience. Doesn't have a formal religious practice but considers herself spiritual and tied to something greater than herself. Doesn't have a silence or meditation practice, but has found meditation tapes somewhat helpful in the past in calming her.

Examination Principles

In addition to the kośa assessments above, the following further describe her initial presentation and build the rationale for the interventions then selected. Keep in mind that, while her case is dramatic, these same findings to a lesser degree are usually present in the more standard joint replacement cases for osteoarthritis.

- **Postural Assessment, Postural Holding Habits, Postural Awareness, and Accuracy:** Marge was surprisingly accurate in sensing her upper body changes to decreased mobility and length of the lateral rib cage on the right, lower right shoulder, and decreased weight bearing in sitting on right ischial tuberosity in sitting. She could not accurately describe the rotation of her pelvis forward or that her right front was in front of the left with the right lower extremity externally rotated compared to the left in sitting or standing. She could sense asymmetry in her gait but, as often occurs, couldn't say what was different side to side and called the short side the opposite of what she demonstrated. Video feedback was provided to allow her literally to see these differences and to her surprise what was actually occurring both statically and dynamically.
- **Breath Assessment:** She was able to note that her breathing was shallow, rapid (16 rpm), chest oriented, and less on the right than left when asked to attend to that. She could also sense her heartbeat and noted accurately that it was regular and steady (72 bpm). She could not perceive motion related to the breathing below her right rib cage but on the left felt it to her waistline.
- **Self-Assessment of the Organs of Sensing:** With direction to perceive, she noted the tongue pushed up against the top teeth, jaw set, soft squint of the eyes with forehead tension and ears feeling pushed forward versus soft and long. She described the skin across her upper back as drawn tight as well as a sense of

"density" and shrink-wrap–like sensation around right groin, lateral hip, and buttock. With direction, she could also feel the pull of skin across the clenched right hand and protracted left scapula. When asked about where it felt like her brain and spinal cord were positioned, she felt like they were lifted and pressed forward (visual imagery for sensing interceptive state of excitability).

Treatment Plan

In conventional rehabilitation, the focus would be on strengthening what was weak and increased mobility where it was needed with gait training. Yoga Therapy broadens the lens to ask, "Where is the suffering and instability of the 'mindstuff' for this person today?" What patterns is she bringing along that lead to that state and what philosophy and technologies might be employed to increase awareness and create new options for action, not only to improve biomechanics, but also to generate stillness in terms of all the kośas reflected by an acquiesced central nervous system, serene and joyful mood, and better movement performance? Her fundamental breathing pattern has been altered for decades, her self-image a challenge, her self-compassion limited, and her central nervous system entrained to heightened vigilance to now include the tachycardia episodes. Also, where within this does she discover the reserve to support her disabled mother in her declining health and increasing need for care? Sidestepping in a Thera-Band loop won't cover it all obviously!

- **Internal "Passive" Exercises:** She'd plateaued in performance because no one had addressed the kośa issues and assessed deficits above. We discussed how once we did that she'd have a platform of stability (yoga) to continue to advance. With some neuro-education, she understood this was the foundation off which she'd proceed even though it didn't feel like the striving and efforting she'd done all her life. She was given very simple practice of bhāvana and Yoga nidrā to use at night that includes visualizing the tissue around her hip blooming back to life with vital circulation, suppleness, and power. These were recorded on her iPhone over her course of visits to build her library at home. She was also given a practice of mudrā to enhance intero and visceroceptive accuracy as well emotional self-regulation as a precursor to small "doses" of 2–3 minute breath-oriented dhyāna (meditation) practices during the day and at night.

- **Manual Therapy/Neuromuscular Reeducation:** In the practices below, manual therapy and reeducation were used to complement and enhance her perceptions rather than to deform or stretch tissue. Touch was used when she couldn't reference spatial positions, when she couldn't initiate motor firing, or skeletally needed loading or unloading to restore postural length and stability. She was particularly responsive to light touch around shoulder girdle, rib cage, and the pelvis for discovering tension patterns and learning how to surrender those, followed by reinitiating desired motor responses once the patterns were broken. This was well received in contrast to the deep tissue deforming touch she'd received before to "break up (sic)" soft tissue.

- **Therapeutic Exercises:** She had previously been doing primarily straight line, open chain conventional strengthening and stretching exercises with external movement attention. The introduction of āsana and prāṇāyāma redirecting attention internally was initially a struggle. We would begin with calming prāṇāyāma of dīrgha breathing (three-part breathing), nāḍī śodhana (nerve cleansing), or a mudrā-supported breath practice such as bhū mudrā (Mother Earth mudrā) for first cakra awareness. Much to her surprise, these "softer" and slower activities generated immediate changes in mobility and performance she thought had all but ceased. Early emphasis on opening the hips and chest with such postures as support matyāsana (fish pose) and supta baddha koṇāsana (reclined bound angle pose), followed by supine with feet against the wall to then standing small versions of the single knee to chest (apānāsana), vīrabhadrāsana I and II (warrior I and II pose) incorporate alignment principles and sensing position and motor sensation side-to-side differences. All of the āsana and prāṇāyāma were very simple, often supported with props learned in the Iyengar tradition and with frequent 1-minute śavāsana sensorimotor integration breaks. Sessions would end with one of the above noted bhāvana or nidrā practices.

- **Directed Therapeutic Activities:** Marge was expected to notice and return with new challenges and discoveries each visit that formed our focus for that day rather than some formulaic plan of care. Pratyāhāra, home exercise discovery, and dhāraṇā from the text were then employed, giving her a template for discovery that she could then employ on her own as well. We would discuss where she perceived the discomfort or inability, what other nonlocal parts of her being might be involved, and then to create situations to explore those limitations more deeply rather than avoid or distress over them. She was very insightful and creative and, as a business problem solver, took quickly to the process. Some of the areas we investigated were her self-consciousness arising from seated surfaces in social situations, facing descending stairs or curbs without rails, not using her cane when she was fatigued, and leaving her mother's company at ease rather than harried. She was very intrigued with how balance postures could be transformed from frustrating failures of performance to introspective experiences of play and self-compassion and how when that happened, her balance actually improved sometimes 100 percent. The author's experience is that in using directed therapeutic activities such as this, the individual's curiosity and adherence levels are enhanced, as well as dropping the fear avoidance around certain activities of daily living (ADLs). They bring to the session what is most important to them (patient values as a part of evidenced-based medicine) and leave with practical, real-world answers to their challenges. Problems become teachers and they are empowered to participate in creating the solutions rather than a dependency on the expert practitioner.

Course of Treatment

Marge was seen six times over a four-month period. She had one six-week break when she was moving her mother into town. She saw her surgeon for her one-year appointment follow-up just before her last visit prior to this writing. The surgeon was very pleased with her gait, her strength, and the radiographic alignment of her pelvis and prosthesis. He asked to see her again in one year and reinforced that it would be at least another year before she should expect to have maximum return. This buoyed her mood and enthusiasm to continue. There were no injuries or setbacks reported during the course. She kept all of her scheduled appointments and eagerly scheduled to continue beyond her last appointment. The author worked with the conventional therapist who worked at the gym to insure appropriate integration and selection of activities and intensities of workouts.

Disposition at This Time

Marge has adopted a softer, longer view to her process that integrates her whole-life experience. Rather than pushing for some perfect outcome, she allows both her own and her mother's limitations to be viewed as opportunities to "exercise" compassion, creativity, and ease. She gets to the gym at least twice a week for her conditioning practice and then uses her various home practices to complement on the off days. She's come to marvel at the relative miracle of her gait versus fixate on the limitations. We've extended follow-ups to every six weeks where we video her gait and tweak her practices as this allows enough time for to report changes and for us to capture performance enhancements. She notes her reactionary behaviors and perception of stress have been reduced dramatically. She laughs more easily, can enjoy times with her mother, and rests better at night. At the last visit, she'd restored her full right hip extension in terminal stance, could sustain vertical upper-body posture throughout gait with symmetric arm swing, and turn rapidly either direction without losing balance, using no assistive device over short distances of 200 feet. She also notes the ability to reinterpret stimuli in her daily life that, in the past, would have generated tension and postural instability, helping her maintain longer periods of equanimity that used to only occur occasionally.

In summary, the pain of her back and knee that necessitated the risky surgery has become a life-changing, life-long practice of enhancing health and joy. This same invitation is available to every individual who is slowed down by joint replacement, whether traumatic or elective. The loss of function and comfort become doorways to expanded consciousness and increased compassion for both self and others when a full spectrum Yoga therapeutic approach is employed to complement conventional rehabilitation. Furthermore, the conventional therapist's experience is enhanced from the monotony of cookie-cutter protocols to an unending exploration of subtlety and triumph while working as a team with the patient/student. This generates a more aware and creative professional, better skilled to ease and prevent future suffering for others and themselves.

Yoga Therapy and the Spine

Eden Goldman, D.C., C.Y.T., Y.T.R.X., E-RYT500

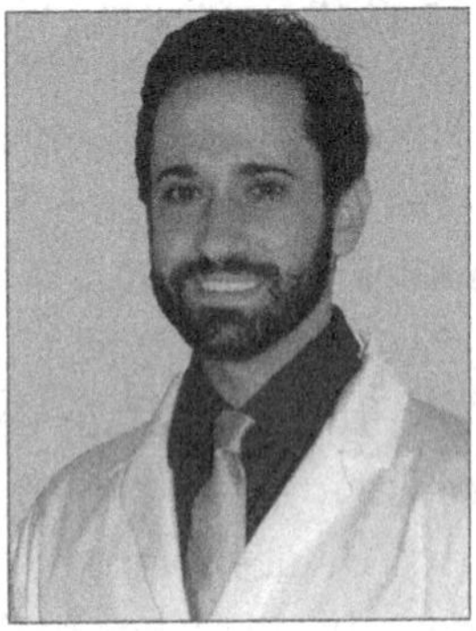

Eden Goldman is a wellness-based chiropractor, certified Yoga Therapist, physical rehabilitation specialist, and owner of the Yoga Doctors Mandiram wellness center in Los Angeles, California. Raised in the tradition and ancient science of Kriyā Yoga, Eden completed his doctorate in chiropractic at the Los Angeles College of Chiropractic. His professional work integrates classical Eastern Yoga therapeutics, Thai massage, and myofascial release bodywork with Western advancements in mind-body medicine, sports science, physical rehabilitation, athletic training, prevention, and chiropractic. Codirector of Loyola Marymount University's Yoga and the Healing Sciences Teacher Training Program and author of *The Secret Art of Adjusting Yoga Poses,* Dr. Goldman has been featured in many publications on Yoga and Yoga Therapy. For more information, please visit www.YogaDoctors.com.

INTRODUCTION

The single most important structure in the human body is the spine. Recognized as the body's wellspring of life and vitality since the time of antiquity, the spine's significance has been well documented. Ancient depictions of the Egyptian Creator God, Ptah, show him holding the Spine of Life in his hands (Brown, 2002). Socrates, the greatest author and sage of the classical Greco-Roman civilizations, went as far as to say, "If you would seek health, first look to the spine" (Lowery, 2011). Traditional Eastern philosophers and Indian Yoga masters also echo similar thoughts and feelings about the spine. Paramahansa Yogananda, author of *Autobiography of a Yogi,* was repeatedly quoted as saying, "The spine is the highway to the Infinite" (Walters, 1990). Even today, the West continues its health-oriented relationship with the spine and the East maintains a spiritual romance with it. This cross-cultural respect for the spine and its contribution to mechanics, medicine, and metaphysics makes it by far one of the most fascinating subjects when it comes to Yoga Therapy and its application to the body.

ANATOMY, ENERGETICS, AND PHYSIOLOGY OF THE SPINE

Typically comprised of twenty-four articulating vertebrae, twenty-three corresponding intervertebral discs, a sacrum, a coccyx, a central cord, and various joints, nerves, bones, muscles, tendons, and ligaments, the adult spine is both an artistic and an engineering marvel in its construction. Structurally, the spine is segmented into five location-based categories:

1. Cervical—the neck, 7 vertebrae
2. Thoracic—the mid back, 12 vertebrae
3. Lumbar—the low back, 5 vertebrae
4. Sacrum—the back side of the pelvis, 1 fused vertebrae
5. Coccyx—the tailbone, 1 fused vertebrae

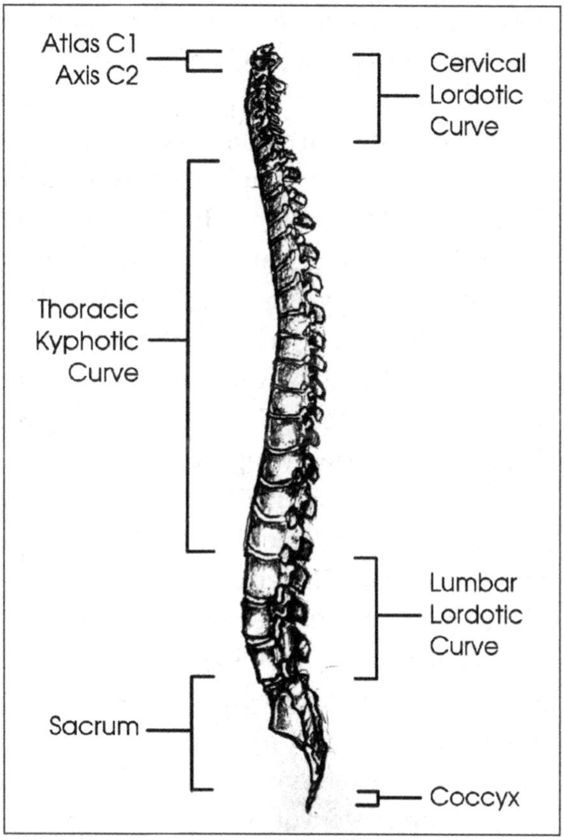

Figure 1. The curves of the spine

To maintain its typical "S"-like shape, there are three main curves observed in the spine as seen in Figure 1. The thoracic spine in the middle of the back is said to have a kyphotic curve. A kyphotic curve, or kyphosis, is known as a primary curve because it is the direction and orientation of the spine at birth after growing in a rounded position for nine months. The two other curves are called lordotic curves. A lordotic curve, or lordosis, is known as a secondary or acquired curve since it is developed after birth through one's life experiences as a child. The cervical lordosis in the neck forms when a baby first lifts its head up at about three to four months. The spine takes this position in order to balance the weight of the head on the small cervical vertebrae in the neck. Comparably, the lumbar lordotic curve is created in the lower back in a similar way at about nine to ten months when a baby first stands on its own two feet. The pelvis and lower spine adjust the curve in order to facilitate the transition from crawling on four limbs as a quadruped to walking as an upright biped on just two legs (Cramer, 2005). The curves are designed to support each other through a variety of actions and tasks encountered in life. Most notably, when the spinal curves are maintained, it is considered the most energy-efficient position for the body to stay upright against the forces of gravity and other extrinsic forces (Richardson, Hodges, and Hides, 2004; Wallden, 2009).

In classical Yoga philosophy, the spine is said to house the three central nāḍīs (channels of energy): iḍā (left channel), piṅgala (right channel), and suṣumna (center channel). The iḍā nāḍī represents the moon, femininity, and the left side of the spine and body while the piṅgala nāḍī represents the sun, masculinity, and the right side of the spine and body (Bharati). They are commonly depicted as two serpents intersecting and interweaving at cakras (energy centers) in the suṣumna nāḍī. The suṣumna houses dormant kundalini energy at its base, and this energy, or consciousness, is "awakened" through the practice of Yoga. Modern yogī physiologists have additionally theorized that the suṣumna nāḍī corresponds to the central canal of the spinal cord in Western terms, and the iḍā and piṅgala nāḍīs run parallel to it on either side, resembling the sympathetic nerve trunks (Glassey, 2011). This depiction of the criss-crossing nāḍīs has been further related to the iconic symbol of Western medicine, the caduceus, as iḍā and piṅgala form the snakes of the caduceus and the suṣumna forms the staff. Thus, the caduceus could be considered a symbol for the entire system of Western medicine as well as kuṇḍalinī śakti (bhāratī).

In describing cakras, Yoga defines them as "major cerebrospinal centers of life and consciousness" (Yogananda, 1995) or "[nerve] plexuses that are the storage places of pranic energy" (Vishnudevananda, 1959). There are usually said to be six or seven main cakras in the spine (depending on whether the crown cakra, or *sahasrāra*, is included) and each have corresponding names, functions, mantras, colors,

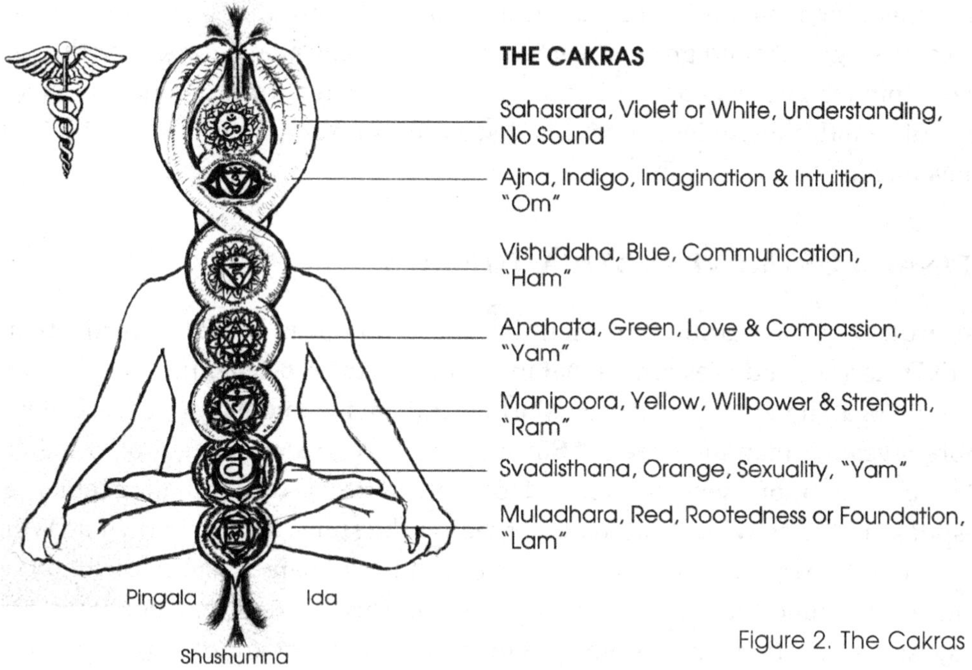

Figure 2. The Cakras

and characteristics associated with them as outlined briefly in Figure 2. Spinal energy exercises called kriyās were brought back into prominence from the caves of the Himalayan mountains in the mid-1800s to teach Yoga practitioners to move energy through their cakras and spines around the six spinal centers of the medullary, cervical, dorsal, lumbar, sacral, and coccygeal plexuses (Yogananda, 1998).

When discussing the spine in terms of chiropractic physiology, its primary function is said to be the protection of the spinal cord and the facilitation of the nervous system. In these roles, the spine is like the trunk of a tree with individual nerves shooting off the central spinal cord like branches off a tree's trunk. These branches, aka the individual nerves, in turn, have smaller and smaller branches that form the basic structure of the nervous systems. Through this complex global messaging network of nerves, the brain connects with the body, organs, and muscles, transmitting signals from the spinal highway to the rest of the body as fast as about 200 miles per hour—or the entire distance of a football field in one second! (Myers, 1995).

In addition to protecting and enabling communication in the body, the spine has other functional duties it is responsible for, including shock absorption (via the discs) from gravity and ground reactant forces, structural integration for the pelvic and shoulder girdles, attachment location sites for tendons, ligaments, muscles, and ribs, and, most relevant to this discussion of Yoga Therapy, flexibility and movement.

SPINAL MOVEMENT IN YOGA THERAPY

Regardless of the tradition or scientific orientation, it is widely agreed upon by both Easterners and Westerners that movement is the most significant spinal function in Yoga Therapy. As ballerina Martha Graham ingeniously stated, "Nothing is more revealing than movement." Since the body learns movement-oriented tasks through repetition, whether refined or not, patterns of adaptation emerge in response to the activities and loads placed on the spine. This is known as Wolff's Law from Western biomechanics (Ruff, Holt, and Trinkhaus, 2006). Muscle contours transform around the spine based on these patterns, posture may become altered, basic spinal functions can become polluted or antalgic (modified due to pain), and pain may result if spinal movements are not properly trained and performed.

So what are the "right" movements? And what should be focused on while training the spine?

When deciding on the right spinal movements in Yoga Therapy, it is based on a number of factors. Initially, it begins with the question "Is there any pain or discomfort?" If there is pain or discomfort and it is affecting or being affected by the spine, then before any therapeutic or yogic treatment can be prescribed additional information must be gathered about the person's history and the source and nature of his/her complaints. As it is in other systems of physical and holistic medicine, when dealing with spinal dysfunctions in Yoga Therapy it is never a one-way-cures-all approach. Each person must be comprehensively and individually assessed. In this way, Yoga Therapy evaluates and honors the unique background, skill set, physicality, and experience of pain or suffering of each individual. Having an understanding of these elements of a person's situation and previous experiences motivates which specific spinal movements, exercises, postures, and sequences can be given at a particular time. The key component is that what is right for individuals differs from person to person and evolves over time as an individual's skills improve and his/her pain and discomfort decreases.

Within Western physical medicine, there are a number of methods of evaluating spinal movement. Traditional orthopedic range-of-motion evaluations are performed most effectively, noninvasively, and reliably with an inclinometer (Wallden, 2009), though a visual estimation from a trained eye will often suffice. The ranges of motion aid in pointing out the direction(s) of spinal movement that may cause pain and discomfort, lack fluidity, and/or need to be improved with training. By isolating specific motions in the spine's three main regions, the different ranges can be assessed by bending either the head or the trunk forward (flexion), backward (extension), to the side laterally (lateral flexion), and rotating from side to side (rotation). The results are compared to the accepted average ranges of motion, which vary between sources, and are observed in the table below:

TABLE 1. RANGES OF MOTION IN THE HUMAN SPINE

RANGES OF MOTION	CERVICAL SPINE	THORACIC SPINE	LUMBAR SPINE
Flexion	60–90	25–45	40–60
Extension	75–90	25–45	20–35
One-Sided Lateral Flexion (L+R)	45–55	20–40	15–25
One-Sided Rotation (L+R)	80–90	30–45	5–18

Table compiled from Peterson, 2002.

While the table above displays the average ranges of motion in the human spine, in Yoga people frequently cultivate a level of flexibility that is so advanced that the chart may not be relevant for a long-time Yoga practitioner.

Looking at it inductively, the table also highlights which movements are preferred in each section of the spine and helps emphasize where it is most advantageous to twist from, bend from, and move from in the spine within a given exercise or asana. The higher the degree of range, the more that section of the spine usually prefers that type of movement. With that in mind, the lumbar spine moves best in flexion, extension, and lateral flexion; the thoracic spine moves best in rotation (due to the connecting ribs restricting other movements); and the cervical spine moves well in all directions to help direct our eyes' gaze to whatever we are doing.

Nevertheless, just like in physical rehabilitation and sports science, spinal movement in Yoga Therapy is not limited to the basic ranges of motion and whether a person can or can't do an action to "x" degree. Properly applied Yoga Therapy evaluates the quality of the spinal movement initiated by the practitioner, which can assist in determining whether a Yoga posture or exercise is appropriate for a person at a given time. It's not just "Can you do it?" It's how you do it; what level of precision, control, ease, breath awareness, and comfort are maintained in doing it; and, can quality spinal movements, a pain-free range of motion, and good form predominate the entire time? Quality movements retrain neurokinetic pathways, establish healthy neurological grooves in the central nervous system's control of the body, and enhance the brain's positive communication with the muscles. In the end, "Practice does not make perfect. Perfect practice makes perfect. Practice just makes permanent" (Morgan, 2009).

If practicing alone or in a group Yoga class without direct one-on-one attention, some subjective questions one might ask about the movements of his/her spine include:

> ***Subjective Feedback:*** Is the movement painful and/or does it re-create my chief discomfort? Do I feel in control of my body? Does my spine feel supported? Does the movement feel good? Can I keep myself safe by performing the movement within a functional training range (FTR) of about 50–80 percent of my maximum effort? Am I able to breathe comfortably, steadily, and rhythmically? Can I breathe in conjunction with my movements? Can I challenge myself without straining myself?

If any of the questions above are answered with a "NO," then a qualified therapist or doctor might be needed to make suggestions and provide treatment, especially if the movement causes pain, numbness, and/or tingling to radiate into the limbs. When working in Yoga Therapy with someone in a one-on-one setting, the therapist/doctor will likely observe the way the movements are being performed as well as when and how pain manifests if it is involved. Together, the practitioner and therapist might consider some of the following objective questions:

> ***Objective Feedback:*** Is the person practicing and moving with good form? Is his/her spine supported by the abdominal muscles and the surrounding intrinsic

musculature? Can the practitioner control and coordinate the inhalations and exhalations during the movement? Are the spinal curves and his/her posture well maintained while transitioning between poses? Are the transitions smooth and safe? Which muscles are chiefly felt during the movements? Where in the spine is the movement being initiated? Can target muscles be isolated and experienced by the practitioner?

If movement is limited or restricted in any way, Yoga Therapy's role for the spine would be wise to "focus on the deficiencies" (Kravitz, 1995) and re-empower those abilities. The initial goal is to objectively identify where there are weak link(s) in the body, not necessarily just where one's symptoms, pain, and tightness are showing up. Increasing one's aptitude in identifying the areas where prana (energy), stability, and/or physical proficiency are compromised or inefficient helps to alleviate pain/discomfort, eliminate dysfunction, and develop better lifestyle habits. In the process, the Yoga practitioner has the opportunity to learn about the interconnectedness of his/her discomfort with physical movements, body coordination, emotions, activities of daily living, self-identity, and posture.

YOGA THERAPY AND POSTURAL SYNDROMES

At their core, physical medicine and Yoga Therapy have one key element that they share irrespective of the style or discipline: posture. "Each and every movement begins and ends with posture" (Liebenson, 1996). When posture breaks down due to an injury or stress, it is known as a postural syndrome. Introduced in the late twentieth century by famed Czechoslovakian neurologist Vladimir Janda, M.D., postural syndromes are developed from muscle patterning and imbalances that occur in response to accidents, sports injuries, falls, repetitive stress, exercise, physical activity, Yoga, and workplace demands like excessive sitting or standing.

In his work, Janda outlined how the body breaks down neuromuscularly with predictable muscle imbalances and systemic dysfunctions that affect the spine and body's overall health (Morris, 2006). He described two specific types of muscles: hypertonic and hypotonic muscles. Hypertonic muscles become shortened, overly toned, excessively tight, rajasic (active), and/or appear to be deceptively strong-looking. These tend to need stretching, relaxation, biomechanical training, and/or massage. Conversely, hypotonic muscles become lengthened, inhibited, weakened, tamasic (inactive), and often lack a full motor response to "turn on." These tend to need strengthening, stabilization, and/or to be functionally activated through a variety of physical and yogic techniques.

Amid this backdrop of hypertonicity and hypotonicity, Janda identified that when the muscles are not in balance and communicating well together two postural syndromes routinely appear known as upper cross syndrome and lower cross syndrome, respectively.

- *Upper cross syndrome*—This affects the upper back and the neck and can cause a hunchback or bird-neck appearance. Hypertonic muscles include the upper trapezius, levator scapulae, and pectoralis major and pectoralis minor muscles; hypotonic muscles include the deep anterior neck flexors, rhomboids, serratus anterior, and the mid and lower trapezius muscles. The condition regularly displays the head being positioned too far forward, shoulder elevation and protraction (reaching forward), altered breathing, abnormal shoulder mechanics, thoracic spine/mid back compression, facial pain, temporomandibular joint (TMJ) problems and/or referred pain to chest, shoulders, and arms.

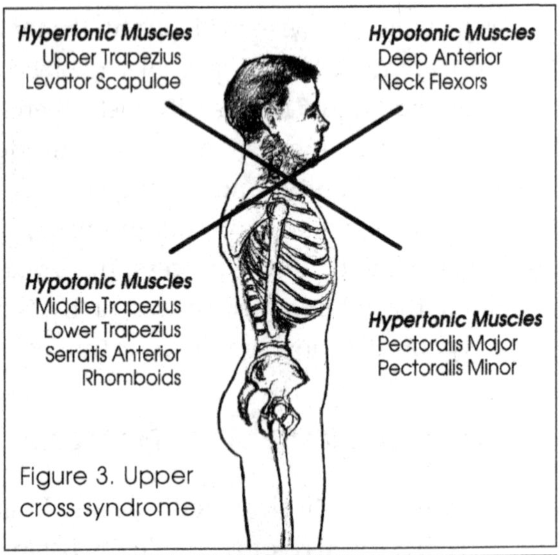

Figure 3. Upper cross syndrome

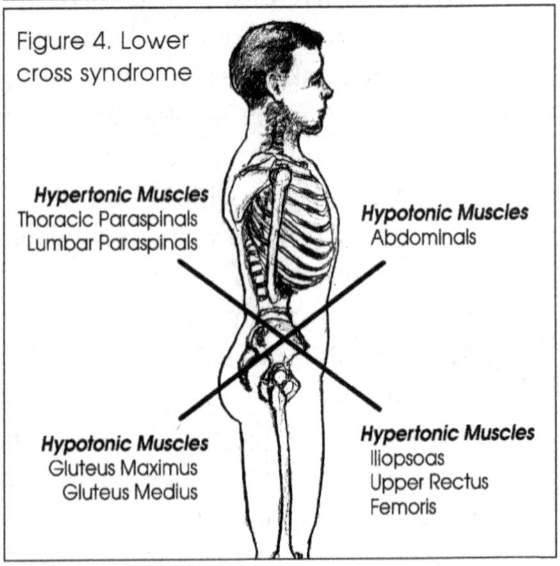

Figure 4. Lower cross syndrome

- *Lower cross syndrome*—This affects the lower back, sacroiliac (SI) joint, and the hips and can cause a pot-belly appearance as well as "gluteal amnesia" (McGill, 2007) in response to excessive sitting (where the gluteal muscles' inhibition is analogous to them forgetting how to do their job). Hypertonic muscles include the iliopsoas, rectus femoris, piriformis, quadratus lumborum, and the thoracolumbar erector spinae muscles; hypotonic muscles include the abdominals and the gluteal muscles as a group. The condition commonly presents with an anterior pelvic tilt, increased hip flexion, compensatory increased lumbar lordosis, and mid back to lower back instability.

In Yoga Therapy, Janda's postural syndromes can be used like road maps to orient practitioners and therapists to areas in the body that have a predictable tendency to become unbalanced and affect the spine's overall health. Moreover, because muscle contractions always require oxygen (even if the muscles are being contracted unconsciously while not in use like in hypertonic muscles), when postural syndromes express themselves in the body it creates physical stress patterns that unnecessarily and uneconomically consume extra oxygen. This additional consumption of oxygen diverts it away from the internal organs, the brain, and other areas of the body that need oxygen too for optimum healing and performance. Ultimately, this means that chronic muscle tension and postural syndromes are not just localized issues in the tissues affecting the spine but are, in fact, global body-wide issues that establish poor and inefficient use of oxygen throughout the body. Understanding Janda's postural syndromes in this way, both locally and globally, can aid in pinpointing areas of weakness/inhibition and tightness/overuse that might require more specific training for the body and/or breath in Yoga Therapy. As the great Yoga master B. K. S. Iyengar said, "Your practice is your laboratory and your methods must become ever more penetrating and sophisticated" (Iyengar, 2006).

THE CERVICAL SPINE

The cervical spine is made up of seven vertebrae and typically gets separated into two categories based on structure and movement: the upper cervicals (C1-C2) consisting of the flexion-extension based atlas (C1) and the rotation based axis (C2) and the lower cervicals made up of C3–C7, which perform all active ranges of motion well. The lordotic curve of the cervical spine is said to be optimal from 40–43 degrees with a normal range consisting of 35–45 degrees (Yochum and Rowe, 2004).

Why is this significant to Yoga Therapy?

Anatomically, the cervical curve's primary function is to support the weight of the head. If the head drifts too far forward increasing the curve or conversely if the cervical curve is reduced, it often becomes a habitual pattern and may result in a permanent change of the neutral position. In a neck that is below the normal range of curve, known as a hypolordotic cervical curve, or a military neck, the lack of curve can create compression on the nerves, breathing deficiencies, and constriction in the blood vessels. In addition, there is the potential for degeneration in the discs and vertebrae, strain in the muscles, and numbness or pain to radiate down the arms. On the other hand, a neck with too much curve, called a hyperlordotic cervical curve, often lacks structural support and can cause forward head posturing, known as anterior head carriage, which is frequently seen in upper cross syndrome. This positioning of the head can put intense pressure on the spinal joints and the surrounding structures if it is not corrected. It is remarkably common in adults, especially in the elderly and in those who sit long hours at a desk or strain while looking at a computer. The recognized long-term effects of forward head posturing can alter endorphin and hormonal production leading to more perceived pain, compress the thoracic cavity limiting one's range of motion, decrease lung capacity by about 30 percent, and add as much as 30 pounds of additional pressure on the neck as shown below (Calliet, 1987).

Figure 5. Cervical Spine Loads *Adapted from (Dalton, 2010)*

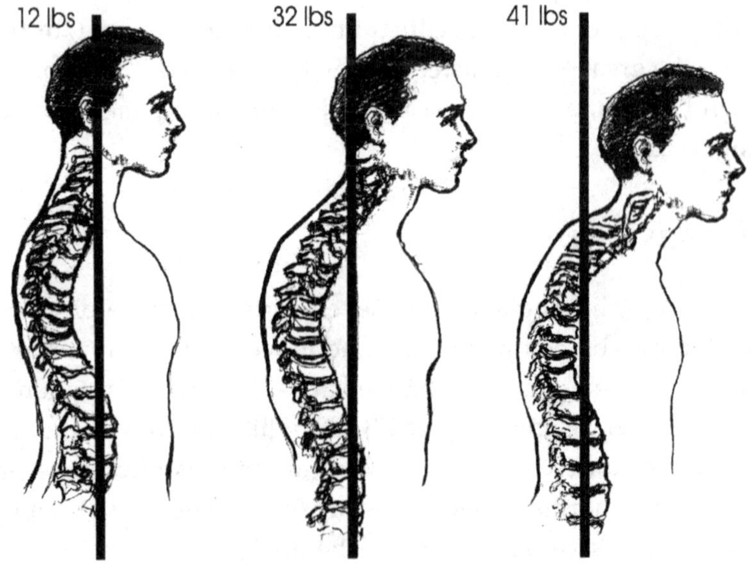

Consequently, being outside the ranges of a normal curve in either direction can create deficiency in a person's awareness, decreases proprioceptive abilities, and forms aberrant substitution patterns of tension, stress, and discomfort in the muscles and joints of the cervical spine.

Fortunately, cervical dysfunctions like anterior head carriage can be effectively treated with Yoga Therapy, patience, and practice. Often overlooked with patients in health care, training the neurology of the neutral position of the head can be a key factor reprogramming the practitioner's proprioception and overall sense of well-being. As Rene Calliet, M.D., put it, "The body follows the head. Therefore, the entire body is best aligned by first restoring proper functional alignment to the head" (Calliet, 1987). Subsequently, a variety of chin-tucking and head-aligning procedures can be applied successfully in the Yoga room to reset the neutral position of the head and reactivate dysfunctional deep anterior neck flexors. This practice features a nodding motion of the head and can be done lying down in śavāsana (corpse pose), standing upright in taḍāsana (mountain pose) against a wall, or in poses like bhujaṅgāsana (cobra pose) and vīrabhadrāsana one (warrior one pose) to give the practitioner both a nonweight bearing and weight bearing experience. Gwendolyn Jull, M.D., found that a reduction in deep anterior cervical flexor muscle activation is associated with increased activation of the superficial hypertonic muscles—the sternocleidomastoid, upper trapezius, and the anterior scalene —indicating a reorganization of the motor strategy (Jull, 2008). When there is a "reorganization of the motor strategy" and muscle substitution patterns occur, the hypertonic muscles will do extra work, fail to relax and remain at rest, and become quicker to get excited and start overworking again while the hypotonic muscles simply fail to "turn on," contribute, and show up to do their jobs as previously described. To change this self-defeating cycle, both sets of muscles must have muscular balance restored.

Since Yoga's essential physical nature is the triumvirate of the decompression of joints, the release of pressure, and the reduction of stress, when too little curve is present a change in the constant compressive force of gravity on the cervical spine may provide the space and release needed in the cervical spinal joints and discs. Posterior to anterior mobilizations of the mid to upper thoracic spine using Yoga asanas, chiropractic adjustment, rehabilitation exercises, and/or a foam roll offers incredible relief to a compressed hypolordotic cervical spine. Additionally, if the level of strain exhibited by the muscles is not too severe, manual traction can be performed by a healthcare practitioner and/or natural gravity-based cervical traction can be applied in Yoga Therapy by inverting the forces of gravity on the body, which assists in decreasing compressive forces. B. K. S. Iyengar introduced this therapeutic technique of gravitational traction to the Yoga world by using two cushioned chairs placed at an appropriate width so that the shoulders and clavicles support the weight of the body as the head dangles in between. Providing that the practitioner's aptitude, skill level, and physiological conditioning warrant the procedure, putting the body upside down with the head free from the floor provides all of the benefits of a traditional headstand, sālamba śīrṣāsana (all limbs standing on the head pose), while alleviating compression and gravity's pressure on the small joints, discs, and vertebrae of the cervical spine. It is a relatively safe option that can be therapeutically applied in Yoga as a substitute for a traditional headstand and has the ability to be used for a variety of chronic cervical spine dysfunctions where compressive force is one of the main issues.

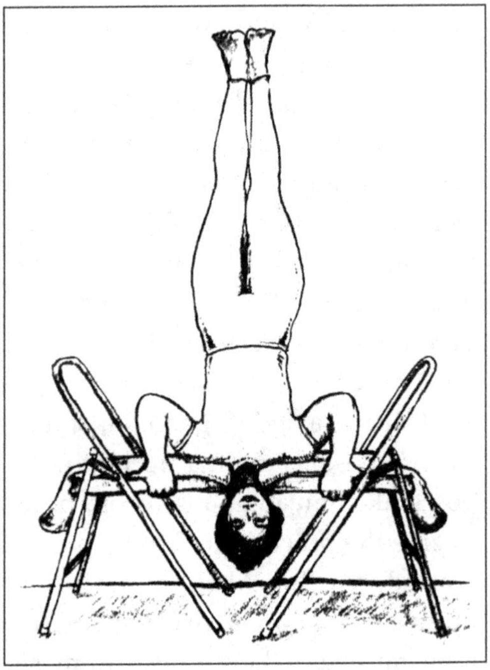

Figure 6. Sālamba Śīrṣāsana (Headstand)

THE THORACIC SPINE

The thoracic spine can be grouped into three sections: upper thoracics (T1–T3), middle thoracics (T4–T8), and lower thoracics (T9–T12). The middle thoracics encompass the apex of the primary kyphotic curve, meaning the spine is the most rounded at T4–T8, which can be seen in Figure 7 on page 299. In my personal philosophy regarding spinal mechanics, the upper thoracics and lower thoracics are functionally unique in reference to the middle thoracics as they are places where the spine begins to transition from the apex of its primary kyphosis to the lordotic curves found in the cervical and lumbar spines, respectively. Jiri Cumpelik, P.T.,

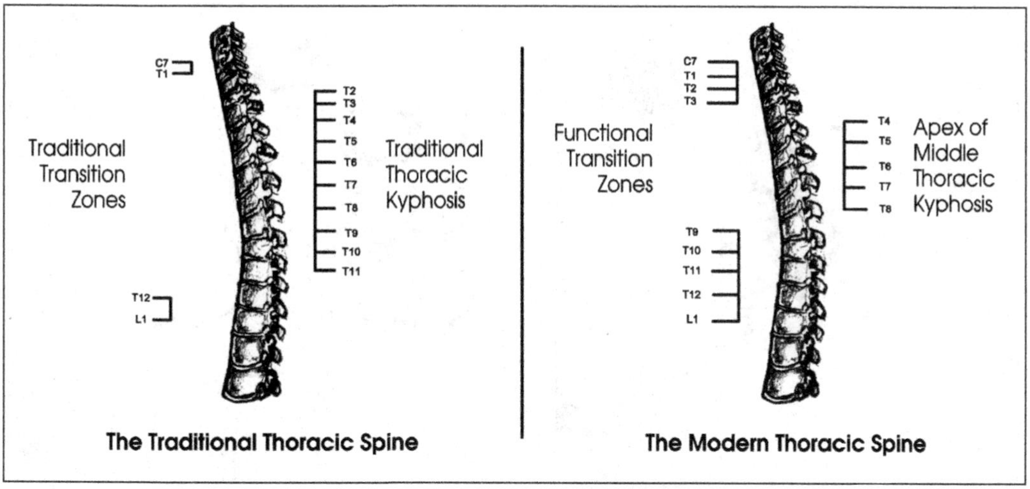

Figure 7. Transitional Zones

says, "In a functional and mobile spine, the physiological movement of the cervical spine starts from T4 and progresses upward, and the movements of the lumbar spine from T6 and go downward" (Cumpelik, 2014). Thus, these areas can be considered extended transitional zones in reference to the traditional transitional zones located at C7–T1 and T12–L1 where weakness and instability injuries commonly occur.

It is easy to infer from this function-based classification that the location of the apex of the middle thoracics at T4–T8 is often a key source of dysfunction in neck, middle, and lower back pain. This is due to the compression and rounded nature of the thoracic kyphosis and the decreased movement of the vertebrae between the scapula, which can be compounded by prolonged periods of sitting in a constrained posture (Liebenson, 2001). "Chairs, desks and computers all conspire with gravity to round our back and shoulders forward . . . slumping, slouching and stooping thus become a programmed habit. The effects of poor posture are seen everywhere and include the loss of energy, headaches, neck or back pain, pinched nerves, etc." (Liebenson, 2010). Releasing tension in the middle thoracics is therefore remarkably important to the entire spine as thoracic, lumbopelvic, and cervicocranial posture have been found to be interrelated as links in a biomechanical kinetic chain as evidenced in the cogwheels picture attributed to the work of Swiss neurologist, Dr. Alois Brügger in Figure 8 on the following page, adapted from (Liebenson, 2001).

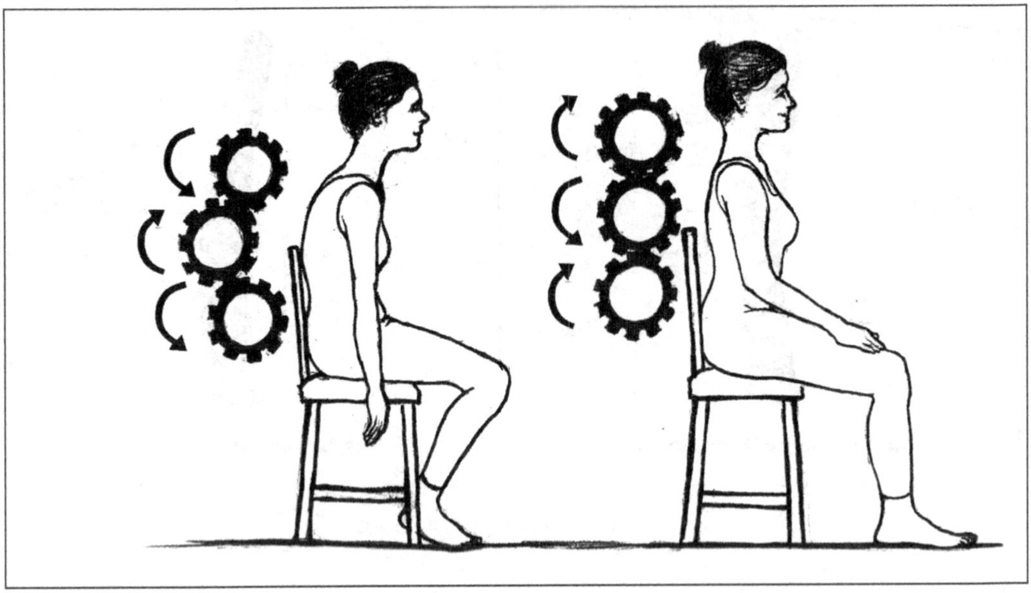

Figure 8. Cogwheels

In the West, clinical dysfunctions of the middle thoracics can be observed mechanically with excessive chin poking, lumbar hyperlordosis, straining in the neck and lower back muscles, and the inability to perform a wall angel posture with good form keeping the hips, shoulders, head, elbows, wrists, and lower back on the wall together with the bent arms. As the foundation for the cervical spine, a lack of motion and accumulation of tension and stress in the middle thoracic region can easily "lock" up the neck above, similar to how a house with a poor foundation shows proverbial cracks in its walls.

The yogic texts further concur with the importance of posture and mobility in the middle thoracic region: "It is slow but sure suicide to walk, sit, rest, talk, or lie down with a caved-in chest. The cells of the lungs become starved thereby, and maladjustments of the vertebrae often occur" (Yogananda, 1925). As a result, Yoga postures were initially designed to simply enable people to sit upright for periods of meditation. The yogis and rishis (sages) of ancient India knew that sitting for long periods of time with a straight spine was a potential problem for people in the thoracic region due to its tendency toward hyperkyphosis, or excessive rounding, in response to gravity and fatigue. To assist with these physical challenges of discomfort and dysfunction in the thoracic spine several effective yogic techniques and rehabilitative strategies/exercises are helpful. Generalized mobilizations of the thoracic spine can be routinely and beneficially found in exercises like catcow, horizontal foam rolling, anahatasana (heart opening pose), Brügger relief position, purushamrigāsana (kneeling sphinx pose), Iyengar/Kolar wall leaning, and isolated thoracic spinal twists. Once the spine has been mobilized, the application of shoulder blade stability exercises focusing on the serratus anterior, mid trapezius, lower trapezius, and latissimus dorsi muscles also give the mid back, thoracic spine, and neck a stronger base and better muscular support for the maintenance of upright posture. Exercises here include serratus punches in ardha kumbhakasana (half plank pose), scapular setting, makarasana (dolphin pose), salabasana (locust pose), Y-exercises, Turkish get-ups, and rotator cuff strengtheners (if discomfort is influenced by shoulder movements). Finally, relaxing, massaging, and/or stretching the superficial hypertonic muscles of the cervico-thoracic region provides one with both immediate and long-lasting relief from pain, stress, and tension when effected.

THE BREATH AND THE SPINE

The emphasis and importance of breathing and pranayama is the most distinguishing feature of Yoga in reference to all other physical and therapeutic disciplines. Surprisingly, many people don't breathe efficiently and unknowingly display signs of dysfunction that affect the spine and its surrounding musculature.

In the body, breathing is an automated function of the nervous system like digestion and other body processes. As with other autonomic activities, we need to breathe to stay alive and we aren't required to pay attention to each and every breath in the process. However, unlike the other autonomic activities, breathing can be consciously regulated with will power and volitional control. If a person can learn to recognize unconscious breathing patterns and establish better patterns, he/she can increase the efficiency of his/her spinal musculature and the awareness of how breathing affects his/her posture. Ultimately, "breath is posture and posture is breath" (Kaminoff, 2008), so "our goal is to instruct the patient [or client] to make them more conscious of their faulty patterns, then how to correct them, so they can practice an exercise repeatedly until it becomes subconscious" (Weingroff, 2010).

As breathing relates to the spine, it has been said that there are several variables and no widely accepted standards of "normal breathing." Nonetheless, there are commonly accepted beliefs in Western medicine (Perri, 2003) where most feel that the abdomen, not the chest, should initiate the breath and it is in a belly-to-chest inhalation and a chest-to-belly exhalation. This is the preferred method of breathing shared by doctors and therapists in cases involving lower-back instability as this manner of breathing can recruit abdominal muscles that might otherwise be inhibited and coaxes them into action. This is also the method of breathing widely taught in the Aṣṭāṅga, Vinyāsa, and Power Yoga traditions.

Interestingly, the "father of modern Yoga," Tirumalai Krishnamacharya (Mohan and Mohan, 2010), modified the traditional belly-to-chest method of breathing in the last decades of his life and began teaching "backwards breathing" according to Western convention as he developed yogic techniques employing chest-to-belly breathing. Chest-to-belly breathing is physiologically logical and takes advantage of the movement and dynamics of the breath when it first flows in and enters the lungs. Leslie Kaminoff, a student of T. Krishnamacharya's son, T.K.V. Desikachar, highlights the scientific aspects of this process in the lungs: "Volume and pressure are inversely related: When volume increases, pressure decreases, and when volume decreases, pressure increases. Because air always flows toward areas of lower pressure, increasing the volume inside the thoracic cavity will decrease pressure and cause air to flow into it. This is an inhalation . . . an inhalation involves the chest cavity increasing its volume from top to bottom, from side to side, and from front to back, and an exhalation involves a reduction of volume in those three dimensions" (Kaminoff, 2007). When performed properly, chest-to-belly breathing creates a wavelike rolling motion in the spine similar to the way a cobra snake undulates. This fluid, natural movement can help facilitate better posture if well-educated and balanced spinal muscles support the action.

When untrained, a chest-to-belly inhale and a belly-to-chest exhale can cause people to recruit and overuse secondary respiratory muscles like the scalenes, pectoralis major/minor, and sternocleidomastoids that substitute and do too much work as seen in situations with dysfunction in the diaphragm or intercostal muscles, physical or emotional stress (when done rapidly or with breathlessness), and in the aforementioned example of the hypertonic muscles of upper cross syndrome. Although secondary respiratory muscles are supposed to assist with breathing in extreme situations (like running a marathon) by pulling the upper rib cage open and, in turn, influencing the expansion of the lungs, they have the tendency to become hypertonic, tight, and overworked when employed as part of a regular breathing pattern. As a result, the secondary respiratory muscles are not advised to be part of a person's overall normal breathing pattern and chest-to-belly breathing is typically not prescribed for those with neck discomfort and/or poor slumping postures. As Tim McCall, M.D., states, "A slumping posture contributes to chest breathing by pushing the lower ribs into the upper abdomen. This limits the diaphragm, which ought to be the primary muscle of respiration, so the chest (and sometimes the neck) muscles take over" (McCall, 2007).

But what if we can teach people how to train chest-to-belly breathing in Yoga Therapy without recruiting the neck muscles?

Then, the chest-to-belly breathing method introduced by Krishnamacharya, which is based on the science of gas exchange and the physics of pressure and volume changes, may have a wider scientific, practical, and yogic application than belly-to-chest breathing.

Regardless of whether breathing is initiated from the belly (like in the West) or from the chest (like in Krishnamacharya's teachings), the key points that constitute a regulated breathing pattern in either style do not change. Like a balloon expanding in all directions, 360 degrees around the spine, proper inhalation technique fills and expands the thorax anteriorly, laterally, and posteriorly, as well as in the four areas of the chest, ribs, abdomen, and pelvis as seen in

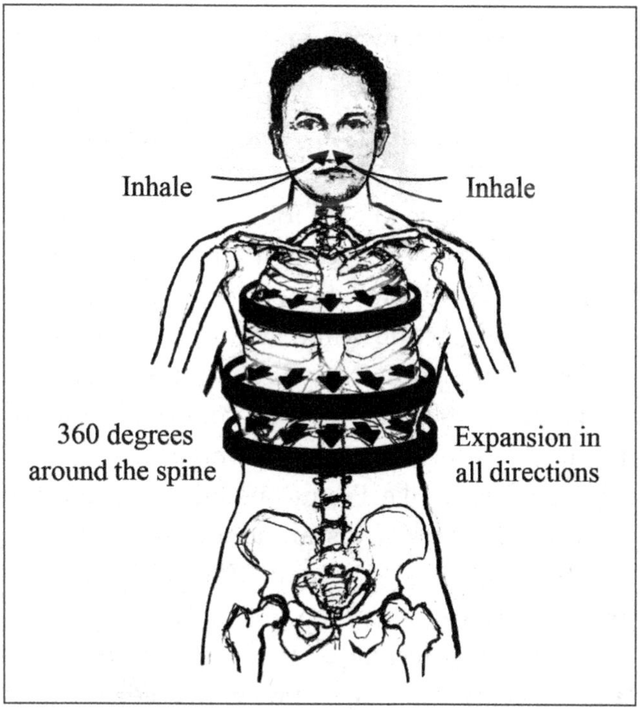

Figure 9. Balloon Respiration

Figure 9. It can be thought of as breathing in the six directions: front, back, left, right, up (to the top of the lungs), and down (to the bottom of the lungs). Whether it was initiated from chest-to-belly or from belly-to-chest on the inhalation, the exhale completes the elimination cycle opposite to the method of inhale. Faulty and/or dysfunctional actions include:

1. Lifting the chest and/or sternum toward the head
2. Lacking a lifting up motion of the lateral ribs
3. Lifting the shoulders toward the ears
4. Excessive engagement/compensation of the upper trapezius, scalenes, or sternocleidomastoids (SCMs)
5. Flaring of the lower ribs
6. Excessive migration of the umbilicus toward the head
7. Abdominal hallowing on inhale breaths (where the abdomen comes in and up instead of protruding out) known as "paradoxical respiration"
8. Underactivity of the lower abdominals and pelvic floor

As yogis have known for centuries, every single breath a person takes affects the structures that connect with the spine. When performed with mindfulness and relaxation, Yoga practitioners can use breathing techniques to improve spino-respiratory function while simultaneously decreasing neck muscle activity and increasing the proficiency of the lungs, intercostals, abdominals, and diaphragm. Thus, breath training may be considered one of the most valuable therapeutic resources in Yoga Therapy and spinal care.

Noted sage-like Prague neurologist and manual medicine specialist, Karel Lewit, M.D., D.Sc., was an advocate of breathing as an integral part of spinal rehabilitation work. He said, "If breathing is not normalized, no other movement pattern can be" (Liebenson, 2007). Below is an adapted version of Dr. Lewit's principle breathing technique that retrains proper spino-respiratory muscle function and can be used in conjunction with other techniques like ujjāyi (victorious) breathing and samavṛtti (equal breathing) prāṇāyāma.

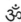

360-Degree Resistance-Based Prāṇāyāma Technique

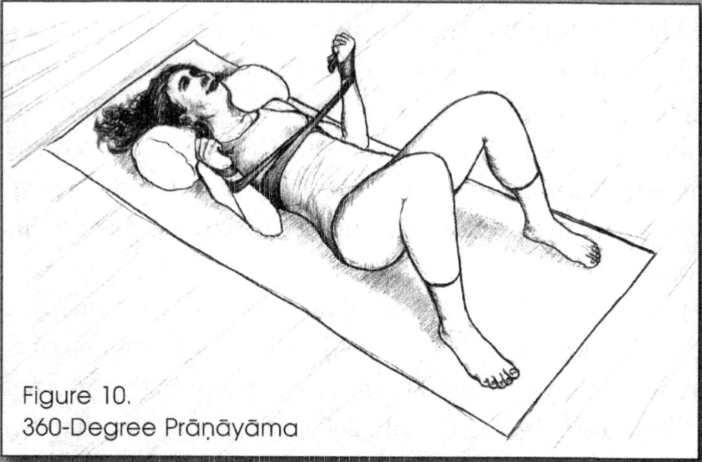

Figure 10.
360-Degree Prāṇāyāma

1. Begin with the spine in a neutral position lying supine on the back with the knees bent.
2. Dig the toes into the floor while keeping the feet flat.
3. Externally rotate the arms and sit them by the side of the body with the palms facing up (known in physical rehabilitation as the Brugger relief position).
4. Elevate the head slightly by resting it on a pillow and press the tongue against the hard palate about 1 inch behind the front teeth (known in Yoga as khecarī mudrā).
5. Place a TheraBand™ or elastic device around the rib cage just below the level of the breasts. Use the hands to pull it tight like a corset to create an appropriate level of resistance for training and double wrap it around the hands on each end for maximum grip.
6. Take a full inhale breath through the six directions in the lungs, intercostals, and diaphragm.
7. Continue breathing deeply while keeping the sternum and the shoulders depressed and go through the list of faulty respiratory actions cited above to correct any associated dysfunctions.
8. Perform as many breaths as needed to improve habitual breathing patterns. (Adapted from Lewit, 1980.)

THE LUMBAR SPINE

The normal adult lumbar spine consists of five vertebrae and five intervertebral discs arranged in a lordotic curve with muscles organized around it in all directions both superficially and deep to provide better support, strength, endurance, and control. As a collective group, the lumbar spine is highly preferential to the movements of flexion, extension, and lateral flexion. It is often injured combining one of these motions with lumbar rotation, especially when under a load, moving too quickly, and/or being in a weight-bearing or an extreme position like many of the Yoga asanas (postures).

Experts estimate that 80 percent of all people will experience back pain in their life (Vallfors, 1985) and this has led to the lower back being one of the most highly researched areas of study in Yoga Therapy, according to the International Association of Yoga Therapists (IAYT) (Lamb, 2006). Many are familiar with the popular study on Yoga for lower back pain by Karen Sherman, Ph.D., M.P.H., sponsored by the National Institute of Health (NIH), that found that Yoga Therapy improved the symptoms of chronic lower back pain when compared to traditional physical therapy exercises and self-help books (Sherman, 2005). Another NIH study performed by Kimberly Williams, M.D., examined people with chronic lower back pain practicing Iyengar Yoga. Over three years, the study showed that those who did Yoga had lifted mood, less pain, and improved function compared to those who received standard medical therapy (Williams, 2009). A study done by Vijay Lad, M.D., found that 80 percent of those practicing Yoga on pain medications for back pain experienced markedly decreased pain compared with 44 percent of those taking only medication. In addition, only 12 percent had recurrences in the Yoga group while 56 percent did in the medication group and the pain medication use of the Yoga group declined by 40 percent (Lake, 2003). Yoga Therapy's proven effectiveness in treating lower back pain is well acknowledged and is discussed in several other chapters of this text.

When considering Yoga Therapy's role in the health, function, and well-being of the lumbar spine, a major component of its success is the application of the concept of spinal stability. Spinal stability comes from the proprioceptive awareness and co-contraction of the abdominal muscles and back muscles as a cohesive unit, not in simply isolating individual muscles like the transverse abdominis (TrA) and multifidii. Spinal expert, Stuart McGill, Ph.D., states that "true spinal stability is achieved with a 'balanced' stiffening of the entire abdominal musculature including the rectus abdominis and the abdominal wall, quadratus lumborum, latissimus dorsi, and the back extensors of longissimus, iliocostalis, and multifidus" (McGill, 2010). This "core" of synergistically engaged muscles and surrounding fascia creates a container of support for the spine. As a result, an internal abdominal pressure (IAP) can be generated in the abdominal cavity to further enhance stability. This pressure can be intensified with the assistance of the diaphragm, which acts on the stability from above in the deepest layers of muscles in the thorax, while the pelvic floor muscles, activated in Yoga through mūla-bandha (the root lock) and ashwini mudra (horse gesture), can provide extra foundational "core" support from below for the lower spine and pelvis. Figure 11 illustrates intra-abdominal pressure together with a balanced system of cooperatively engaged muscles.

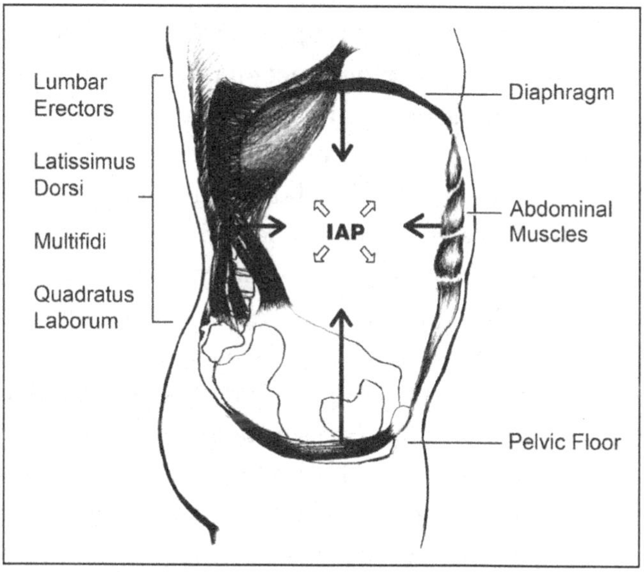

Figure 11. Intra-Abdominal Pressure

In terms of positioning, the safest and most mechanically justifiable approach to enhancing lumbar stability through exercise ensures a neutral spine posture (McGill, 2006). A neutral spine is the position of an individual's spine where every joint is held in an optimal position to allow an equal distribution of force through the entire structure (Howard, 1995). From a Yoga Therapy perspective, spinal neutrality is where there is the least amount of stress and strain in the spine and the greatest amount of calmness, ease, and comfort. Therefore, the oft-given instruction in general Yoga classes to "drop the tailbone down and under," which clearly and forcibly takes the practitioner out of neutral, is an ineffective long-term strategy to stabilize the lower back and/or reduce hyperlordosis. In the right situation or for a desired intention, anterior or posterior tilting of the pelvis may prove to be more valuable than staying in neutral in order to target a stretch into a severely tight or restricted muscle (like the psoas in a lunge stretch) if no other means of accessing and isolating it is available. But, if dropping the tailbone becomes a programmed habit in the spine, it can lead to the chronic destabilization of the lower back by taking the spine out of neutral. To reduce hyperlordosis while maintaining a neutral spine, a physical maneuver called a sternal crunch can be applied, which facilitates the anterior upper abdominal muscles. It is performed by dropping the front ribs toward the back ribs, doing a mini-crunch with the sternum, and engaging the upper abdominal muscles while keeping the shoulders relaxed and lateralizing the breath to keep the diaphragm expansive. Especially for people who have lower back pain and/or sit excessively, the additional reactivation of the powerful posterior chain muscles (the glutes and the hamstrings) through exercises like clamshells, glute bridges, crab walks, gym ball curls, standing functional reaches, and/or modifications to traditional asanas may also assist in supporting a neutral curve.

Another significant topic in Yoga Therapy that relates to the lumbar spine is continued use of the abdominal hallowing procedure, uddīyāna bandha (the belly lock) as a core stability technique. Yet, historically, uddīyāna bandha, where the belly is brought in maximally toward the spine, was never designed for spinal stability. The ancient Yoga masters developed this technique to enhance the way that prāṇa and energy is moved through the spine when practicing advanced prāṇāyāma techniques and kriyās (spinal energy exercises). While uddīyāna bandha can sometimes be taught to new Yoga practitioners to help them learn how to feel and engage the abdominal muscles while in a nonload position like lying on the back, modern rehabilitative medicine has repeatedly shown that the abdominal hallowing procedure is the most mechanically ineffective stabilization maneuver for control of spine motion and stability (Lederman, 2010) when compared with abdominal bracing and a natural spine strategy. Similarly, it has been reported that "the instability of the hallowing position reduces the potential energy of the spinal column causing it to fail at lower applied loads" (McGill, 2009), and "there seems to be no mechanical rationale for using abdominal hallowing . . . to enhance stability" (Grenier and McGill, 2007). Alternatively, a technique known as abdominal bracing, where the muscles are co-contracted and engaged with minimal to moderate effort by pressing outward from the innermost layers of the core, has been shown to create extra support around the spine and enhance intra-abdominal pressure and, in turn, spinal stability. In research evaluations, bracing improved stability over hallowing (Lederman, 2010) and "bracing creates better patterns that better enhance overall stability" (Grenier and McGill, 2007) when compared to abdominal hallowing. The top contra-indication for abdominal bracing, though, is if a Yoga practitioner has a preexisting spinal compression issue that gets worse with increased pressure around the spine like a disc protrusion or a neurologic spinal problem with radiating symptoms into the limb(s). If properly applied, the aforementioned sternal crunch and abdominal bracing techniques can become well programmed long-term habits that promote healthier function in the abdominal muscles and enhance the general stability of the lumbar spine.

DIRECTIONAL PREFERENCE LOWER BACK PAIN

In the movement sciences and Yoga Therapy, many spinal conditions can be subcategorized for easier reference. Gordon Waddell, M.D., states that 94 percent of back pain is mechanical back pain, 5 percent is due to spinal nerve root irritation and 1 percent is due to more serious pathology (Waddell, 2004). This is extremely encouraging because it highlights that the vast majority of people can be affected, treated, and/or co-treated (with a doctor or therapist) using basic body mechanics and spinal rehabilitation techniques found in movement disciplines like Yoga Therapy.

Correspondingly, mechanical back pain can be broken down even further. Studies suggest that one of the best methods of subclassifying mechanical back pain is to organize the conditions based on pain pattern and directional preference (Wernecke, 2011). The term pain pattern refers to what is known as the centralization or decentralization of a person's radiating symptoms of pain, numbness, and/or tingling into a limb. Centralization means that the radiating symptoms in the limb are retreating and moving more centrally toward the spine. Decentralization means that the symptoms begin in the spine and are decentrally moving away from the spine toward the limbs. Decentralization is usually thought to be more serious and severe and may signal the need for assistance from a qualified therapist familiar in working with neurologic conditions. The term directional preference refers to the fact that there are spinal disorders that are biased toward certain movements and radiating pain, numbness, or tingling may be alleviated or exacerbated through either flexing or extending the spine. Dr. Rick Morris, D.C., has termed this system of cataloguing conditions by pain pattern and directional preference with the aptly named terms: *flexion faults* and *extension faults* (Morris, 2009).

Flexion Faults

These are back problems that increase and become more debilitating and decentralized when a person performs flexion exercises like forward bends (standing, sitting, or lying down), sitting in a chair or at the computer, putting on pants/shoes/socks, mārjāryāsana (cat pose) in cat-cow, apānāsana (supine knees to the chest pose), and/or halāsana (plow pose). The Yoga Therapy treatment that is usually advised includes McKenzie extension exercises like cobras, belly sphinxes, standing back bends, gluteal bridges, locust pose vinyāsas, supermans, etc., which decrease the pressure on the discs and nerves when properly applied. Specific diagnostic examples of flexion faults include most disc protrusions and bulges, piriformis syndrome, vertebral fractures, degenerative disc disease, and sciatica.

Extension Faults

These are back problems that increase and become more debilitating and decentralized when a person performs extension exercises like backbends, walking, standing, ūrdhva dhanurāsana (upward-facing bow pose), or even laying down on the stomach. The Yoga Therapy treatment that is usually advised includes Williams flexion exercises like paścimottanāsana (seated forward bend pose), uttānāsana (standing forward bend pose), supine knees to chest, etc., and core work, which decreases pressure on the vertebrae, the vertebral joints, the spinal cord, and the muscles that open the spinal canal. Specific diagnostic examples of extension faults include spinal stenosis, facet joint syndrome/joint imbrication (where the joints are compressed into each other causing extra pressure in the joint capsules), spondylolisthesis (where one vertebra slips forward in relationship to the vertebrae below it), pregnancy, and lumbar erector muscle hypertrophy.

While the above general classification system is a safe and effective guide for creating a distinct division between conditions based on pain pattern and directional preference, an evaluation by a qualified health professional is always advised if the complaint is acute and/or if pain, numbness, or tingling exist. Ultimately, pain and discomfort often decrease from not just knowing what to do, but, even more important, what *not* to do with our bodies. Quite regularly, the "counter pose," or the opposite movement of the one that causes pain and discomfort, has incredibly curative latent properties. In this way, Yoga Therapy can assist in developing greater postural awareness, in identifying certain conditions that have a preference for a certain direction of movement, and in setting up an environment that optimizes one's healing potential.

SCOLIOSIS

Scoliosis has been a common spinal misalignment since the beginning of recorded civilization. It appears in cave paintings of prehistoric man and the famous Greek physician, Hippocrates, was said to have treated scoliosis with braces in the fourth century BCE (Miller, 1990). Fortunately, for people who are afflicted with this condition today, healing remedies like Yoga Therapy can provide incredible support.

Architecturally, scoliosis is a lateral curvature of the spine, typically in the thoracic region, and there are two kinds: functional scoliosis and structural scoliosis. A structural scoliosis is genetic and the resulting curve is subject to the anatomical limitations and growth of the body. It is the harder of the two to treat using Yoga and movement therapy and can be caused by many things including a hemivertebae (a wedge-like vertebra that doesn't grow to the same size as the others), a block vertebrae (where two or more spinal segments fuse and grow into one), a decrease in melotonin levels, a short leg, hormonal changes in children who have an early growth spurt, and idiopathic/unknown reasons (Cramer, 2005). On the other hand, a functional scoliosis is due to the imprecise development of the skeletal muscles and connective tissues that support the spine. This kind of scoliosis could be due to a number of factors such as one's work environment, lifestyle, and previous injuries—as well as acquired mechanical patterns and postural habits. When the degree of curve is minor in a functional scoliosis, it can usually be managed with physical rehabilitation and Yoga Therapy. While a curve up to about 5 to 10 degrees is considered to be normal in adults, a minor scoliosis is a curve of 10 to 20 degrees. These slightly scoliotic people frequently find Yoga Therapy and other complementary therapies like chiropractic, acupuncture, massage therapy, and osteopathy to be very useful in managing day-to-day discomforts that arise. A serious scoliosis requiring more extreme procedures like external bracing ranges from 20 to 40 degrees and the most severe scoliosis cases occur when the curve exceeds 40 degrees, where surgical bracing and vertebral fusion are considered so that the vital organs housed within the rib cage and spine are not compromised.

When talking about Yoga Therapy's role in treating scoliosis, there are several ways in which the spine can be approached whether it is functional or structural scoliosis. Studies suggest that the effects of psychological stress actually have a large impact on the spine and result in an increase in spinal compression (Davis, 2002). Since at its core scoliosis is based on the compressive force of gravity acting on the spine, Yoga Therapy's emphasis on relaxation and calmness, one of its most attractable hallmark features, gives it far-reaching implications in the psycho-somato-emotional effects of scoliosis. By reducing stress via activities like conscious breathing, prāṇāyāma, and individualized āsana, Yoga Therapy can assist in relieving the subjective compressive feelings and stress experienced by the practitioner. Some additional physical exercises/āsanas that may be helpful to consider in working with scoliosis include triangle pose, lying sideways on a bolster, śalabhāsana (locust pose) variations, seated chair twists, supta padangusthasana (reclined hand to foot pose) (Miller, 2006), hinging at the hips and folding the torso off the end of a table (with the body being supported from below by blankets stacked on a chair) (Schatz, 1992), horizontal foam roller exercises, and physical therapy swords where the practitioner reaches across his/her body and does a maneuver akin to pulling a sword from its sheath (Liebenson, 2005). The use of even just one or two of these Yoga Therapy procedures, if they are the correct exercises for that particular practitioner's body, will go a long way in easing the discomforts caused by a scoliotic spine.

CONCLUSION

For thousands of years, yogis have philosophized, "Health is a state of complete harmony of the body, mind, and spirit" (Iyengar, 2006), and modern medicine, ironically, is rediscovering this approach. When applied to the body and, more specifically, to the spine, health is the perfect balance of intrinsic and extrinsic forces in a cooperative, well-communicating, and organized system. In our bodies, we experience this balance unconsciously both on and off the mat as neurokinetic patterns in the central nervous system that hardwire neurons and muscles together to form our spine's basic postural habits. Whether in an āsana, sitting in a chair, standing up, or even lying down, these habits are made up of sensitivity-based responses to the proprioceptors in the joints, tendons, and muscles that tell us where we are in space and give us the opportunity to make changes and recalibrations. Training this "sixth sense" of awareness and our proprioceptive abilities in Yoga Therapy rewires our neurokinetic pathways and reinforces more conscious and educated postural choices and muscle patterning.

Fundamentally, Yoga Therapy is the philosophy, art, and science of adapting Yoga techniques to treat the various dysfunctions and ailments of the body. Applied to the spine, it has significant potential in its role in the modern landscape of preventive medicine. Whether it is remembering to get up and stretch every 20 to 30 minutes while sitting at one's desk, or learning core techniques, or keeping the head in alignment to decrease muscle tension and stress, or learning what *not* to do in Yoga to maintain a healthy spine, many of the pains we experience in the spine can be prevented through the proper application of Yoga Therapy. This was foreshadowed by the great sage, Patañjali, in Sūtra 2.16 of his 2,000 year old, *Yoga Sūtras,* when he said, *"Heyaṁ duḥkham anāgatam* . . . Prevent danger and suffering before it arises" (Satchidananda, 1990).

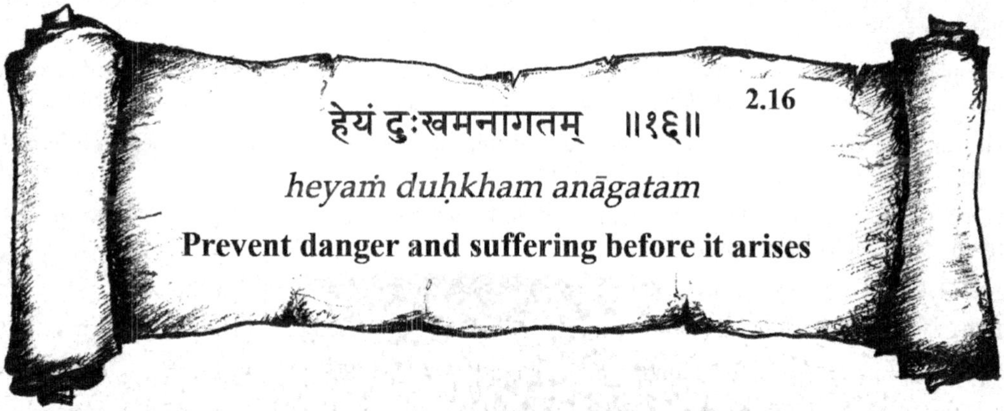
2.16
हेयं दुःखमनागतम् ॥१६॥
heyaṁ duḥkham anāgatam
Prevent danger and suffering before it arises

At its essence, Yoga is not about straining, it is about sustaining. It is not about achieving, it is about accepting. It is not about showing off, it is about tuning in. It is not about *looking* good, it is about *feeling* good. The more these concepts are reinforced, the more intelligent choices are made. Better choices lead to better habits, which lead to better posture, and eventually to a healthier spine and lifestyle. Remembering these ideals, Yoga Therapy can help people discover the positive aspects of spinal health and wellness naturally inherent within the practice.

REFERENCES

Bharati, S. J. "Kundalini Awakening." n.d. Traditional Yoga and Meditation of the Himalayan Masters. SwamiJ.com. Web. Accessed 4 July 2011. http://www.swamij.com/kundalini-awakening-2.htm.

Brown, V. "The Concept of the Djed Symbol." 2002. Pyramid of Man. Web. Accessed 4 July 2011. http://www.pyramidofman.com/Djed/.

Calliet, R. M. *Rejuvenation Strategy.* New York: Doubleday and Co., 1987. Print.

Cramer, G. D. *Basic and Clinical Anatomy of the Spine, Spinal Cord and ANS.* St. Louis: Elsevier Mosby, 2005. Print.

Cumpelik, J. "Bringing the Prague School to You." 2014. Rehab Chiropractor. Web. Accessed 12 Apr. 2014. http://www.rehabchiropractor.com/jiri/.

Dalton, E. P. "Foward Heads = Funky Necks." 2010. Erik Dalton's Myoskeletal Alignment Techniques. Web. Accessed 9 July 2011. http://www.daltonarticles.com/public_html/ForwardHead FunkyNeck.html.

Davis, K. G., et al. "The Impact of Mental Processing and Pacing on Spine Loading." *Spine* 27.23 (2002): 2645?2653. Print.

Glassey, D. D. "The Nerve, Meridian and Chakra Systems and the CSF Connection." 2011. Heal Touch: Life, Energy and Healing. Web. Accessed 7 July 2011. http://www.healtouch.com/csft/life_energy.html.

Grenier, S. G., and S. M. McGill. "Quantification of Lumbar Stability by Using 2 Different Abdominal Activation Strategies." *Archives of Physical Medical Rehabilitation* 88.1 (2007): 54–62. Print.

Howard, A. P. "Neutral Spine." In-Balance.com. 22 Aug. 1995. Web. Accessed 7 July 2011. http://www.in-balance.com/NEUTRAL.HTM.

Iyengar, B. K. S. *Light on Life: The Yoga Journey to Wholeness, Inner Peace and Ultimate Freedom.* Kutztown, PA: Rodale, 2006. Print.

——. *Light on Yoga.* New York: Schocken/Knopf, 1995. Print.

Jull, G. E. *Whiplash, Headache and Neck Pain.* Philadelphia: Churchill Livingstone, 2008. Print.

Kaminoff, L. *Yoga Anatomy.* Champaign, IL: Human Kinetics, 2007, pp. 5–6. Print.

——. "The Anatomy of Breathing and Yoga." *Yoga Therapy Rx* (pp. 1–20). 2008. Loyola Marymount University, Los Angeles.

Kravitz, L., and R. Andrews. "Fitness and Low Back Pain." *IDEA Today* 13.4 (1995): 44–52. Print.

Lake, N. "Back Builders." *Yoga Journal* (May/June 2003): 24. Print.

Lamb, T. "Yoga and the Back and Neck." International Association of Yoga Therapists. 18 Apr. 2006. Web. Accessed 6 July 2011. http://www.iayt.org/site_vx2/publications/Bibliographies_General/back.pdf.

Lederman, E. "The Myth of Core Stability." *Journal of Bodywork and Movement Therapies* 14.1 (2010): 84–98. Print.

Lewit, K. P. "Relation of Faulty Respiration to Posture, with Clinical Implications." *Journal of the American Osteopathic Association* 79.8 (1980): 525–529. Print.

Liebenson, C. D. "Abdominal Exercises Made Simple." *Journal of Bodywork and Movement Therapies* 11.3 (2007): 199–202. Print.

——. "McKenzie Self-Treatments for Sciatica." *Journal of Bodywork and Movement Therapies* 9 (2005): 40–42. Print.

——. "Mid-Thoracic Dysfunction: A Key Perpetuating Factor of Pain in the Locomotor System." Dynamic Chiropractic. 12 Sept. 2001. Web. Accessed 5 July 2011. http://www.dynamicchiropractic.com/mpacms/dc/article.php?id=18210.

——. "Postural Exercises on the Foam Roll." *Journal of Bodywork and Movement Therapies* 14.2 (2010): 203–205. Print.

——. *Rehabilitation of the Spine: A Practitioner's Manual,* 2nd Ed. Baltimore: Lippincott, Williams and Wilkins, 2007. Print.

——. "The Czech School of Manual Medicine: Studying with Lewit and Janda." Dynamic Chiropractic. 18 Nov. 1996. Web. Accessed 5 July 2011. http://www.dynamicchiropractic.com/mpacms/dc/article.php?id=39448.

Lowery, J. D. "What Is Health?" Peace of Life Chiropractic. 2 Jan. 2011. Web. Accessed 11 July 2011. http://peaceoflifechiropractic.wordpress.com/2011/01/02/what-is-health/.

McCall, T. M. *Yoga as Medicine: The Yogic Prescription for Health and Healing.* New York: Bantam, 2007. Print.

McGill, S. P. *Designing Back Exercise: From Rehabilitation to Enhancing Performance.* Waterloo: Back Fit Pro, Inc., 2010. Print.

——. "Exercises for Spine Stabilization: Motion/Motor Patterns, Stability Progressions and Clinical Technique." *Archives of Physical Medicine and Rehabilitation* 90.1 (2009): 118–126. Print.

——. *Low Back Disorders: Evidence Based Prevention and Rehabilitation,* 2nd Ed. Champaign, IL: Human Kinetics, 2007. Print.

——. "Lumbar Spine Stability: Mechanism of Injury and Restabilization." *Rehabilitation of the Spine.* Baltimore: Lippincott, Williams and Wilkins, 2006, p. 102. Print.

Miller, E. B. "Yoga for Scoliosis." *Yoga Journal* 1990. Web. Retreived on July 6, 2011. http://www.yogajournal.com/practice/1060

——. "Back to Back." *Yoga Journal* (May 2006): 74–83. Web. Retreived on July 6, 2011. http://www.yogajournal.com/health/2118

Mohan, A. G., and G. Mohan. "Memories of a Master." YogaJournal.com. 2010. Web. Accessed 25 Feb. 2014. http://www.yogajournal.com/wisdom/2590.

Morgan, W. D. "Cross-Fitness Injury Prevention: Protecting Lumbar Disc in Squatting Motions." *Dynamic Chiropractic* 32.9 (2009): 1–4. Print.

Morris, C. D., et al. "Vladimir Janda, M.D., Ds.C.: Tribute to a Master of Rehabilitation." *Spine* 31.9 (2006): 1060–1064. Print.

Morris, R. D. (2009). The Low Back and the Yoga Practitioner. *Yoga Therapy Rx* (pp. 1–16). Los Angeles: Loyola Marymount University.

Myers, D. G. *Discovering Psychology*, Fourth Edition. New York: Worth Publishers, 1995. Print.

Penn State. "Body's Built-In Computer Helps Recovery from Sports Injury." ScienceDaily. 15 October 1998. Web. Accessed 5 July 2011. www.sciencedaily.com/releases/1998/10/981015075931.htm.

Perri, M. D. "Pain and Faulty Breathing: A Pilot Study." *Journal of Bodywork and Movement Therapies* 8 (2003): 297–306. Print.

Peterson, D. D. *Chiropractic Technique: Principles and Procedures*, Second Edition. St. Louis: Mosby, 2002. Print.

Richardson, C. H., P. W. Hodges, and J. Hides. *Therapeutic Exercise for Lumbopelvic Stabilization*. London: Churchill Livingstone, 2004. Print.

Ruff, C. H., B. Holt, and E. Trinkhaus. "Who's Afraid of the Big Bad Wolff?: 'Wolff's Law' and Bone Functional Adaptation." *American Journal of Physical Anthrolpology* 129.4 (2006): 484–98. Print.

Satchidananda, S. *The Yoga Sutras of Patanjali: Commentary on the Raja Yoga Sutras*. Yogaville: Integral Yoga Publications, 1990. Print.

Schatz, M. M. *Back Care Basics: A Doctor's Gentle Yoga Program for Back and Neck Pain Relief*. Berkeley: Rodmell Press, 1992. Print.

Sherman, K. E., et al. "Comparing Yoga, Exercise and a Self-Care Book for Chronic Low Back Pain." *Annals of Internal Medicine* 143.12 (2005): 849–856. Print.

Vallfors, B. "Acute, Subacute and Chronic Low Back Pain: Clinical Symptoms, Absenteeism and Working Environment." *Scandinavian Journal of Rehabilitative Medicine Supplement* 11 (1985): 1–98. Print.

Vishnudevananda, S. *The Complete Illustrated Book of Yoga*. New York: Julian Press, 1959. Print.

Waddell, G. D. *The Back Pain Revolution*. London: Churchill Livingstone, 2004. Print.

Wallden, M. N. "The Neutral Spine Principle." *Journal of Bodywork and Movement Therapies* 13.4 (2009): 350–361. Print.

Walters, J. D. *The Essence of Self-Realization*. Nevada City: Crystal Clarity Publishers, 1990. Print.

Weingroff, C. P. "DNS in Performance." CharlieWeingroff.com. 28 May 2010. Web. Accessed 10 July 2011. http://charlieweingroff.com/2010/05/dns-in-performance/.

Wernecke, M. W., et al. "Association Between Directional Preference and Centralization in Patients with Low Back Pain." *Journal of Orthopedic and Sports Physical Therapy* 41.2 (2011): 22–31. Print.

Williams, K., et al. "Evaluation and Efficacy of Iyengar Yoga Therapy on Chronic Low Back Pain." *Spine* 34.19 (2009): 2066–2076. Print.

Yochum, T. R., and L. J. Rowe. *Essentials of Skeletal Radiology*, Third Edition. Philadelphia: Lippincott Williams & Wilkins, 2004. Print.

Yogananda, P. *Yogoda or Tissue-Will System of Physical Perfection*. Boston: Sat-Sanga, 1925. Print.

——. *Autobiography of a Yogi*. Los Angeles: Self-Realization Fellowship, 1998. Print.

——. *God Talks with Arjuna: The Bhagavad Gita*, Second Edition. Los Angeles: Self-Realization Fellowship, 1995. Print.

PART TWO

DIVERSE APPROACHES TO YOGA THERAPY

Integrative Restoration iRest® Yoga Nidrā: Healing in Wholeness

Richard C. Miller, Ph.D.

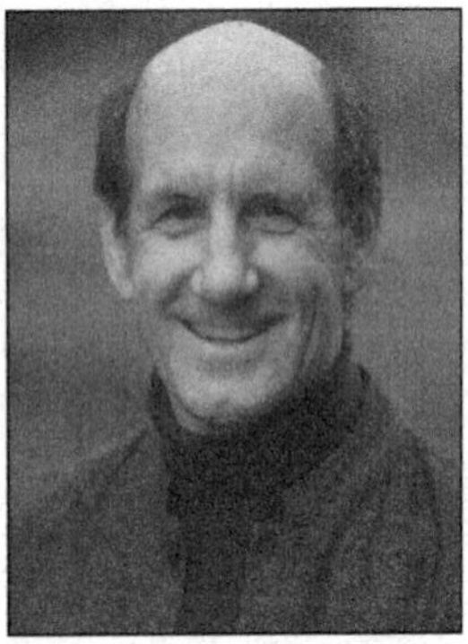

Richard Miller is a clinical psychologist, researcher, Yogic scholar, and spiritual teacher who's devoted his life to integrating Eastern and Western traditions of awakening and psychology. He's the founding president of the Integrative Restoration Institute, cofounder of the International Association of Yoga Therapy, and founding president of the Institute for Spirituality and Psychology. Richard authored *Yoga Nidrā: The Meditative Heart of Yoga* and *The iRest Program for Healing PTSD: Yoga Nidrā Meditation for Deep Relaxation and Overcoming Trauma;* conducts trainings and retreats internationally; and engages in research on the iRest Yoga Nidrā Meditation protocol he's developed for health, healing, and awakening.

INTRODUCTION

Yoga nidrā is a transformative practice derived from the ancient East Indian non-dual tantric (*tan* "to extend" and *tra* "to liberate") teachings of meditation. The practice is comprised of a series of inquiries, which are designed to extend our understanding of and liberate the mind's penchant to divide what's whole into separate parts. Yoga nidrā supports psychological, physical, and spiritual healing, and awakening to the unchanging peace and equanimity that is fundamental to our essential nature. The practice affirms our unitive Yoga (wholeness with all of life), regardless of our circumstance or nidrā (state of consciousness).

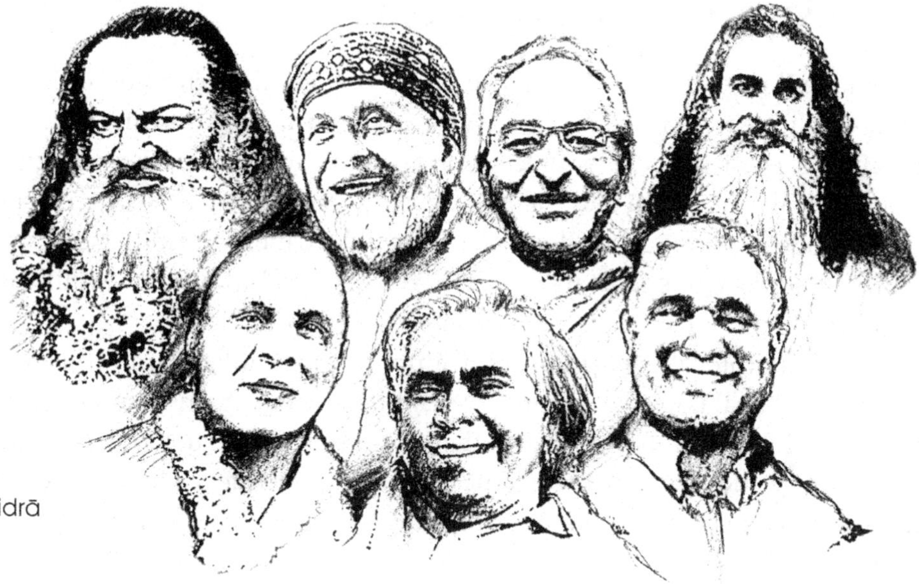

Yoga Nidrā
Yogis

The teachings of Yoga nidrā are not concerned with philosophical intellectualism or secondhand information. Instead, the practice is concerned with our firsthand knowing of who and what we are, free of psychological, cultural, and philosophical conditioning. Yoga nidrā is designed to put us in the driver's seat of our healing and awakening, rather than relying on outside authorities. Various yogis have revitalized the practice of Yoga nidrā into the current century including Swami Sivananda and his disciples, Satyananda Saraswati (Bihar School of Yoga), Swami Satchitananda (Integral Yoga), and Swami Vishnudevananda (Sivananda Yoga Vedanta Center), as well as Swami Rama (Himalayan Institute) and his disciple, Swami Veda Bharati (Swami Rama Sadhaka Grama), and Sri Brahmananda Saraswati (Radhaswami School of Surat Shabd Yoga), among others.

Source texts that address the underlying principles of Yoga nidrā include the *Trika-Shasana* as found in the *Śiva Sūtras;* Tantra in such texts as the *Mahānirvāṇa;* Vedanta in writings including the *Māṇḍūkya and Taittirīya Upaniṣads* and the *Tripura Rahasya,* and the teachings of Yoga as found in *Yogataravali* and the *Yoga Sūtras of Patañjali* with its emphasis on pratyāhāra (restoration of the senses to their natural functioning) wherein the mind's propensity to identify with its projections is transcended and we realize and learn to live from our underlying unitive nature even as we go about experiencing a world of separate objects.

INTEGRATIVE RESTORATION—iREST

Integrative Restoration, or iRest is a modern-day secular rendition of Yoga nidrā. Unlike traditional forms of Yoga nidrā that incorporate cultural and religious symbolism, the iRest protocol respects our age, culture, occupation, religious, and philosophical orientation and mental, physical, and spiritual health. iRest doesn't impose philosophical, cultural, or ideological doctrines. Instead, iRest consists of secular inquiries that enable us to restore our essential health and well-being, and awaken us to our innate interconnection with all of life.

The iRest protocol is *integrative* as it supports the healing of unresolved physical and psychological issues. It's *restorative* as it restores the body-mind to its inherent felt-sense of peace and equanimity that is present no matter our ever-changing circumstances. iRest is both the perspective of, and the means for, unfolding transformation, healing, and awakening at all levels of life: physical, psychological, and spiritual.

RESEARCH ON iREST

Research reveals iRest as both a supportive program as well as a standalone protocol for healing physical and mental concerns such as stress, anxiety, sleep issues, chronic pain, depression, posttraumatic stress (PTS), exhaustion, and compassion fatigue (Miller, et al., 2014). Based on iRest research, the Surgeon General's Pain Management Task Force has endorsed Yoga nidrā as a Tier-1 approach for pain management, and the Defense Centers of Excellence have recommended iRest for continued studies as a complementary medicine for the treatment of PTSD (Schoomaker, 2010; Defense Centers of Excellence, n.d.).

Research on iRest has been, and continues to be, conducted by the Department of Defense and Veterans Administration as well as at military and veteran hospitals, homeless shelters, chemical dependency units, and in university settings. iRest has been studied with active duty military and veterans experiencing posttraumatic stress disorder (PTSD), chronic pain, traumatic brain injury (TBI), and sleep disorders. It has also been used by hospital staff experiencing insomnia and compassion fatigue; couples seeking to increase resiliency and marital enrichment; school counselors and college students to decrease stress and increase resiliency; patients going through cancer treatment or experiencing multiple sclerosis to help manage stress;

people experiencing chemical dependency; couples wishing to increase their fertility; and those experiencing homelessness. As a result, iRest is now being integrated into programs at active duty military and VA facilities, hospitals, clinics, homeless shelters, chemical-dependency units, recreation centers, universities settings, and Yoga and meditation centers (Miller, et al., 2014). In these various settings iRest is being utilized as both a standalone program and a supportive protocol in conjunction with other programs such as Yoga Therapy, psychotherapy, physical therapy, and allopathic medicine.

iREST FOR THE WEST

As a secular form of meditation, iRest is uniquely suited for Westerners and for individuals from cultures all over the world. The protocol has been translated into many languages to support participants in other cultures including Spanish, French, German, Hebrew, Arabic, and Farsi (Miller, et al., 2014). Often likened to deep relaxation, iRest is, in actuality, a comprehensive meditation protocol that teaches tools designed to help us live in harmony with our body, mind, and emotions through the variety of circumstances that life brings so that we feel intimately connected with ourselves, others, and the world around us as we go through life. The iRest protocol is comprised of a series of ten inquiries that practitioners use to explore, heal, and transcend physical, mental, and emotional issues that otherwise give rise to separation, distress, pain, and suffering. iRest research participants report specific improvements across a variety of measures (Miller, et al., 2014) including:

Decreases in:

- Depression
- Anxiety
- Stress
- PTSD
- Insomnia
- Perception of chronic and acute pain

Increases in:

- Ability to have restful and restorative sleep
- Well-being and serenity
- Joy, vitality, purpose, and meaning in life

- Interpersonal, peer, and marital relationships
- Comfort and ability handling situations they can't control
- Perceived control over their lives
- Ability to handle chronic issues such as PTSD, pain, and stress

iRest is designed to restore the body, mind, and senses to their natural functioning. This allows us to naturally experience our interconnectedness with all of life as we go about our daily routines. Embodying and living our natural state of interconnectedness enables us to welcome, explore, and transcend levels of identification that otherwise uphold our perception of separation and suffering.

These levels, or sheaths, of identification include the physical and energy body and the sheaths of emotion, cognition, and ego identification. The practice of iRest doesn't entail assessment, diagnosis, or treatment. Rather it's concerned with enhancing our ability to explore our fusion with and limitations that ensue from our overidentification with these sheaths, or *kośas,* that bind attention and keep us bound in subject-object separation, reaction, and suffering. The practice of iRest leads to the emancipation of attention from fusion with these sheaths so that we can be responsive, rather than reactive, with our emotions, thoughts, and actions within ourselves and in the world around us.

SEPARATION AND WELCOMING

The stages of iRest are designed to help us explore our identification with the belief of being a separate self or ego-I, which creates inner and outer division and feelings of separation, disharmony, and constriction. The belief in separation generates within us a feeling that "something's missing," "wrong," or "off" in our life. When the ego-I thought fuses with this feeling, we believe that something's wrong with our basic sense of self. Living fused with the belief of being a separate self gives rise to reactive division and reaction to our reactions. When we're angry, we're angry that we're angry, even as we try to be calm, cool, and collected. When we feel guilty, we feel guilty about feeling guilty. Reactive patterns are defensive strategies, which occur when we believe we should be other than we are, and this moment should be other than it is.

iRest suggests that the way out of our cage of reactivity lies in learning to welcome each moment just as it is, and our self, just as we are. Welcoming lies outside of reactive emotions and conditional beliefs. It doesn't involve analysis, judgment, conclusion, or other movements based on impositions by a conditioned mind that wants things to be other than how they are. Welcoming allows us to take perspective and sense actions that are in harmony, rather than in reaction, with the moment. iRest enables us uncover our "perfect" response to each moment that allows us to feel that our lives have meaning and purpose and our actions are in harmony with the entire universe.

SUBJECT-OBJECT DUALITY

In everyday living we tend to emphasize the objects that are in our awareness: sensations, emotions, cognitions, and our felt-sense of being a separate self. Here, we live in subject-object duality, as a subjective observer to what we're observing, as a "welcomer" to what we're "welcoming." But there arrives a stage during iRest where attention is freed from these objects and turns upon itself, where awareness and welcoming are emphasized, free of subject-object duality.

When attention turns upon itself, the observer becomes the observed. Here, we experience ourselves as a neutral spaciousness in which polarities of observer and observed, and welcomer and welcomed lose their driving force and dissolve into *"being observing," "being welcoming."* We shift from being a noun (subject) to being a verb (process). As we shift perceptually into "being," conceptual beliefs are no longer nourished and the felt-sense of separation dissolves into our underlying ground of unitive wholeness.

STAGES OF INQUIRY

The stages of iRest (as shown in the table below) are simple yet take time to integrate because of the tenacity of our personal, familial, and cultural conditioning. It takes time to welcome, assimilate, and transcend entrenched patterns of perceiving imposed by our conditioned mind. While the stages of iRest are never fixed and can be engaged in any order, it's useful to learn iRest in a systematic way before utilizing the protocol in a free and spontaneous manner.

TABLE 1. STAGES OF iREST

STAGE	PURPOSE
1. Heartfelt Mission	Affirming what gives value, purpose, and meaning to our life
2. Intention	Affirming vows that support actualizing our Heartfelt Mission
3. Inner Resource	Affirming an inner sanctuary of security, resiliency, and well-being
4. BodySensing	Welcoming physical sensations
5. BreathSensing	Welcoming natural rhythms of breathing and energy
6. Feelings & Emotions	Welcoming opposites of feeling emotion
7. Thoughts	Welcoming opposites of thoughts and beliefs
8. Joy	Welcoming happiness, love, equanimity, peace, and joy
9. Wholeness	Recognizing our unitive wholeness
10. Integration	Integrating iRest into all aspects of daily life

STAGE ONE: AFFIRMING OUR HEARTFELT MISSION

"It is the intensity of the longing that does all the work."

—KABIR

We begin iRest by locating the felt-sense of our Heartfelt Mission by inquiring: *What are the core values that provide meaning, purpose, and value to my life? What is it that motivates me to be fully engaged with life? What is it that life wants of me as its unique and perfect expression.*

It's important to discover, experience, and embody our deepest Heartfelt Mission during our lifetime. Our Heartfelt Mission is connected to our desire for intimacy, wholeness, authenticity, and understanding the underlying mystery of life. It is connected to our longing to be spontaneous, compassionate, kind, and loving. During this initial stage of iRest we welcome and affirm our Heartfelt Mission into the foreground of our conscious mind, not as a future possibility, but as already true. Instead of saying, *May I feel whole, healthy, and free,* or *May I feel loved,* we instead affirm, *I am wholeness, health, and freedom in this and every moment,* or *I am love itself.* We affirm the reality of our Heartfelt Mission as the actuality of this moment so that it evokes an attitude of aliveness, right now.

Our Heartfelt Mission is not intellectual. It arises from deep within as a "bottom up" process that emerges from life expressing itself through our body-mind as core actions that instill purpose, meaning, and value to our lives. Living our Heartfelt Mission reconciles "my will" with "thy will" wherein we feel not just that *I'm living life,* but that *Life is living me.*

STAGE TWO: SETTING OUR INTENTION

"If you believe you can or you can't, you're right!"

—Henry Ford

During stage two we inquire, *What are intentions that support the actualization of my Heartfelt Mission?* Robust intentions serve as gyroscopes or magnetic compasses that keep us on course. Like the banks of a river, they keep us flowing in the right direction and enable us to navigate our journey of living our Heartfelt Mission, keeping our course straight and true, no matter our state of mind or body.

Intentions can be short- or long-term, each designed to support our realizing particular goals. These include healing physical pain or trauma, confronting reactive emotions or beliefs, and/or rearranging diet and lifestyle to assist us in actualizing our life's purpose.

Like the Heartfelt Mission, intentions are "bottom up" processes that emerge from life itself, expressing through our body-mind, which we formulate as present-tense affirmations. Instead of saying, *May I be aware,* we affirm, *I am awareness itself.* Instead of saying, *I will stop smoking,* we affirm, *I am a nonsmoker.*

STAGE THREE: EXPERIENCING OUR INNER RESOURCE

"Our work is to keep our hearts open in hell."

—STEPHEN LEVINE

During iRest we may encounter strong emotions, beliefs, traumas, and unresolved psychophysical issues. At times we may feel disoriented as we explore various levels of our psyche. We may experience fear or anxiety, a sudden loss of ground as if we're in free fall, or archetypal feelings of terror or aloneness. Therefore, it's helpful to have in place our Inner Resource, an inner sanctuary, or safe haven, which provides us with the felt-sense of indestructible security, ground, and resiliency, and restful equanimity and well-being, which we feel and experience as present no matter our circumstance.

Throughout iRest, we nourish our Inner Resource as we encounter and heal challenging emotions, beliefs, and memories from unresolved incidents in our life such as loss, trauma, accidents, and/or physical, psychological, or sexual abuse. The Inner Resource is our inner refuge, which helps us navigate existential fear and anxiety that can arise along the way, as we heal our beliefs in separation and recognize our inherent unitive wholeness.

During iRest, should we feel overwhelmed by some inner or outer circumstance, we take refuge in our Inner Resource. Here we rest in the felt-sense of security, ground, well-being, and confidence, which we then take back with us as we continue to face and resolve core issues that otherwise distract attention from the deeper inquiries that the practice of iRest reveals.

STAGE FOUR: BODYSENSING—WELCOMING SENSATION

"When we live in innocent, unconditioned listening
our body goes spontaneously into deep peace."

—JEAN KLEIN

During BodySensing, we rotate attention through the physical body noting, feeling, and welcoming sensations, wherein the body is realized to be an expansive field of radiant sensation. As with each stage of iRest, we aren't trying to fix, alter, or change our experience. Whether sensation is strong or weak we're learning to welcome the "what is" of it, without intention to fight, fix, change, or "go beyond" what's arising. iRest draws its strength from the understanding that everything that changes goes through five natural phases of transformation: birth, growth, stability, decay, and death. Like bubbles rising to the surface of a lake, everything ultimately transforms, revealing our appropriate response to each moment of life.

Messengers

During BodySensing the physical body is welcomed into awareness as vibrant sensations, which are recognized as messengers, or pointers to their underlying causes to which we can take appropriate actions. BodySensing is soothing to the nervous system and invites deep relaxation and the felt-sense of well-being into the body and mind. As such, it is a form of mindfulness training. Its practice develops focused attention, develops the mind's ability to remain undistracted, and supports concentration and one-pointed attention.

There are literally billions of events occurring in the body at any given moment. Our body is constantly sending us "messengers," which are informing us of how we're feeling and how we need to respond. For instance, when we mistakenly touch a hot pan, our hand instantly jerks away as the mind registers, *Ouch, that's hot!* These messengers of sensation (as well as emotions and cognitions) inform our bodymind how to respond to each situation, person, or life event. We can miss these messengers when we don't take time to sense our body. If we don't pay attention, eventually the body will have to shout at us with physical or mental symptoms such as a stomachache, sore back, anxious feeling, or depression.

BodySensing reawakens our capacity to register the body's subtle cues. For example, one student noticed an unfamiliar sensation in her armpit during BodySensing, which led her to discover early-stage cancer that was removed before chemotherapy was deemed necessary. When we can sense and welcome subtle cues, we're able to take appropriate actions, which is one of the many advantages of practicing BodySensing and the various stages of iRest.

STAGE FIVE: BREATHSENSING—WELCOMING BREATH AND ENERGY

"One who understands the breath quickly tastes the ecstasy of liberation."

—GORAKSASHÂSTRA

BreathSensing is a form of mindfulness training that helps us become aware of how our body is breathing in relationship to what we're experiencing. Like BodySensing, BreathSensing supports recognition of subtle movements, or messengers of information, within our body-mind. Here we observe how body, mind, and breathing are a unified experience. For instance, when the body is tense, breathing can become short, irregular, and shallow, activating the sympathetic fight-or-flight response. When the body is relaxed, breathing can become deep and rhythmic, activating the parasympathetic rest/renew response. In addition, BreathSensing nourishes our mind's ability to remain undistracted and one-pointed.

BreathSensing releases tension stored in the body, especially around the area of the chest, diaphragm, abdomen, and pelvis. This enables us to access information to recognize, process, and integrate sensations, emotions, and cognitions so that we can feel at ease, compassionate, and caring toward our self and others.

STAGE SIX: WELCOMING OPPOSITES OF FEELINGS AND EMOTIONS

"Out beyond ideas of wrong-doing and right-doing is a field. I'll meet you there."

—RUMI

During this phase of iRest we learn to recognize the constantly changing world of feeling and emotions, which are comprised of opposites such as warm/cool, tense/relaxed, happy/sad, fearful/courageous, etc. As opposites are welcomed, they are recognized as pointers, or messengers, to their underlying unity, which reveals deeper levels of understanding.

TABLE 2. OPPOSITE STATES OF CONSCIOUSNESS

Happy	⟷	Sad	Courageous	⟷	Fearful
Relaxed	⟷	Tense	Cool	⟷	Hot
Comfort	⟷	Discomfort	Pride	⟷	Shame
Peaceful	⟷	Anger	Sharp	⟷	Dull
Easeful	⟷	Anxious			

Feelings such as comfort/discomfort, hot/cold, dull/sharp, as well as emotions such as anger/peaceful, anxious/easeful, or shame/pride are exquisite messengers. They provide us with rich sources of information on how we should respond to the world around and within ourselves so that we're able to stay in harmony with ourselves and the world around us. When we touch a hot stove, pain arrives to warn of danger. When expectations are thwarted, irritation arises alerting us to reexamine our underlying beliefs. In and of themselves, feelings and emotions are neither good nor bad, neither right nor wrong. They're simply messengers that provide information.

Our task is to welcome the legitimacy of our feelings and emotions so that we can understand appropriate and harmonious responses that enable us to be well adjusted and fully functioning human beings.

iRest helps us to be proficient at recognizing the variety of feelings and emotions we experience as we navigate life. We need to be sensitive to the entire range of feelings and emotions, and to welcome rather than repress, deny, or, in some cases, even express them. iRest is a process that helps us recognize and respond to our feelings and emotions rather than becoming fused with and reactive to them.

STAGE SEVEN: WELCOMING OPPOSITES OF COGNITION—THOUGHTS, BELIEFS, IMAGES, AND MEMORIES

"Thoughts change, not you."

—Ramana Maharshi

During iRest we learn to welcome every experience that life brings as changing facets of our underlying wholeness. Our mind may resist this understanding by exclaiming, *"How could this be a facet of wholeness?"* Doubt is only one of the ways the mind divides what is in reality whole and projects a sense of separation. During this phase of iRest, we learn to recognize beliefs that maintain identification through our beliefs of limitation and separation. Cognitions of thought and image are welcomed, without aversion, attachment, or grasping, and allowed to go through their natural stages of transformation as changing objects unfolding in awareness.

The Law of Opposites

Like emotions, as cognitions arise, their opposites also co-arise. Opposites are never separate. They are complimentary polarities arising within a unified field of awareness. When we identify with only one-half of a pair of opposites, e.g., separation versus nonseparation, grief versus joy, or shame versus potency, we remain fused in our experience. By welcoming and experiencing opposites of cognition, we're able to gain insight into, and heal our misperceptions that keep suffering in place.

During iRest, each cognition is paired with its opposite as a way of assisting their full disclosure into awareness. *I'm unlovable* is paired with *I'm love, itself. I'm not good enough* is paired with *I'm always doing the best that I know how.* We cannot stop life's tumultuous waves of experience, but we can learn to surf them. The practice of iRest is our surfboard, teacher, surfing lesson, and ability to surf all rolled into one.

As opposites are acknowledged, welcoming replaces refusing, psychophysiological integration unfolds, well-being arises spontaneously, and we're able to experience inner peace and equanimity even in the midst of conflict. True healing takes place when we cease trying to rid ourselves of our experience and instead welcome the full range of opposites that comprise our moment-to-moment experience.

STAGE EIGHT: WELCOMING JOY, BLISS, LOVE, AND WELL-BEING

"We grow old because we stop laughing."

—Chuck Gallozzi

As attention is liberated from being fused with cognitions, psychological movements of attachment, aversion, and grasping are naturally released, and well-being, equanimity, peace, love, joy, and even bliss naturally arise. For most people joy, peace, and equanimity are relative experiences, coming and going, dependent upon the changing conditions of life. We are conditioned to believe that joy is dependent upon possessing some object, be it money, job, lover, lack of disease, or even enlightenment. Our search for objects or experiences that will bring lasting happiness always misses the mark. Ironically, it is our searching that takes us away from experiencing everlasting peace, well-being, and joy, which are already innately present within.

Discovering Inherent Joy

During this eighth stage, iRest helps us investigate Joy as our inherent presence or beingness, wherein equanimity, peace, and joy can be discovered to exist independent of changing states of consciousness. We may begin by sensing an inner sense of pleasantness, and then gradually build our ability to experience pleasure, happiness, joy, well-being, bliss, and imperturbable peace and equanimity. It's truly amazing to discover that there doesn't have to be a reason to feel joyful and equanimous. Joy is already inside us waiting to be welcomed to the forefront of our consciousness.

Joy Is Good Medicine

We all know moments of joy and equanimity, even if they are few and far between. It's common knowledge that joy raises our spirits and relieves stress. Scientific research reveals that joy keeps us healthy and helps heal disease (Lemonick, 2005). Joy, even in small doses, affects our entire physiology including the respiratory, cardiovascular, muscular, central nervous, endocrine, and immune systems (Berk and Tan, 1995). Joy releases oxytocin, serotonin, and endorphins, natural chemicals that enable us to feel an inner sense of well-being and everything else unfolding in our experience.

BRAIN REGIONS ALTERED BY PTSD

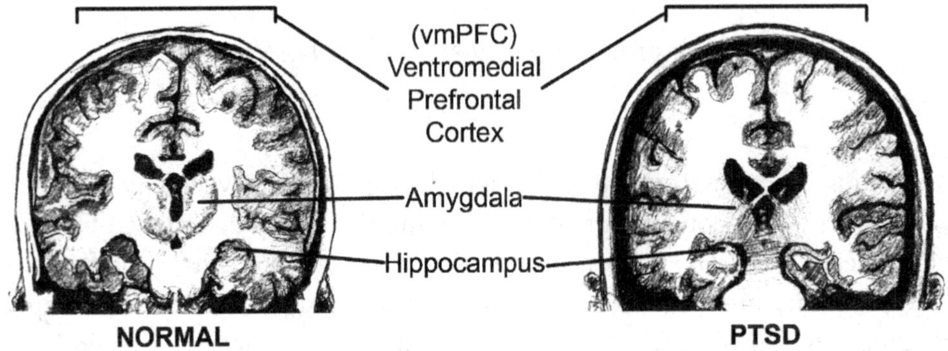

Understanding joy as a potent healing force is not new. In ancient Greece, hospitals were built near amphitheaters where patients could attend comedies to facilitate healing (Sesana, 2013). Modern medicine is now conducting research that demonstrates the healing power of joy and how it can change the shape and function of the brain and nervous system (Nilsen).

People who are joyful and optimistic are at reduced risk of cardiovascular and pulmonary disease, diabetes, hypertension, colds, and upper-respiratory infections. They are likewise found to have reduced levels of cortisol, which is produced by the adrenal glands in response to stress and is known to suppress immune function (Sesana, 2013). Brain tissues of people experiencing long-term depression and PTSD undergo structural changes including reductions in size of the hippocampus and increases in the size of the amygdala, as well as increased activity in the amygdala and decreased activity in the left-frontal cortex.[1] Fortunately, researchers have also discovered that the brain is highly plastic and constantly changes throughout our lifetime.[2] As people heal through depression and PTSD, the size of the hippocampus increases and the amygdala decreases. Additionally, there are decisive left-lateral shifts toward increased frontal cortex activity and reduced activity within the amygdala and right frontal cortex.

True Joy

iRest takes us beyond psychophysiological-induced states of happiness. It invites us to experience joy and equanimity independent of particular situations or objects.

During iRest we welcome "relative" joy into our body-mind and use it as a pointer to a deeper unchanging, or absolute, joy that is the source from which all relative states of happiness arise.

At first, we welcome constructive states of emotions and thoughts as antidotes to their opposites. Experiencing constructive states changes our psychophysiology and increases our ability to experience constructive states of consciousness (see Table 2 on page 329). iRest then invites us to recognize how all states of consciousness are changing appearances pointing to the ground in which they arise, awareness, which can be recognized by its subtle but unmistakable quality, which signals our transition into the ninth stage of iRest.

STAGE NINE: WELCOMING OUR WHOLENESS

"Before I am 'this' is who I am."

—NISARGADATTA MAHARAJ

iRest sharpens our ability to witness sensations, feelings, emotions, and thoughts as they arise. Witnessing is a neutral stance wherein we place no judgments upon what we experience. Instead, we observe as a neutral witness to all that we perceive. Witnessing allows us to gain perspective and see the larger picture that often escapes us when we're embroiled in an emotional reaction. As we become established in witnessing, we realize that sensations, feelings, emotions, and thoughts are transitory and constantly changing. To the degree we react, we become slaves

---

1. The hippocampus is essential for appreciation of memory and the context of events. The hippocampus provides information about context and helps govern emotional responses so that they are appropriate to the context. In both depression and PTSD the hippocampus actually shrinks due to the presence of high levels of cortisol. When depression is treated with antidepressant medication, it prevents the atrophy of the hippocampus.

People with a history of severe aggression exhibit atrophy or severe shrinkage of the amygdala. The amygdala is needed for anticipating negative consequences, and people prone to pathological extremes of rage are unable to foresee the consequences their rage will have. There is actual atrophy of the frontal lobes in individuals who exhibit antisocial behavior.

2. Neuroplasticity is the understanding that the brain continually changes as a result of our experiences, whether through fresh connections between neurons or through the generation of new neurons. Our quota of happiness can be enhanced through mental training because the very structure of our brain can be modified.

to our emotions. As we develop the capacity to witness and welcome emotions, without repressing, refusing, or reactively expressing them, we recognize appropriate responses. Then, having served their purpose, the sensations, emotions, and thoughts continue through their cycle of transformation and ultimately dissolve. By our willingness to truly welcome and fully experience what is, we're able to observe the "what is" transform without our becoming reactive. In fact, the word *experience* means "to live through," leaving no trace behind (*Merriam-Webster*, 2009).

Separation

The mind's identification with being a separate witness, however, creates a division of subject and object, witness and witnessed, which supports our felt-sense of separation and obstructs our perception of our interconnectedness with the underlying wholeness of life. During this ninth stage, iRest invites us to turn the witness upon itself. Here, there is a natural collapse from being a separate witness into "being witnessing." This dissolves separation and reveals our innate ground of unconditioned and unitive wholeness.

During this stage of iRest, we are invited to feel ourselves "as" being. We feel ourselves as the spacious field of being-awareness in which all experiences arise. At this point, welcoming is turned away from its objects, and into "being welcoming," where we feel ourselves as nondual wholeness that is without opposite, as the space of being-awareness in which all opposites arise.

As we relax into "being," we experience our underlying innate peace and harmony that is always present. Being may be likened to a blank screen upon which the movie of life appears. Depending upon the contents of each scene, we laugh or cry, but the screen upon which the movie is projected remains untouched by the film. Being remains untouched by experience and exists in every moment of life as unchanging equanimity.

This phase of iRest reveals that our innate nature is unconditioned, unchanging, and spontaneously arising. As we transition back into our everyday life, we carry this understanding with us. As we interact with people, work, sleep, eat, and play, we retain the equanimity and peace of being. Each time we engage iRest, we are nourishing and strengthening our connection with our underlying essence of equanimity and harmony, which provide us with a steady, balanced, and serene anchor that is recognizable during every moment of life.

STAGE TEN: WELCOMING EVERYTHING JUST AS IT IS

"I have shown you the path.
It is now up to you to travel the path."

—BUDDHA

The essential experiences and understandings of iRest can be learned through individual and/or group sessions, as well as through Mp3 guided recordings. iRest is an approach that supports our ability to embrace, respond, and live each moment of life. Whether walking, talking, eating, working, playing, interacting, or resting, the practice of iRest helps us experience ourselves as a changeless mystery of equanimity, peace, stillness, wholeness, and well-being within which our changing sensations, emotions, thoughts, and images are arising.

iRest Yoga Nidrā culminates in our ability to live our unconditioned freedom of equanimity and peace in the midst of the circumstances of life. Here, the five senses and mind function naturally, doing their job of projecting separation, while our awakened "sixth sense" simultaneously perceives unconditioned nonseparation. The world of separate objects continues to arise, but the mind no longer perceives only a dualistic reality of separate objects. We live beyond the duality of concepts and identification with the ego-I, even as the duality of concepts and the ego-I continue to arise. We recognize our unconditioned freedom whether the body-mind is awake or asleep. This is the culmination of iRest Yoga Nidrā and the path of Yoga.

CONCLUSION

Ancient in its formulation as a timeless practice of meditation, the teachings of Yoga nidrā are designed to be adapted to our individual needs, respecting the changing epoch we live in. Secular by design and research proven, iRest is a modern-day application of Yoga Therapy that is continuing the ancient teachings of Yoga nidrā and meditation. iRest is being practiced as a standalone and complementary supportive program, across countless settings worldwide, with a range of individuals who are facing a variety of mental and physical health-related challenges as well as those seeking to enhance resiliency, well-being, spiritual awakening, and enlightenment.

The nonprofit educational foundation Integrative Restoration Institute (IRI) sponsors trainings and certifies iRest teachers and trainers worldwide. For further information on research, classes, workshops, trainings, and iRest Teacher Certification, please visit IRI's website: www.iRest.us.

REFERENCES

Berk, L., and S. A. Tan. "Eustress of Mirthful Laughter Modulates the Immune System Lymphokine Interferon-Gama." *Annals of Behavioral Medicine* (Supplement). Proceedings of the Society of Behavioral Medicine's 16th Annual Scientific Sessions, 1995, p. C064. Print.

Berk, L., S. A. Tan, and W. Fry. "Eustress of Humor-Associated Laughter Modulates Specific Immune System Components." *Annals of Behavioral Medicine* (Supplement). Proceedings of the Society of Behavioral Medicine's 16th Annual Scientific Sessions, 1993, p. S111. Print.

Berk, L., et al. "Neuroendrocrine and Stress Hormone Changes During Mirthful Laughter." *American Journal of the Medical Sciences* 298.6 (1989): 390–396. Print.

Berk, L., et al. "Eustress of Mirthful Laughter Modifies Natural Killer Cell Activity." *Clinical Research* 37 (1989): 115A. Print.

Berk, L., et al. "Humor Associated with Laughter Decreases Cortisol and Increases Spontaneous Lymphocyte Blastogenesis." *Clinical Research* 36 (1988): 435A. Print.

Defense Centers of Excellence (DCoE) for Psychological Health & Traumatic Brain Injury. "PTSD: Treatment Options." n.d. Web. Retrieved June 21, 2013. http://www.dcoe.mil/ForHealthPros/PTSDTreatment Options.aspx.

Horvatin, T. "In Search of the Healing Theatre of Ancient Greece." Centre for Playback Theatre, New Paltz, NY, 2010. Web. PDF available at http://www.playbacktheatre.org/wp-content/uploads/2010/04/greece-horvatin.pdf.

Integrative Restoration Institute. iRest Yoga Nidra Research and Programs. 2014. Web. Retrieved 1 Mar. 2014. http://www.irest.us/programs/irest-research-and-programs.

Lemonick, M. "The Biology of Joy." *Time* magazine. 9 January 2005. Web. Retreived on June 21, 2013. Available at http://content.time.com/time/magazine/article/0,9171,1015863-1,00.html.

Merriam-Webster Dictionary. "Experience: Something personally encountered, undergone, and lived through." Dictionary entry. Springfield, MA: Merriam-Webster, Inc., 2009.

Miller, Richard, et al. A complete listing of published papers and posters on research studies using iRest Yoga Nidra are available at www.irest.us/irest-research-and-programs.

Nilsen, D. L. F., compiler. A list of 350+ scientific research papers on laughter. Laughter Online University. n.d. Web. http://www.healinglaughter.org/blog/350-scientific-research-papers-on-laughter/.

Schoomaker, E. B. "Pain Management Task Force: Providing a Standardized DoD and VHA Vision and Approach to Pain Management to Optimize the Care for Warriors and Their Families." Final Report. Office of the Army Surgeon General, May 2010, p. 43. PDF available at http://programs.rockpointe.com/content/online/painassembly/downloads/Pain-TaskForce-Report.pdf.

Sesana, L. "The Ancient Greek Theater at Epidaurus." *Washington Times* 23 August 2013. Print.

Integrative Yoga Therapy

Joseph Le Page, M.A.

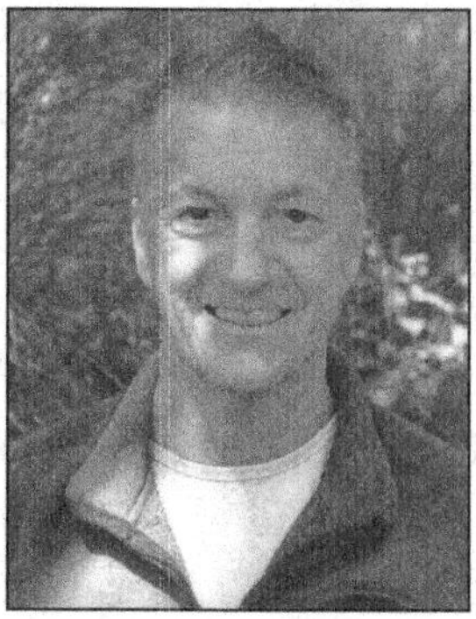

Joseph Le Page is the founder of Integrative Yoga Therapy (IYT) and IYT's training programs. A pioneer and leader in the field and a Kripalu-trained Yoga teacher with a master's degree in teaching from the School for International Training, Joseph has taught Yoga psychology at Sonoma State University and at Antioch University. He is a graduate of the Phoenix Rising Yoga Therapy Training program and has been a speaker at major conferences including Yoga Journal, the International Association of Yoga Therapists, and the Kripalu Center for Yoga and Health. Together with his wife, Lilian Le Page, Joseph directs IYT and the Enchanted Mountain Center for Yoga and Health in Brazil and is the author of the *Yoga Teacher's Toolbox* and *Mudras for Healing and Transformation*.

INTRODUCTION

Integrative Yoga Therapy (IYT) was founded in 1993, and, over the past twenty years, more than 3,000 students from around the world have completed IYT's Professional Training Programs. These programs are grounded in a unique ten-step therapeutic process, forming a complete healing program that is successfully being used in a variety of healing environments, including hospitals and clinical settings. IYT's experiential approach to learning allows students to integrate in-depth information through the creative process while using a wide variety of Yoga tools. These tools and techniques are used to design therapeutic programs for specific groups and for one-on-one Yoga Therapy sessions.

The IYT approach to Yoga Therapy is based on the model of the five kośas. This model comes from the *Taittirīya Upaniṣad* of approximately 3,000 years ago. The five-kośa model serves as a map of the human being for guiding the spiritual journey and also as a guide to global health and healing. *Kośa* can be translated as "sheath" or "layer" and refers to the multiple dimensions of our being, our five "bodies": physical, energetic, psycho-emotional, wisdom, and bliss. A less frequently used, but equally important, translation of the word *kośa* is "treasure," referring to all dimensions of our being as treasures waiting to be unfolded and understood through the practices of Yoga (SpokenSanskrit, 2011). Each of the names of the kośas is followed by the word *maya,* which in this context, means "consisting of." Through this model, therapists acquire an embodied understanding of the tools and techniques used in Yoga Therapy so they are able to design and implement easily accessible practices for their program participants. The exploration and integration of the five kośas naturally leads us to the recognition of our own true being whose nature is freedom and unity. This recognition of our true Self is the essence of the Yoga journey and needs to be integrated into all of the ways that we perceive Yoga as a vehicle for health and healing. A brief overview of the kośas will allow us to see their importance within the practice of Yoga Therapy and for our IYT therapists.

ANNA-MAYA-KOŚA: PHYSICAL BODY

Anna means "food." The anna-maya-kośa is the material dimension of our being that is sustained by food. It encompasses the anatomy and physiology of the body as well as the five elements (earth, water, fire, air, and space) that form the matrix of our body and all of creation. By deepening awareness of our physical being, the bodily systems and the five elements come into balance more easily. This balance lays a firm foundation for awakening and integrating the other dimensions.

At the level of the physical body, IYT practitioners gain an in-depth understanding of anatomy and physiology for each system of the physical body and the most common health conditions associated with them. Balance or imbalance in each system is assessed using evaluation tools centered on the five kośas, using specific Yoga techniques to address imbalance at each level of being. The mechanics of movement are studied, including healthy range of motion for each of the joints in the body, so that the most common musculoskeletal problems can be assessed along with the benefits and contraindications of Yoga techniques for each of these areas.

Trainees in our system also gain proficiency in modifying and teaching Yoga postures to a wide variety of individuals and groups relevant to their special needs, including the use of props. An in-depth understanding of Ayurveda is foundational for adapting all of these skill sets for individual needs, including āsana (posture), prāṇāyāma (breathing), mudrā (gesture), Yoga nidrā (relaxation), and meditation.

PRĀṆA-MAYA-KOŚA: ENERGY BODY

Praṇa is the life force energy that permeates all of creation, including our physical bodies. The prāṇa-maya-kośa is that aspect of our being composed of vital energy. The breath is a primary vehicle for receiving and distributing prāṇa throughout our subtle anatomy, which includes the cakras (energy centers), the prāṇa vāyus (energy currents), and the nāḍīs (energy channels). The free flow of prāṇa is essential for the nourishment of the physical systems as well as for cultivating balance in the mind and emotions. As we balance the energy body, it allows the physical systems to be fully nourished at a subtle level. Attuning to the energy body also allows us to see that we are more than our physical being, thereby reducing stress and tension.

At the level of the prāṇa-maya-kośa, IYT practitioners gain an understanding of how unhealthy breathing patterns reflect patterns of stress and how to eliminate these patterns, allowing the mind-body to come back into balance. Thirty prāṇāyāma techniques, organized into ten families by level of difficulty, are taught along with preparatory exercises to awaken the breath. These prāṇāyāmas are adapted to the specific needs of individuals and special focus groups using the framework of *Ha* (sun) and *Tha* (moon), the range of Yoga techniques from calming to energizing.

IYT trainees develop an in-depth understanding of prāṇa in the form of the five prāṇa vāyus (movements of energy), which nourish specific systems of the body with vital energy. Detail is given in the use of āsana, prāṇāyāma, mudrā, bandha, and imagery to restore optimal circulation to each vayu. Knowledge of prāṇa enhances the ability to channel prāṇa consciously to specific regions and organs of the body for balancing the energetic dimension and, subsequently, for rebalancing the physical being.

Along with the five kośas, the cakra system serves as a primary model for understanding whole person wellness. Trainees develop the ability to locate the cakras experientially, learning how to sense balance and imbalance in each, and how to apply Yoga techniques to promote overall well-being. All of these methods for exploring the energy body are supported by the science of mudrā, an essential facet and practice in IYT.

MANO-MAYA-KOŚA: PSYCHO-EMOTIONAL BODY

Manas means "mind," and the mano-maya-kośa is the psycho-emotional dimension of our being that is made up of thoughts and feelings that compose the personality. This kośa tends to be one of the most challenging aspects of our being because it is the field in which we experience the full range of feelings from happiness to suffering. As we embrace our psycho-emotional being without judging or rejecting our thoughts and feelings, we naturally live with greater lightness and ease to support physical healing.

At the level of the mind and emotions, trainees in the IYT certification program gain an in-depth understanding of the stress response on each system of the body as well as the most effective Yoga techniques for stress reduction in relation to the systems affected. This includes recognition of what constitutes a healthy stress response and the identification of how symptoms progress, leading to the chronic stress response and development of a stress-related illness.

As part of this global understanding of stress, illness, and wellness, the nature of emotions is explored within the context of Yoga psychology and trainees develop skills for working appropriately with emotions that may arise during a Yoga Therapy class or a one-on-one session. Yoga nidrā and other relaxation techniques are practiced regularly to facilitate experiential understanding of how these tools promote balance at the level of the mano-maya-kośa by reducing overall stress and bringing equilibrium to emotional ups and downs.

VIJÑĀNA-MAYA-KOŚA: WISDOM BODY

Vijñāna means "higher wisdom," and the vijñāna-maya-kośa is the dimension of our being that allows us to witness, understand, and eventually release limiting beliefs. As these beliefs are released, patterns of thought and emotion associated with them dissolve naturally, allowing us to experience a greater sense of freedom and ease, which supports physical health and healing.

Yoga philosophy is the foundation of Yoga Therapy. As trainees develop skill in working with the various tools and techniques of Yoga, they also gain a broad understanding of traditional Yoga texts, in particular, the *Yoga Sūtras* and the *Bhagavad Gītā*. These texts offer a vision of how mind-body health is a reflection of our growing awareness and integration along the spiritual journey and serve as a pathway to wisdom and, ultimately, spiritual liberation.

ĀNANDA-MAYA-KOŚA: BLISS BODY

Ānanda means "bliss," and the ānanda-maya-kośa encompasses our inherent positive qualities naturally unfolding as limiting beliefs are released. These essential qualities include equanimity, contentment, joy, limitlessness, wholeness, and inner peace. The blissful experiences awakened during meditation and other spiritual practices are expressions of the ānanda-maya-kośa. As we awaken our inherent positive qualities, any sense of defectiveness, self-judgment, or self-criticism is released, allowing us to live with greater harmony. Recognizing our own inherent positive qualities also allows us to see these traits in others. Uniting with our essential being in the form of these positive qualities is healing in the ultimate sense from the Integrative Yoga Therapy perspective.

During the IYT certification program, trainees explore a wide range of spiritual states as expressions of our authentic being as core beliefs are released. Through these experiences and realizations, people gain an appreciation of how these positive qualities, including love and compassion, influence physical health and healing.

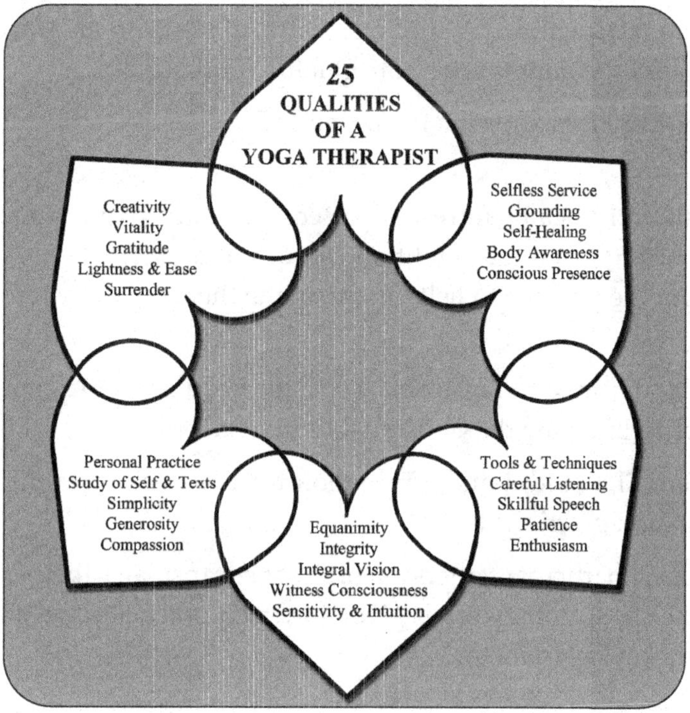

THE INTEGRATIVE YOGA THERAPY TEN-STEP PROCESS

One of the foundations of Integrative Yoga Therapy is its unique ten-step Yoga Therapy process. Variations of this ten-step process are used in both individual Yoga Therapy sessions and programs for special focus groups. This ten-step process is outlined below and the individual steps are referenced later in this chapter in the section on the twenty-five essential healing principles.

1. **Check-in.** The Yoga Therapist checks in with the students to see how their week has been and reviews the mudrā, affirmation, and breathing techniques from the previous week.
2. **Educational Theme.** The Yoga Therapist introduces a theme in order to awaken a specific "Core Quality," or facet of healing, such as the importance of body awareness, posture, or breathing.
3. **Awareness Exercise.** A guided awareness exercise follows the introduction of the theme, allowing students to explore a particular Core Quality.
4. **Sharing.** Students share their experiences with the group.
5. **Mudrā and Affirmation.** A specific mudrā, along with an affirmation, is presented in order to support the Core Quality for that class.
6. **Breathing Exercises.** Specific breathing techniques are introduced to support healing.
7. **Warm-Ups and Yoga Postures.** Yoga sequences are given that are appropriate for the specific group or condition. Mudrā and affirmations are interwoven throughout the practice to help integrate the theme directly into the mind and body.
8. **Yoga Nidrā (Guided Relaxation).** A specific Yoga nidrā technique is presented each week to integrate the Core Quality more deeply.
9. **Meditation.** The mudrā and affirmation for the week form the foundation of the meditation practice.
10. **Closing.** Each participant offers a word that encapsulates their experience, integrating the class. Homework is given in which practicing the mudrā and affirmation is a key component.

As the class flows through these ten steps, the therapist is able to facilitate health and healing at all dimensions of being from the kośa model: physical, energetic, psycho-emotional, wisdom, and spiritual.

THE INTEGRATIVE YOGA THERAPY TEN-WEEK PROGRAM

IYT therapeutic group programs are normally ten weeks in length and are based on the model of the five kośas. Initial classes focus on the physical body, followed by awareness on the breath and energy body. Later classes explore the mind and emotions through themes such as stress and culminate with a discussion on deeper human and spiritual values. The IYT Healthy Heart Program, offered since 1994, uses the ten-week program shown in the table below.

Each class within the ten-week program focuses on a specific theme related to mind-body-spirit health with a special focus on hypertension and the cardiovascular system. Each theme is introduced in a short lecture format and brought to life through an experiential exercise. The theme is then woven throughout the class and reinforced by a home-study assignment to integrate the theme into daily life. Each theme builds on information from previous weeks and forms a progression following the model of the five kośas. The intention of the weekly themes is to integrate the twenty-five essential healing principles that underlie the program. The Yoga techniques serve as a vehicle, the Yoga Therapist as a guide, and the changes in health parameters are a reflection of the extent to which these healing principles are integrated.

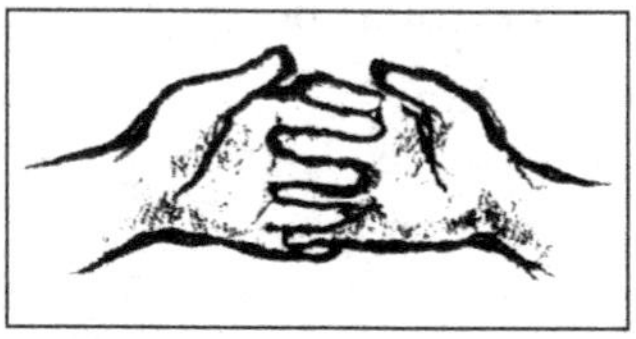

Week 1: Visualizing optimal health
(Overview)
"I visualize a new dawn of perfect health."
Core quality: New possibilities

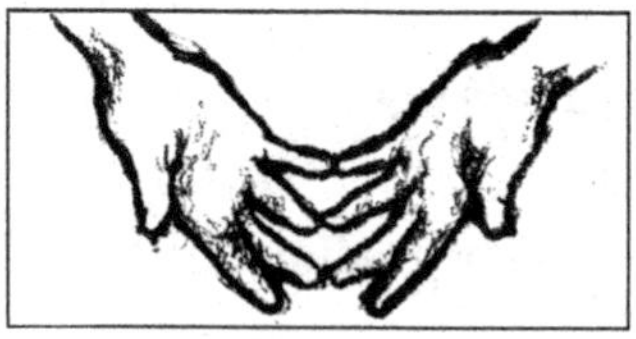

Week 2: Stress reduction
(Overview)
"I am completely relaxed and at ease."
Core quality: Relaxation

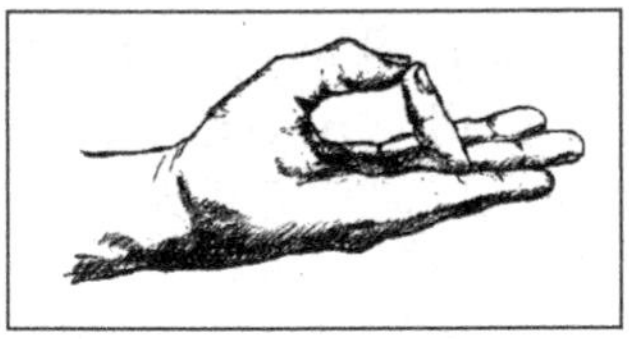

Week 3: Body awareness
(Anna-maya-kośa—Physical body)
"I trust and honor my body."
Core quality: Healthy embodiment

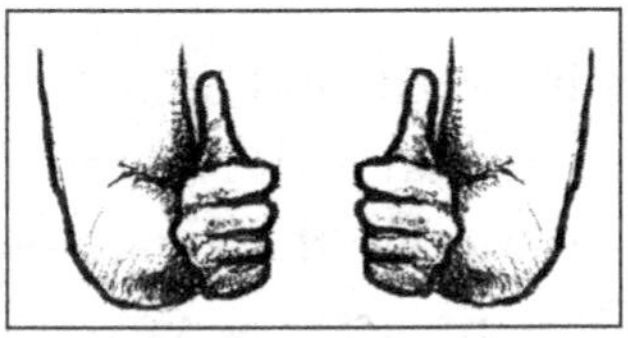

Week 4: Correct postural alignment
(Anna-maya-kośa—Physical body)
"My body and spine are naturally aligned."
Core quality: Optimal alignment

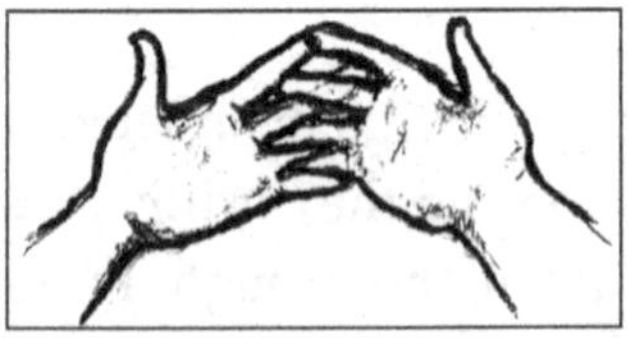

Week 5: Optimal breathing
(Prāṇa-maya-kośa—Energy body)
"My breath flows freely and easily."
Core quality: Breathing completely

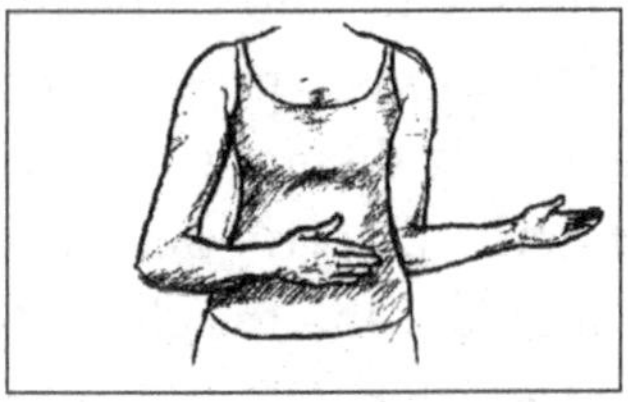

Week 6: Self nourishment
(Prāṇa-maya and Mano-maya kośas—
Energy and Psycho-Emotional bodies)
"I awaken to my own spring of inner healing."
Core quality: Self-nourishment

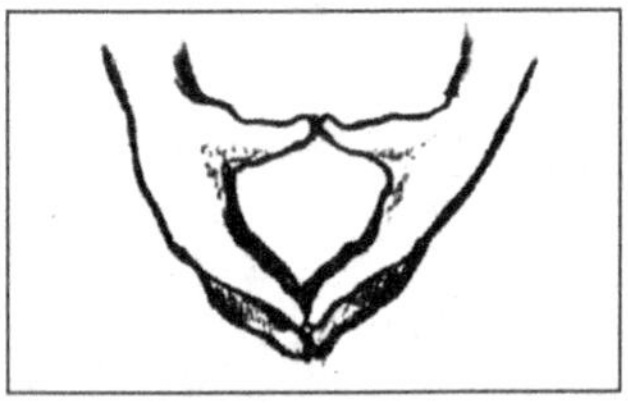

Week 7: Awakening the senses
(Mano-maya-kośa—Psycho-Emotional body)
"I awaken my senses to live each day
more vibrantly."
Core quality: Living more fully

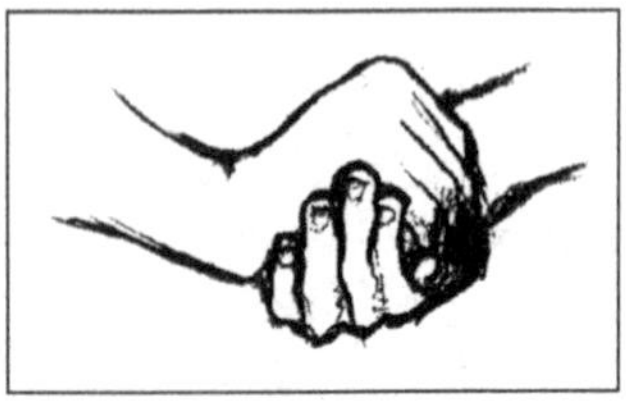

Week 8: Gratitude
(Mano-maya and Vijñāna-maya kośas—
Emotional and Wisdom bodies)
"I treasure each moment of life as a precious gift."
Core quality: Gratitude

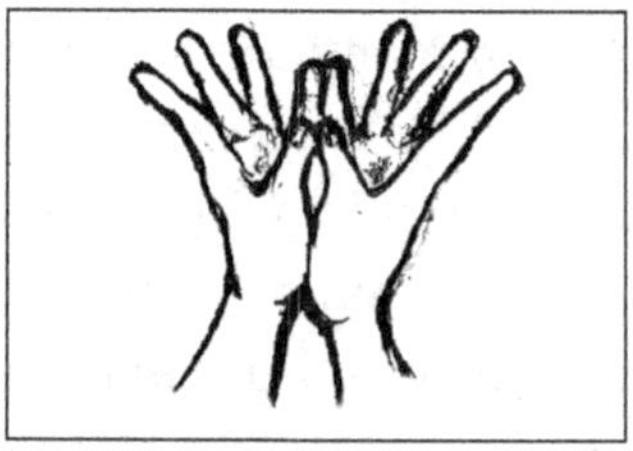

Week 9: Opening the heart
(Vijñāna-maya-kośa—Wisdom body)
"My heart beats in synchrony with the heart of all beings."
Core quality: Compassion

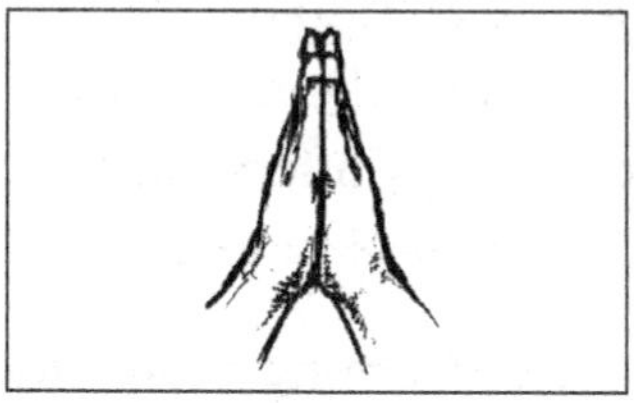

Week 10: Life's deeper meaning
(Vijñāna-maya and Ānanda-maya kośas—Wisdom and Bliss bodies)
"I align with my life's deeper meaning."
Core quality: Purpose and meaning

HEALING THE WHOLE PERSON: THE TWENTY-FIVE ESSENTIAL HEALING PRINCIPLES

Over the years in IYT, we have observed certain essential elements whose cultivation are fundamental to the success of Yoga Therapy programs. The following twenty-five essential healing principles are organized within the model of the five kośas, with five principles identified at the level of each kośa. These principles are awakened within the ten steps of the IYT class structure along the unfolding of the ten-week program. The principles are relevant to all Yoga Therapists and practitioners regardless of the tradition in which they have studied and have a direct impact on students and clients who have selected Yoga Therapy as part of their wellness program.

Healing Principles at the Level of Anna-Maya-Kośa: Physical Body

1. **Enhanced Body Awareness.** Through our programs, participants develop a deeper, fuller connection to their own bodies. This allows a friendship to develop for them in an area that may have been seen as a place of conflict or pain. Enhanced body awareness allows students to sense balance and imbalance more easily and also supports healthy posture and alignment. The body awareness portion of our program (3), along with breathing exercises (6) and the warms-up and Yoga postures (7), help support the cultivation of greater body awareness.

2. **Experiential Understanding of the Systems of the Body.** For many participants, their bodies are objects and they receive information about their bodies from the medical community. Most have never explored the systems in which their symptoms occur. Through Integrative Yoga Therapy, practitioners attune to the body systems experientially and also expand the capacity for self-regulation, introducing them to the possibility of self-healing. The weekly educational themes (2) familiarize them with the systems of the body related to the focus of their particular program and the awareness exercises (3) allow them to explore these systems. The Yoga nidrā section (8) at the end of class offers them an opportunity for self-healing within the body systems they have explored.

3. **Optimization of Posture and Release of Chronic Muscular Contraction.** One of the clear benefits of our Yoga Therapy programs is the release of chronic muscular contraction along with a strengthening and balancing of all main muscle groups of the body. This naturally leads to healthier posture, and we have found that the experience has been that most participants find relief from areas of chronic pain. We have also observed pain relief in conditions that affect the entire body such as fibromyalgia. The steps of the program involving breathing and posture (6 and 7) have an obvious impact, but muscular relaxation and pain also find relief and benefit from the mudrā and affirmation portion (5) of class. In addition, Yoga Nidrā (8) can be specifically oriented to release muscular tension and relieve pain.

4. **Supporting Optimal Physiological Functioning.** Yoga techniques support optimal physiological functioning in a wide variety of ways. The breathing techniques (6) enhance lung capacity and increase oxygenation of the body systems. The postures (7) work through the "squeeze and soak mechanism," whereby areas are first compressed, then stretched back open, enhancing circulation and removing toxins. Mudrā, introduced in step five and repeated throughout the program, are also an excellent means of directing breath and awareness to specific areas, organs, and systems of the body.

5. **Balance of the Five Elements.** Both Yoga and Ayurveda are based in Sāṁkhya philosophy. Within the vision of Sāṁkhya, imbalance in the three guṇas (rajas, tamas, and sattva) creates imbalance at all levels of being, including the five elements that comprise the physical body. Once participants are taught to maintain

a feeling of balance within the five elements within their own bodies, all portions of the class can be used to enhance this sense of balance. The final meditation (9) is especially important for integrating this balance of the five elements.

Healing Principles at the Level of Prāṇa-Maya-Kośa: Energetic Body

6. **Experiential Knowledge of the Breath.** For students coming into our Yoga Therapy programs, the breath is normally a completely unconscious function, except when obstructed. Through the breathing exercises (6) and synchronization of breath and movement during warm-ups and postures (7), participants reestablish healthy breathing patterns. Developing mastery of yogic breathing techniques also supports an enhanced sense of self-regulation and self-esteem. As the experience of the breath moves beyond the respiratory system itself and students begin to sense the subtle breath, it serves as a bridge to the subtle body.

7. **Balance Within the Subtle Body: Prāṇa Vāyus and Nāḍīs.** From a Yoga perspective, balance within the subtle body is essential for health in the physical body. This balance is especially important at the level of the prāṇa vāyus and the nāḍīs. Each of the five prāṇa vāyus (energy channels) nourishes a particular system or systems of the physical body. These prāṇa vāyus can be presented to participants as flows of nourishing energy that support the process of healing. Mudrā and affirmation (5) are especially important in sensing and balancing the flow of the prāṇa vāyus. By introducing and exploring the polarities of sun and moon through the framework of activity and rest, balance in the major nāḍīs can be introduced and cultivated.

8. **Balance in the Cakras.** The practice of traditional Haṭha Yoga, with its focus on the body, emerges directly from the Tantric tradition (Singleton, 2010). A study of āsana reveals that one of the principal inspirations within their origin and evolution is the opening of the cakras. The cakras are a map of the entire Yoga journey from basic survival needs to awakening, leading to the transformation of the body into a sacred temple of spirit. Balance within each of the cakras has a vital role to play in our health at all levels of being, including the physical body. Cakra work can be presented effectively within Yoga Therapy programs, even with individuals who have no previous experience with spirituality or the subtle body. This is done by framing the exploration as an ability to sense aliveness

and vitality in particular areas of the body. The educational theme (2) and awareness exercise (3) can be used to introduce these concepts. They can then be reinforced through the mudrā (5), warm-ups and postures (7), Yoga nidrā (8), and meditation (9).

9. **Integration of Body and Mind Through the Breath.** The synchronization of breath and body naturally creates a sense of integration at all levels of being. It can produce positive feelings that help relieve sensations of discomfort and pain, both physical and emotional. Creating a sense of calm and ease, synchronizing breath and body allows participants to release feelings of depression and anxiety. The integration of movement and breath also helps participants connect with the more subtle dimensions of their being so that life issues and problems become less pressing, allowing stress to be released.

10. **Pranic Healing.** Once participants have developed a familiarity and friendship with their breath and the flow of energy through their bodies, they can begin to direct this energy consciously as a support for healing. Within our programs, we incorporate slow-motion movements, called Kum Nye, from Tibetan Yoga into posture practice (7). These movements are specifically designed to cultivate and channel healing energy to specific areas of the body. During Yoga nidrā (8) and meditation (9), this subtle healing energy can be directed to specific systems of the body.

Healing Principles at the Level of Mano-Maya-Kośa: Psycho-Emotional Body

11. **Learning to Relax.** For those facing health challenges, learning to relax can be difficult. Oftentimes, illness creates a state of vigilance. There can also be a sense of anxiety about how their condition could progress and how their lives could be affected. Individuals who have lived with chronic health challenges may also develop a kind of emotional armoring in which they have shut down to sensations and feelings as part of their coping mechanism. All the steps in the class structure are important for learning to relax. The awareness exercise (3) allows participants to move into their bodies. The sharing within the group (4) allows them to express and release tension and feelings. Specific mudrā (5) are used to support the relaxation process. The effect of these gestures is

enhanced by affirmations that are repeated out loud and silently. Specific breathing exercises (6), such as "ha" breathing and kāki prāṇāyāma as seen in the inset section below, help release stress and tension. Warm-ups and postures (7) release tension from every area of the body and slow motion movement exercises (7) help relax even those participants who are most guarded and resistant. All of these relaxing effects are consolidated in Yoga Nidrā (8) and integrated during meditation (9). Students affirm their relaxation in the closing (10) as they share words, such as "calm," "tranquil," "relaxed," and "peaceful."

"Ha" Breathing and Kaki Prāṇāyāma

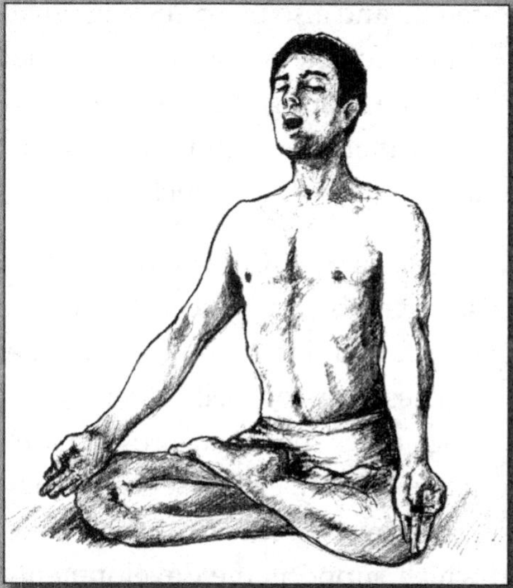

There are several variations of "ha" breathing. The most basic form is to lift the shoulders toward the ears in slow motion while passively inhaling. Exhale through the mouth with a long sigh—*Ahhhhh!*—while gradually softening the shoulders away from the ears. Repeat three to five times. "Ha" breathing may also be done with more shoulder movement on the exhalation: lift the shoulders toward the ears in slow motion while passively inhaling. Exhale through the mouth with a short, rapid exhalation using the sound of "ha" while relaxing the shoulders downward. Repeat 3–5 times. It is not unusual for this breath to evolve into a breath of laughter, which is an excellent way to release stress.

Kaki prāṇāyāma is a cooling breath that utilizes kāki mudrā (forming a beak with the mouth). This opening creates a type of straw through which the breath is drawn. Inhale through the mouth and exhale through the nose.

12. Sense of Community. Throughout the ten weeks of the IYT program, a sense of community develops in which students and teachers become a support group. This sense of support is important in all stages of illness—and especially important after initial diagnosis when an individual may feel isolated. After the ten-week program, there is an ongoing follow-up program in the form of a gentle Yoga class that extends this group support. In some cases, the same group is together as much as five years after their initial program, continuing to support each other in the healing process. This sense of community is especially cultivated during the check-in at the beginning of class (1), the sharing (4), and the closing (10).

13. **Expression of Feelings.** During group sharing (4), participants share in pairs and/or in the full group based on their experience in the awareness exercise (3). They are supported in this process through guidance in nonjudgmental listening and also in expressing what they are feeling in the moment. This process allows for the release of emotional tension and stress. Participants also report that the sharing skills developed during the ten weeks of the program help to cultivate better coping methods and communication skills with their families and communities, which also assists in reducing stress.

14. **Increased Self-Confidence.** Many participants coming into our program are suffering both physically and psychologically. Some sense themselves as failures for having become sick. Others have been dealing with feelings of defectiveness and low self-esteem long before the onset of their illness. Because the Yoga exercises in our program are adjusted to the level of the student, participants quickly gain a sense of confidence and competency. They also develop significant abilities to autoregulate their breathing and their level of relaxation, which supports the development of self-esteem. The ability to share (4) their experience and their progress weekly in the group also supports enhanced self-confidence. Final sharing (10) supports them in confirming their progress and enhancing self-esteem. The enhanced self-esteem among participants is so palpable that it can even be seen in their posture.

15. **Reduction of Symptoms of Anxiety and Depression.** There are very few Yoga Therapy situations in which we encounter individuals with a single condition. For example, in our Healthy Heart Program, a large number of participants are also diagnosed with depression and/or anxiety. Participants who have anxiety and/or depression often report a decrease in symptoms over the

course of the program. We have also conducted several programs entitled "Repainting the Rainbow of Your Life," specifically for anxiety and depression, with positive results. All facets of the program contribute to symptom reduction in anxiety and/or depression and the increasing ability to remain in silent meditation is key.

Healing Principles at the Level of Vijñāna-Maya-Kośa: Wisdom Body

16. **Clearly Defined Goals for Healing.** When students come into the program, there is often a sense that healing is something that is done to them by the medical community. Over the ten weeks of our program, this vision begins to shift as they recognize the importance of self-healing at all levels of being. As this new vision develops, they create a plan or direction for healing, not only in terms of their posture and breathing, but also in terms of their attitudes, relationships, and values. The educational theme (2), awareness exercise (3), and sharing (4) components are especially important in facilitating this change in vision. The mudrā and affirmations (5) allow this new vision to be integrated.

17. **Releasing Core Beliefs.** When participants begin our Yoga Therapy program, most have never explored the systems of belief that underlie their behavior, thoughts, and feelings. They see the personality as relatively fixed although susceptible to minor adjustments. Through the program, participants gradually come to see that they have choices and options in the way they respond to all life situations and even to their own thoughts and feelings. As they learn to develop a greater level of objectivity, they recognize that they can perceive and actually choose how to respond. This release of core beliefs begins by their learning to relax in situations that normally would have created tension. This ability to release core beliefs is introduced within the educational theme (2) and awareness exercise (3). Change, itself, occurs during sharing (4) and especially during Yoga nidrā (8), where shifts of perspective are integrated into one's personality.

18. **Redefining Challenges.** When participants come into the program, their tendency is to see life as relatively black and white in terms of the things they like and the things they don't like. One of the things they don't like are the side effects experienced in chronic illness. Over the course of the program, this way

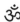

of seeing begins to gradually shift as they take responsibility for their own health. Through this process, life challenges and issues come to be seen more as opportunities for transformation and learning. Redefining challenges as opportunities reduces the level of stress and its subsequent effects. The mudrā and affirmations (5) and breathing exercises (6) are especially important because they can be used any time the person meets a challenge and chooses to respond rather than react.

19. **Learning at All Levels of Being.** As participants come into our Yoga Therapy programs, they are normally familiar with learning as a mental process. Along the ten weeks, they come to understand that learning is a process of global transformation at physical, psychological, and spiritual levels. The educational theme (2), awareness (3), and sharing (4) introduce approaches to transformation, such as better posture and better breathing, along with more positive attitudes and beliefs. These new ways of seeing are supported through mudrā and affirmation (5), integrated into the breath through breathing exercises (6), and brought into the body through warm-ups and postures (7). Learning occurs at subconscious levels in Yoga nidrā (8) and meditation (9), while the benefits of the entire practice are reinforced and absorbed at all levels during the closing (10), where each participant shares a single word that summarizes their experience.

20. **Exploring Life's Deeper Meaning.** Many participants coming into our therapeutic classes have often been too busy with their daily routines to take time to reflect on their life's meaning. Illness can change priorities, creating the motivation for individuals to see themselves and life in new ways. An important part of the IYT programs is creating a space in which participants can reflect on and define the things that make life worth living. These vary widely and range from hobbies to sports to family to religious beliefs. What occurs in this exploration is that participants visualize how they could bring these things into their lives more regularly and also identify the obstacles that keep them from appreciating life more completely. Even more important, over the ten weeks, many participants learn how to attune to a place of peace and happiness within their own being that requires nothing from the external world, yet gives them a deeper sense of meaning. All components of the program support this process, but meditation (9) is especially important in attuning to that place of inner peace and inherent meaning.

Healing Principles at the Level of Ānanda-Maya-Kośa: Bliss Body

21. Cultivating Values. Within Yoga philosophy, cultivating values and positive qualities in the form of the yamas and niyamas is an essential part of the practice. For many participants in our Yoga Therapy classes, the study of these yogic values gives their lives a sense of meaning and also provides a framework for dealing with challenges that cause stress. The affirmations (5) present a unique quality to be cultivated during each weekly session, while the mudrā provide an easy point of reference to remember these qualities and practice them throughout the week. These mudrā and affirmations are repeated at regular intervals throughout all segments of the class and are also given as homework.

22. The Body as a Source of Positive Sensations Rather Than Pain. For those with chronic illness, coping with discomfort and pain requires tremendous amounts of time, energy, and even financial resources. This can lead to an attitude of unease or even antagonism toward one's own body. Throughout the ten-week program, participants learn that the body is also a source of positive sensations and feelings, even of blissful feelings. These positive sensations are awakened through the mudrā (5), breathing exercises (6), and through slow-motion movements during the warm-ups and Yoga postures (7). Combining breath and movement is especially helpful for awakening positive sensations in the body.

23. Integration of All Facets of Being. Using the model of the five kośas, all facets of one's being are explored at different points over the ten weeks. This movement through the kośas cultivates an overall sense of integration and harmony, which is a hallmark of Yoga practice. This enhanced sense of integration and harmony, in and of itself, helps release stress. This integration of all five kośas also supports healing because there is an expanded awareness that is developed. Even if their symptoms don't change at the level of the physical body, the practitioners' sense of who they are expands greatly so that they see these symptoms within a larger framework.

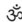

24. Living in the Present Moment. The very nature of the human mind is movement in time, scanning the past to remember threats, and projecting into the future to avoid danger and optimize possibilities. This leaves very little time for actually living in the present moment. For those with chronic illness, this movement away from the present moment can be even more pronounced as a temporary escape from pain. Anxiety about the progression of their condition can draw them into a future orientation while ruminating about what they may have done wrong can cause individuals with chronic illness to become stuck in the past. The Yoga Therapy program, through the body awareness exercise (3) and sharing (4), brings participants back into their bodies and into the present moment by focusing on "what is" and finding the best way to work with it. Breathing exercises (6) and postures (7) also support students in coming back into their bodies and into the present moment. As students embrace the present moment, they are able to recognize that even though pain may be present, positive sensations and experiences are also available.

25. **Awakening Spirituality.** Most participants coming into our therapeutic programs have some form of religious orientation, but very few have ever had spiritual experiences. Over the course of ten weeks, as we move from the physical body toward the higher dimensions of being, students become more comfortable with spirituality. In the second half of the program, as we begin to explore life's deeper meaning, spiritual experiences often occur, allowing students to see themselves and their spiritual life in new ways. Our focus on respect for all religious traditions allows these experiences to be channeled and integrated within each individual's understanding of spirituality. These experiences offer hope and a sense of meaning that require no changes in their external environment. The positive nature of these experiences has the power to reduce stress and promote a positive attitude, which supports health and healing.

All twenty-five healing principles are integrated throughout the ten-week program. In IYT, mudrā and affirmation (5) are the common threads that weave them all together and are especially powerful tools for cultivating these principles and integrating them into daily life.

MUDRĀ AND YOGA THERAPY

Mudrā are gestures of the hands, face, and body that promote physical health, psychological balance, and spiritual awakening. The Sanskrit word *mudrā* can be translated as "gesture," "seal," "attitude," or "signature." Mudrā are gestures that evoke psychological and spiritual attitudes, each with its own specific quality or "signature." The word *mudrā* is derived from two root words: *mud,* which means "delight," "pleasure," or "enchantment," and *rati,* which means "to bestow" (SpokenSanskrit, 2011). Mudrā bring forth our own inherent delight and enchantment, which are always present and waiting to be awakened.

There are several categories of mudrā. These include facial gestures that serve to awaken subtle spiritual energies, full-body mudrā that enhance and maintain the flow of subtle energy for extended periods, and hand gestures. Hand gestures are the most widely used form of mudrā, both in classical Indian dance and as a vehicle for healing and awakening. Mudrā play an important role in every facet of Integrative Yoga Therapy's methodology:

- Mudrā allow students in our IYT certification programs to sense and explore experientially all facets of Yoga psychology, including the kośas, cakras, prāṇa vāyus, nāḍīs, and the eight limbs of Yoga.
- In one-on-one Yoga Therapy sessions, mudrā offer an almost infinite range of possibilities for supporting health and healing by directing breath awareness and energy to specific areas and systems of the body.
- In group Yoga Therapy sessions, mudrā are used to awaken and support the main theme or Core Quality of each week. Mudrā are used together with affirmations; these are repeated throughout the class to reinforce the theme and to give each class a specific intention and identity.
- Mudrā are ideal for practice outside individual sessions and group Yoga Therapy programs because they can be practiced any place, at any time, and provide a way to maintain the healing benefits of Yoga Therapy quickly and easily between sessions.
- Traditionally, hand mudrā have been recommended for a wide range of health conditions. They are among the most versatile and universally accessible of all the tools and techniques of Yoga.

Mudrā as Vehicles for Health and Healing Through the Five Kośas

The power of mudrā to support health and healing rests in their ability to cultivate balance and harmony within all dimensions of our being.

Anna-Maya-Kośa: At the physical level, mudrā direct breath and awareness to particular areas of the body, enhancing our awareness and deepening our ability to recognize and respond to the body's messages more easily. Mudrā also support optimal breathing. In mudrā practice, the gesture itself guides the breath and has the ability to change the speed, focus, quality, and location of our breathing almost instantly. As mudrā bring awareness and breath into specific areas, a massaging effect is created that increases circulation to the areas where the breath is directed.

For deepening awareness of the anna-maya-kośa, join the thumbs of each hand to the tips of the ring fingers and extend the remaining fingers. Rest the hands, palms facing upward, on the thighs. This is pṛthivī mudrā (Gesture of the Earth).

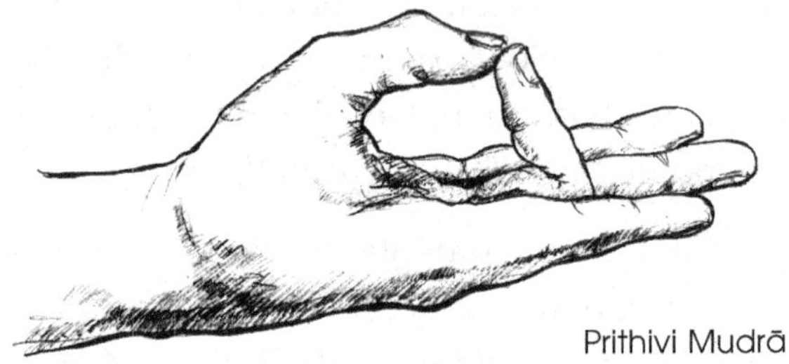

Prithivi Mudrā

Prāṇa-Maya-Kośa: As mudrā expand and channel the breath, they also promote balance within our subtle anatomy—the cakras, prāṇa vāyus, and nāḍīs. The breath is a primary vehicle for prāṇa (life force energy). By channeling the breath into specific areas of the body, mudrā enhance our sensitivity to the flow of subtle energy, removing energy blockages and thereby reestablishing the free flow of prāṇa.

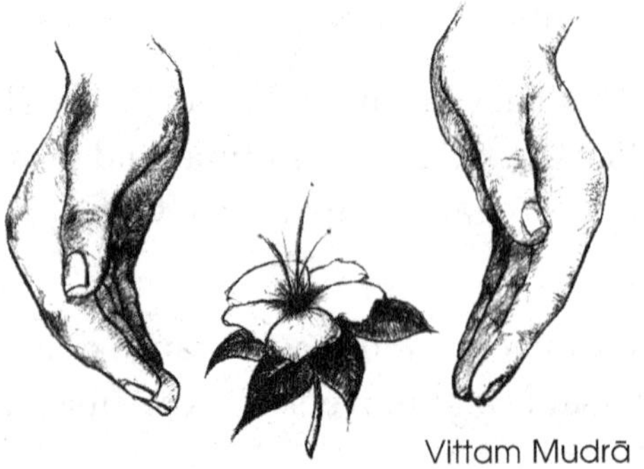

Vittam Mudrā

To experience the flow of energy that is the prāṇa-maya-kośa, hold the hands about twelve inches apart with the palms facing each other, slightly cupped, in front of the lower abdomen. Allow the hands to gently expand away from each other on the inhalation and to rest back toward each other on the exhalation. This is vittam mudrā (Gesture of Vital Energy).

Mano-Maya-kośa: At the psychological level, mudrā evoke moods and feelings that range from calming to energizing. There are specific gestures for instilling relaxation and serenity, such as jalāśaya (peaceful lake). Others, including vajra-pradama (unshakable trust), enhance enthusiasm, optimism, and vitality. Mudrā, like kubera (wealth) or svasti (well-being), can support the cultivation of a wide range of psycho-emotional qualities, including self-confidence, courage, and self-esteem.

Pūrṇa hridaya mudrā (Gesture of the Open Heart) helps us become more comfortable with our psycho-emotional being, the mano-maya-kośa, by enhancing our ability to embrace thoughts and feelings more easily. Hold the hands in front of the heart with the palms facing each other, fingertips pointing upward. Interlace the tips of the fingers inward with the right index finger closest to the heart. Stretch the thumbs downward to touch at their tips, so that a heart shape is formed.

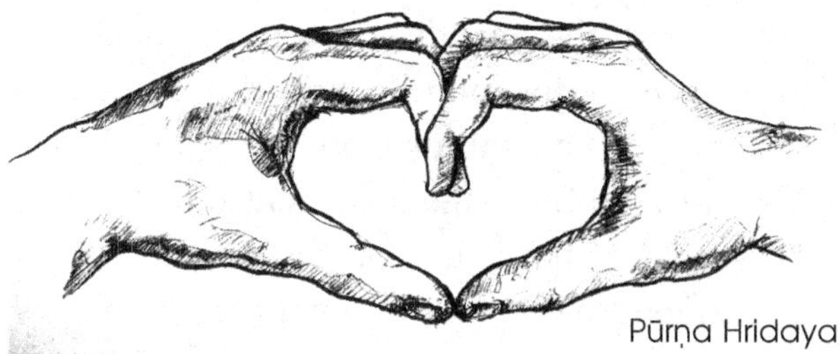
Pūrṇa Hridaya

Vijñāna-Maya-Kośa: Mudrā also support us in perceiving and releasing the limiting beliefs that sustain challenging thoughts and feelings by developing tools that bring awareness of our priorities that give life more meaning.

To awaken the inner witness, moving into the vijñāna-maya-kośa, touch the pads of the index fingers to the tips of thumbs on the same hand and extend the other fingers straight out. Bring the hands together in front of the chest with the pads of the middle, ring, and little fingers touching the same fingers on the opposite hand. The thumbs touch along their length and the tips of the index fingers touch so that they form a line parallel to the earth. This is citta mudrā (Gesture of Witness Consciousness).

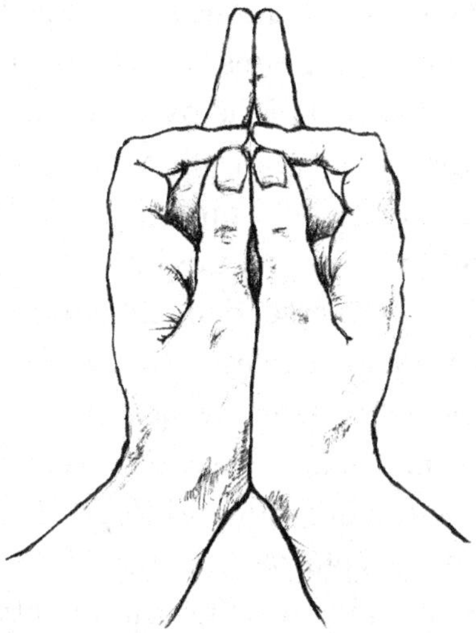
Citta Mudrā

Ānanda-Maya-Kośa: As limiting beliefs are released, space is created for the unfolding of our innate positive qualities. The integration of all of these Core Qualities naturally reveals our true nature that can be experienced as freedom and unity.

For a sense of lightness and ease that is the bliss body, the ānanda-maya-kośa, touch the tips of the index, middle, and ring fingers to the tips of the thumbs on the same hand. Extend the little fingers straight out and rest the backs of the hands on the thighs. This is haṁsi mudrā (Gesture of the Inner Smile).

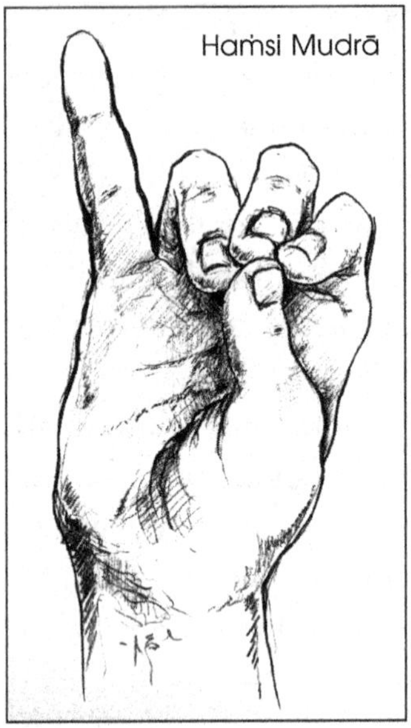

CONCLUSION

Yoga Therapy is one expression of the evolution of the Yoga tradition. Integrative Yoga Therapy is one facet within this growing field. By placing the structure of our training programs as well as our treatment programs within the framework of the five kośas, IYT helps reinforce an essential foundation of Yoga Therapy as the appropriate application of Yoga techniques for health and healing within all dimensions of being. Through our development of a ten-step educational methodology within ten-week programs, IYT plays an important role in reminding us that Yoga Therapy is essentially an educational process. In defining the twenty-five essential healing principles within the framework of the five kośas, Integrative Yoga Therapy helps to show how this educational process is also a journey of healing. Through extensive exploration of the art and science of mudrā, IYT helps elucidate how the breadth and depth of Yoga techniques can be expanded, making them suitable vehicles to be used in Yoga Therapy and in life. And finally, by elaborating upon and practicing the twenty-five qualities of a Yoga Therapist, IYT upholds another essential foundation of Yoga Therapy: that we are all both teachers and learners along the journey of Yoga.

REFERENCES

SpokenSanskrit. Online Sanskrit-English Dictionary, version 4.2. 2011. Web. Retrieved 15 Aug. 2011. http://www.spokensanskrit.de.

Singleton, M. *Yoga Body: The Origins of Modern Posture Practice.* New York: Oxford University Press, USA, 2010. Print.

IYENGAR YOGA THERAPY

Kofi Busia

•••••••

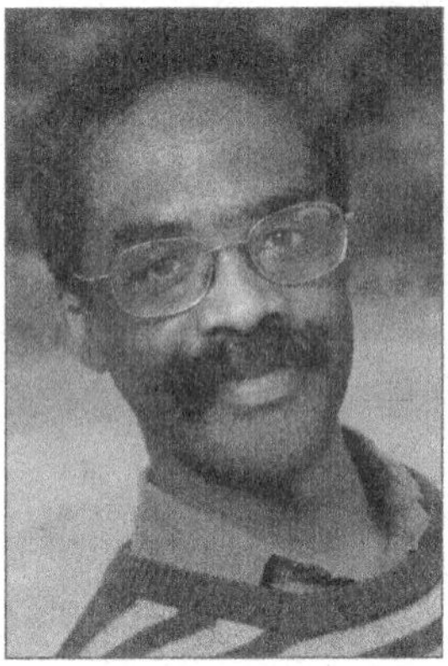

Kofi Busia is one of the world's foremost teachers in the Iyengar tradition. He has been teaching for nearly forty years and has held an advanced Iyengar teaching certificate for more than thirty-five years. He began his study of Yoga as a student at Oxford and has taught professionally ever since. From the 1970s through the mid-1980s, Busia studied directly with B. K. S. Iyengar on a regular basis at the Ramamani Iyengar Memorial Yoga Institute in Pune, Maharashtra, South India. A scholar and teacher in Sanskrit and Indian philosophy, Busia is editor of *Iyengar: The Yoga Master* and is currently working on a translation and commentary of the *Yoga Sūtras of Patañjali*.

"Yoga teaches us to cure what need not be endured
and endure what cannot be cured."

—B. K. S. IYENGAR

INTRODUCTION

What are people's expectations of me when they seek me out as an "Iyengar Yoga Therapist" and what are my expectations of them? These mutual expectations and the treatment regimen they imply are outlined in the health diagram on page 361. Whether we are the givers or the receivers of Iyengar Yoga Therapy, it is virtually the definition of our joint human condition that health and happiness have the tendency to oscillate. As Iyengar himself clarifies in the above quote, it is our lot to learn to live with such ups and downs. Health, then, is rather more like a melody.

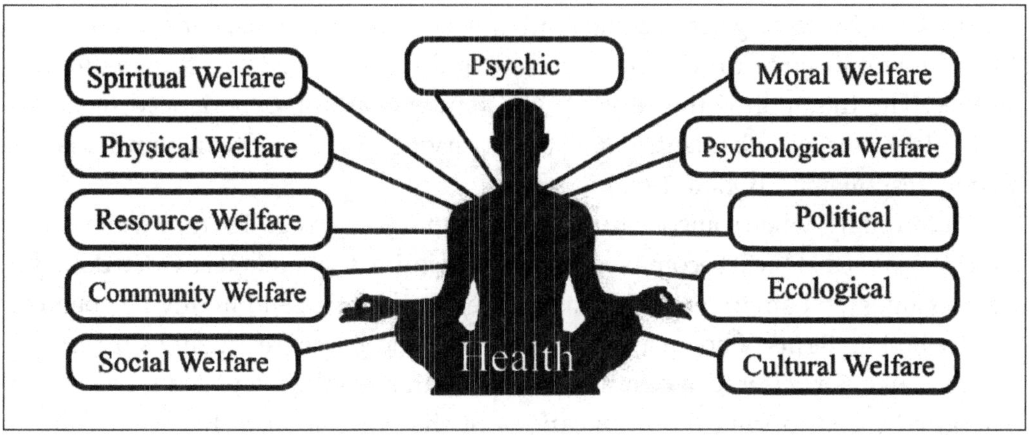

We must learn like well-trained singers to align ourselves with a series of steady, but melodious notes through all such vicissitudes.

Although Yoga is multifaceted and defies easy categorization, our emphasis here is on a branch of Yoga: Iyengar Yoga Therapy. The Iyengar approach to wholeness centers on the practice of āsana or physical posture, yet it does so in a more precise and therapeutic way. This practice intersects—controversially, in some eyes—with the modern Western and explicitly biomedical approach to sickness, which insists that health and sickness result from scientifically explainable biological processes. With this in mind, as an Iyengar Yoga Therapist, I align myself with that imperative and provide a variety of individualized therapeutic options for my clients.

THE ROOTS OF THERAPY

We begin by considering the word *therapist.* It is a more modern rendering of the older "therapeutist" derived from the Greek *therapeutikos.* A close Greek synonym is *diakonos,* which gives us the word *deacon,* which is defined as someone who waits on, is a messenger for, or ministers to another. The *Chambers Dictionary of Etymology* even more helpfully tells us that it is related to *enkonein,* which means "be quick and active, especially in service" (Barnhart, 1988). The word *therapy* comes from *therapeia* and *therapeutes* or "one who ministers." It was most commonly translated into Latin as *ministerium.*

Thomas Oden, in his book *Kerygma and Counseling,* says: "More particularly, it means attentive, caring service, the kind of heedful, scrupulous, conscientious care that one would hope to receive in private and intimate matters, such as medical service. The therapon is the servant who renders careful, experienced, watchful, meticulous, skilled, obedient, painstaking service to the one to whom he is intimately responsible" (Oden, 1966).

Accordingly, when someone turns to me as an Iyengar Yoga Therapist, one of their expectations is that I will become something of an intimate attendant as Oden describes. I am to minister. I am to render a considerate, confidential, and highly personalized service both in terms of how I approach him/her and in the treatment I suggest.

We can get a better idea of our joint expectations of the proposed Iyengar Yoga Therapy by considering the implications of the word *melody.* Evolved from the Greek *melodia,* its primary ingredient, which was not originally a musical term, is *melos.* This refers to the collected body of humans and/or animals . . . essentially all sentient beings when they are understood as an organic entity. In this sense, *melodia* is a kind of "sung tune" that emerges, conjointly, from all beings. The number of beings may be so many that I as an Iyengar Yoga Therapist and the person who seeks me out may appear to be two separate individuals. However, we are all one melody. The person to whom I am ministering and I create a collaborative focus on the melody we both will improvise together. Consequently, my role as the therapist is to help anyone who turns to me to find his/her own distinctive voice. Through practice, we craft a set of postures and practices that assist him/her in discovering and aligning with his/her individual life-song.

IYENGAR YOGA THERAPY IN THE WEST

It is important to have a clear understanding about the goals of any Iyengar Yoga Therapy interaction. Exact definitions like those listed above facilitate analysis and direction, but, if the terms become too explicit, they become confining obstacles. Unnecessarily rigid boundaries do not gel well with the mishmash of life's fluid vagaries. Yet, if the terms are understood too broadly, there is the risk of losing focus and diluting therapeutic potential. Another danger is that the ignorant can masquerade as knowledgeable; the incompetent as experts. We therefore need to understand the concept of the health we are trying to promote both narrowly and broadly.

Our goal may be "health," but defining it is somewhat problematic. The World Health Organization famously tried to do so by saying: "Health is a state of complete physical, mental and social well-being and not merely the absence of disease or infirmity" (World Health Organization, 1946).

This is a very grand, but also a much criticized definition. While it proposes that health is some kind of wholeness or completeness, it simultaneously raises a lot of questions. The "complete physical, mental and social well-being" it suggests is frankly unattainable. For example, a particular difficulty with the industrialized West is that people live far longer than in the past. Scientific and technological advances allow access to therapies, services, and techniques (like Yoga Therapy) that were simply unavailable in a prior age. People now expect to be cured of things they at one time had no choice but to quietly endure. We, of course, cannot ignore modernity's impact, but, as the "health diagram" makes clear, some health issues are ancient and transcendent. Yoga's cosmogony and conceptualization of wholeness and completeness differs radically from Western medicine's more biomedically directed approach, so we begin there, in the "health diagram," in physical welfare.

THE PHILOSOPHIC BACKBONE OF YOGA THERAPY

The *Yoga Sūtras of Patañjali* define *Yoga* as *yogaścittavṛttinirodhaḥ* or "wholeness consisting of a complete grasp and command over the process of being and becoming aware." Yoga's abiding declaration is that the human animal is a part of prakṛti (nature), infused by puruṣa (spirit). The human life is an expression of puruṣa dharma. *Dharma* is notoriously hard to define, but we can think of it in this context as an effort to find the laws of nature, as they pertain to how I should relate to those laws as a willing and active being. Gravity makes objects fall, and sometimes I can see the object is going to hit my foot and hurt it. I can cuss and swear, but it is unlikely that that accords with dharma. Alternatively, I can think that it is not nice this has happened but accept it quietly and with good grace because it just seems more fitting, given that unavoidability. Each life therefore is, or should be, a practical and experiential attempt to grasp the true nature and method for being of an in-dwelling spirit.

Yoga insists that it is the dharma or unique inevitability of human beings to be composed of, and ultimately be responsible for, consciousness. It is also their dharma, a part of the "is-ness" or "beingness" of things, that they should recognize themselves as participants in a consciousness drama through being encased in bodily form. To view the physical body as a mere expression of scientific imperatives limits that true being within and promotes dukha (suffering). Over-identification with the physicality of the body also gives too much emphasis to the inherent unconscious drive for separation from spirit while engaging in sensory stimulation. Iyengar Yoga's view is that, taken by itself, the strictly biomedical approach diminishes true health and must align itself with something broader. Whatever may be Yoga's views, we cannot ignore the biomedical approach. The physical body cannot survive without its ever on-going physiology and its constant string of metabolic processes. Therefore, resource welfare is placed next to physical welfare in the "health diagram" and this covers everything the body needs to maintain itself. It includes food and nutrition, embraces house and home, recognizes all the supplies needed to survive, and appreciates the energies needed to attain them.

Yoga is very clear that the first step in attaining health is to seek samādhi (enlightenment) and find the light of the knowledge of the true Self within. In his *Light on the Yoga Sūtras of Patañjali,* Iyengar describes this by saying "asana is perfect firmness of body, steadiness of intelligence, and benevolence of spirit" (Iyengar, 2002). Health is not something passive. It is a positive radiation of well-being. So, how do we facilitate any needed transformation in Iyengar Yoga Therapy?

I once helped a lady with many niggling aches. She had a particularly painful and tender shoulder, carpal tunnel issues, and a longtime history of low-grade headaches. It was relatively easy to determine that the resource welfare issues stemming from her job were greatly and negatively impacting her health. We gradually healed the woman working—through āsana—on her resource welfare. During the time we trained together, the office she worked in was increasingly being computerized, and she thought that she was both too old and too unintelligent to be retrained. Consequently, she was terrified that she would be considered to be expendable and replaced with someone younger with the relevant computer skills. This impacted her community welfare also shown in the "health diagram" earlier in this chapter. Constant conflicts with her coworkers with whom she had to interact to aid her resource welfare added to her overall sicknesses and insecurities. This formed as a part of her healing ambition. A regimen of gentle standing poses, twists, and hip and chest openers greatly improved her vasodilation, gradually strengthened her physical and psychological welfares, and removed her aches. The ensuing steadiness gave her a new perspective. Her improved psychological welfare gave her a palpable feeling of lightness and enhanced her overall sense of health and well-being. She eventually got the self-confidence to enroll in some evening classes on her own dime and time. As her confidence and skills increased, so did her health. Her conflicts at work disappeared, and she was soon keyboarding and databasing with the best of them.

As the quote from Iyengar and the WHO definition both make clear, health is considerably more than simply "not being sick." Medicine may be the conscious attempt by a ministering healthcare practitioner to restore physiological and metabolic functioning, but therapists try to do more. Therapists explore the interface between medicine, healers, and sufferers . . . and the ineffable sense of well-being linking them. A true therapeutic interaction is something more than being given a pill or an injection because therapy cannot really be offered to someone who merely passively receives it. Therapy requires an active participant.

THE DISTINGUISHING FEATURES OF IYENGAR YOGA

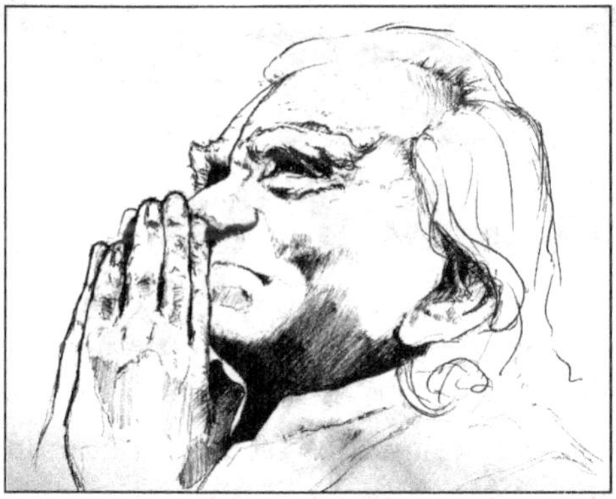

B. K. S. Iyengar

Iyengar Yoga really began when B. K. S. Iyengar began to teach in Pune at his Guru Krishnamacharya's insistence. Yoga had greatly benefitted him, and he wanted to understand how and why it had done this. His Guru had sent him to Pune to teach because he was one of the few who had even a smattering of English, but he was not confident in his fluency. His lack of experience in teaching, combined with his occasional loss of words, encouraged him to spend long hours practicing and observing what he was doing, so he could follow the *Yoga Sūtras* and teach from a direct personal experience. From that grew the three characteristic components of this Yoga system: They are like a melody and emphasize 1) an alignment of the body with effort to develop a technique that always hits the "right note" and commonly uses the instruments of props like blocks, blankets, and straps, which were invented and pioneered by Iyengar, to provide better support for the joints and body in Yoga āsanas; 2) an appropriate sequence of poses to make entire and healthful melodious phrases that gradually harmonize the body; and 3) a timing or recommended interval that each note should be held, in the same way that it is both the length of notes and the intervals between them that makes each melody distinct. My role as a therapist in this discipline is to study āsanas and sequences and the effects of those "notes," so I can help my client gradually learn to improvise and develop the techniques, sequences, and timings that bring him/her to radiance in good health.

THE ROLE OF THE IYENGAR YOGA THERAPIST

Iyengar Yoga Therapy is a proven complementary treatment for modulating the cardiac parasympathetic system, for those suffering from carpal tunnel syndrome, osteoarthritis, and a host of other ailments (Khattab, et al., 2007; Garfinkel, et al., 1994; Garfinkel, et al., 1998). As an Iyengar Yoga Therapist, I help my patients with my specialist knowledge on how to use alignment and props within posture to eliminate suffering in these conditions and many others. At their core, the words *patient* and *patience* have the same Latin root: *pais* and *pati.* While "to be patient" is still recognized as meaning "to endure calmly," the more medically oriented "to be a patient" eventually used the same word to refer, more specifically, to anyone enduring the suffering associated with medical treatment.

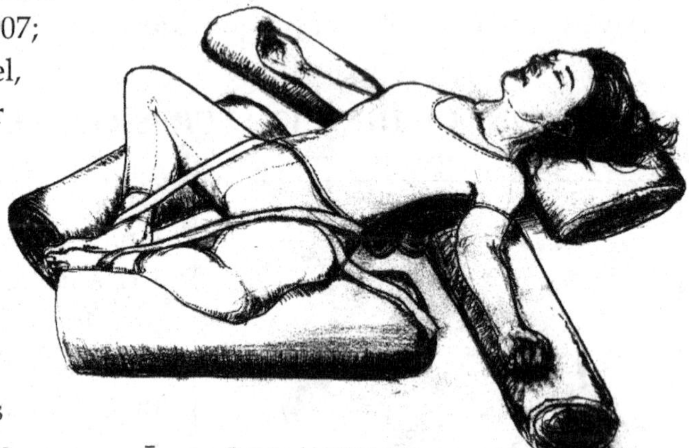

Āsana Props Harmony

Oliver Basso, writing in the *British Medical Journal* in 1999 highlights the essential passivity of the patient's accepted role: "The word *patient* means 'one who endures a doctor or other health professionals.' This is because one is merely ill until a representative of the health profession appears. Only then does one become a patient. Thus, contrary to common belief, a patient is not someone enduring an illness but someone enduring a doctor!" (Basso, 2003).

Yoga and Western medicine often take radically different approaches to health. Iyengar Yoga's view is that health is a relationship to the dukha (suffering) that life inevitably brings. Health is the ability to find an abundant and profound joy in the face of our ultimate extinction and requires that a patient come to understand more about existence, both personal and cosmic. Iyengar Yoga Therapy uses the body's fund of physical welfare to persuade our consciousness to align itself with all the other welfares that extend beyond the mortal frame. True health demands that of us. It necessitates that we extend out to our manifest divinity.

THE IMPORTANCE OF SPIRITUAL WELFARE

As the "health diagram" shows, spiritual welfare is a vital part of overall health and an essential aspect of Yoga Therapy. Since social, community, and political welfare are all also an intrinsic part of health, we can go beyond Iyengar Yoga and learn from the story of Rita and Doug Swan. When their sixteen-month-old son, Matthew, was screaming in pain as he lay dying from meningitis, the Swans enacted what they knew about spiritual welfare. As Christian Scientists, they refused to call a doctor. They believed that their son could only have sickened because either he, or they, or all of them together, lacked sufficient faith in God. Driven by their concept of community welfare, they summoned their church healers to pray over their infant son. Unfortunately, by the time Rita relented and rushed Matthew to hospital, he was beyond help and passed away.

Rita Swan then reassessed her notions of the psychic, psychological, spiritual, political, and social welfares. Her views on health shifted dramatically. She wrote *The Last Strawberry*, a book outlining her experiences, and formed the nonprofit organization Children's Health Care Is a Legal Duty (CHILD) to campaign for the rights of other children being denied medical care through the religious motivations of their parents or other caretakers.

As is well known, Yoga means union. Few therapists would extend spiritual welfare so far that they would allow someone to die for a religious belief. Yet, in Yoga's eyes, the root of all suffering is indeed psychic, religious, and spiritual. It is ahaṁkāra (individuation) and, just as important, dharma (here meaning that ineffable psychological property that makes us realize, and want to accord with, the life-drama transmitting itself through us) insists that our lives are not separate. Fundamentally, Yoga's ideas on psychic and spiritual welfare are that the entire community sickens when its individual members do not embrace one another with those bonds of unity.

REMOVING SUFFERING

We all have a right to define our own vision of suffering. We also have the right to find the best way to alleviate it. The woman mentioned earlier who had work-related shoulder discomfort was fortunate that her shoulder pains were totally alleviated by our treatment. Had she felt any lingering soreness, her suffering would have been worsened by—if not directly caused by—her inner turmoil and the subsequent disconnect she experienced from her deficiencies in resource and community welfare. Due to that inner turmoil, she initially lacked the psychic drive needed to prevail in her quest for health. She, however, was able to create it as she began to understand her own personal health. The work of healing is always ongoing and transcends physical welfare.

What makes us "fully human" is our contact with dukha (suffering) and our ability to reduce our suffering. As an Iyengar Yoga Therapist, I have specialist knowledge, not merely about how to use āsana and alignment to promote physical welfare, but also in the underlying and more cosmic issues of karma and dharma. The former becomes what we can see we can do to play our full part in the expression of the laws of total being, including the inexpressible and spiritual, that are the latter.

The essence of any Yoga-as-therapy is vairāgya (detachment) and the insistence that the impact of pains and discomforts of all kinds can be persuaded to recede in consciousness so they cease being a drain on our overall energy. Any regimen of āsanas needs to address and express that reality and that view of health.

The psychic welfare that helps us to find and to implement our curative processes influences our psychological health and is a vital part of our overall health. The individual's community and social welfares that help to clarify what health is, and then promote that vision to its members, are equally vital to health since they influence our psychological welfare. As an Iyengar Yoga Therapist, I convey that, even though we are physical and biological beings, it does not divert us from appreciating that we are simultaneously moral, social, cultural, spiritual, and a host of other beings. We cannot yet cure cancer, for example, but Iyengar Yoga Therapy can still help relieve the inner fears and turmoil that can accompany someone's knowledge that he/she has just been diagnosed with a possibly terminal illness. Yoga can enhance the inner light of joy, of peace, and well-being of any individual or circumstance where people are willing to seek health together and an improved quality of life.

CONCLUSION

A theory on the origin of disease is impossible without a partner theory on the origin of life. Yoga is predicated on the notion that our true spirit can never be confined. Yoga's essential message is that we are all beings of consciousness . . . and nothing but beings of consciousness. To be healthy is not simply to be free from loss and limitations. It is to see health's consequences and potentialities within ourselves. Sometimes health means that we should protest against whatever is looking to limit and confine us. As Iyengar puts it, "Yoga teaches us to cure what need not be endured" (Busia, 2007).

Iyengar Yoga Therapy believes that true health is powerfully radiative. It is always in the body somewhere, and, in its arrangements, it is always seeking to emerge. Iyengar Yoga Therapy reduces discomfort, keeps the body moving, and settles the mind. It helps us heal by approaching our true essence through our body and recommends to us to align with these truths:

Developing consciousness in our given manifestation of being alleviates suffering and transforms us into instruments for limitless joy and gratitude.

I, as an Iyengar Yoga Therapist, do my best to help those who come to me. I help them to find a more harmonious and melodious expression of themselves through my given range of āsanas and other accoutrements of my trade familiar to me through my own practice. I study everything I can possibly study in regard to anatomy, physiology, and their associated subjects within Western health. Moreover, I also contemplate karma, duḥkha, dharma, saṁtoṣa (that positive and willing radiance of contentedness in being and good health that Iyengar described in the quote given earlier), kaivalya (that source of certain knowledge in wellness of being, and in what to do next to maintain it, that emanates from the inner well-spring of good health it connects us to), vairāgya (detachment)

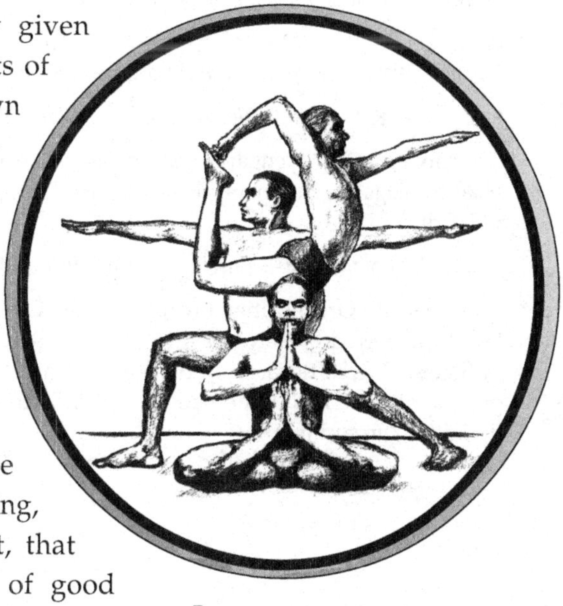

Āsana as Temple

and their associated Eastern concepts. I do my best to see them at work in my own life so I can be a resource and assist others in seeing them in theirs.

As Iyengar puts it, "The body is my temple, āsanas are my prayers" (Busia, 2007). And, as an Iyengar Yoga Therapist, when a patient stands before me and is desirous of being relieved from suffering, it is my duty to find the cause and which āsanas or "states of being" will relieve his/her suffering (and mine as well). In this way, we continue through the great journey of existence together as only one melody, one temple, and one prayer.

REFERENCES

Barnhart, R. K., Ed. *Chambers Dictionary of Etymology.* Edinburgh: Chambers/W. Wilson Company, 1988. Print.

Basso, A. *Aphasia and Its Therapy.* New York: Oxford University Press, USA, 2003. Print.

Busia, K. *Iyengar: The Yoga Master.* Boston: Shambhala, 2007. Print.

Garfinkel, M., et al. "Evaluation of a Yoga-Based Regimen for Treatment of Osteoarthritis of the Hands." *Journal of Rheumatology* 21.12 (1994): 2341–2343. Print.

Garfinkel, M., et al. "Yoga-Based Intervention for Carpal Tunnel Syndrome: A Randomized Trial." *Journal of the American Medical Association* 280.18 (1998): 1601–1603. Print.

Iyengar, B. K. S. *Light on the Yoga Sutras of Patanjali.* London: Thorsons, 2002. Print.

Khattab, K., et al. "Iyengar Yoga Increases Cardiac Parasympathetic Nervous Modulation Among Healthy Yoga Practitioners." *Evidence-Based Complementary and Alternative Medicine* 4.4 (2007): 511–517. Print.

Oden, T. *Kerygma and Counseling.* Philadelphia: Westminster Press, 1966. Print.

World Health Organization Preamble to the Constitution of WHO as Adopted by the International Health Conference, New York, 19–22 June 1946; Signed on 22 July 1946 by the Representatives of 61 States. Official Records of the World Health Organization, no. 2, p. 100, and entered into force on 7 April 1948. WHO International. Web. Retrieved 20 March 2013. http://www.who.int/about/definition/en/print.html.

KUNDALINI YOGA THERAPY AS TAUGHT BY YOGI BHAJAN®

Shanti Shanti Kaur Khalsa, Ph.D.

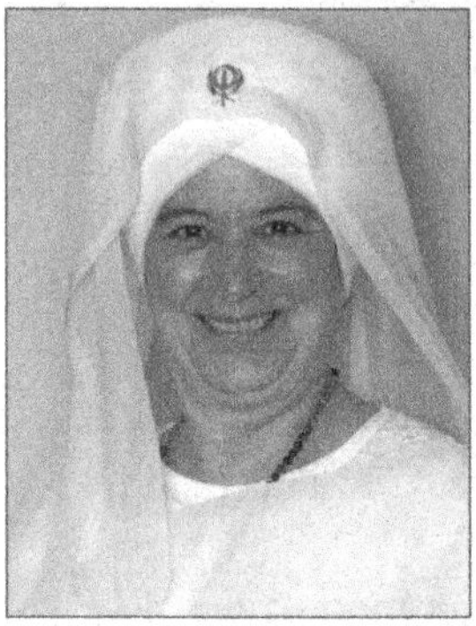

Shanti Shanti Kaur Khalsa has brought the ancient teachings of Kundalini Yoga to the people and into modern medicine since 1971. She began to teach people with chronic or life-threatening illnesses in 1986, under the guidance of her teacher, Yogi Bhajan, who brought Kundalini Yoga to the West and taught it openly for the first time. Dr. Khalsa is the director of the Guru Ram Das Center for Medicine and Humanology in Espanola, New Mexico, which is dedicated to bringing Yogi Bhajan's teachings into twenty-first-century health care. She is a charter member of the International Association of Yoga Therapists and served on the team that developed IAYT Educational Standards for Yoga Therapy teacher training programs worldwide.

INTRODUCTION

"The process of self-healing is the privilege of every human being. Self-healing is not a miracle, nor is it a question of being able to do something that most people can't. Self-healing is a process that occurs through the relationship between the physical and the infinite power of the soul. It is a contract, a union—that is the science of Kundalini Yoga."

—YOGI BHAJAN (OCTOBER 7, 1974)

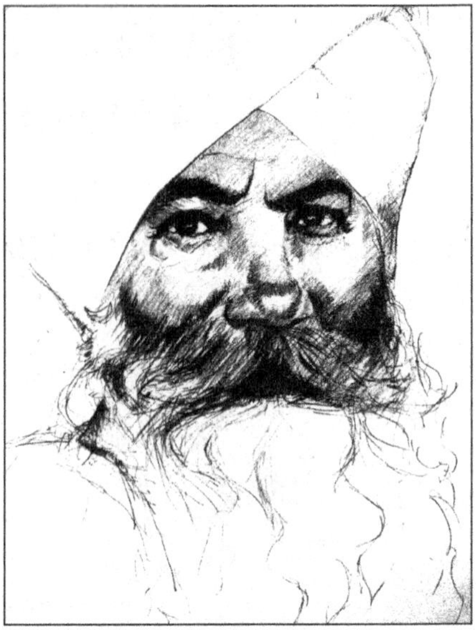

Yogi Bhajan

Kundalini Yoga, as taught by Yogi Bhajan, like most yogic lineages and traditions, is not inherently a therapeutic method. It originated as a practice for healthy people to experience their excellence. When we train to teach this form of Yoga, we learn to teach it to healthy people, not to people with life-threatening or chronic health conditions. Under the guidance of Yogi Bhajan, his students developed ways to deliver the practices of Kundalini Yoga to support health recovery. This is what we now call Kundalini Yoga Therapy.

The seed for teaching Kundalini Yoga with a therapeutic intention was planted in me during a lecture in 1985 in Los Angeles, California, when Yogi Bhajan stated, "The body has the capacity to immune itself." This resonated with me and awakened my curiosity. How can we create a stronger immune system through the practice of Yoga? The question was not simply academic. The planet was at the beginning of the AIDS epidemic that now, more than thirty years later, continues. As a Kundalini Yoga teacher, I wondered, *Can the practice of Kundalini Yoga benefit a person living with HIV?*

Under the direction of Yogi Bhajan, I investigated what was medically known at the time about the immune system and what it needs in order to function optimally. This information was matched with specific Kundalini Yoga techniques and kriyās (sets of yogic movements for a specific purpose) to meet those needs. They were taught in a progression of instruction over six weeks toward improved capacity and endurance.

In October 1986, the first classes for people with HIV and AIDS began. There was still no medical treatment, and clinical trials of azidothymidine (AZT) had just started. Students were under great duress, in fear, and/or outright ill from their weakened immune systems, opportunistic infections, and the experimental AZT treatments they were receiving. Like modern clinical trials, it was an empirical process, and we were testing and refining our therapeutic practices on live patients. We had no idea how the students would respond in actual classes or if the practice of Kundalini Yoga would lead to improved health outcomes. The belief that we have within us what we need to be well was the basis of our approach, and this belief moved us forward. As Yogi Bhajan said, "All healing is based on a relationship. The fundamental relationship is to your Self and Soul. You are missing nothing. You are complete within yourself." (*Aquarian Wisdom*, Bhajan Y., 2004)

The practice of Kundalini Yoga and meditation seemed to provide participants with what they needed: the release of pain, stress, and fatigue; increased vitality and endurance; and a strengthening of the body's natural defense. In the years following, hundreds and hundreds of HIV positive students gained improved health through a Kundalini Yoga program we called "Immune Fitness." Most participants experienced reduced anxiety and depression, had fewer symptoms and side effects from treatment, stabilized and improved their immune markers, and regained their health. Many lived long past their prognosis. In addition, their consciousness changed. They regained hope for their future and began to live as if they would get well . . . and many did! Some early participants of our program are still alive and well today.

This is the original story of the application of the ancient practice of Kundalini Yoga to modern therapeutic purpose. At the time, we did not call what we did Yoga Therapy. Under the guidance of my teacher, I was simply teaching to people with serious medical conditions. However, I was teaching differently than when I taught to healthy people. It took us about two years to identify and to codify what was different about *what* was taught and *how* it was taught, and we now recognize that there are particular differences that distinguish a Kundalini Yoga *teacher* from a Kundalini Yoga *Therapist*.

WHAT DISTINGUISHES KUNDALINI YOGA AS A THERAPY?

When I started teaching to people with health conditions, other teachers in the Yoga community cautioned me, "You can't teach Kundalini Yoga to ill people; it is too hard, too vigorous, too strenuous." These words, though well intended, came from the perspective of a Yoga *teacher* teaching to healthy people. When we teach Kundalini Yoga for health recovery, we do not teach in the same way. We teach as a Yoga *Therapist*. Teaching Kundalini Yoga therapeutically requires a different set of skills from those needed to teach to people who are basically healthy. In each situation, the techniques or practices of Kundalini Yoga are the same, but it is the selection, application, and manner of teaching that is different.

We do not teach Kundalini Yoga to a diagnosis, a condition, or a disease. We teach Yoga to the person who has the condition. This means that we relate to each student as a unique individual. We assess how they are experiencing the condition, including their strengths and capacities—not just their limitations—so that we can best select the Yoga and meditation that will assist them in getting well. Through the application of deep intuitive listening and observation, we pay close attention to the student's experience and select those yogic methods that meet the student's needs. The Kundalini Yoga Therapist gives verbal cues and supports the student to be comfortable in his/her body, to slow down, to pause, to listen, and to connect with him/herself.

Yogi Bhajan recognized the importance of the psychology of the person in recovering from illness. In the spring of 1987, he requested that I explore and discover what he termed the mental mentality of eleven conditions that he listed and to develop a yogic approach for each. Our programs began to incorporate a strong psychological component and expanded to include courses for people recovering from all forms of cancer, chronic fatigue, fibromyalgia, stroke, heart disease, diabetes, arthritis, psychological conditions, such as depression and anxiety, and life transitions.

For nine years, I had a private practice in Los Angeles teaching Kundalini Yoga for health recovery. In 1995, Yogi Bhajan gave the vision for a nonprofit organization to bring Kundalini Yoga into health care, and so, I moved to a small town near Santa Fe called Espanola, New Mexico, to be the center's founding director. Though the center is based in a rural community, our reach is international; wherever there is a Kundalini Yoga teacher, we provide programs. We currently train teachers to become Yoga Therapists throughout the United States and in seventeen countries throughout the world.

Teachers in our tradition consider Kundalini Yoga to be a sacred science. It is a system based on the practice of moving prāṇa (life force, or vital energy) by the praṇī (the person). The sacredness of the person is awakened through this practice and brought into action through the physical body.

KRIYĀ IN KUNDALINI YOGA THERAPY

"If there is a place in you that you feel is not functioning properly, you have the capacity to circulate this pranic energy to it. Focus your mind on that place and you will find such a beautiful action happening and within a second, everything will change."

—YOGI BHAJAN (APRIL 23, 1969).

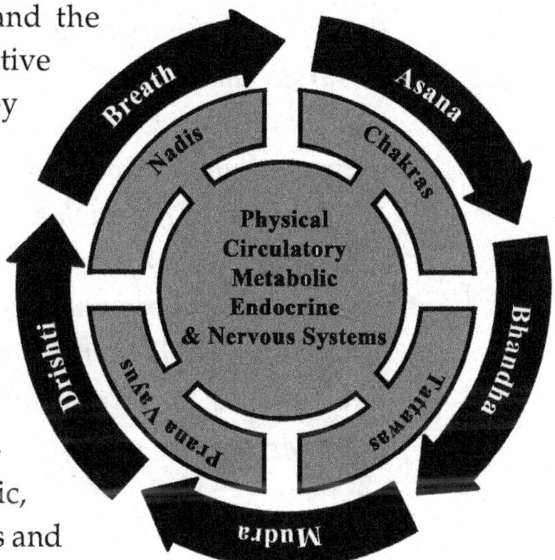

Kriyā Chart

The rhythmic targeted movement of kriyās and the application of breath with movement are distinctive in the practice of Kundalini Yoga as taught by Yogi Bhajan. *Kriyā* means "completed action" and consists of a predetermined series of one or more exercises or postures in combination with prāṇāyāma and mantra (the repetition of specific sounds) to affect various nerves, glands, or organs with an outcome greater than the sum of its parts. Each kriyā acts as a recipe combining breath, posture, bhanda (constriction at one of the three diaphragms—pelvic, rib cage, or throat), mudrā (position of the hands and fingers), mantra, and dṛṣṭi (where the eyes are focused during meditation). Each kriyā has a specific effect on the physical structure and physiology of the person practicing.

In addition, Kundalini Yogis understand that healthy body function is influenced by the subtle anatomy of nāḍīs, cakras, guṇas, tattvas, and prāṇa vāyus. Nadis are the pathways through which prana flows. Cakras are eight concentrated circles of energy along the center of the body from the base of the spine to the crown of the head and beyond. Each cakra has specific qualities and characteristics. The three guṇas are qualities of energy found in various proportions in each person. When these qualities are out of balance then illness or dis-regulation of the human system arises. The five main tattvas are considered the basic elements of the physical body. The five main prāṇa vāyus are qualities of vitality and movement of prana within the body. The prāṇa vāyus regulate inspiration, digestion, absorption, elimination, integration, and cohesion.

Kriyā engages both physical and subtle anatomy in a process of invocation of prāṇāyāma (the process of breath and breathing techniques) and pratyāhāra (the process of inner and outer alignment or synchronization): holding two opposites to lead to integration and regulation of the being.

THE PRINCIPLES OF KUNDALINI YOGA THERAPY

"The whole body structure relates to my elevation, my beingness, the delivery of my purpose on the planet as a soul. Disease comes from structural change or misalignment. The body and its bones have no screws or bolts to keep it together. It is held together by tissue and by muscle and kept in continuity through the fascia. When you move one part, all moves, all benefits. In life we have our stress response patterns where certain muscles get acted upon and others don't. As life becomes unbalanced, so does the body. Inflammation and low, inefficient, lymphatic and blood circulation result. The structure and the physiology are interrelated through neurochemistry, endocrine balance, and blood chemistry. These are the gas to the car; as with a car, if one part is missing the whole thing goes off."

—Yogi Bhajan (July 2, 1984).

Here are a few of the principles or ways of thinking therapeutically as a Kundalini Yoga teacher that Yogi Bhajan taught:

1. Teach to the student, not to the diagnosis.
2. Start with what is right and you will never go wrong.
3. Match the Yoga to the student, not the student to the Yoga.
4. Do not teach by formula; never apply the general to the specific or the specific to the general.
5. Teach to relax.
6. Raise vitality.
7. Start from where the student is; accept the student as they are in each moment.

In each individually tailored program and in curriculums for group classes for people with specific health conditions, the practice of Kundalini Yoga and meditation addresses the source and symptoms of the condition, complications, and the side effects of treatment. No matter what the diagnosis, we notice that the range of effects and outcomes of Yoga practice contribute to a more complete recovery with less debilitation and shorter duration.

THE EVOLUTION OF KUNDALINI YOGA THERAPY

In the contemporary field of Yoga Therapy, we speak in two languages: the language of yogic traditions that include the ancient concepts, principles, and practices, and the language of Western medicine and scientific inquiry. We live, serve, and teach in both worlds.

What brings most contemporary westerners to Yoga practice covers trends about 10–12 years apart. When Kundalini Yoga was introduced to the west by Yogi Bhajan in November 1968, those who came sought self-awareness and spiritual development. Through most of the decade of the 1970s, people came to Yoga classes in the many traditions taught in the west for these same reasons. Through the 1980s and early 1990s, people mostly came for fitness. Through much of the 1990s and into the first decade of this century, people came to relieve stress. Since the early 2000s and into the present day, people have come to the practice of Yoga with the expectation it will fix something. The amount of Yoga Therapy research that has been done over the past thirty years supports this expectation.

For the first two decades of teaching therapeutically, we did not call what we did Yoga Therapy. We did not even have a definition for it. Yogi Bhajan prescribed caution in the language we used because at the time there was insufficient research to support the practice of Yoga as a therapy. There was not much vocabulary for us in the language of Western medicine. Yet, now that the landscape is significantly changed because of the explosion in Yoga Therapy research, we are using the descriptor of Yoga Therapy to describe our trainings and the approach we take when teaching Yoga to a population with health conditions.

We borrowed from the International Association of Yoga Therapists concepts of Yoga Therapy to form our definition. Kundalini Yoga Therapy is the process of empowering individuals to progress toward improved health and well-being through the application of the philosophy and practice of Yoga. This includes Yoga and meditation practice, yogic psychology, self-reflection, and yogic recommendations on lifestyle and diet.

Skill, technique, and knowledge are necessary but not sufficient to create an effective Yoga Therapist. We view the skills, competencies, and consciousness of a Yoga teacher, a Yoga Therapist, and a yogic healer as distinct from each other, though there is overlap. A Yoga teacher instructs healthy people in the practices of Yoga and uses directive or command language. A Yoga Therapist has the basic training of a Yoga teacher with additional specialized skills, knowledge, and competencies to work with a person with a health condition toward recovery. He/she uses invitational language, inviting and suggesting the person take an action. A yogic healer invokes healing through his/her presence and intention. He/she uses the language of silence and stillness.

A Kundalini Yoga Therapist embodies all three characteristics and draws on the three identities and skill sets to create an environment for their students to flourish. In each role, we start with the belief that the student has within them the resources to be well; we hold the person as whole and healthy. Our purpose is to release or dissolve anything that may impede what is already right with them and strengthen the students' access to their inner guidance and hidden potential.

RAISE VITALITY FIRST

Instruction in Yoga practice and information by themselves do not lead to transformation or health recovery. Getting well rarely follows a linear process and frequently a student will assess their current circumstances and decide they don't have the resources to get well. It looks like the illness is bigger than they are and making change is just too difficult.

The person with the diagnosis needs to set their mind—their mental frequency —to raise vitality, to raise the śakti energy (subtle inner power) in order to overcome the obstacles to health recovery. This is one reason we put attention to yogic psychology and apply principles of health behavior change in all of our Kundalini Yoga Therapy programs.

Kundalini Yoga practices support what we have come to call *adaptive competence.* This is the ability to respond to the changing challenges inherent in getting well again. These include self-efficacy, resilience, the ability to manage setbacks, flexibility, endurance, a felt connection to inner guidance, and one's support for change.

As in most traditions, therapeutic Kundalini Yoga programs are most successful when tailored to the individual student, even in a group class setting. There may be fifteen women with breast cancer in the class, yet each brings a different experience of the condition and each has different needs. In addition, we recognize that getting well presents one set of challenges. Staying well presents another. The design of the programs takes this into account and incorporates methods to both change the somatic signature and support new habits.

HOW KUNDALINI YOGA THERAPY IS DELIVERED

Within these parameters, there are three methods of program delivery a Kundalini Yoga Therapist employs:

1. Private instruction with the diagnosed person and a friend or family member of the person's choice. This model is shared by most Yoga and Yoga Therapy traditions. The difference in Kundalini Yoga Therapy is that we take a systems approach and include the additional element of social support.
2. Group classes with students with the same condition, and friends and family members included. This model expands the experience of support for both the person with the diagnosis and the friends, family, and loved ones they invite to join them in class. There may be a belief among participants that being with others with the same diagnosis brings mutual understanding, that others in the class "know what I am going through." Content is specific to the diagnosis, and the curriculum avoids any yogic method contraindicated. In Kundalini Yoga Therapy, we teach across the condition to what is in common with the students and the students' abilities.
3. Group classes with students with mixed conditions, and friends and family members are included. This is a model based on the work of Jon Kabat-Zinn, Ph.D. As he describes in his book *Full Catastrophe Living: Using the Wisdom of Your Body and Mind to Face Stress, Pain and Illness* (Kabat-Zinn, 1990), Dr. Kabat-Zinn noticed that, when people learn how to relax, their health improves no matter what the diagnosis. People with diabetes, cancer, heart disease, and chronic pain all come together. In these classes, there is no focus or attention given to a specific diagnosis. Rather, emphasis is on stress reduction and building relaxation skills. Light movement, breath, meditation, Yoga nidrā,

and śavāsana comprise the course content. (Yoga nidrā and śavāsana are related yet distinct practices that bring about a state of deep relaxation with awareness.)

LEARNING FROM "THE SPECIAL SIX"

When I was in training, one of my colleagues observed that we learn most of what we will ever need to know from working with just six students. It may take us hundreds of students to meet "the special six," but the lessons we learn from them apply to most all of our cases. Since 1986, I have been what we now call a Yoga Therapist and I can attest to my colleague's observation. No matter what the diagnosis, there are principles in common in treating people through the practice of Yoga.

A regular Kundalini Yoga class and a therapeutic class both include breath, movement, mantra, meditation, and deep relaxation. However, the structure and content of a therapeutic Kundalini Yoga class differs from a regular Kundalini Yoga class. In a therapeutic class, there are three to four relaxation periods compared to one in a regular class, and the pace of the session flows to meet the pace of the student. In a regular class, the teacher instructs and the students are expected to match the instruction. In a therapeutic class, the Yoga is matched to the student; there is no attempt on the part of the teacher to match the student to the Yoga. The teacher gives the student what the student can do to begin. There is no need to modify any practice if we teach from the student's starting point. Starting from where the student is provides a base for the student to build self-efficacy and self-mastery; both qualities are necessary for change.

When working with students individually, a Yoga Therapist needs to understand the condition from the medical diagnosis, his/her own yogically based assessment, and the student's experience of the condition. Through a conscious interview process and mindful observations, he/she assesses the student along these fundamental guidelines:

1. Breath and posture
2. Flexibility and range of motion
3. Strengths and limitations of the student: physical, mental, and emotional
4. Medically diagnosed condition and course of disease progression

5. Co-occurring conditions and cofactors
6. Contraindications for the condition and for the particular person with the condition
7. Stage level of the illness or condition, if appropriate
8. Side effects of medical treatment
9. Person's personal experience of the condition
10. Person's personal objectives and comfort level
11. Social and family support

This is a lot of information, and not all of it needs to be collected during the first session. Nor will all of it be directly factored in to the treatment plan. Gathering it, however, is extremely important for the Yoga Therapist. It informs the means of fulfilling the first two treatment goals we have with every session, no matter what the diagnosis: to raise vitality and to engender capacity for calm. When dealing with chronic or acute illness, we must first cultivate prāṇa (energy) and sukha (ease). These two factors are necessary for the student to leave feeling better, to restore hope, to set in motion what the body needs to get well, and to provide the energy and ease for starting and maintaining the habits necessary to stay well. We cannot solve the problem or get well from the condition of illness preserving the person's initial state of being or consciousness. We need to shift the frequency and raise the śakti (the person's vitality and experience of personal power) of agency in their recovery first.

TOOLS AND METHODS OF THE KUNDALINI YOGA THERAPIST

The first tool of the Yoga Therapist is awareness. In Kundalini Yoga Therapy, we consider the practice of Yoga Therapy akin to meditating on a mandala where there are many entry points. A mandala is a circular symbol representing the universe and is used as a focal point for meditation. Mandala means circle and typically the mandala image is arranged around a central element. The image seems to "radiate" out from a central point in a tightly balanced, geometric composition. Each mandala has at least four entry points. Following the mandala as metaphor for the practice of Yoga Therapy, the Yoga Therapist meditates on the client, listening, looking and feeling for the central element and the entry point for that individual. The art of an intake interview is to listen deeply, to see and feel, and to sort for that person's starting points, which consist of what is important to them, what their needs are, and their areas of motivation. This information guides the Yoga Therapist in ways that will best meet the student's needs.

The next tool is acceptance. Acceptance is an ancient yogic concept that is also a paradox. For something to be different than it is, it must first be accepted as it is. We call it the *Paradox of Change.* We want the condition to be different; yet, to get there, we must accept it. This means the therapist is quiet and still inside him/herself so that preconceived ideas, assumptions, or conclusions drawn from previous experience with others of the same diagnosis don't interfere with the current situation. The Yoga Therapist pays attention to the person as he/she is in that moment and identifies that person's starting point. Acceptance is no small thing; it is in fact, the basis for full recovery.

The first intention of the Yoga Therapist is not to change the student, but to accept him/her in a way where the student deeply feels the therapist's acceptance and empathy to the situation. It is this compassionate understanding that creates trust on the part of the student and the internal ease that is a condition for change to happen.

Then, we teach the person (and whomever they brought to the session for support) to relax. Deep relaxation addresses many aspects of recovery, including structural, physiological, emotional, and energetic. Likely there is fear, discomfort, pain, and other sensations that create inner disturbance. Likely the person has been through other approaches before he/she came to the Yoga Therapist and holds a thought that he/she may not get well. The person needs to experience some level of self-command or else he/she will continue to feel powerless. Teaching him/her to relax provides this experience.

Deep relaxation, or Yoga nidrā, is an essential skill for recovery from any condition. It is one of the first things we teach, and it is woven throughout all subsequent instruction. If it is the only technique that is learned or practiced, it is so effective across the elements of health recovery that it may be sufficient, in itself, to create change.

RESOLVING LIMITATIONS TO ACCESS ONE'S HEALING POTENTIAL

"Total harmonious relaxation cures the body.
To achieve this there must be coordination between the
three facets of ourselves: body, mind and soul."

—YOGI BHAJAN (APRIL 9, 1988).

To a Kundalini Yogi, one of the origins of illness is unresolved inner conflict. From the first session and continuing into the series of sessions, the Kundalini Yoga Therapist explores and identifies what may be causing the person's inner conflict and considers how to address it. The Yoga Therapist explores the person's limitations—the restrictions and inner conflicts—and applies yogic techniques to release the limitations and dissolve the conflict in order to open the person to his/her natural healing potential.

It may take until the second or third session, but once the needs of the person are clarified and agreed upon, the Yoga Therapist identifies what Yoga, meditation, and lifestyle approaches best meet these needs and mobilizes his/her inner resources. He/she then shapes the collected material into a treatment plan with a weekly progression to build skill and mastery based on the person's learning needs.

A key point is that we don't have to solve every problem, practice everything there is to practice, make every habitual change there is to make, and/or do everything exactly right in order to get well. The value in making small, simple steps is that these are more likely to be maintained than taking big leaps. Two principles Yogi Bhajan taught to apply are:

1. A little bit goes a long way.
2. Doing something is better than doing nothing.

Kundalini Yoga Therapy includes the whole of Yoga in an integrated practice of Yoga's various elements. Movement plays an essential role in creating structural, physiological, emotional, and energetic transformation so the body and being can recover. To a Kundalini Yoga Therapist, this involves an understanding of the process and application of prāṇāyāma, mantra, kriyā, and deep relaxation. The tension and stress that impair structural, circulatory, metabolic, endocrine, and nervous system function are released with the practice of specific kriyās and breath techniques. Neural and structural pathways open and ojas (the subtle essence that is responsible for vitality) and the five main prāṇa vāyus (qualities and movement of energy) work more fluidly, providing access to one's natural healing capacity.

As Yogi Bhajan said, "The pelvic bone is where the breath of life is triggered and where the breathing power of the pranic body is found. The lungs are cleansing processors, the diaphragm is the aid to that process, and it is through the spinal column that the energy flows." He continues, "The inside organs need to be moved, not just your muscles. The inner organs must be stimulated. . . . They must understand and reorganize their supplies." (*Aquarian Wisdom*, Bhajan Y., 2004)

According to Yogic tradition, the following prāṇāyāma mantra meditation from Kundalini Yoga as taught by Yogi Bhajan is practiced when the practitioner would benefit from a calm mind, increased vitality, balanced parasympathetic and sympathetic nervous systems, improved immune function, and deeper experience of inner strength. It is called the Healthy, Happy, Holy Breath, and we always begin Kundalini Yoga practices with tuning-in.

TUNING IN

Before practicing any kriyā or meditation from Kundalini Yoga as taught by Yogi Bhajan®, we chant the ādi mantra, *Oṁ namo guru dev namaḥ,* at least three times. This helps us tune in to our divine teacher within, provides us with a protective link to the "Golden Chain" of masters of the tradition, and assures us clear inner guidance for the practice of Kundalini Yoga. The words of the mantra are from the Gurmukhī language and mean "I bow to the infinity within me, to the divine teacher within." *Oṁ* is translated as the infinite within the finite, or the creator within the creation. *Namo* is reverent greetings. *Guru* is the giver of the technology or the teacher. *Gu* means darkness; *Ru* means light. *Guru* is that which dispels darkness and awakens the light within. *Dev* means transparent, or nonphysical.

To make the check-in more effective, sit on the floor or in a chair and lengthen and align the spine and neck. Slightly tuck the chin in and place the palms of the hands together flat at the center of the chest with the fingers pointing upward. Press the sides of thumbs lightly, yet firmly, into the center of the sternum.

Close your eyes. Inhale deeply through the nose. Initiate the sound of *Ong* from the navel and let the sound resonate through the cranial bones and out the nose as if you are blowing a conch. On the same breath, slide into the sound of *Namo*, making the *Na* sound short and the *Mo* sound extended. Continue with the sound of *Guru* on the same breath (you may sip in a half breath through the mouth, after Namo, if needed) raising the pitch about a third tone higher on *Dev*. Finally, finish the mantra with the final *Namo*, exhaling all the remaining breath. Inhale deeply and repeat for a total of at least three repetitions. Remain still afterward for between 20 and 30 seconds, then open your eyes, and begin the first practice. (Khalsa, 1996).

THE HEALTHY, HAPPY, HOLY BREATH

To practice the Healthy, Happy, Holy Breath, sit on the floor or in a chair and lengthen and align the spine and neck, keeping the chin slightly tucked in. Place the hands in jñāna mudrā (seal of knowledge), with the tip of the index finger touching the tip of the thumb, leaving the other fingers straight. Place the back of the hands on the knees with the elbows straight and the palms facing up. With the eyes closed, inhale deeply through the nose, gently retain the breath, and mentally recite, "Healthy am I, Happy am I, Holy am I" three times (*Aquarian Wisdom*, Bhajan Y., 2004). On the exhalation, recite the words once aloud. Inhale and continue repeating the sequence for 3 to 11 minutes. To end, take a deep breath in, release it, and relax.

THE POWER OF MANTRA

> *"Mantras are not small things, mantras have power.*
> *They are the mind vibration in relationship to the Cosmos.*
> *The science of mantra is based on the knowledge that sound*
> *is a form of energy having structure, power, and a definite*
> *predictable effect on the cakras and the human psyche."*
>
> —Yogi Bhajan

From a yogic perspective, we understand that everything is vibration or frequency. Mantra, a specific application of sound, is an accessible method to transform and penetrate frequency. Making the sounds out loud creates movement, releases stress, and builds vitality even when the movement of the body is restricted due to pain, injury, and/or surgery. We can create movement in lymphatic circulation through chanting out loud; we create movement in structural, psychological, physiological, and recurring conditions all through the applied use of sound. Almost every Yoga tradition uses sound, and, with Kundalini Yoga, it is inherent within each kriyā as a way to distribute and equalize energy.

Each health condition has its own psychology that can be impacted and transformed through sound. Chanting out loud regulates breath rhythm. Most people who have health conditions need to breathe deeper and slower but many have a challenge doing this. Chanting can help do it for them. It releases the restrictions to deep breathing while raising vitality, creating calm, and improving mood. We can penetrate, break down, and turn around the vibrational frequency of the ill health condition through the specificity of mantra. The recitation of mantra dissolves inner conflict and emotional and physical pain through transformation of frequency.

All mantras inherently have the power to change one's vibration and frequency. However, each mantra does have a specified effect. The art of the Yoga Therapist is to select the sound current that meets the particular need. The most frequently used mantras in Kundalini Yoga Therapy are Sat Nam, which can be translated as "Truth is my identity" and "Har" and its variations, which tap into the hidden capacities and healing energy of the person.

CASE STUDY

One of the earliest Yoga Therapy students I had was Frank, a physicist and engineer. The finest achievement of his life was that he was on the team that landed the first Apollo mission to the moon in 1969. He was proud of his participation in that, and it meant a great deal to him.

When Frank came to me, he had stage-4 lung cancer. He found Kundalini Yoga Therapy through the recommendation of a friend, who told him he needed to address the stress of his diagnosis and medical treatment. He was anxious and depressed, tired all the time, had sleep disturbances, and experienced nausea and other side effects of his Western medical experience. His breathing was shallow, and he had limited mobility in his upper body due to a recent surgery and resulting lymphedema.

Frank was skeptical and quizzical at the same time. He asked a lot of questions and, in the first few sessions stated he was not quite sure what to make of the whole "Yoga thing." We began by having him practice a prāṇāyāma-based meditation known as "pauri kriyā" to release stress and build self efficacy, as well as a simple tapping kriyā known as "Tapping Series for Lymphatic Circulation." This improved his sleep, vitality, and mood and allowed him more comfort and ease in his body. Over the course of the next six months, our work together included an advanced prāṇāyāma technique called the "One Minute Breath" that the yogic traditions indicate increases natural killer cells and improves lung function. Descriptions of pauri kriyā and the One Minute Breath can be found below. As his range of motion and endurance improved, Frank practiced Kundalini kriyās and meditations to improve immune function, build self-efficacy, and deepen his access to his inner guidance. He modified his diet and habits of daily living to build his reserve energy, restore ojas and balance, and strengthen the five main prāṇa vāyus.

Frank's self-reflection practice helped him identify a key unresolved inner conflict. When he retired from NASA, he left his identity and most of the friendships he had made over the decades. Nothing in his current life filled the void, and he was conflicted about the decisions he had made to move to another city, to decline the consulting package he was offered, and to retire. He now thought he had done these things because "that is what you are supposed to do at my age," and he felt these actions did not reflect his soul's purpose. Somewhere inside himself he believed he was done with life, yet this is not what he wanted. He shared with me in session, "I still have a lot of life in me, and I want to live it."

It was at this point that Frank made a conscious decision to get well and to do what he understood would support that process. He knew that his prognosis was poor, yet he reminded himself that he was not a statistic. While there was no guarantee that his new health behaviors would put him in the percentile of those who recovered from stage-4 cancers, his well-being was significantly improved, and therefore the behaviors were worth continuing.

He used his self-reflection practice to uncover a new purpose. Frank loved children, and he loved parties. He started a children's party business where he played a host, a clown, and a game leader. He told me, "My new business unlocks so much joy! I am having the time of my life." Within eight months of starting Yoga Therapy, Frank recovered and the cancer went into remission. Through the rest of his life, Frank remained cancer free.

PAURI KRIYĀ

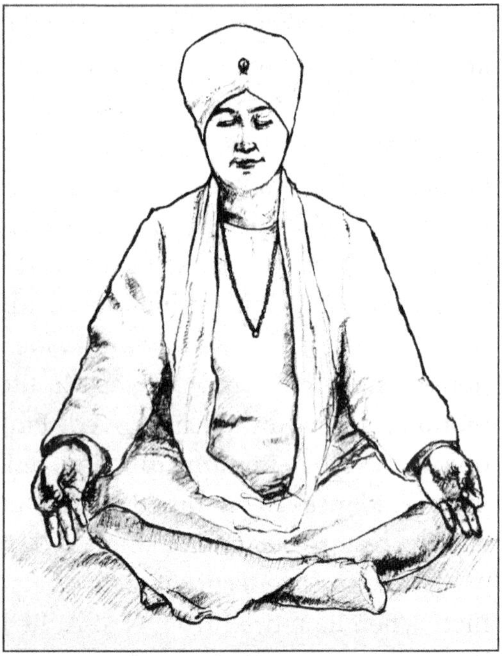

Pauri Kriyā posture

This concentrative meditation has been shown to be effective in research on the effects of meditation on self-efficacy beliefs. To perform the technique, sit comfortably with your spine aligned and your hands resting on the knees with the palms facing up and the elbows straight. With the eyes closed, inhale by dividing the breath into eight equal, separate parts, like sniffs. On the first segment of the eight parts, silently repeat the sound of *Sa,* on the second silently repeat *Ta,* on the third repeat *Na,* on the fourth repeat *Ma.* Silently repeat *Sa* on the fifth, *Ta* on the sixth, *Na* on the seventh, and *Ma* on the eighth part of the eight-part inhalation.

While you breathe and silently repeat the sounds, move the fingers of each hand in the following sequence: On *Sa* press the tips of the index finger and thumb firmly together, on *Ta* press the middle finger and thumb tips, on *Na* press the ring finger and thumb tips, and on *Ma* press the little finger and thumb tips together.

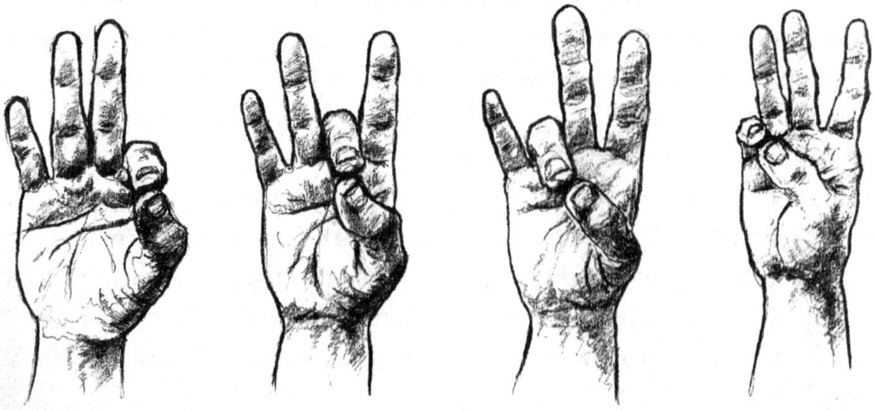

Pauri Kriyā Hand Positions

To exhale the breath, recite, *Sa Ta Na Ma, Sa Ta Na Ma,* in a monotone. Coordinate the pressing of the thumb tips to the fingers with the corresponding sounds, just as you did during the silent eight-part inhalation. Continue this sequence for 3 to 11 minutes.

If you notice your mind wandering, simply return your attention to the breath, sound, and finger sequence of the meditation. At the end of the meditation, inhale in one long breath, retain your breath briefly, and exhale in one long breath. Conclude by relaxing your posture and opening your eyes.

ONE-MINUTE BREATH

The secret to this advanced meditation is to remain relaxed physically and mentally. Begin by sitting comfortably with the spine aligned and your hands on your knees with the palms facing up and the elbows straight. Close your eyes and feel your entire body relaxed and at ease. Let your breath become slow and deep.

Slowly inhale to the count of 20. You may repeat the mantra *Sa Ta Na Ma* five times or use another method to help you keep count. Retain the breath for a count of 20, then slowly exhale to a count of 20. Inhale slowly and repeat the sequence. It is normal for the body to make adjustments throughout the practice. Be patient with yourself as you build skill. Start slowly, perhaps counting to 5-5-5 or 10-10-10 instead of 20-20-20, and build your practice over time from 3 to 31 minutes.

At the end of the meditation, inhale in one long breath, retain your breath briefly, and exhale in one long breath. Relax your posture and open your eyes.

CONCLUSION

When Yoga Therapy began as a modern field in health care in the late 1980s, there was little research on the application and outcomes of Yoga practices on medical conditions. Now there are new studies reported every week from research conducted all over the world. Through the years, we have conducted outcome studies on our programs as a way of evaluating their effectiveness. Our first study in Kundalini Yoga Therapy measured the effects of meditation practice on self-efficacy beliefs for people who are HIV positive, and we had favorable results. In 1994, I earned a Ph.D. in Health Psychology from Columbia Pacific University for this research.

When we train Kundalini Yoga Therapists, we draw on the results of modern

Yoga Therapy research to inform the practice of traditional Yoga. The Guru Ram Das Center for Medicine and Humanology, which Yogi Bhajan and I currently direct, conducts our own program outcome studies and supports the research of other Kundalini Yoga Therapists. To date, we have outcome measures and/or actual research data on the following:

1. Meditation effects for people living with HIV
2. Meditation effects for chronic insomnia
3. Meditation effects for reversing cognitive impairment
4. The effects of alternate nostril breathing on heart rate and angina
5. A six-week program for stroke recovery
6. A seven-week program for people with type 2 diabetes
7. A one-week program for recovery from posttraumatic stress disorder
8. A twelve-week program for generalized anxiety disorder

The current focus of our work at the center is training Kundalini Yoga teachers to become Kundalini Yoga Therapists. Training programs are offered in seventeen countries to prepare teachers to teach safely, therapeutically, and effectively.

The knowledge, experience, techniques, and skill of the Yoga Therapist are only part of what makes the work with clients successful. Intuitive, deep listening, inner stillness, inclusion, the ability to be with ambiguity, sensitivity, and compassion are additional factors. In our Kundalini Yoga Therapy trainings, special attention is given to the personal development of the consciousness of the teacher to engender awareness, intuition, compassion, deep listening, sensitivity, humility, endurance, and grace.

The 1,000-hour, three-year program prepares trainees to teach Kundalini Yoga to people with a wide range of health conditions, including chronic and life-threatening illness, psychological conditions, and those preparing for death. We build on participants' basic Yoga teacher training to deepen and expand the application of yogic philosophy, yogic technique, and habits of conscious living toward health recovery. Deep attention is given to the therapeutic application of prāṇāyāma, dṛṣṭi (where one focuses the eyes during meditation), mudrā, āsana, and bandha (to lock, to hold, or to tighten). There are three main bandhas that are applied in Yoga practice and a fourth that integrates them: bhāvana (mental image), svadhyāya (self-reflection), the rhythmic, targeted effects of kriyās, and Yoga nidrā.

Trainees learn to take a systems approach to include friends, family members, and the healthcare team. Trainees also learn to understand and work with the condition itself, as well as its complications, to manage contraindications and side effects of medical treatment. They learn Yoga and meditation research methods and how to track outcomes and conduct data collection. Within their scope of practice, we cover working in hospitals, clinics, and other medical settings, collaborating with health professionals in a team approach, professional ethics, marketing, business, and legal aspects of a Yoga Therapy practice.

The heart of our training in Kundalini Yoga Therapy is understanding and working with the client's process of change and developing sensitivity to the Yoga and to the needs of the student. For, as Yogi Bhajan said, "Yoga, with its every system, is going to prevail. We clearly see this trend. . . . Yoga is a science for all humanity. It is the custodian of human grace and radiance. It holds a great future for every human being. It brings mental caliber for purpose and prosperity of life. The future of Yoga is bright, bountiful and blissful." (*Aquarian Wisdom*, Bhajan Y., 2004)

REFERENCES

Bhajan, Y. Yogi Bhajan Lecture Archive. Lecture by Siri Singh Sahib Bhai Sahib Harbhajan Singh Khalsa Yogi Ji. Location unknown. 7 Oct. 1974. Web. Available at http://fateh.sikhnet.com/sikhnet/articles.nsf/fed9a32db02c04088725667 1004e06c3/8d50e43c5a0dd309872576fd007d1763!OpenDocument.

——. Lecture. 23 Apr. 1969.

——. Lecture. 2 Jul. 1984.

——. Lecture. 9 Apr. 1988.

——. Pauri Kriya, personal communication, 1990.

Bhajan, Y. *Aquarian Wisdom*. Espanola, New Mexico, 2004.

Kabat-Zinn, J. *Full Catastrophe Living: Using the Wisdom of Your Body and Mind to Face Stress, Pain and Illness*. New York: Delta, 1990.

Khalsa, S. P. K. "Adi Mantra," "One Minute Breath," and "Healthy, Happy, Holy Breath" are from *Kundalini Yoga: The Flow of Eternal Power*, by Shakti Parwha Kaur Khalsa. Los Angeles: Time Capsule Books, 1996.

YOGA THERAPY CASE REVIEW: CHRONIC INSOMNIA

Subjective Findings

Marta was a thirty-seven-year-old woman who presented with chronic primary insomnia experienced over the previous six months. She had difficulties falling asleep, taking three hours or more each night to get to sleep. She would often wake up tired, indicating the sleep she did get was not even that restful. Marta reported, "I drag myself through the day and dread going to bed at night. I have been staying up later and later thinking that when I finally do get to bed I will be so tired that I will fall right asleep, but this isn't what happens. No matter what time I go to bed, it still takes me about three hours to fall asleep. Sometimes I don't sleep at all. And I still have to get up at 6 a.m. to get to work on time. While some nights I get as much as five hours of sleep, it feels like I barely sleep at all."

Before coming for Yoga Therapy, Marta had gone to a sleep lab where she received testing and the diagnosis. There were no apparent cofactors or evident medical causes such as sleep apnea. The sleep lab physician gave her a sleep hygiene routine that included standard advice: avoid caffeine, alcohol, and nicotine for at least five hours before bedtime; sleep in a quiet, dark, cool, well-ventilated room; minimize exposure to light before and during sleep; establish a soothing bedtime routine; keep a consistent bedtime and awakening time; exercise early in the day; and eat lightly early in the evening. She reported that she followed the guidelines and still had trouble falling asleep.

Marta was wary of prescription sleep medication because of potential side effects and dependency. She had tried various herbal and nutritional supplements and over-the-counter remedies with no noticeable benefit. She stated, "I want to be able to sleep on my own. But nothing I do makes it better. I read somewhere that Yoga and meditation might help." So, although Marta expressed she was hopeful, she came to the first session frustrated, discouraged, fretful, fatigued, and anxious.

Objective Findings

Breath Assessment: Marta's breathing was shallow, rapid, and irregular. Her pelvic and thoracic regions were restricted, and the muscles of the spine, neck, shoulders, and rib cage were tight. She spoke in quick bursts and moved around in her chair and had challenges getting comfortable while standing. As Marta described her situation, she sighed and yawned frequently.

Physical (Anna): Marta held patterns of restriction in the psoas, diaphragm, pelvis, and thorax while walking, breathing, standing, and sitting. Her body movements and speech patterns indicated chronic anxiety, worry, and the ill effects of long-term stress.

Energetic (Prana), Spirit (Ananda), Cognitive (Vijana): Marta had been suffering from low prāṇa (energy) for some time. She was worried, tired, irritable, unable to think clearly, and had difficulty completing tasks, staying focused, or carrying a consistent train of thought. Marta drank five to seven cups of coffee every day and consumed three "5 Hour Energy" drinks to get through the day. In addition to feeling "lousy" most of the time, Marta had little energy to enjoy her life. "Some days I just want to give up," she told me. Since Spirit, or vitality, and the elevation of the flow of thought both depend on the quality and level of prāṇa, these are all reported here together during assessments.

Emotional (Mano): "I don't think of what my mind does as anxiety," Marta explained. "I don't feel anxious. I have a lot of demands at work. Not sleeping is just stress, that's all." Upon further inquiry, she described a protracted and contentious divorce in the months leading up to her sleep disturbance. Her home was at risk, she was in considerable debt, and she was afraid that her dream of having children was dissolving along with the marriage. She lost the steady financial support of her husband and took on a position at work that brought her an increase in monthly income but required more of her than she had to give at the time. Marta was concerned that she might lose her job due to poor performance. "I always feel I am behind, and I just can't catch up." Yes, she was stressed; she was also anxious and depressed about her current ability to provide for herself; and she was fearful of her future. She was living in a chronic state of survival and felt angry, defeated, and hopeless.

Assessment

Marta was experiencing more emotional distress than she had identified on her own. She always saw herself as strong and did not recognize or acknowledge the financial and emotional toll the divorce took on her. She only had a few tools to deal with the challenges she faced and the result was chronic hyperarousal, which led to her chronic insomnia. Evidence from Western medical research supports this conclusion: "Primary insomniacs suffer from a disorder of hyperarousal and . . . the elevated arousal produces the poor sleep and other symptoms reported by patients. It is therefore suggested that new treatment strategies directed at reduction of arousal level be considered in these patients" (Bonnet and Arand, 1997).

From the yogic perspective, Marta's anxiety, depression, and hyperarousal are conditions of chronically low prāṇa. Her habits of daily living reduced prāṇa and ojas, and she did little to replenish them herself. The shock and stress of the divorce and increased workload further pulled on her reserves. Self-care dwindled for Marta as she poured her time and energy into work. She did not eat properly, had no regular exercise or self-reflection, spent hours in front of a screen each night, and her time with friends and family had substantially diminished.

In our view, Marta needed to restore rhythmic balance and restful sleep, she needed to rebuild her prāṇa and ojas, and her nervous and endocrine systems needed to be reset.

Treatment Goals and Action Plan

The treatment goals for Marta included:

1. Restore rhythmic balance in the nervous and endocrine systems so that Marta can relax and sleep.
2. Alleviate anxiety and depression.
3. Form new habits of daily living so that treatment goals are maintained.
4. Restore the prāṇa vāyus and ojas so that new habits are maintained.

The first step in our plan of action was to arrange support for Marta to develop a personal practice. By her own admission, she was unable to do anything more than what she was already doing to get by. "I am just too tired," she said. Yet, Marta agreed to ask a friend to practice with her in order to get started and stay motivated. The friend was also invited to the second session.

Marta was to resume the sleep hygiene routine the sleep lab physician gave her with the addition of the following Yoga and breathing practices. We kept the home practice brief, simple, and accessible for the first two weeks, which was enough to provide effective results. As recommended by ancient yogic teachings and by Western research on chronic insomnia, "Treatments for insomnia, such as relaxation, exercise training, and some medications, have in common a shift away from sympathetic nervous system dominance and toward parasympathetic activation. As such, these treatments may provide long-term benefits over and above short-term improvement in reported sleep quality" (Bonnet and Arand, 1998).

Marta had no contraindications for Yoga practice. Her home practice for the first two weeks consisted of a variation of mārjāryāsana (cat pose) paired with bitilasana (cow pose), sūrya bhedana (left nostril breathing) and bālāsana (child's pose).

To breathe more deeply and completely, Marta needed to open the thoracic and pelvic regions of her body and lengthen and release tension in the psoas. She practiced a rhythmic variation of cat-cow for 3 minutes on each side, where one leg was extended out and up on the inhalation into cow pose, and the knee was brought toward the nose on the exhalation into cat pose. Next, she sat in sukhāsana (easy pose) for her left nostril breathing practice. Closing the right nostril with her right thumb or index finger, Marta breathed long and deep out of the left nostril for a period of 3 minutes. After her breathing practice, Marta lengthened her torso forward over the legs and rested her forehead on the floor in child's pose to calm the mind and relieve tension in the body. Child's pose can be performed with the hips on the heels or in this way with the legs crossed in sukhāsana. Finally, Marta was instructed to extend her arms in front or by her sides and to breathe slowly and deeply for 3 minutes.

Marta's practice was initially recommended for a half hour to an hour before going to sleep. Although she set her bedtime as 10:00 p.m., she had her friend come to her townhouse at 7:30 p.m. so they could practice together. The intention was to first establish the new habit with support. In a few weeks or so, the pattern of hyperarousal would be sufficiently diminished, and she would be better rested so she could practice at 9:00 p.m. on her own. By the third week, Marta was breathing more deeply and completely. Her speech pattern slowed, and she was more still. Moreover, she was falling asleep more quickly and readily. This helped her feel more energy, calmer, and more hopeful about her situation. She still relied on caffeine as a backup; however, she was down to three cups of coffee per day and, at that point, had stopped consuming energy drinks altogether.

With these gains, Marta was prepared to reset her nervous and endocrine systems and rebuild ojas and prāṇa. Her home practice assignment changed. She now practiced the Kundalini Yoga kriyā for Calmness and Anti-Anxiety followed by the Shabad kriyā prāṇāyāma meditation. The kriyā for calmness and anti-anxiety provides breath and movement sufficient to release stress, yet is not so stimulating that it keeps Marta up at night. Shabad kriyā works on a 22-beat breath cycle to reset internal rhythms and has been taught as a Yoga Therapy for sleep for thousands of years.

COURSE OF TREATMENT

We met twice a week for the first three weeks, until Marta was more consistent with her personal practice. Then, we met once a week for the next six weeks in order to support the establishment of new habits followed by meeting once a month for the remainder of the year in order to maintain the habits.

Once Marta was falling asleep readily and sleeping for six to eight hours a night, she no longer felt overwhelmed at work and had energy to spend time with her friends and family. The anxiety and depression were substantially alleviated, and she was happier and felt better. She began to make lifestyle changes too that would give her endurance and more consistent energy. She stopped caffeine and began to reduce and then eliminate sugar. She introduced ghee into her diet and increased fresh fruits and vegetables.

Some obstacles in this case were that Marta first needed to release tension in key areas of her body so that she could shift her stress-response breathing pattern. The home practice assignment for the first two weeks prepared her for deeper breathing work of the kriyā and meditation. A bigger challenge was to reduce the time she spent in front of a computer or television screen each night. The light from countless hours in front of her technological devices upset her neural and endocrine balance and kept her in a state of hyperarousal. Nevertheless, it was such an entrenched habit of having a television, computer, or handheld device on for many hours each night that it took about ninety days for Marta to get a handle on it. Her solution was to turn off every device at 7:30 p.m. *no matter what,* and she was advised to not return emails or check her social media in the middle of the night.

Marta continued the kriyā for Calmness and Anti-Anxiety and Shabad kriyā prāṇāyāma meditation for four months. Over time, the hyper-arousal pattern ceased and the internal rhythms of her nervous and endocrine systems were restored. Now, when she overworks or is stressed, it is simple for Marta to reset herself for sleep. "When I can't sleep now all I have to do is three to five left nostril breaths and I'm out. If I need more, I do seven to fifteen minutes of Shabad kriyā. It's really, really effective!"

CALMNESS AND ANTI-ANXIETY SERIES

This series is an excellent example of how an exercise series can be not too strenuous, but result in very calming and relaxed state of being. We would typically begin the practice with the tuning-in technique described in the chapter "Kundalini Yoga Therapy as Taught by Yogi Bhajan" in this text. The series will balance prāṇa and apāna (incoming and outgoing energy), increase lung capacity, and is said that it will allow you to control your thoughts and senses, while the breath meditation is for calmness.

1. **Meditation with Whistle Breath.** These first six exercises are a kriyā. Come sitting comfortably cross-legged, with the chest high, and the chin level to the ground and slightly tucked in. Gently close the eyes and focus at the root of the nose. Inhale through puckered lips with a whistle and exhale through the nose. It can take practice to whistle while you are inhaling. If you cannot whistle, inhale slowly through puckered lips and exhale through the nose. Concentrate on the whistling sound at the brow point with long, slow, and deep breathing. (5 minutes)

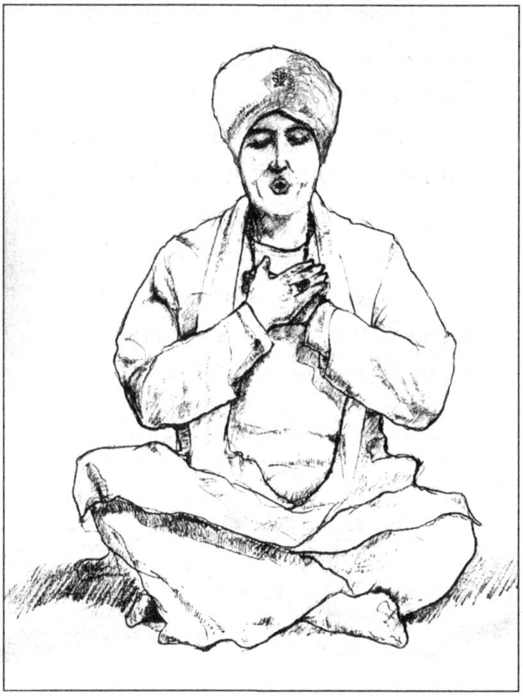

Meditation with Whistle Breath

2. **Cobra Pose with Whistle Breath.** Come out of the seated position and lie flat on your stomach. Bring the chin on the ground with the palms down on the mat underneath and slightly forward of the shoulders. Have the legs together with the tops of the feet on the floor. Now, inhale and raise the head up and the chest up while smoothly pushing yourself up. Make sure the arms are shoulder-width apart, elbows are a little bent, fingers are pointing forward, shoulders are rolled back and down, chest is high, and the head is back. The whole pelvic area is on the ground. You can be resting comfortably on the forearms in salamba bhujaṅgāsana (sphinx pose) if it is more comfortable for you. Exhale with a whistle. Continue inhaling through the nose and exhaling through puckered lips in a whistle. Concentrate on the whistling sound with long, slow, and deep breathing. (3 minutes)

3. **Nose to Knees.** Roll over onto your back and draw the knees up to your chest. Wrap the arms around the knees while lifting the head up and place the nose in between the knees. Keeping the mouth closed, make the sound *hung* emphasizing and lengthening the *ng* sound. If the neck is tired, rest it on the mat briefly, and then bring it back between the knees when you are ready. Continue inhaling through the nose and exhaling by making this sound. (2 minutes)

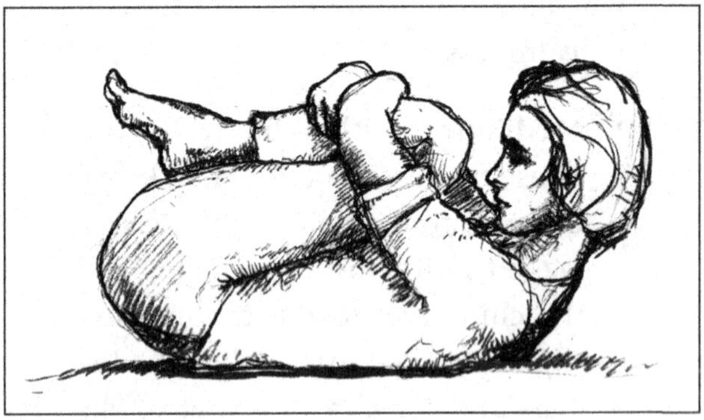

Nose to Knees

4. **Relaxing Easy Pose.** Relax on the back with the legs crossed as though you were sitting up in a comfortable cross-legged position. Place the arms by the sides with the palms up and with normal and relaxed breathing. (5 minutes)

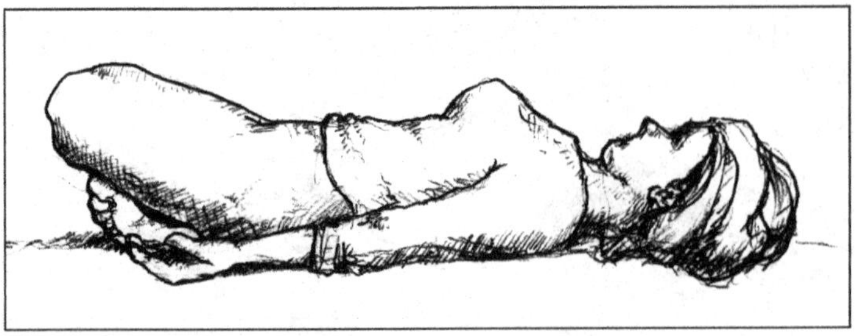

Relaxing Easy Pose

5. **Washing Machine.** Draw the knees up to the chest and rock yourself up. Sit comfortably cross-legged. Bring the hands on the shoulders with the fingers in front and the thumbs in back. Inhale and twist the torso left and then exhale and twist the torso right. Keep the chest up high and let the head travel with the shoulders. (1 minute)

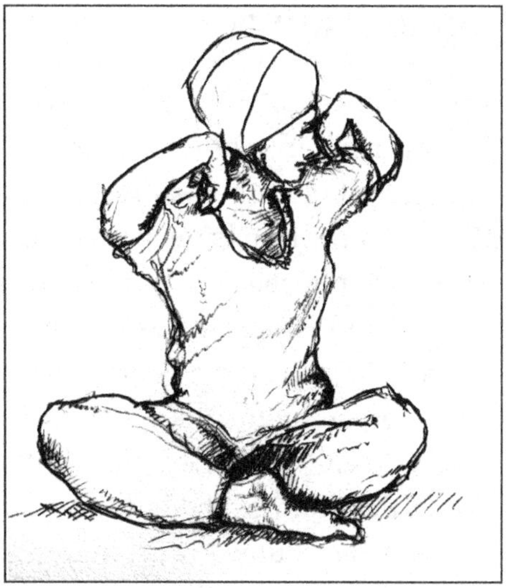

Washing Machine

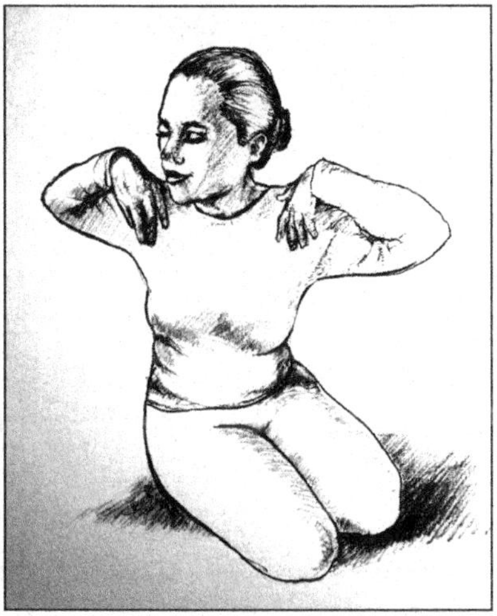

6. **Washing Machine Sitting on Heels.** Continue the same exercise sitting on the knees and heels. (1 minute)

Washing Machine
Sitting on Heels

7. **Baby Pose.** Sit back on the heels and place the forehead on the ground. Have the arms, by the sides, near the ankles, with the palms resting up. If this places too much pressure on the head or neck, then have the forearms resting on the ground in front of the head. Allow the shoulders to relax and breathe normally. (3 minutes)

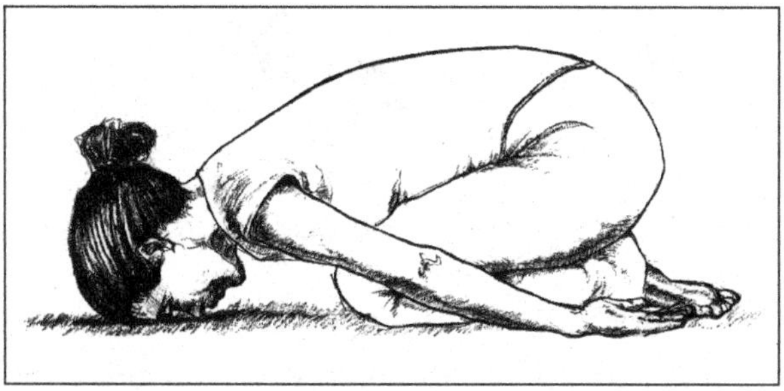

Baby Pose

SHABAD KRIYĀ

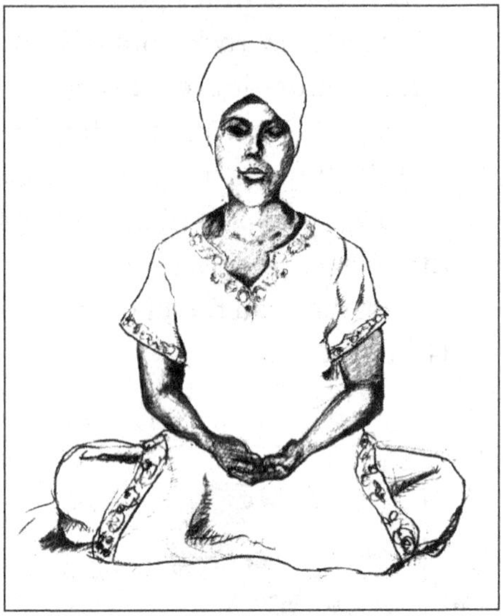

Shabad Kriyā

Effectiveness of this meditation is in the 22-beat rhythm. The best time to practice it is nightly before bed as regular practice of the technique brings deep and relaxed sleep. Sit in a comfortable posture with the spine aligned and supported as needed. This may be cross-legged on the floor or in a chair with both feet flat on the floor. Place the hands in your lap with the back of the right hand resting in the palm of the left. Both palms face up with the thumbs touching and pointing forward as seen in the picture to the right. The eyes are partially open. The gaze is downward, along the sides of the nose, eventually resting and focusing on the tip of the nose while keeping both sides of the nose in equal view. The pineal and the pituitary glands and the area between them are balanced by this eye focus. You may feel a slight pressure at the frontal lobe.

Inhale in four equal parts, mentally vibrating the mantra *Sa Ta Na Ma,* with one syllable for each part of the inhalation. Gently retain the breath; do not strain. Mentally vibrate the sound of the mantra for four cycles while holding the breath for a total of 16 beats. Exhale completely in two equal strokes with the mental sound, Wahe Guru. To end, inhale deeply in one long breath. Close the eyes and totally relax all focus and muscular activity in the eyes. Lengthen both arms overhead and shake the hands vigorously for about 10 seconds. Exhale and relax. Begin practice with 3 to 7 minutes and build up to 15 minutes.

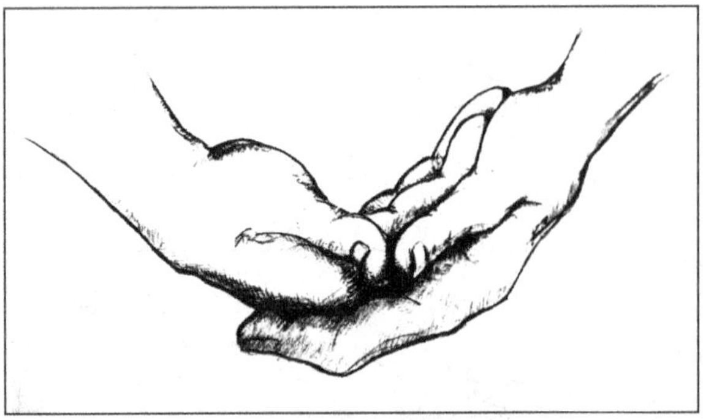

Shabad Mudrā

According to yogic tradition, this breath rhythm and sound combination regenerates and balances the natural rhythm in brain, neural, and endocrine function. Western research supports its application in the treatment of chronic insomnia as reported by Harvard researcher, Sat Bir Singh Khalsa (Khalsa, 2004).

REFERENCES

Bonnet, M. H., and D. L. Arand. "Hyper-arousal and Insomnia." *Sleep Medicine Reviews* 1.2 (1997): 97–108. Print.

——. "Heart Rate Variability in Insomniacs and Matched Normal Sleepers." *Psychosomatic Medicine* 60.5 (1998): 610–615. Print.

Khalsa, S. B. "Treatment of Chronic Insomnia with Yoga: A Preliminary Study with Sleep-Wake Diaries." *Applied Psychophysiology and Biofeedback* 29.4 (2004): 269–278. Print.

Khalsa, S. P. K. "Adi Mantra" from *Kundalini Yoga: The Flow of Eternal Power.* Los Angeles: Time Capsule Books, 1996. Print.

Khalsa, N. S. (2010). "Calmness and Anti-Anxiety Series" from *The Art, Science and Application of Kundalini Yoga, 3rd edition.* Dubuque, IA: Kendall Hunt Publishing, 2010. Print.

Khalsa, G. S. K. "Shabad Kriya" from *Meditation Manual for Intermediate Students.* Espanola: KRI Publications, 1975. Print.

PHOENIX RISING YOGA THERAPY

Michael Lee, M.A., Dip. Soc. Sci., E-RYT 500

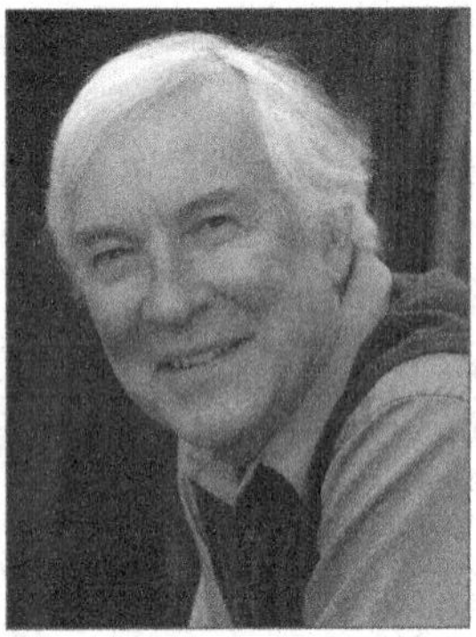

Michael Lee first became interested in the transformative power of Yoga in the early 1980s based on personal experiences with his practice and study with various teachers in Australia and the United States. He moved to the United States from Australia to live and teach at the Kripalu Center for Yoga and Health in Lenox, Massachusetts, in 1984. Combining his Yoga experience with his background in education and humanistic psychology, he completed a dissertation on the therapeutic benefits of Yoga for life-related issues and gained a master's degree in holistic health education from Norwich University in Vermont in 1986. Shortly thereafter, he developed Phoenix Rising Yoga Therapy, which today has more than 2,000 trained practitioners worldwide.

HISTORY AND DEVELOPMENT OF PHOENIX RISING YOGA THERAPY

In the mid 1970s, I worked as a lecturer at the Administrative College of Papua New Guinea in Port Moresby and then as a consultant for South Australian Government in Adelaide, Australia. Exploring areas of humanistic psychology and developing training programs that focused on changing behavior, I held a deep interest in how people change and transform in life. I had attended courses at the Australian National University led by faculty who were trained at the Esalen Institute in Northern California with Fritz Perls and at the Tavistock Institute in England. These programs were considered to be on the leading edge of experiential educational practice with regard to behavioral change.

At the same time, I began to embrace the discipline of Yoga, attending daily classes at the nearby Satyananda Ashram in the Adelaide Hills, and quickly determined that my Yoga practice seemed to be facilitating change in my own life. In my experiences at work, I found that simply talking about "change" may help people initially with new behaviors. However, the outcomes were usually short lived. On the other hand, awareness gained from a deep mind-body connection similar to what I was learning in my Yoga practice seemed to support, not only lasting change, but transformation at a personal level. I was determined to explore this further.

In 1984, I was granted a scholarship by the South Australian Government to study in the United States for a year to examine the viability of new program development based on Eastern philosophies and practices. I chose an independent study master's degree program through Vermont College of Norwich University. My focus was self-study in Yoga Therapy engaging the question, "Can yogic practices and a yogic lifestyle support transformation and change at a personal level in terms of both physical and mental health?"

During my study I lived, practiced, and worked at the Kripalu Center in Lenox, Massachusetts, initially as a student and then as a member of the teaching faculty. It was during this time that I experienced an unforgettable event that changed my life and also gave birth to Phoenix Rising Yoga Therapy.

Here is my story of change:

A friend was using the wall to support me in the triangle posture on my right side when my body began to quiver uncontrollably. I witnessed an intense red-blue, burning sensation in my right hip and believed I had pressed into the posture as deeply as I could, feeling pain that wasn't really physical pain. My mind was shouting, *Get out of here. Stop now! What are you doing? Get on with it.* I was definitely at an edge between the known and safe bodily experience and the unknown, "unsafe" territories. The escalating sensations in my right hip were becoming almost unbearable when my attention shifted from what was happening in my body to what was taking place with my mind. I was becoming more and more agitated and wanted to release out of the posture.

Placing his hand gently against my chest, my friend embraced my growing resistance by simply being fully present to my experience. He didn't reassure or try to calm me. He was just there. This enabled me to surrender again and again into what was happening in the moment, to deepen my breath and simply witness the strange noises emanating from my mouth and throat. The hot, fiery, red burning poured out of my hip like a volcanic eruption. My whole body vibrated, and I felt warm tears streaming down my face without knowing what they were about or why they were there.

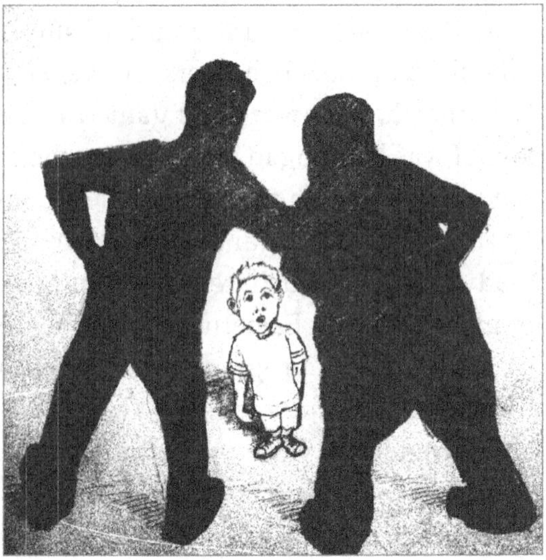

My body began to feel very small as I reexperienced myself as an eight-year-old boy standing on a school playground about to be beaten up by a group of older boys. The terror of that frightened child penetrated every cell of my being as I continued to release emotionally, feeling out of control. Yet, paradoxically, I was totally safe at the same time. I felt a loving presence emanate from deep inside, reassuring me that the experience could be fully engaged. Incredulously, the sensations passed almost as easily as they had come, and I released out of the posture feeling very different. Internally, I felt stiller, quieter, and suspended in a sense of timelessness. I was very *present*—to the moment and to myself. Serenity had replaced the terror.

Afterward, I recall "integrating" the experience using some of the tools I had become familiar with in my work as a change agent. I asked myself questions like *What really happened? What did I feel? What is the significance of this experience? How does this affect my life? What aspects of this experience show up in other areas of my life? In what situations have I felt this fear before?* I was able to begin to see how I had carried my experience as an eight-year-old child into my life practice and noticed the limitations it had created in me. I quickly resolved the issue and began to live my life from that day on with a different core belief around issues of power and the fear of intimidation.

Looking around the Kripalu ashram, I realized that many of my Yoga colleagues there had experienced an "emotional release" in their practices at various times. I also learned that, for many, the experiences they had, while sometimes very powerful in nature, could not be easily integrated into their life experience or used in helpful ways. My own personal experience and subsequent resolution and change led me to develop a process that made use of both the deeper levels of awareness that come to me in Yoga experiences as well as the open-ended processes that I had learned from my work in education and humanistic psychology. And so, Phoenix Rising Yoga Therapy was born.

At this time, I also began working at the nearby DeSisto School in Lenox, Massachusetts, a boarding high school for troubled teens. With the support of the school's director, the late Michael DeSisto, I developed a Yoga-based "Wellness Lifestyle" program for the school. Students in the program attended daily Phoenix Rising Yoga Therapy classes and individual sessions. They explored a yogic lifestyle in a special dormitory set up for the program and also received weekly Gestalt-based therapy sessions from the school's psychotherapy staff. Making rapid progress in dealing with emotional issues and finding resolution, these students seemed to do so more quickly than many of their peers who were not participating in the special program. Although no formal research was conducted, several of the psychotherapists working at the school at the time praised the effectiveness of the Yoga Therapy program and recommended it to students.

I was encouraged by this progress at the DeSisto School and continued to develop my work using this Yoga-based mind-body approach and began to see individual clients for Yoga Therapy sessions in both Stockbridge, Massachusetts, and New York City. Before long, many of my Yoga teacher colleagues were asking me to teach them the work I was developing. They wanted to be able to create the same kind of integrated transformational experience for others in one-on-one sessions. So, I launched the first Phoenix Rising Yoga Therapy Training, and seven people registered for the six-day program held over three weekends in Trenton, New Jersey, in April 1987.

As Phoenix Rising Yoga Therapy evolved, I witnessed many people getting in touch with a deeper self that reflected their inner wisdom. They seemed to become aware of the hidden, unconscious aspects of themselves that colored their perceptions and influenced their actions and choices in life. Deep physical, emotional, and spiritual shifts gave them the courage to face self-limiting fears and, in so doing, effect long-lasting and profound change in their lives. Clients changed careers and addresses, ended destructive relationships and self-destructive behaviors, and moved on with greater openness and capacity to change their life experience. They realigned their lives to reflect what they discovered waiting for them at the core of their being as it was revealed to them during their Phoenix Rising Yoga Therapy sessions.

The modality has continued to evolve and grow, gaining recognition in the mainstream of the medical and psychotherapeutic communities of the world. The services Phoenix Rising practitioners offer today are being seen as adjunct therapy in the treatment of various medical and psychological conditions. Phoenix Rising Yoga Therapy is a simple and profoundly effective tool for expanding awareness and supporting people in their quest for greater authenticity and wholeness.

DEFINITION OF YOGA THERAPY WITH THE PHOENIX RISING APPROACH

Life provides us with the opportunity for all to unfold in accord with our "true nature." Phoenix Rising Yoga Therapy offers process-based practices that facilitate this unfolding. Phoenix Rising teacher and scholar of Yoga philosophy, Jen Munyer, makes the following connections between the Phoenix Rising Process and the traditional roots of Yoga:

> The Phoenix Rising Yoga Therapy process invites clients to use presence and focused relaxed awareness on several aspects of their immediate experience including their breath, their body in āsana (posture) held at a point of therapeutic tolerable discomfort (their "edge"), the many layers of their emotions that arise and the thoughts that get sparked by their experience in all layers of their being. The *Taittirīya Upaniṣad* references these layers of being, or the 5 kośas (sheaths) that cover the soul. With refined awareness to these layers, a client is able to gain valuable and meaningful information about themselves ranging from insight into their saṁskāras (imprints left on the subconscious mind from past and present experience) to their behavioral tendencies that influence their present behavior, posture and way of being/vāsana. While a client might be able to do this on their own through practice, the power of having their experience witnessed by a practitioner mirroring to them their vijñāna kośa (the layer of being that has the capacity to receive all experience free from judgment) accelerates the client's ability to access their own deeper layers of wisdom. (Munyer, 2012)

The final and most important aspect of a Phoenix Rising Yoga Therapy session is a guided meditation (also known as "integration"), which supports the client in integrating all the awareness gained through his/her experience. In Sūtra 2.26, Patañjali suggests that viveka (discernment) is the means for the avoidance of avidyā (ignorance or misidentification with the Real). This final meditation in a Phoenix Rising session is a process of discernment that guides the client directly to their own source of wisdom, acceptance, and truth. This wisdom is then used by the client to access his/her highest state of mind—their *buddhi*—the aspect of mind that, in its most clear and refined form, can offer action steps that correspond to the soul's wisdom and desire. The vijñāna kośa is directly informed from both ānanda-maya-kośa (bliss body or the realm of where our deepest and most true impressions of self are stored) and the divine consciousness of soul. By receiving wisdom from this aspect of his/her being, the client is able to create meaningful and profound changes in his/her life that come directly from his/her capacity to discern his/her own soul's directions and messages.

From a modern Western perspective, Phoenix Rising Yoga Therapy draws its foundational base from the work of Carl Rogers (therapist and educator) and Malcolm S. Knowles (educator). Rogers declares, "Experience is, for me, the highest authority. The touchstone of validity is my own experience. No other person's ideas, and none of my own ideas, are as authoritative as my experience. It is to experience that I must return again and again, to discover a closer approximation to truth as it is in the process of becoming in me" (Lee, 1999).

This statement is in concert with what the great saints Sri Aurobindo and Patañjali saw with regard to the nature of being human. Phoenix Rising Yoga Therapy uses a mind-body process to support the individual in becoming aware of and learning from his/her unique experience.

Malcolm Knowles was a highly influential figure in education in the second

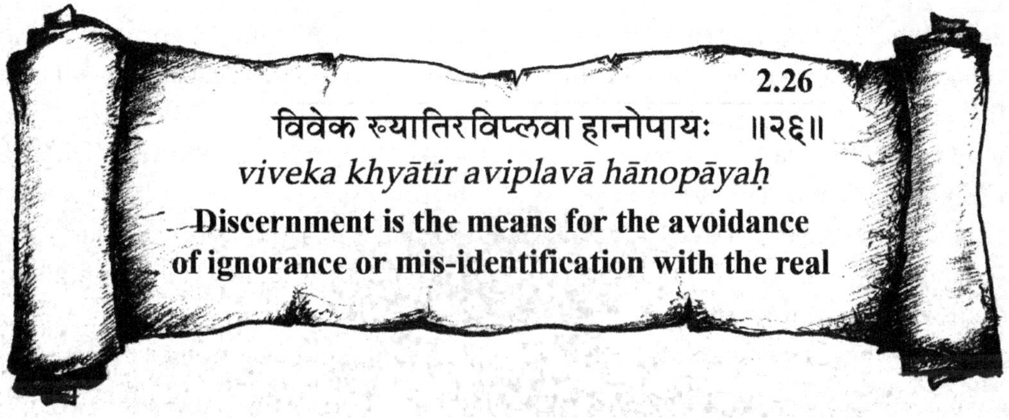
2.26
विवेक ख्यातिरविप्लवा हानोपायः ॥२६॥
viveka khyātir aviplavā hānopāyaḥ
Discernment is the means for the avoidance of ignorance or mis-identification with the real

half of the twentieth century. His work was a significant factor in reorienting adult educators from "educating people" to "helping them learn." He believed, "Adults should acquire a mature understanding of themselves. They should understand their needs, motivations, interests, capacities, and goals. They should be able to look at themselves objectively and maturely. They should accept themselves and respect themselves for what they are, while striving earnestly to become better" (Rogers in Ingleby, et al., 2010).

Phoenix Rising Yoga Therapy could thus be defined as a process by which one gains a more mature understanding of oneself with the capacity to look upon oneself with greater acceptance, compassion, and the ability to transform by bringing that awareness to action in life.

METHODS AND PHILOSOPHICAL CONCEPTS UNDERLYING PHOENIX RISING YOGA THERAPY

The Phoenix Rising approach to Yoga Therapy is based on both ancient yogic teachings and modern mind-body processes that enhance one's life in body, mind, and spirit. While many forms of Yoga Therapy might use the term *client-centered,* meaning that the approach gives focus to the needs and wants of the client, Phoenix Rising Yoga Therapy takes this even further. Phoenix Rising Yoga Therapists are trained to guide a "process" and do not offer "prescriptions" or advise a client on how he/she should conduct his/her life. The processes that they facilitate are designed in such a way that the client is very easily able to discern what works for them in their lives in all dimensions . . . and also what does not work. The Phoenix Rising integration process helps the client then decide what they might want to do about whatever they have become aware of and what is the highest priority. At the same time, the process itself has intrinsic benefits and by-products regardless of the content. Clients often report feeling more grounded, more centered, more focused, more aware, and generally less stressed and better able to cope with life. Over time, clients begin to naturally apply the processes to daily life. They are able to take in the experience of a given moment for what it is and notice any judgment or label they might apply to it. They become more accepting of what is going on in their world and more empowered to change.

Many new students in training in Phoenix Rising Yoga Therapy face two immediate challenges. First, they are required to let go of their concept of themselves as the "doer" and take on the role of "facilitator." They learn how to guide a "dual process." In one area, they are directive and the other nondirective. They skillfully and professionally guide the physical form of the experience along with the inner process. They then must learn how to "get out of the way" as the client engages this process. The therapist then shifts to practice a form of deep loving presence without interference or trying to "steer" the client in any particular direction. The nondirective part of the dual process in Phoenix Rising Yoga Therapy is yogic in origin based on the ideal of the "inner guru" and the notion that we already know what we need to know—we simply need to be present enough to allow it to surface. Carl Rogers was not known as a yogi but had the same deep faith in the potential and power of human beings to transform. He said, "In my early professional years I was asking the question: How can I treat, or cure, or change this person? Now I would phrase the question in this way: How can I provide a relationship which this person may use for his own personal growth?" (Rogers, 1961).

One study by Aspy and Roebuck showed evidence that the Rogerian approach gave rise to increased scores on self-concept measures, indicating more positive self-regard, gains in creativity scores, greater spontaneity, and use of higher levels of thinking (Gordon, 2006).

Because of this approach, Phoenix Rising Yoga Therapy is seen as an appropriate modality for supporting healing related to the myriad of "lifestyle" disorders and psychoemotional issues. Clients often report the disappearance of physical pain associated with these conditions after receiving sessions or classes or attending groups guided by Phoenix Rising practitioners. It is an ideal approach for stress management because of its capacity to empower the client to take charge of his/her life in new and effective ways.

Through practitioner-assisted Yoga postures and a dialogue process that is both open-ended and nondirective of the outcome of the session, the client is facilitated through an experience of him/herself in the present moment. And whatever happens in the present moment physically, emotionally, intellectually, and spiritually finds richness in relationship to the bigger picture of how that client is being in the world in daily life with work, play, family, and relationships. Using focused breathing and the opportunity to verbalize the in-the-moment experiences—thoughts, emotions, sensations, and memories—clients experience a connection as well as a deeper attunement to their own internal guidance.

In the one-on-one Phoenix Rising Yoga Therapy session, the client is usually guided through several therapist-assisted or supported Yoga postures accompanied by client-directed dialog to support focused awareness. The key distinction is that the therapist does not provide "content"—only "process" directions. For example, in many guided inner process experiences, Yoga teachers tend to focus on language that relaxes the client or that takes him/her to a calming environment. A traditional talk therapist might direct a client's attention to a specific feeling or event. The Phoenix Rising Yoga Therapist does neither. Instead, he/she will simply direct the client's awareness to his/her moment-to-moment experience and only intervene directly in the process if safety becomes an issue. The Phoenix Rising Yoga teacher or group facilitator guides a similar "dual process" experience for clients in a class or group setting in such a way that each person in the room is offered the opportunity to engage his/her own unique experience and explore moment-to-moment awareness as he/she engages it. Surprisingly, when the conditions are right and they are able to let themselves fully into their experience, clients discover themselves in deeper and deeper layers of awareness. Through this process of awareness and discernment, clients have the opportunity to release old undigested experiences, traumas, personal beliefs, and out-of-date habits and patterns, enabling them to move more fully into life with new perspective and personal efficacy.

AREAS OF EXPERTISE AND APPROACH

Phoenix Rising clearly falls into the psychospiritual domain of Yoga Therapy. At the same time, there is a distinct physical part to the work and the client's body is a key element in the process. It is used, however, more like a doorway to the fuller experience of self than as an end in itself. Rather than treating a specific condition, physical or mental, Phoenix Rising Yoga Therapists guide a process with the client as a key participant. The most significant skill set required for practitioners in this kind of approach centers on their capacity to facilitate an experience for the client while keeping their own interpretations, beliefs, and values at bay. To do this well, practitioners are in touch with their own bodies, are comfortable in using their body as a key source of awareness, are experienced and comfortable in supporting a physical experience (assisted āsana), are skilled at facilitating an inner process that engages the client's unique experience without interference and/or input from the practitioner, and creates an overall safe container for the client for the entire experience. Phoenix Rising Yoga Therapist, Renne Reusz, states it this way:

There is no intent to fix you in a Phoenix Rising Session. Instead, you are met in the moment, with no judgment or criticism, no matter how (seemingly) wrong, weak, strange, stupid, or bad "things" are. There is allowance and space for all parts of you to show up, and essentially to let you be yourself. Can you imagine what this would be like—to be met just as you are, with no need to change or fix anything, imperfections and all?

Deep down I believe this is what we all need, to be witnessed, in this moment, for all that we think and do. As humans, we seem to have an inherent need for connection with others. We need to be seen as our authentic selves and to be welcomed with an open heart. But for many of us, bearing our intimate selves feels vulnerable, so it is only when we are met in that space, where safety and love reside, where unfinished and irregular are not only welcome, but regarded as objects of beauty, that we can shed the protective skin to expose our ever-evolving, unique selves. This is the realization of Phoenix Rising Yoga Therapy—to be an unconditional, supportive presence to your process. (Reusz)

"The curious paradox is that when I accept myself just as I am, then I can change."

—C.R. Rogers, 1961

ILLUSTRATIVE CASE STUDY

Ed was a man in his late forties. He had been a Yoga student for a few years when he decided to have a Phoenix Rising Yoga Therapy session. He decided it was time to deal with an issue that his Yoga practice had so far not been able to change. During his intake information prior to his first session Ed was asked what he might like to get from his experience. What was it he was looking to receive from Yoga Therapy? He quickly declared that he wanted to be happier and happy more of the time. His therapist asked him to say a little more about his desire, and Ed went on to explain that, ever since his teen years, he noticed that most of the time he felt unhappy but didn't really know why. He said that a friend had recently inquired if he was "okay" because his facial expression suggested sadness a lot of the time.

The first session began with a brief body scan. In the Phoenix Rising approach, this means the therapist directs the clients attention to various areas of their body and asks him/her to focus awareness there briefly and to report what he/she notices. No attempt is made by the practitioner to interpret the information. At the end of the scan, the client is asked to reflect on what was most noticeable. The client may be invited to tell the practitioner a little more about whatever it is he/she notices. This is done purely to deepen the client's awareness. Ed reported that he felt a lot of discomfort in his upper back, particularly around his shoulders. He also felt a tenderness and somewhat vulnerable feeling in his chest. When asked what area of his body he might like to explore in his first session (and possibly subsequent sessions), he said he would like to focus on his upper body, mostly his chest and shoulders.

For the next two weeks in two sessions a week apart, Ed engaged various assisted postures with his therapist's support and focused on the sensations he experienced, most of which were in his upper body. These upper body and mostly chest-opening postures were chosen collaboratively with Ed at the beginning of each session when he was guided through a brief body scan. As the sessions progressed, he became more familiar with the approach and with focusing his awareness and answering his therapist when she asked "What's happening now?" His responses flowed more easily as the process developed, and he became more detailed as he grew more comfortable with this way of working. At times, his therapist would ask him to "Tell me more," and he would go into a little more detail with his descriptions. His responses were sometimes concerning the physical sensations and sometimes the feelings. At other times, he would observe himself thinking about a past event or current concern. After both his first and second sessions, he reported feeling more relaxed and "walking taller."

In his third session, Ed's therapist supported him in an assisted cobra posture with his hips engaged on the floor and his chest elevated and open at the front. She guided his breath to establish the posture at a tolerable "edge" and encouraged him to allow his breath to just "fall out" with each exhale. After a few minutes of further dialog, Ed began to become agitated. When asked, "What's happing now?" he exploded with an outburst of anger saying, "I want those bastards to get off my (expletive) back!" His therapist asked him to say more. He elaborated. His emotions also shifted from anger to sadness as he began to sob. She gently eased him out of the posture and guided him into the child's pose pressing on his back to counterstretch the previous posture, all while staying physically and inwardly present to him. After a brief transition, he returned to a seated position, and his therapist began to guide the integration part of the session.

During this part, Ed related what had happened during the session and how it related to his life story. He talked about how as a young boy his father had often been anxious about Ed's performance in several aspects of his life. His father seemed to be disappointed with him no matter what Ed did. He did well at school, but it was never good enough. At sports, he was barely average in talent and his father did not think much of his efforts, but he still played. His grandfather had treated him similarly and even once told him that he was just like his father—not very good at anything much. Later in college the story was the same. He graduated but not with any kind of distinction. He got a job, and he quit after a few years when he hadn't really progressed very far in the organization. The same happened with his next job and the next. He became a freelance technical writer, and, by working long hours and staying focused, he could manage to make a living though he didn't much like the work. He had maintained a distant relationship with his father, who would occasionally ask when he was going to find a real job. When his therapist directed him to focus inward and seek guidance from his "higher self" around what had transpired, he said, "I am free! Free at last of the expectations of my father and grandfather. Free to be me—no matter what I do with my life. My body has set me free!"

During subsequent sessions, Ed allowed the body sensations and awareness in the moment to take him into connection with other areas in his life that had been impacted by his inherited self-limiting beliefs. He set his own "homework" after each session around things in his life that he wanted to change as a result of his new knowledge. A few months later he switched jobs and became a landscaper. He'd always loved gardens and remembered times when he had shared this love with his mother. He seemed happy with the change and, after about six months of weekly sessions, declared that he had achieved his goal. He was experiencing a happier life for most of his days. He also looked different and noticed this physical change internally as well as externally. He felt taller, no longer sensed restriction in his back, and felt like his chest led his body in forward movement with soft strength rather than vulnerability. He visited his aging father and sought ways to support him in his waning years without any expectation of acceptance. Ed knew from the inside that he was indeed worthy of the life he was living regardless of anyone's approval.

RESEARCH AND LITERATURE

Many elements of the practice of Phoenix Rising Yoga Therapy are supported by current and historical research, particularly in relation to the bridge between Yoga Therapy and psychotherapy as tools for self-awareness and transformation. In Harold Coward's book, *Jung and Eastern Thought,* he explores Jung's fascination with Eastern philosophy and examines underlying energy systems comparing prāṇa with Freud's notion of the unconscious. He saw a primary connection between Yoga and therapy in that both traditions seek self-improvement through self-awareness.

In Phoenix Rising Yoga Therapy, the relationship between Yoga Therapist and client is considered essential to the effectiveness of the work. Research has shown that regardless of technique, the single-most influential factor in reported success is a feeling of empathy, safety, and understanding that exists between therapist and client (Lambert, 1992). This research indicates that it is the therapist's role to facilitate such a relationship that will, in turn, foster personal growth in the client.

The Phoenix Rising Yoga Therapy community is committed to objectively examining the therapeutic modalities and interventions used by its practitioners. Starting in 2009, a large-scale research project was designed and conducted with Phoenix Rising practitioners in their group and individual sessions. Results of the work suggested that individuals who participate in Phoenix Rising group or individual sessions experience decreased depression and anxiety symptoms and concurrently report increased personal awareness (Racanello, 2012). Additionally, when designing the Phoenix Rising Group Facilitator Training Program in 2003, I gathered my own informal research into the effects of my Eight-Week Stress Reduction Program with the initial trial group. To run some controls, I invited graduates of the new training program to collect predata and postdata from participants in subsequent groups using a standardized research symptom checklist. Results collected from over 200 participants showed that 80 percent of participants reported a reduction in stress-related symptoms following the eight-week program.

CONCLUSION

Yoga Therapy is a broad field of study. Within its scope are modalities ranging from those that focus more on the physical body to therapies whose intention is to offer a holistic approach to life enhancement. Some Yoga Therapies diagnose or offer to fix a specific problem. Phoenix Rising Yoga Therapy instead facilitates a process. That process enables individuals to make changes in their lives at all levels of being and brings them into greater balance and harmony, fulfilling one of the major tenets of Yoga. This is done through the body, through simple dialogue, witnessing, and validation—processes that find their roots in both traditional yogic theory and elements of psychological and educational theories compatible with yogic philosophy. The results have impact and people change their lives and themselves. Overwhelmingly, they appreciate those changes. The results are similar to more traditional forms of Yoga Therapy, but the way of getting there is different. Phoenix Rising Yoga Therapy offers a process rather than a prescription. Different approaches serve different needs and, as a community, Phoenix Rising Yoga Therapists applaud the diversity found within the profession of Yoga Therapy and look forward to the opportunity to collaborate with those pursing different approaches to healing, health, and well-being.

REFERENCES

Angot, M. *Taittiriya-Upanisad avec le commentaire de Samkara.* College de France, Paris, 2007. Print.

Aspy, D., and F. Roebuck. "Our Research and Our Findings." C. Rogers, *Freedom to Learn: A View of What Education Might Become.* Columbus, OH: Charles E. Merrill, 1969. Print.

Aurobindo, Sri. *Essays on the Gita.* Pondicherry, India: Sri Aurobindo Ashram Publication Department, 2000. Print.

——. (1972). *The Upanishads.* Pondicherry, India: Sri Aurobindo Ashram Publication Department, 1972. Print.

Casey, J. T., and C. Chapple. *Reconciling Yogas: Haribhadra's Collection of Views on Yoga.* New York: State University of New York Press, 2003. Print.

Coward, Harold. *Jung and Eastern Thought.* Sri Satguru Publications, 1991. Print.

Fowler, J. D. *The Bhagavad Gita: A Text and Commentary for Students.* Eastbourne: Sussex Academy Press, 2012. Print.

Gordon, G. *Building Engaged Schools: Getting the Most Out of America's Classrooms.* New York: Gallup Press, 2006. Print.

Ingleby, E., et al. *Learning to Teach in the Lifelong Learning Sector.* New York: Continuum International, 2010. Print.

Iyengar, B. K. S. *Light on the Yoga Sutras of Pantanjali.* London: Thorsons, 2002. Print.

Kirschenbaum, H., and V. R. Henderson, Eds. *The Carl Rogers Reader.* New York: Houghton Mifflin Harcourt, 1989, p. 25. Print.

Knowles, M. S. (1975). *Self-Directed Learning: A Guide for Learners and Teachers.* Englewood Cliffs: Prentice Hall/Cambridge, 1975. Print.

Knowles, M., E. F. Holton, and R. A. Swanson. *The Adult Learner: The Definitive Classic in Adult Education and Human Resource Development,* 6th ed. Burlington, MA: Elsevier, 2005. Print.

Lambert, M. J. "Psychotherapy Outcome Research: Implications for Integrative and Eclectic Therapists." *Handbook of Psychotherapy Integration,* J. C. Norcross and M. R. Goldfried, Eds. New York: Basic Books, 1992. Print.

Lee, M. *Phoenix Rising Yoga Therapy—Bridge from Body to Soul.* Deerfield Beach, FL: Health Communications, 1997. Print.

——. "Phoenix Rising Yoga Therapy." *Beyond Talk Therapy: Using Movement and Expressive Techniques in Clinical Practice,* D. J. Wiener, Ed. Washington, D.C.: American Psychological Association (APA), 1999.

——. *Turn Stress into Bliss: The Proven 8-Week Program for Health, Relaxation, Stress Relief.* Gloucester, MA: Fair Winds Press, 2005. Print.

Munyer, Jennifer. *Phoenix Rising Yoga Teacher Training Manual.* Bristol, VT, 2012.

Racanello, A. "The Effectiveness of Phoenix Rising Yoga Therapy." Graduate Center Research, Educational Psychology, City University of New York, 2012. Print.

Rogers, C. R. *Counseling and Psychotherapy.* Boston: Houghton Mifflin, 1942. Print.

——. *Client-Centred Therapy: Its Current Practice, Implications, and Theory.* Boston: Houghton Mifflin, 1951. Print.

——. "The Necessary and Sufficient Conditions of Therapeutic Personality Change." *Journal of Consulting and Clinical Psychology* 21.2 (1957): 95–103. Print.

——. *On Becoming a Person: A Therapist's View of Psychotherapy.* Boston: Houghton Mifflin, 1961. Print.

——. "Significant Learning in Therapy and in Education." *Educational Leadership* 16 (1959): 232–243. Print.

——. *Freedom to Learn: A View of What Education Might Become.* Columbus, OH: Charles E. Merrill, 1969. Print.

——. *Freedom to Learn for the 80s.* Columbus, OH: Charles E. Merrill, 1983. Print.

PŪRṆA YOGA THERAPY'S APPROACH TO HEALING

Aadil Palkhivala, N.D., J.D.

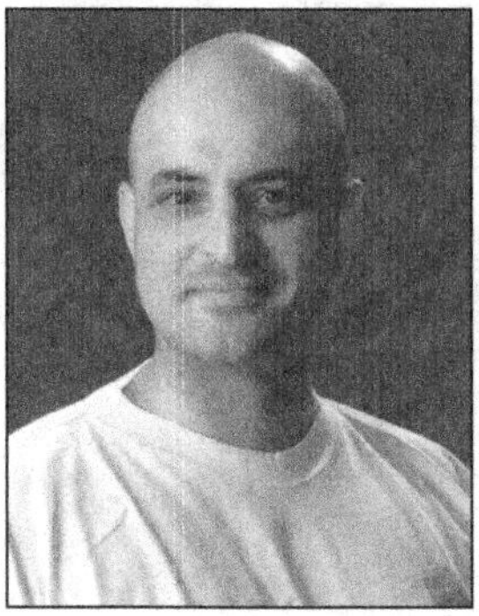

Aadil Palkhivala and his wife, Savitri, are the founders of Pūrṇa Yoga, a holistic synthesis of Yogic traditions based on the works of Sri Aurobindo and The Mother. Born in Bombay, India, Aadil's experience of holistic healing began observing Iyengar's classes at the age of three, commenced with formal study with him at the age of seven, and, at the age of twenty-two, he was the youngest person ever to be awarded Iyengar's advanced Yoga teacher's certificate. Nearly thirty years later, Aadil is recognized as one of the world's top Yoga teachers. He has a bachelor's degree in physics and math from St. Xavier's College, University of Bombay, a postgraduate degree in law from Golden Gate University, and is the author of three teacher training manuals as well as *Fire of Love: For Students of Life and Teachers of Yoga,* a book that seeks to restore the essence of Yoga. Constantly educating himself in his passion for teaching the "whole Yoga," Aadil is also a federally certified naturopath, a certified Ayurvedic health science practitioner, a clinical hypnotherapist, and a certified Shiatsu and Swedish bodywork therapist. He has written extensively for *Yoga Journal* as their lead "āsana expert" columnist and as the writer of the "Teacher's Column" on *Yoga Journal's* website.

INTRODUCTION TO PŪRṆA YOGA

The uniqueness of Pūrṇa Yoga's approach to the practice of Yoga and to therapy comes from its core belief that all parts of the human being need to be addressed for healing to happen. This belief is born from the Yoga of the great sage, Sri Aurobindo, which he called *Pūrṇa Yoga,* or its English translation: Integral Yoga.

Pūrṇa Yoga and its therapeutic expressions address the various aspects of the human being by taking a myriad of forms, each with its own lineage. Until the client is ready to connect with Spirit and solve all his/her problems, the Pūrṇa Yoga Therapist has a wide variety of tools to offer the client from various modalities. The āsana and prāṇāyāma lineage grows from my work with B. K. S. Iyengar. The meditation lineage comes from my wife, Savitri, and Sri Aurobindo. The philosophy lineage stems from the sacred yogic texts and teachings of the Vedas, the four purusharthas, the Bhagavad Gītā, Patañjali, and Sri Aurobindo. The nutrition and lifestyle lineage grows out of Ayurveda, ancient Chinese nutritional herbology, and my studies in modern nutrition as a licensed naturopath.

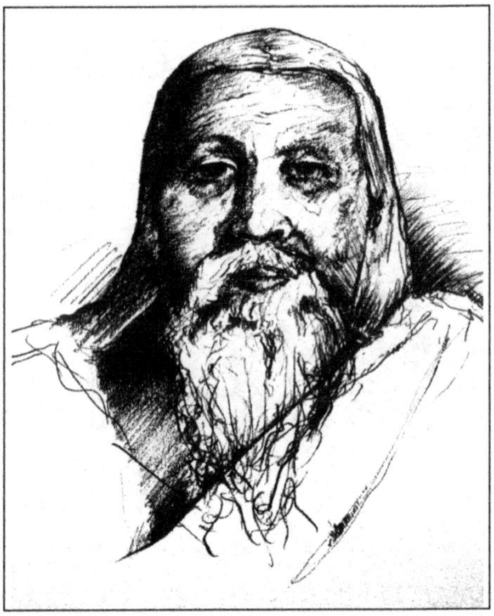

Sri Aurobindo

Each of the therapeutic modalities of Pūrṇa Yoga thus has its own unique character and can be explored with greater depth and appreciation.

MEDITATION

Traditionally, meditation has been a beautiful and reliable way to calm the brain. In Pūrṇa Yoga, meditation is an active process, not a passive one. The meditation techniques we use in Pūrṇa Yoga are simple and add something vital to the experience. These techniques can be accomplished by anyone and comprise a system in which students and clients actively use their hands to move energy and Light into and through the body—helping them connect with Spirit. The hands are also used to collimate the energetic emanations of the brain, thereby making the brain both still *and* focused. This is the process that Patañjali called dhāraṇā (concentration). The mental focus is then used to connect with one's inner intuition, which in turn communicates with the conscious mind of the client creating the process that Patañjali called dhyāna (meditation). Today, scientific minds postulate that the fundamental particle is not a particle at all, but a photon (Arkangel, 2010). This means that not only does light affect matter, it IS matter. In meditation, working with light is working with the building blocks of the material universe. Since the body is a microcosm of the universe, meditation in Pūrṇa Yoga thus integrates the body's building blocks with those of the universe. The meditation techniques we use were received by Savitri in inspired meditations over the past few decades and can be practiced in a relatively short time, making it possible for a person to fit them into a busy schedule. (Check out an example of one of the meditation techniques in the "Intention, Breath, and Movement of Light" section of this chapter.)

Why does meditation sometimes achieve healing when āsana cannot? Clients who practice āsana with precise alignment often show dramatic improvement in their symptoms, including pain relief, yet the symptoms gradually return when the practice is discontinued. In such instances, the practice of āsana becomes merely a Band-Aid, another way of treating symptoms rather than causes. In other cases, the āsana practice that would be required to heal a problem cannot be done because another problem precludes it. For example, one client of mine had a very sluggish thyroid condition called hypothyroidism. The āsana practice we generally require for hypothyroidism is the practice of sarvaṅgāsana (shoulderstand) and its entire cycle. However, my client could not do sarvaṅgāsana or the cycle because of a reversed cervical curve, a condition in which sarvaṅgāsana is contraindicated. Therefore, healing could not be brought about through the modality of āsana. It was through practicing meditation that the client discovered the cause and cure of her condition. The cause was a blockage in the throat cakra, the vortex of communication and expression. Thus, my client's throat problems began to clear up when she learned to open her throat and voice her feelings despite the chronic resistance from her cantankerous spouse. Her cervical curve returned and now she can do both sarvaṅgāsana and śīrṣāsana (headstand). This, of course, helped her thyroid tremendously, and she is now off medication under the supervision of her doctor.

Some Pūrṇa Yoga students come to our studios only for the meditation classes. Our "mothership" studio is in Bellevue, Washington, where students and clients have been coming for twenty-one years. I have personally observed several of these students move from sickness to health without any other practices except the practice of meditation.

ĀSANA

The Pūrṇa Yoga approach to āsana has the familiar outward look, but a different inward intention and dimension. Our approach to āsana and prāṇāyāma is based on precise alignment in form, but this is combined with a clear sense of the *intention* behind the action, the *movement of breath* through the body, and the *guided flow of Light* energy.

My own chronic pain taught me the vital importance of these inward dimensions of āsana. In 1981, I was teaching in London. One evening, I severely ruptured two vertebrae in my back (L4-L5 and L5-S1) by simultaneously lifting a heavy crate overhead while twisting. I was bedridden for two months and had to wear a custom-made steel brace that separated my rib cage from my pelvis to prevent pressure on the discs. The doctors in London said I would probably never bend forward or backward again and that surgery was the best option, which I didn't consider to be an option at all. I flew back to India, supine, using five adjacent airline seats because I could not sit up. I treated this injury with āsana for the next three decades. Every time I practiced the series for the lower back, the pain would go away, my spine would realign, and I would eventually feel fine. Yet, inevitably, my back would "go out" again just a few months later.

It took me three decades to realize that āsana alone was not a lasting solution to my problem, but only a temporary fix. What brought about this realization was that I had begun a serious practice of meditation with Savitri. The meditation techniques she developed helped me realize how to move the breath in the body and what intention to hold during the practice. I also understood what color of light to meditate upon during the practice of āsana while focusing on the lower back. In the last five years, I have not had a serious recurrence of my back pain. I now realize that traditional āsana practice alone lacks the power to heal unless it is combined with intention, breath, and the Light of the Soul. In Pūrṇa Yoga Therapy, meditation and āsana are inseparable partners in healing.

APPLIED PHILOSOPHY

Philosophy, as we define it, is the exploration of the connection between beliefs and reality. A key part of the therapeutic process in Pūrṇa Yoga is the exploration of the client's thoughts and beliefs and the client's resulting actions or inactions. Diseases do not just happen or occur randomly; they are often caused and invited by our negative patterns of thinking and/or our lack of integrity. In Pūrṇa Yoga, we observe and examine our beliefs and patterns of thinking, focusing primarily on the thoughts, words, and actions in day-to-day life, for these can manifest as joy or disease.

Can whiplash be caused by patterns of thinking? I once had a client who came to me because of complications arising from a severe whiplash. I asked her to explain the circumstances of the accident that caused her injury. She said she had been sitting at a red light and a car hit her from the rear. In the ensuing discussion, I learned that she had suffered another whiplash a year before. She had been sitting at a stop sign and a car crashed into her. After investigating further, I learned that she had experienced a third whiplash just two years before that! Again, it was caused by another car crashing into her stationary vehicle. Once we discussed this remarkable pattern of events, she burst into tears and admitted that she felt completely stuck in her life. Her getting hit while she was stopped and "stuck" in her car was simply her outer world mirroring her inner world. She had rejected many chances to make changes and move forward. Remarkably, without doing a single āsana or a single meditation technique, her whiplash pain was largely gone by the time she finished crying. She had never before made the connection between the accidents and her thoughts and that empowered her to make changes. By being ignorant of the cause of her problem, she could not heal it. She resolved to move forward in her life at every opportunity. Notwithstanding the disappearance of her symptoms, I gave her a program of āsana that would further support her and return her cervical spine to its natural curve.

2.3

अविद्यास्मिता राग द्वेषाभिनिवेशाः क्लेशाः ॥३॥

avidyāsmitā rāga dveṣābhiniveśāḥ kleśāḥ

The afflictions are ignorance, I-am-ness, attachment, aversion, and the fear of impermanence and death

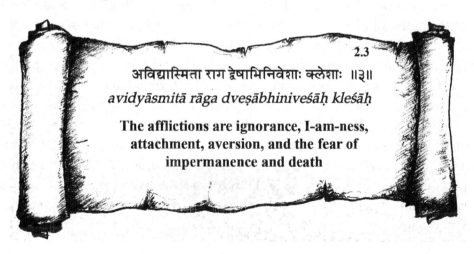

For serious students of Yoga, a study of philosophy is invaluable. When I feel that my life is not progressing, I turn to the kleśas, the five obstacles of the mind articulated by Patañjali in Sūtra II.3 of the *Yoga Sūtras.* Instead of fumbling around and searching for a belief or philosophy that can serve me, I use something that has proven its effectiveness for thousands of years and examine where I may be stuck. The five kleśas are:

1. Avidyā—Ignorance (of reality through observation with conditioned perception)
2. Asmitā—Ego (self-importance and self-involvement)
3. Rāga—Attachment
4. Dveṣa—Aversion
5. Abhiniveśa—Fear of Impermanence (often translated as the fear of death)

NUTRITION AND LIFESTYLE

In Pūrṇa Yoga Therapy, we believe that many diseases are the inevitable result of choices we have made about what we put into our body and what we put our body into. Healing comes from inside out, but also from outside in. The outside-in approach is called contextual healing. This means that the client's lifestyle contextually affects his/her health and happiness.

We inform our students and clients in Pūrṇa Yoga about the possible consequences of their nutrition and lifestyle choices. Toxins in our diet (such as artificial chemicals/fertilizers, GMOs, and pesticides) and toxins in our water (such as fluoride and chlorine) can cause chaos in the body and lead to disease (Fletcher, 2006). Similarly, the toxins in our environment—the formaldehyde in our furniture (National Cancer Institute, 2011), the paint on our walls containing volatile organic compounds (Levin, 2011), the plastics that have estrogen mimickers (Biello, 2008)—all of these can lead to extreme confusion in the cells and disease. Recently, I had a client who had been diagnosed with Parkinson's disease. After inquiring into the patterns of his lifestyle, we were able to connect his symptoms to a chemical he used for cleaning his bathroom. I suggested a program that he followed diligently for two months and he was soon walking without his walker.

As a Yoga Therapist, I have found it crucial to share with clients that antiperspirants may contribute to breast cancer or Alzheimer's disease (Mercola, 2012). The unhealthy parabens and the blocking of perspiration prevent the lymphatic system from removing toxins from the armpits. Also, antiperspirants are laced with microcrystalline aluminum, which, when inhaled all day, can pass through the nasal passages into the brain. Aluminum has been shown to be one of the causal factors for Alzheimer's disease (Graedon and Graedon, 2013). No matter how much Yoga the client does, the disease is not likely to vanish completely until he/she stops using the antiperspirant in the context of his/her lifestyle. Healing cannot be accomplished if the cause is not removed and/or treated. In this example, we would let our Yoga students know that, while the application of a deodorant is a necessary courtesy to one's fellow students, the use of antiperspirants is the opposite of courtesy to one's own body.

The idea of context includes the work environment (fluorescent lighting has adverse effects on the nervous system) and relationships (loving relationships help bolster the immune system). Moreover, our context includes our relationship to money and wealth, the colors we choose to wear (wearing black has been shown to diminish one's immune system), the work we do, the music we listen to, the programs we watch, the sunlight we allow or disallow into our lives, and so on. There is a glut of information available today on all matters of health and lifestyle, and much of it is incomplete, incorrect, misleading, or confusing. In Pūrṇa Yoga, we attempt to guide our students through the labyrinth of information to help them create contexts that promote health and happiness.

IS IT YOGA?

Is it Yoga or is it just good therapy? Some people might argue that our focus on context and lifestyle takes us too far beyond the traditional boundary of Yoga, and too far beyond the role of the Yoga teacher. Is it really the role of the Yoga teacher to be concerned with antiperspirants and fluorescent lights? Why bother? Just follow Patañjali!

Different times have different necessities. Patañjali did not write his words under fluorescent lights or drink fluoride in his water! *Yoga, to be alive, must evolve and adapt.* The truths that were valid 2,000 years ago must be updated and revised according to the times. Pūrṇa Yoga is concerned with health. Thus, we take information and insights from the ancient world and therapeutically adapt and apply them to our modern world. After all, what is ancient now was once modern, and what is modern now will be ancient 2,000 years from now!

THE ROLE OF THE CLIENT AND THERAPIST

Before we look more specifically at how we diagnose and treat a client, we must discuss and clarify the respective roles of the therapist and the client.

There are five criteria for successful healing according to Pūrṇa Yoga:

1. The client must have the urge to be well.
2. The client must have the willingness to change.
3. The client must be given appropriate and specific guidance for the condition.
4. The client must consistently apply or practice the therapeutic guidance.
5. The client must have patience.

The only responsibility of the therapist is criterion #3. The first rule of healing is that you can't heal anyone. The client is the one who heals.

These days, I only accept clients who want to get better. The sad truth is that many clients do not truly want to do what is necessary to get better. Some have a vested interest in being sick, whether this be a financial advantage (disability payments), emotional advantage (to get sympathy), or psychological advantage (changing habits is challenging). Some simply find it more convenient to be degenerating than regenerating.

How do I discern between an authentic and an inauthentic urge to get better? I ask the client, "Are you willing to do what I suggest each and every day for a period of months? It will involve making changes that may make you uncomfortable. Are you willing to make these changes? Are you serious?"

As we explore these questions, I carefully observe the client. I look at his/her face and body language. I listen to his/her tone of voice. Is the person tentative or totally committed? It is my job to determine if there is a genuine desire to be well because only from that place can treatment really begin.

HOW WE APPROACH DISEASE

In Pūrṇa Yoga, we believe that neither a disease nor a person needs to be treated. What needs treating is an imbalance.

All disease is a manifestation of an imbalance of some kind. These imbalances may be in the energy meridians of the body or in the musculoskeletal system. The imbalance may be a manifestation of a disparity between what I am doing and what I believe I should be doing. Or between what I truly believe and what I force myself to say. There are many such imbalances. If there is an imbalance in the prāṇa-maya-kośa (subtle body), this will manifest as disease in the physical body. The energetics of the organic system must be considered. For example, when the second and third cakras are not spinning correctly, one feels depleted and disempowered. In the example given above, the throat cakra (responsible for expression and communication) was not spinning properly. Since the throat energy was not flowing from the cakra, it manifested as a blockage in the thyroid and the cervical curve. Long before it manifests, a disease usually exists *in potentia* in these sorts of imbalances and disparities. The disease manifests when we don't attend to the signals and signs that have been informing us of these imbalances. These signs of imbalance indicate that we are out of sync with our nature, not living our dharma (true purpose), and not connected with our Source, our Spirit.

The fundamental cause of all problems in our lives—whether it be a conspicuous and disappointing lack of happiness or the painful presence of a condition such as cancer or arthritis—is a separation from our Source. Most treatment methods do not permanently heal because they do not dare to address this essential issue. Yoga, in its essence, does exactly that. Yoga makes the healing Light of the Spirit flow into the consciousness of the mind, through the nervous system, and into the organs, muscles and bones of the human body.

ASSESSMENT FOR SACROILIAC AND LOWER BACK PAIN

How would a Pūrṇa Yoga Therapist treat a common malady? Let us consider a hypothetical client who comes in with severe sacroiliac and lower back pain. The therapist determines whether the patient is willing to commit to a program for a number of months. Many therapists fail to ask this question because they are afraid of losing patients who come wanting "a quick fix."

Then, the therapist asks questions related to the injury: What are your fears? Do you feel that you don't have control over yourself or the essentials in your life? The lower back holds emotions related to issues of control. A lack of control creates destabilization of the S-I joint and lower back. A lack of control also may cause some to try to grab control, which then freezes the muscles in the lower back. The muscles between the vertebrae (intervertebral muscles) respond to these subconscious thoughts of fear and uncontrollability. Thus, the therapist must probe into the client's subconscious issues.

At this point, the therapist has only begun to gather information. Much more information will be needed before a program is suggested.

In terms of physical evaluation, the therapist would ask the client to walk back and forth several times. *Which side is tighter? Which hip is higher? Which foot is more externally rotated?* The therapist is looking for physical imbalances. The patient is then viewed in taḍāsana (mountain pose) from the side to check whether the pelvis is tipped forward (anteriorly) and the lumbar spine is in excessive lordosis. These indicate overly tight illiacus muscles and/or overly tight psoas muscles. The therapist records all of these facts and takes the client through the Pūrṇa Yoga Hip Opening Series as a diagnostic tool. This indicates to the therapist whether the following hip movements are in balance: extension and flexion, adduction and abduction, internal rotation and external rotation.

The Pūrṇa Yoga Therapist must also ask questions about diet. Foods that create an acid ash (leaving the system acidic after digestion) invariably cause inflammation. Foods that leave an alkaline ash reduce inflammation and therefore ameliorate pain and chronic tension. Members of the nightshade family (especially eggplant) are notorious for causing inflammation. Other perpetrators of inflammation include refined sugar and artificial sweeteners, gluten-rich foods, red meats, corn, processed food, GMO products, hydrogenated oils, caffeine, alcohol, carbonated beverages, and synthetic chemicals. A person can do āsana all day and not experience freedom from pain if they are consuming foods or food-mimicking substances that cause inflammation. Environmental toxins such as formaldehyde (from furniture and carpets) also cause inflammation. Stress, insufficient sleep, and lack of exercise all contribute to inflammation.

The therapist further inquires about the client's lifestyle. *What parts of your life make you happy? What parts concern you? Do you feel your life is fulfilling and meaningful? Do you have regrets? Do you have a fulfilling, happy relationship? Are you stressed by your spouse, or by an urge to have one, or by an urge not to have one?* Notably, a question that some may consider rude, irrelevant, and un-yogic, *How is your financial life?* It is the number-one cause of stress in our society today! The therapist then asks questions that relate to the physical world. *What kind of chair do you use at work? How do you sit? Do you enjoy your work? Do you work in a stressful environment?*

Looking deeper energetically, the three cakras involved in S-I issues are the first, second, and third cakras. These represent stability, creativity, and power. The therapist also asks questions that have bearing on these three issues. When does your lower back pain act up? When you have lower back pain, what kinds of emotions, thoughts, feelings, and stories preceded the pain? Do you feel anxious about anything in your life?

Finally, the spiritual dimension is questioned. *Do you feel spiritually fulfilled? Do you feel connected with God? Do you feel your Soul is with you? Do you feel guided from the inside? Do you feel your decisions come from an inner authenticity or simply from rational analysis?*

All of these are potentially important questions in the therapeutic process.

METHODOLOGY FOR RELIEVING SACROILIAC AND LOWER BACK PAIN

Once the diagnosis is complete, the Pūrṇa Yoga Therapist reaches into his/her "tool bag" and pulls out healing modalities and approaches that are relevant to the situation.

In this hypothetical case dealing with the sacroiliac joint and lower back pain above, the therapist is likely to start by treating the musculoskeletal system. The therapist would possibly teach this client the Pūrṇa Yoga Hip Opening Series, making the necessary adjustments to balance out the imbalances that were diagnosed. For example, if external rotation comes easily in his/her hip, but the internal rotation does not, the client would be asked to spend a specific amount of extra time doing the internal rotation. The therapist would check the student periodically and make the appropriate adjustments.

While each situation is always approached individually, the next candidate for treatment would be the Pūrṇa Yoga Lower Back Series. This series releases the hip flexors and tension in the erector spinae and the quadratus lumborum muscles while also releasing tension at the origins of the hamstrings.

TWO LOWER BACK RELEASES FROM THE LOWER BACK SERIES

Release 1, Stage 1: Lie on your back on a sticky mat as shown in the figure below with your feet together and on a wall, heels touching the floor, and your body perpendicular to the wall. Slowly bend your knees and wiggle toward the wall until your knees are about 10 inches off the floor. Then press your right foot into the wall and bed your left knee into your chest, holding the top of the shin with both hands as shown.

Release 1,
Stage 1

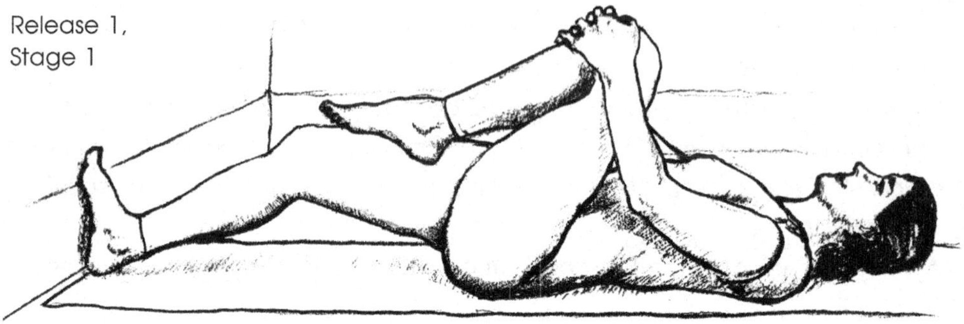

Release 1, Stage 2: Exhaling, slowly straighten your right leg, trying as much as possible to remain stuck to the sticky mat and sliding as little as possible. Hold this position for two breaths and then bend the right knee once again. Release the left leg and let the left foot drop to the floor. Slowly return to stage 1 on the other side and repeat. Doing both sides is one repetition. Repeat Release 1 three times, changing sides each time. This will gently release and readjust the sacroiliac joint.

Release 1,
Stage 2

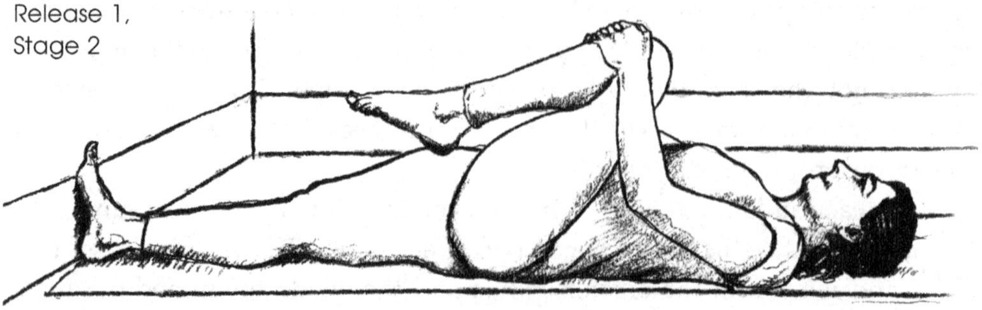

Release 2: The method is the same as for the previous exercise except that, instead of holding the shinbone, you hold the foot with both hands as shown in the figure. Please keep the knee that is held by the hands in between the arms and keep it bent at about 90 degrees. If you find it difficult to hold the foot, you may use a strap around the foot and hold it with both hands, one on each side. Repeat Release 2 also three times. This will help release the lower back muscles.

Release 2, Stage 1

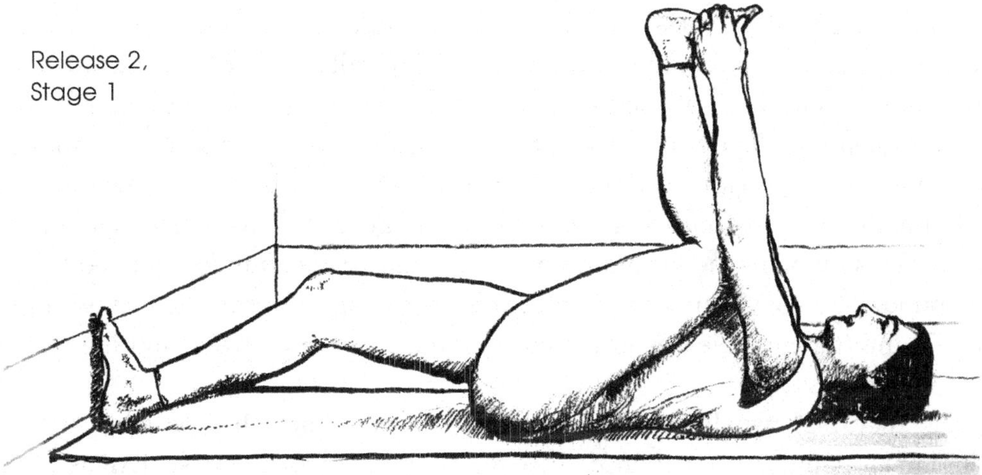

Release 2, Stage 2

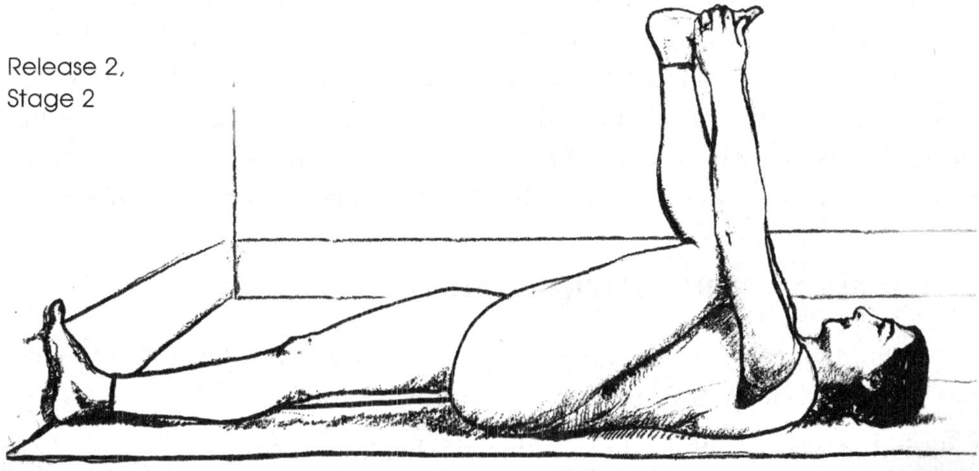

INTENTION, BREATH, AND MOVEMENT OF LIGHT

Once the client has learned the outward forms of the āsana from the Pūrṇa Yoga Hip Opening Series and the Lower Back Series, it is time to integrate intention, breath, and movement of Light. Pūrṇa Yoga Therapy incorporates these inward elements based on the information gathered from the diagnostic inquiries. That which the student wants more of (stability, creativity, power) is attached to the inhalation. The student breathes these qualities in while imagining a light-colored light. Light pink often works well for the lower back. That which causes stress is attached to the exhalation and a dark color. Typically, the therapist guides the client's breath into tense muscles on the inhalation using the light-colored light. On the exhalation, the client is asked to pull out the dark color from the muscles. This causes psychological and physical transmutation of energy in those muscles. Additionally, a bījā mantra may be used to enhance the vibratory effect of the breath. (This involves the humming of certain consonant sounds followed by the *mm* sound. The consonants vary according to the specific cakras. For example, softly humming *yum* releases heart tension, diaphragmatic stress, and intercostal muscles hardness.)

The therapist usually also recommends an alkaline-ash-producing diet to reduce the inflammatory response in the muscles. There are many such diets available and reputable ones can be found online. I recommend consuming dark green leafy vegetables, turmeric, flaxseed oil, most berries, cruciferous vegetables (e.g., broccoli, cabbage), avocados, freshly made vegetable and fruit juices, and Sunrider herbal foods. Lemon juice, stevia, or Sunrider's Fortune Delight could also be added to the water to facilitate and assimilate better hydration. Since pesticides and fertilizers are known toxins, Pūrṇa Yoga Therapy always recommends a diet consisting of only organically grown food, as fresh and as local as possible.

OTHER PŪRṆA YOGA THERAPY METHODOLOGY

Due to limitations of space, further techniques that Pūrṇa Yoga Therapy might train and/or teach the above client include, but are not limited to:

- Sitting on a chair without aggravating his/her lower back pain
- Walking by lifting the pit of the abdomen and relaxing the buttocks

- Ways of achieving balance in the six hip movements
- Various meditation techniques to relax stress in the emotional body
- Attuning the energetic body so that energy flows harmoniously into the physical body
- Eliminating, reducing, or countering toxins in the work and home environments
- Developing a regular exercise and sleep schedule
- Applying yogic philosophy to day-to-day life, especially with regard to issues of control and power, anxiety, regrets and fears
- Creating harmonious relationships
- How to make choices that create income streams and relieve thought patterns that perpetuate lack and impoverishment
- Revealing and then transforming the habitual stories and patterns that resist change and prevent the release of pain
- Recognition that we are not merely mind and body and that it is only in Spirit that we find fulfillment and healing

CONCLUSION

For the person who doesn't merely want to cover up his/her symptoms but has a genuine desire to heal from the very core of his/her being, who realizes that his/her pain is simply a reminder that he/she is off track, who desires to lead a more fulfilling life, and who wants his/her Spirit to be his/her guiding light—for this person, Pūrṇa Yoga is a gentle and powerful offering.

REFERENCES

Arkangel, C. "Could the Photon Be the Sole Elementary Particle?" Naked Science Forum. 10 Sept. 2010. Web. Retreived July 14, 2013. http://www.thenakedscientists.com/forum/index.php?topic=34413.0.

Biello, D. "Plastic (Not) Fantastic: Food Containers Leach a Potentially Harmful Chemical." ScientificAmerican.com. 19 Feb. 2008. Web. Retreived July 14, 2013. http://www.scientificamerican.com/article/plastic–not–fantastic–with–bisphenol–a/.

Fletcher, A. "12 Reasons to Reject Fluoridation and Chlorine." Naked Science Forum. 4 Apr. 2006. Web. http://www.thenakedscientists.com/forum/index.php?topic=3934.0.

Graedon, M. S., and T. Graedon. "Studies Support Link Between Aluminum and Alzheimer's Disease." Chron.com. 7 June 2013. Web. http://www.chron.com/news/health/article/Studies-support-link-between-aluminum-and-4586632.php.

Levin, H. "5 Ways to Free Your Home of Dangerous Chemicals." Money Crashers Blog: My Money, U.S. News & World Report. 2 February 2011. Web. http://money.usnews.com/money/blogs/my-money/2011/02/02/5-ways-to-free-your-home-of-dangerous-chemicals.

Mercola, J. (2012). "99% of Breast Cancer Tissue Contained This Everyday Chemical (NOT Aluminum)." Mercola.com. 24 May 2012. Web. http://articles.mercola.com/sites/ articles/archive/2012/05/24/parabens-on-risk-of-breast-cancer.aspx.

National Cancer Institute. "Formaldehyde and Cancer Risk." FactSheet. 10 June 2011. Web. http://www.cancer.gov/cancertopics/factsheet/Risk/formaldehyde.

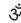

STRUCTURAL YOGA THERAPY AND AYURVEDIC YOGA THERAPY

Mukunda and Chinnamasta Stiles

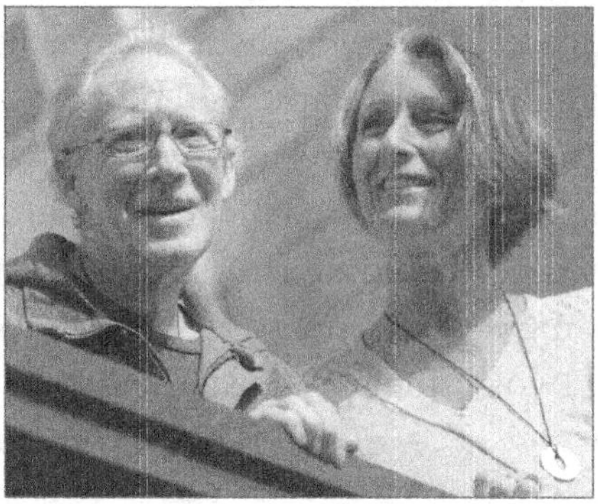

Mukunda Stiles is the creator/author of many texts, including *Structural Yoga Therapy, Ayurvedic Yoga Therapy,* a concise yet devotional rendition of the *Yoga Sūtras of Patañjali,* and *Tantra Yoga Secrets—18 Lessons in Tantric Consciousness.* Chinnamasta Stiles, his Devi, edited *Tantra Yoga Secrets* and has written several articles on nutrition and Ayurvedic Yoga Therapy. As this book was being edited, Mukunda Stiles left his body vessel. His beloved, **Chinnamasta**, held him in her arms beyond his last breath on February 18, 2014. As requested by Mukunda, Chinnamasta will share his teachings and legacy with those who are willing to step into profound transformation, just as they had done sitting side by side, teaching together. She has an extensive background in deep healing with Yoga, Ayurveda, and Tantra in private and group settings. Chinnamasta offers teachings from their home base in San Francisco, California, and to spiritual seekers worldwide. Their websites are www.Yogatherapycenter.org and www.shivashaktiloka.com.

INTRODUCTION

The Structural Yoga Therapy and Ayurvedic Yoga Therapy methods are both deeply rooted in the *Yoga Sūtras of Patañjali,* the original textbook of Classical Yoga. This ancient text helps us make sense of life, aids in the development of self-knowledge, and helps us understand the cycles of what brings us pain and suffering.

Ultimately, the *Yoga Sūtras* detail that which leads us to peace and harmony, which is the goal of optimal wellness. Step one of Rāja Yoga's classical eightfold path laid out by Patañjali proclaims "ahiṁsa," or "do no harm." There is apparent similarity to the code of medicine established by Hippocrates that requires physicians to pledge to "do no harm to anyone" (Hippocrates, 2004). True health, both physical and mental, is restored once one finds his/her way from harm to harmony because only then can all functions of the body and mind return to balance.

Since its inception in 1976 over thirty-five years ago, our school and our graduates have served a variety of health conditions using our dualistic approach and we have found incredibly beneficial results. Our Yoga Therapy methodology goes further than simply treating the symptom. Structural Yoga Therapy's scope is to address and reduce muscular and skeletal pain while Ayurvedic Yoga Therapy's scope focuses on finding the root causes of diseases, including stress, inflammation, tumor, or congestion, among others and bringing the body-mind-heart back to balance. The following is an explanation of these two systems of Yoga Therapy.

STRUCTURAL YOGA THERAPY

Structural Yoga Therapy (SYT) is a systematic approach to freeing normal range of mobility (ROM), reestablishing muscle tone and alleviating joint pain. Although this system appears to be centered on the physical body, it has far-reaching implications for the subtle bodies as well. Back in 1973, a Hollander named Nikolaas Tinbergen won the Nobel Prize for studying how posture affects every system of the body, not just the neuromuscular system composed of the joints, bones, ligaments, muscles, and nerves, but all of the other physiological systems (Tinbergen, 2013). This means that a change in posture will be reflected in changes in other systems, including the endocrine system, immune system, cardiovascular system, and respiratory system. A perfect example would be elevated shoulders, which often

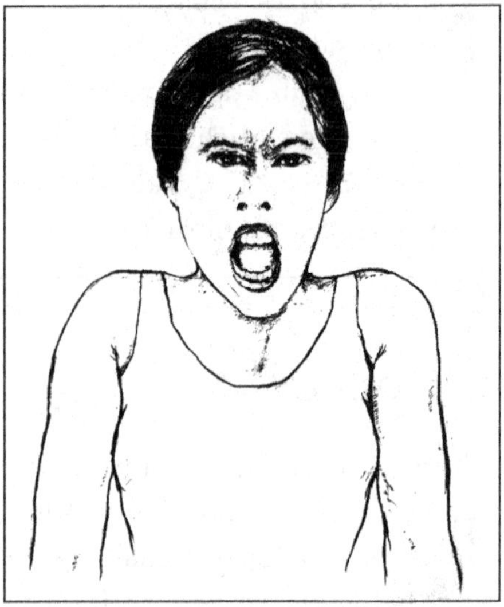

Elevated Shoulders

reveal whether someone is "uptight" or stressed, and both are characterized by high cortisol levels and a weakened ability to resist disease. On the other hand, rounded shoulders may tell us if someone is depressed because when someone is depressed his/her chest tends to collapse more often, he/she will usually smile less, experience a decrease in endocrine production, and have the tendency to underbreathe or breathe in such a way as to make the respiratory system less efficient. These repeated patterns continue the cycle of the issue. In situations like these, Yoga Therapy's intervention helps to integrate the individual on all levels. Through the study of postural language, we can gain a wealth of information expressed through the physical body that can be used to gauge the efficiency of the various systems and the effectiveness of our communication and therapy.

BODY-READING ASSESSMENTS

Reading body language is instinctive; it is something we each do subconsciously as a way of "tuning in" to others and ourselves. Each of us does this in our own way to get a better sense of one another. One form of body reading involves evaluating muscular tension. Postural changes may occur simply as a response to stress. When someone says, "You look stressed out," he/she is reading your postural cues. A stress-related condition may have prevailed so long that the individual does not realize that the associated muscular tensions have created postural changes that have gone ignored. Consequently, messages from those muscles tend to go unnoticed. Ultimately, freedom from tension allows us to more naturally express happiness and health. By changing our posture with Yogāsanas and other practices, Yoga Therapy initiates these positive changes. We are not overly concerned about what happens in our outer life when we do Yoga. Our focus is on the joy of the practice and on becoming more sensitive and aware of the encouraging warning signs of approaching dis-comfort and dis-ease.

Although "perfect posture" is somewhat subjective and illusive, postural imbalances do create musculo-skeletal tension to which we unconsciously adapt. Commonly, our adaptation involves a lack of awareness of the muscular tensions and the associated messages they reflect. We have learned to live with our aches and pains, accepting them as normal, and we teach our children to expect the same. Many postural abnormalities, such as knock knees, minor scoliosis, high shoulders, and/or fallen arches were either predisposed from birth or were shaped by our upbringing. One does not need to be professionally trained in body reading to notice these deviations from the norm. Such abnormalities are often due to heredity or developed through childhood observations that are then molded into habits. "In a worldwide survey of postural habits, Gordon Hewes showed that we sit, kneel, stand, recline in ways that are socially determined . . . [and] it is now clearly established that human posture, physique, motor habits, and body image, as well as emotions and thought patterns, are culturally shaped" (Leonard and Murphy, 1995). What gets lost in this context is the human capacity for transformation. To change our posture without a change in consciousness is not the goal of Yoga. Classical Yoga is rooted in transformative experience. How you transform the underlying patterns that created your aches and pains will determine how you transform from a body predisposed to stress to one that is composed of harmony. In Structural Yoga Therapy, we feel that any pathological condition or stress can create a change in muscle tension and posture. By identifying these specific tensors, a Structural Yoga Therapist can prescribe Yoga postures and breathing exercises customized and tailored to fit a client's particular situation. For many students, Yoga practice becomes a long-term commitment no longer tied to disease symptomology.

A cardinal rule of Structural Yoga Therapy is "If it's not broke, don't fix it."

What we mean by the application of this great motto is if there is no pain or discomfort associated with the region of a postural change, do not try to change that posture. Of course, bring attention to the area and make certain that your practice increases your awareness of postural differences that you weren't aware of before body reading. But don't worry about them. Many postural changes are due to the body's attempt to find balance following a trauma, accident, injury, or long-term stressor. The trauma may have been emotional or even psychic and can create postural change. All in all, be aware of the uniqueness of your body because you are not only physically different from anyone else but you also have your own personal way of responding to situations in life.

In the real world, bodies are infinite in their variety of shape and size. Everyone's experience varies when practicing Yoga postures. Your unique postural alignment and how you have learned to react to tension will differ markedly from others. Yoga training with accurate and compassionate instruction will change not only what you feel but it will also teach you how to attend to the sensations of your body. As these changes take place, you find that your goals also change. You may want to pursue a different direction than what originally brought you to Yoga.

It's been our experience in Structural Yoga Therapy that you can find more of yourself through Yoga than any other discipline, so we first attempt to get to know the body and its current posture.

In Yogāsana, we often encounter students who are very flexible and have excessive mobility by nature. Hypermobility must also be assessed. These students with hypermobility are initially drawn to Yogāsanas because they are good at it. Yet, genetic hypermobility gets many Yoga practitioners into trouble. This is especially true when holding poses for a long duration or when a person finds him/herself repeating the same or similar postures too frequently. It is at these times when hypermobile joints tend to become overused. The surrounding muscle tissue can begin to lack muscle tone, firmness, and stamina. This lack of proper muscle use leads to "locking" the ligaments to compensate for the lack of stability in the joint. A locked joint, while providing stability, lacks mobility and the ability to adapt to change in position as well as changes in life. The overstressed ligaments will also hide the lack of strength or engagement in the muscles that support the joint and they will get deformed and hypermobile over time.

Skeletal shape is another important component of body reading and is essential to individualizing instruction that helps one find comfort in yogāsana. In our male-dominated Yoga world, structural differences between men and women are often overlooked or not even recognized. Traditionally, Yoga was a male pursuit and most of the great teachers throughout history have been men. This often results in modern forms of Yoga that are appropriate for men and do not adapt to the unique concerns of the female frame. This means female Yoga students are trying to follow alignment instructions and Yoga principles that were intended for men's bodies. For women, following this male version of alignment designed to suit the needs of narrower hipped frames stresses the medial knee, lateral pelvis, and the sacroiliac joints during standing poses.

Another common body reading for women is the presence of a carrying angle in which the upper arm is not properly aligned with the lower arm. When the upper arms are placed palm up in supination, the upper arms are supposed to run parallel in mild shoulder flexion even though the forearms deviate about 10 degrees. The tendency is to ignore this difference and keep to the standard alignment protocol of placing the hands directly under the shoulders in dog pose, stick pose, handstands, and similar motions. This frequently causes strain and pain in the elbows, shoulders, and/or cervical joints. Unknowingly, women are often instructed to ignore the stressful responses coming from their bodies and push through it to the aligned, "accepted" visual image of the pose.

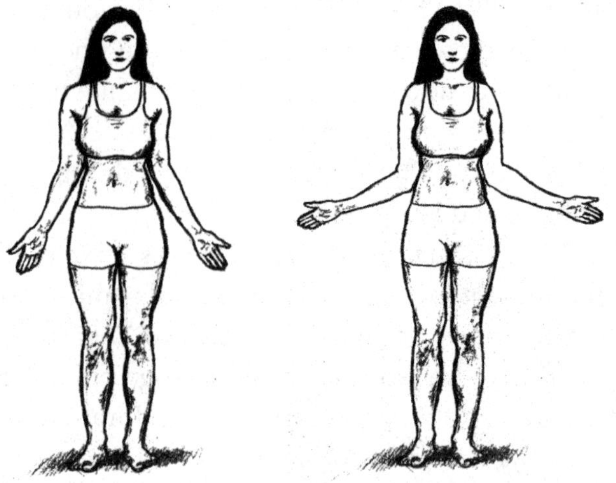

Normal Carrying Angle of Elbows

Excessive Carrying Angle of Elbows

There are obvious dangerous implications for corrections that standardize yogāsana practices given to students with misaligned skeletal conditions and varying skeletal shapes. At the present time, there is also an unwillingness on the part of the Yoga community at large to acknowledge that skeletal misalignments and uncomfortable reactions in āsanas (postures) typically need immediate attention and require personal adaptation for the practitioner. "Pushing through the pain" is too often wrongly advocated. Well-intentioned Yoga teachers also give medical advice and general recommendations for health conditions without any progressions for future changes in the symptoms of the situation. Thus, students may be told that doing a specific pose perfectly will alleviate their pain without any formal training in Yoga Therapy or a healthcare discipline. Effective Yoga Therapy recommendations need to change over time to match the progress of the recipient. Professor Krishnamacharya coined a phrase, "adapt to the individual," which forms the essence of Yoga's therapeutic methodologies and is our approach to yogāsana in Structural Yoga Therapy. If the recommendations given by a trained Structural Yoga Therapist do not make a significant level of change in three weeks, then more specialization or a referral to another, more appropriate, healthcare provider may be needed. To maximize its effectiveness, true Yoga Therapy follows a formal assessment with a qualified therapist and is given one-on-one to get to know the nature, structure, and health issues of the practitioner.

ĀSANA GUIDELINES IN STRUCTURAL YOGA THERAPY

Structural Yoga Therapy is especially beneficial for chronic pain and is not recommended for acute pain.

The following principles govern the experience of correct āsana from the standpoint of Structural Yoga Therapy:

1. Adjust your body for comfort regardless of how it may begin to lose the "picture perfect" image of the pose that is shown when following your teacher or photos from Yoga books.
2. Always make an effort to extend your spine.
3. Calm the physical and psychic effort required to hold the posture.
4. Make a conscious scan of your body to relax all those areas of unnecessary tension and become ecological in using only those parts required to attain and sustain the posture.
5. Maintain steady, rhythmic, natural breathing through the nose and an awareness of the changes in your breath's movement patterns.
6. Distinguish the feelings of contraction and pain from those of simply stretching to refine your body's awareness.
7. Coordinate your movements into and out of the postures in a relaxed, yet alert manner harmonized with your breath.
8. Move with an awareness of the position of your body without visual cues (a subcortical function called proprioception) and develop the process of pratyāhāra (focusing and withdrawing the senses from external objects).
9. Isolate the movements of major muscle groups so that the postures can be done with a minimum of effort. Make adjustments for changes in your body's alignment as your strength and flexibility improves.

RANGE OF MOTION (ROM) AND MUSCLE TESTING (MT) ASSESSMENTS

The manual used in the Structural Yoga Therapy training program shows the normal ranges of mobility for each joint motion, as illustrated by a simple series called the Joint Freeing Series (JFS), which can be seen in the figure below.

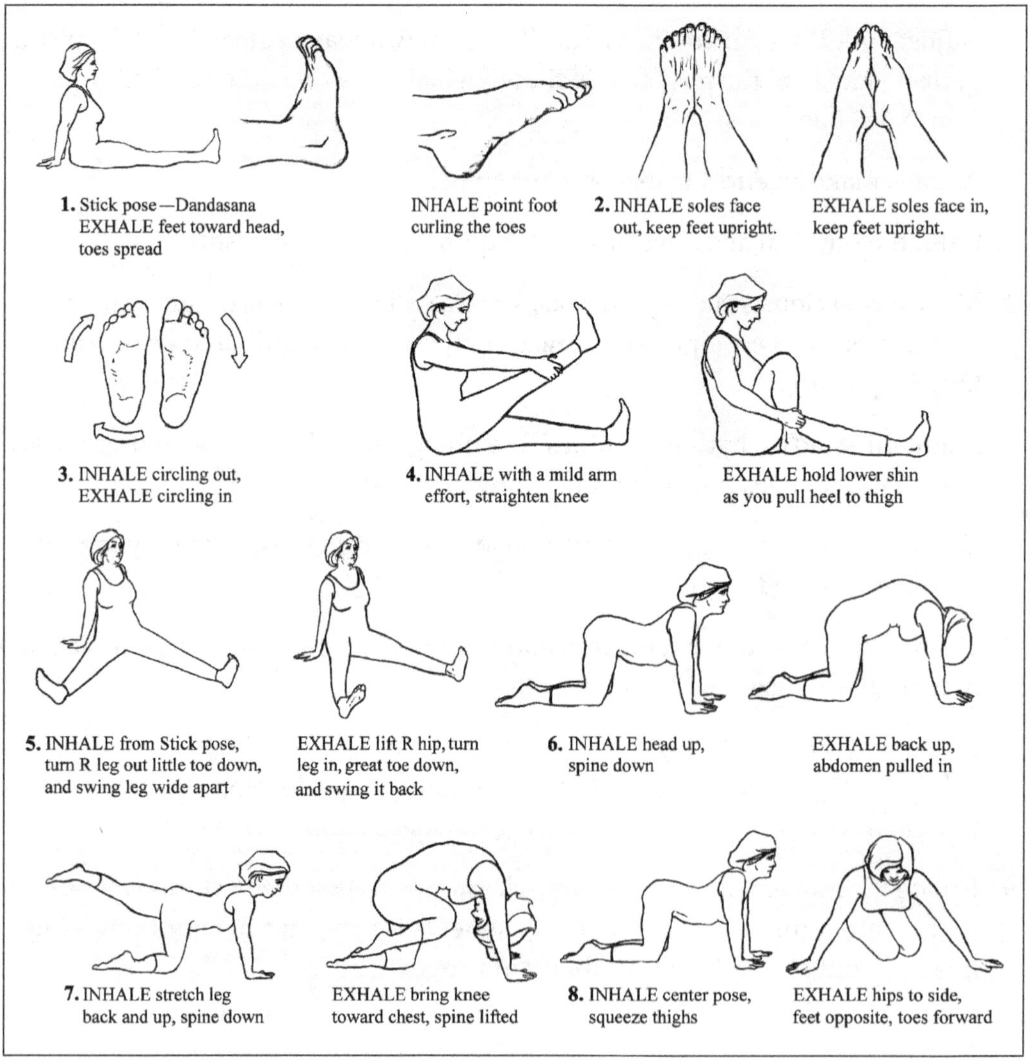

Joint Freeing Series (Pavanmuktāsana)

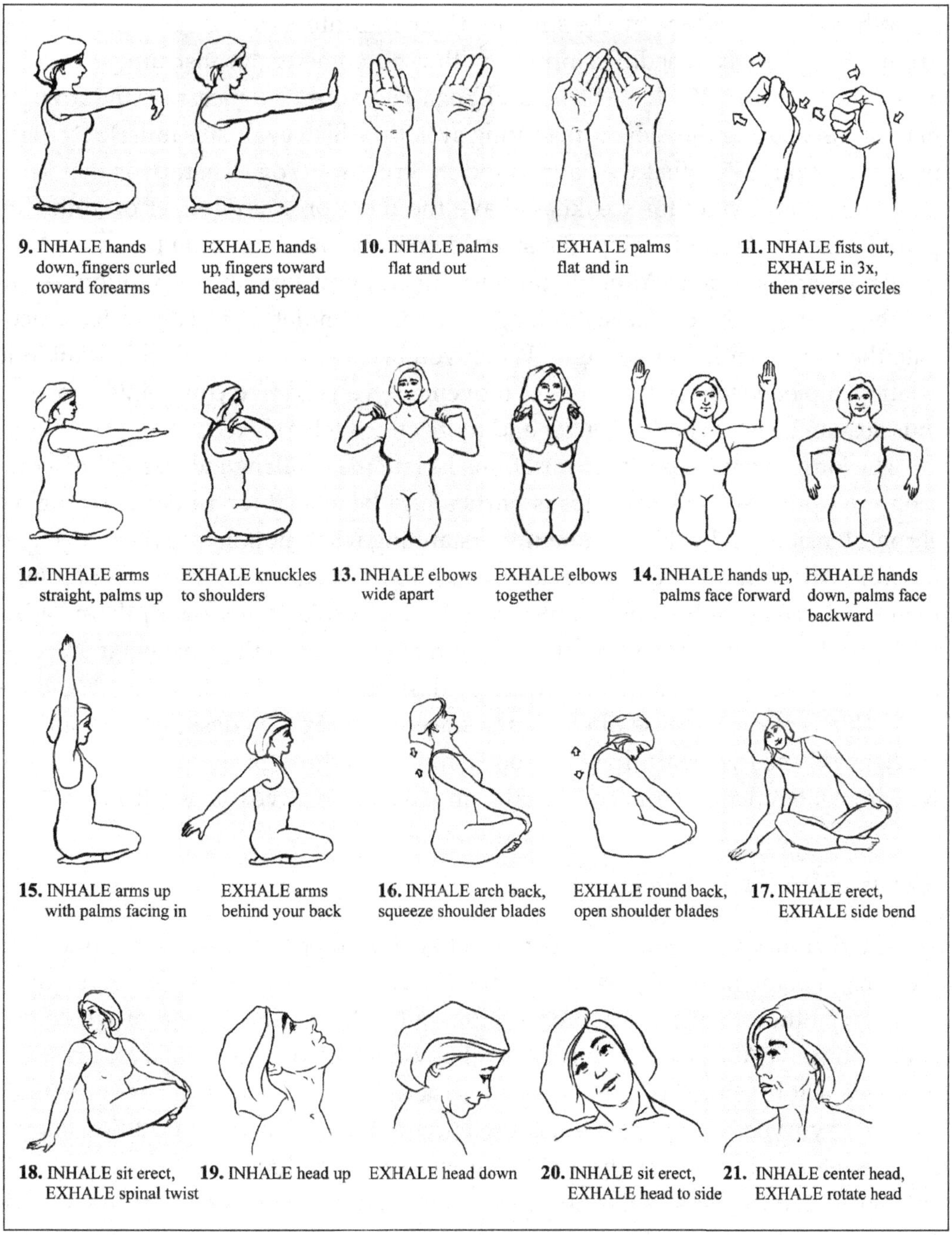
9. INHALE hands down, fingers curled toward forearms
EXHALE hands up, fingers toward head, and spread
10. INHALE palms flat and out
EXHALE palms flat and in
11. INHALE fists out, EXHALE in 3x, then reverse circles
12. INHALE arms straight, palms up
EXHALE knuckles to shoulders
13. INHALE elbows wide apart
EXHALE elbows together
14. INHALE hands up, palms face forward
EXHALE hands down, palms face backward
15. INHALE arms up with palms facing in
EXHALE arms behind your back
16. INHALE arch back, squeeze shoulder blades
EXHALE round back, open shoulder blades
17. INHALE erect, EXHALE side bend
18. INHALE sit erect, EXHALE spinal twist
19. INHALE head up
EXHALE head down
20. INHALE sit erect, EXHALE head to side
21. INHALE center head, EXHALE rotate head

Joint Freeing Series

When the JFS is done by the student, these indicators can reveal what muscles are likely to be weakened. Performed with a goniometer, an instrument used to accurately measure ROM, the Structural Yoga Therapist next measures the strength of the muscle using the Meyerding rating system, which evaluates muscle strength on a scale from 1–5. What we have found in Structural Yoga Therapy is that Yoga programs that correct for weakness have the most profound effect on relieving pain. Therefore, strengthening, not stretching, is the most common factor we train in alleviating joint pain. After all, muscles function by antagonistic motions—that is, when one muscle contracts, its antagonist must completely relax in order to activate the full potential for strength. When you become conscious of this symbiotic relationship between the two sides of movement, you can free your joints and your muscles can be made both stronger and more effectively relaxed.

The joint-freeing poses and variations isolate the challenge to strengthen commonly weak muscles. This series is particularly beneficial for students who have chronic tensions and pain. Without understanding what motions are restrained and learning what underlying muscles are weak, students will continue to avoid toning their weakened muscles and compensate for that weakness by overutilizing adjacent muscles. As the body uses what is habitual rather than the weakened muscles, postural misalignments regularly continue despite more attempts at health and fitness. This is at the expense of efficiency since our body was designed for optimal efficiency. When we learn how our body functions through the practice of Yoga, we can regain greater harmony with the underlying creative forces within us.

AYURVEDA AND YOGA

Yoga and Ayurveda belong to each other like a brother to his sister, the breath to the body, a plant in its soil. Taken in context, each one nourishes the other; removed from each other, they can exist for a while but will lack the feeling of wholeness and continuity. Although Yoga has been known in the West for just over one hundred years, it has only been in the past few decades that Ayurveda has come to be studied. Ayurveda and Yoga are sister sciences of the Indian Vedic tradition known as the Sanātana Dharma, paths to the Eternal Truth (Panikkar, 2006). The teachings are considered timeless as they apply to everyone in all cultures and times. Classical Yoga and Ayurvedic practices have the potential to bring about a lasting change in people's lifestyles, health, and overall outlook on their life's purpose.

David Frawley, a preeminent authority on Vedic culture, has written that "Ayurveda is the Vedic science of healing for both body and mind. Yoga is the Vedic science of self-realization that depends upon a well-functioning body and mind" (Frawley, 1999) and builds upon the foundation of Ayurveda. Ayurveda needs Yoga because it is unfulfilling to the human psyche as it evolves toward self-realization. The practice of the two sciences as a lifestyle is necessary for the achievement of their independent goals.

AYURVEDA'S FOUR GOALS OF LIFE

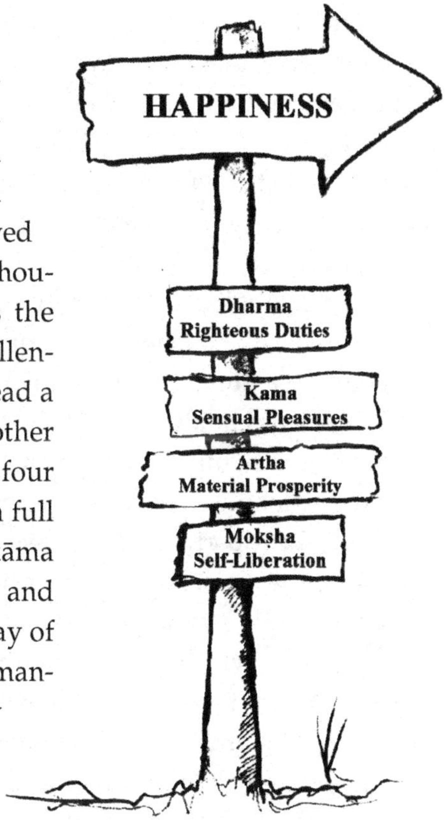

Yoga and Ayurveda both developed during a cultural period of India's history that was broad in its perspective of the significance of human existence. Similar to how Patañjali wrote down the *Yoga Sūtras* around 200 BCE, Ayurveda enjoyed a long history of medical and health studies for thousands of years before being written down as the *Caraka Saṁhitā* toward the end of the first millennium. The prime directive of this culture is to lead a fulfilling life. According to the teachings of another Ayurvedic text, the *Sanātana Dharma,* there are four avenues thata must be fulfilled in order to live a full and happy life: dharma (righteous duties), kāma (sensual pleasures), artha (material prosperity), and mokṣa (self-liberation) (Panikkar, 2006). This way of life requires one to perform duties in a virtuous manner, to maintain the health and vitality necessary to fulfill one's desires, to acquire and possess the material wealth necessary for social position, and to pursue peace of mind and spiritual liberation. For the yogi, the objective is to promote the spiritual progress of the individual through deepening sādhana (practice) as the means to mokṣa (liberation). For the ayurvedist, the goal is to balance the doṣas (subtle principles) so that health may be maintained or restored, moving back from vikṛti (the current imbalance) toward prakṛti (the natural constitution present at birth).

THE FORCES AND ELEMENTAL QUALITIES OF AYURVEDA AND YOGA

In Ayurveda, five basic elements of creation—earth, water, fire, air, and ether—manifest as the three biological energy forces, called doṣas. These three qualities are vāta (composed of air and ether), pitta (composed of fire and water), and kapha (composed of earth and water). The three doṣas can be seen as the vitalizing forces of life; when they are in balance, health and clarity are the natural outcome. When out of balance, the doṣas cause disease, decay, and death. This is their nature. "It is important to remember that these descriptions reflect the pure aspect of each constitutional element; however, no individual constitution is made up solely of any one element. Rather, each person is a combination of all three elements, with a predominant tendency toward one or more" (Lad, 1985). Health of the body produces a by-product of vitality and emotional health. This creates a tendency for mental health. Svastha (true health) is a coming home to your Self. To the yogi, health is not merely determined by the physical body, nor is it created by physical exercise alone. The yogi's aim in health is to quiet dis-ease and bring the primal qualities and five basic elements into equilibrium to promote a state of spiritual balance called sattva guṇa (harmony). For the ayurvedic practitioner, the goal is to balance the three doṣa qualities, vāta, pitta, and kapha, which are seen as the primary driving forces in maintaining and creating health and well-being.

In Yoga and Ayurveda, the universe is seen as manifesting three fundamental biological properties. Vāta possesses creativity that expresses itself as movement in which the elements of air and space are predominant. In the yogic and ayurvedic literature, vāta's biological property is refined into its higher subtler form of energy called prāṇa, which governs rhythm, motion, and sensitivity of the mind. Pitta represents transformation, which expresses itself as energy or vitality through the elements of fire and water. Tejas is a refined form of pitta that creates discernment, the higher function of mind. Kapha is known for preservation and receives nourishment through the elements of water and earth. Ojas is the refined form of kapha, providing the foundation of all nurturing qualities that become the immune system, breast milk, and the placenta.

Lacking or having an excess of a doṣa is experienced physically and energetically. For example, a lack of vāta would be directly experienced as a tendency to speak very little, while an overabundance of vāta would be experienced as excessive talking. A lack of pitta would be expressed as a complete loss of appetite, while an excess of pitta would be experienced as excessive thirst and hunger. A lack of kapha is experienced as a feeling of emptiness in the head and the heart, while an excess is experienced as heaviness and weight gain. The information conveyed by an expert Ayurvedic Yoga Therapy practitioner is not merely one more alternative method to be free of diseases. By learning to read the digestive process, skin, facial expressions, tone and pitch of the voice, observe the changes in respiration, reading the twelve radial pulses, and other diagnostic skills, the Ayurvedic practitioner gains a way to perceive the instantaneous manifestations of life. Ayurveda shows us how changes in diet, lifestyle, exercise, and the spiritual practices of Yoga promote health and longevity. It directs us to live a life of fulfillment as stated in *Caraka Saṁhitā—Sūtrasthānam,* "The body and mind constitute the substrata of diseases and happiness [i.e., positive health]. Balanced utilization [of time, mental faculties, and the objects of sense organs] is the cause of happiness" (Sharma and Dash, 1976).

AYURVEDIC YOGA THERAPY

In Ayurvedic teachings, it is frequently unclear whether there is a need to increase or decrease the doṣa that is imbalanced. For that reason, two people who have the same diagnosis may have a prescribed practice very different from one another. In the most prevalent approach of Ayurvedic Yoga Therapy, an Ayurvedic practitioner strives to decrease the qualities of a doṣa that has been elevated. Other methods focus on increasing the opposite quality in a different doṣa. This is the method for relieving the primary attributes of each doṣa as described in one of the original treatises on Ayurveda, the *Caraka Saṁhitā* (Sharma and Dash, 1976). Finally, a third approach is to focus attention to doing yogāsanas resulting in a balanced state of the doṣa. Thus, positive attributes such as strength, stamina, patience, open heart, and humility will predominate. The great yogī and revolutionary philosopher, Sri Aurobindo, said, "Yoga is condensed evolution" (Aurobindo, 1984). In our philosophy, the client is encouraged to develop a relationship with the body based on personalizing the teachings with discrimination, "detachment and consistent earnest effort" as described in the *Yoga Sūtras* I.12 (Stiles, 2002).

Ultimately, the practice of any aspect of Yoga has the ability to either imbalance or balance the body and doṣas, especially yogāsana. Our constitution depends on

1.12

अभ्यास वैराग्याभ्यां तन्निरोधः ॥१२॥

abhyāsa vairāgyābhyāṁ tan nirodhaḥ

The arresting of the mind's fluctuations comes about through consistent earnest effort and detachment

the configuration of doṣas; they influence our body's function and guide our emotional and psychological reactions. As external conditions change like time of day and weather, changes in diet and lifestyle might be necessary to maintain balanced health. Different Yoga poses as well as different methods to do familiar poses may also be used to regulate internal changes and provide balance to the doṣas.

In Ayurvedic Yoga Therapy, āsanas can be classified according to their location and the doṣa they balance. The seat of vāta is the pelvic cavity and colon organ, and sitting poses have the ability to stimulate or balance vāta doṣa. The seat of pitta is the abdominal cavity and the small intestine, and twisting and back-bending poses whose major affect is on the abdomen and middle back can positively affect pitta doṣa. The seat of kapha is the chest and the stomach, and poses like setu bandhāsana (bridge) and sarvaṅgāsana (shoulderstand) can help affect kapha doṣa.

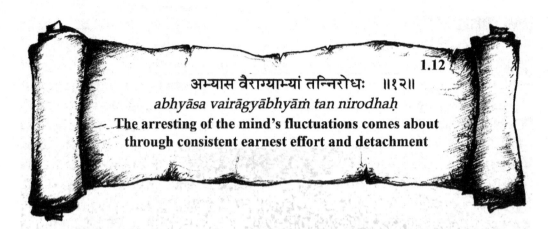

More important than where yogāsanas work in our anatomy is how they are practiced in Ayurvedic Yoga Therapy. A balanced vāta-predominant student would seek a long-term practice that emphasizes relaxation and spirituality that could be studied for a lifetime. An unbalanced vāta would tend to jump from one method to another, seeking to solve their current problems or stress before moving on to something more *en vogue*. A balanced pitta-predominant student would seek a practice that is stimulating and has enough variety to keep him/her from getting bored. However, an unbalanced pitta would do this practice intensely until a repetitive motion injury or inflammation developed, then switch to another activity altogether like rollerblading. A balanced kapha-predominant student would seek a method that appeals to his/her sensitive and devotional nature that is also challenging to his/her desire for physical fitness. An unbalanced kapha would come for Yoga class to lose weight but would stop if he/she became tired or depressed.

Svatmarama Yogi, the author of the fourteenth-century manuscript, *Haṭha Yoga Pradīpikā*, believed that removing disease-producing obstructions from the natural functioning of prāṇa (energy) helped to stimulate healing. What follows are some ways to deepen the breath, restore the body, and balance the particular doṣas using Yoga Therapy.

YOGA THERAPY FOR VĀTA

Vāta constitutions need a container to hold themselves in balance. A major problem for them is being a "leaky bucket" and losing prāṇa. The first and most obvious way to create a container is by regulating one's lifestyle. Relaxation, prāṇāyāma (breathing techniques), and meditation practices affect the subtler qualities of vāta, and, if emphasis is placed there first, it can create a grounded personality. A regulated lifestyle that seeks to balance biological rhythms with eating, relaxation, exercise, and working is most important. In Yoga's repertoire, we have practices for balancing the vāta qualities within us to promote natural biological rhythms like menstruation, elimination, sexual expression, speech, sleep, digestion, and physical motions to calm the mind and elevate intuition.

Vata predominant Yoga practitioners need to practice poses that focus on the pelvic region and the colon, which are the main sites of vāta. A vāta-balancing practice would place primary emphasis on developing sensitivity through inquiry practices. Asking, "What do I feel?" and "Where do I feel it?" does more to balance vāta than anything else. The deeper a vāta can go inside, the better. The most useful poses for vāta promote freedom in the major joint areas of the lower body—the hips, lumbar spine, and knee joints. Forward-bending poses are good but should not be forced or held in a prolonged fashion. Some vātas are naturally flexible and must be cautioned not to promote any excessively increased ranges of motion, which can diminish their prāṇa. Balancing poses such as those in vṛkśāsana (balancing tree), garuḍāsana (eagle), and naṭarājāsana (dancer king pose) will increase concentration and be good for restoring vāta.

Āsanas are best done by vātas with rhythmic, steady, and regular breathing. It is good for vāta to discipline their memory by learning sequences that build upon previous week's training. Prāṇāyāma is more important for vāta predominant practitioners than for pittas or kaphas as it soothes their sensitive nature, which is more prone to disturbances than the other doṣas. Ujjāyi prāṇāyāma (victorious breathing) forms the core of the vāta prāṇāyāma practice. Variations such as anuloma viloma (alternate nostril breathing)—also known as nāḍī śodhana (purification of the subtle channels) are useful in balancing vāta (Mutktibodhananda, 1998).

YOGA THERAPY FOR PITTA

The pitta quality is enhanced by cooperation and sharing activities. Pitta quality will especially enjoy partner Yoga practices done in a lighthearted manner. Pitta needs Yoga practices that maintain their digestive fire and warm personality, yet temper their tendency toward inflammatory conditions. In Yoga's repertoire, we have practices for balancing the pitta qualities, thus promoting natural biological functions of digestive assimilation, eyesight, skin, liver function, and increasing one's mental property of discernment.

Pitta predominant Yoga practitioners would be wise to focus on Yoga poses like spinal twists and those that apply beneficial pressure to the navel region and the solar plexus. These provide a massage to the area of the liver, spleen, small intestines, and pancreas, which is good for pitta doṣa. Backbending poses, including bhujaṅgāsana (cobra), dhanurāsana (bow), and salabhasana (locust), stimulate pitta when it is deficient or sluggish and are best practiced in moderation or by going in and out of the poses with mild exertion. Milder poses such as viparīta karaṇī mudrā (inverted action), sālamba sarvaṅgāsana (shoulderstand), and halāsana (plow) are supportive in restoring serenity to pittas when their lifestyle has become too demanding. When the body/mind becomes too hot, pittas should practice a cooling type of breathing called śītalī prāṇāyāma (see figure at left) where the tongue is curled and the lips are pursed. This will go a long way in quieting down the fiery nature of pittas.

Śītalī Prāṇāyāma

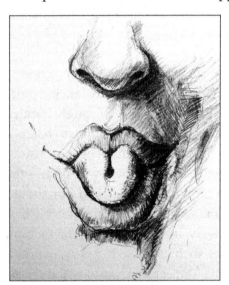

YOGA THERAPY FOR KAPHA

Kapha-imbalanced people may have a sluggish digestive system and/or a slow metabolism. By performing practices that affect the region of the abdomen, kaphas can help to increase their digestive fire. The focus for treating kapha is promoting strength and stamina along with cleansing practices to detoxify the system. In Yoga's repertoire, we have practices for balancing the kapha qualities, thus promoting natural biological functions of the heart, cerebrospinal fluid, lubrication of the joints, mucous membrane, respiration, sensual pleasure, and memory.

Kapha predominant Yoga practitioners ideally practice vigorous exercises with regular discipline. In the Yoga regimen, this includes daily practice of sūrya namaskāra (sun salutations). For kaphas, the program needs to be physically challenging and done with effort to develop strong arms, chest, and upper back with a focus on developing muscular strength in the lower trapezius and latissimus dorsi muscles. Poses that are particularly beneficial for them include sarvaṅgāsana (shoulderstand), setu bandhāsana (bridge), siṁhāsana (lion), matyāsana (fish), mayurāsana (peacock), and vīrabhadrāsana (warrior). People with the tendency toward kapha imbalances usually benefit from holding their Yoga poses longer than vāta- or pitta-predominant types. This helps focus their mind and body on actions that purify them and increase stamina. Along with Yoga, we usually advise them to exercise throughout the day by walking in nature, working in the garden, or swimming. Being in a natural environment is particularly beneficial for kapha doṣa as it helps to maintain their connection with the earth and the cycles of nature. Kapālabhātī prāṇāyāma regularly practiced will assist kaphas in keeping excessive mucous to a minimum. Heating prāṇāyāmas, such as bhastrikā and sūrya bhedana, are recommended as well. Uddīyāna bandha can be emphasized once a kapha has mastered the basics of prāṇāyāma and has a consistent practice. This will help to maintain the strength of the diaphragm and heart muscles. Both a physical Yoga and a devotional practice are necessary for kapha. Devotion without physical discipline will make kapha stagnate; physical exercise without devotion is just simply hard work, leaving kapha feeling dry. Kaphas need to follow their heart more than any of the other doṣas. Scholar Joseph Campbell gave excellent advice to kaphas when he told his PBS viewers, "Follow your bliss."

CONCLUSION

People tend to joke about how difficult life can be since we were never given an owner's manual for self-care. Yet, Ayurveda provides just such an "owner's manual" by presenting us with timeless teachings that inform our decisions in living a more fulfilling lifestyle. In support, Classical Yoga helps us by providing detailed guidelines on how one can free the positive potentials of the mind and live a fulfilling spiritual life. For the yogi, the means to the goal of health, or to "live within the Self," is to become "freed from the primordial forces of suffering."

Dr. Vasant Lad, the world's foremost exponent of Ayurveda today, has said that Ayurveda and Yoga are sister sciences, implying that they share a similar worldview and descended from the same root. Yet, these sisters are clearly not twins. They take different directions in fulfilling their objectives. From our perspective, Ayurvedic teachings provide the foundation for physical health, and Yoga helps to improve our structural relationships with the body while also developing our spiritual side. When they are carefully studied and developed into a personal lifestyle through guidance from an experienced teacher, Yoga Therapy and Ayurveda are practices that together lead to harmony.

REFERENCES

Aurobindo, Sri. *The Synthesis of Yoga.* Pondicherry, India : Sri Aurobindo Ashram, 1984. Print.

Frawley, D. *Yoga and Ayurveda.* Twin Lakes, WI : Lotus Press, 1999. Print.

Hipprocates. *Of the Epidemics.* Whitefish, MT: Kessinger Publishing, 2004. Print.

Lad, V. *Ayurveda, the Science of Self-Healing.* Wilmont, WI : Lotus Press, 1985. Print.

Leonard, G., and M. Murphy. *The Life We Are Given.* New York: Jeremy Tarcher/Putnam Books, 1995. Print.

Muktibodhananda, Swami. *Hatha Yoga Pradipika.* Jharkland: Bihar School of Yoga, 1998. Print.

Panikkar, R. *Espiritualidad Hindu: Sanatana Dharma.* Barcelona: Editorial Kairos, S.A., 2006. Print.

Sharma, R. K., and V. B. Dash. *Agnivesha, Charaka Samhita.* Varanasi, India : Chowkhamba Sanskrit Services Office, 1976. Print.

Stiles, M. *Yoga Sutras of Patanjali.* Boston, MA: Red Wheel/Wiser, 2002. Print.

Tinbergen, N. "Nikolaas Tinbergen—Nobel Lecture: Ethology and Stress Diseases." Nobelprize .org. Nobel Media AB 2013. Web. 11 Apr 2014. http://www.nobelprize.org/nobel_ prizes/ medicine/laureates/1973/tinbergen-lecture.html.

SVASTHA YOGA THERAPY AND AYURVEDA: HOLISTIC WELL-BEING

A. G. and Ganesh Mohan

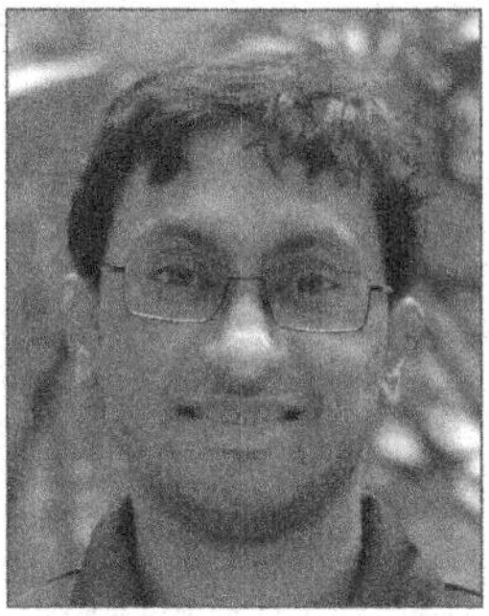

Svastha Yoga Therapy and Ayurveda was founded by the Mohan family to carry on the work of the great yogī Tirumalai Krishnamacharya. **A. G. Mohan** was one of the few personal students of Professor Krishnamacharya through the last eighteen years of the master's life. His wife, Indra, started teaching and practicing Yoga just one year after A. G. began. Their daughter, Nitya, apart from practicing Yoga from childhood, is an expert in Indian classical music, Vedic chanting, and the use of sound. **Ganesh**, their son, pictured at left, is a physician trained in modern medicine and Ayurveda. Together with his father, A. G. Mohan, Ganesh cowrote the book *Krishnamacharya* (Shambhala, 2010), and he currently leads Svastha's work on Yoga Therapy.

KRISHNAMACHARYA

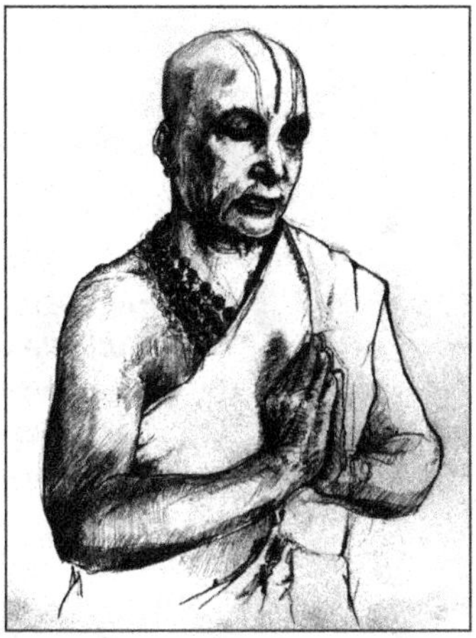

Tirumalai Krishnamacharya

Much of Yoga today has derived and evolved from the teachings of the yogī Tirumalai Krishnamacharya (Ruiz, Fernando Pagīs. "Krishnamacharya's Legacy." *Yoga Journal*, 2001). Krishnamacharya traveled across the breadth of India in the early 1900s, immersing himself in traditional studies, to eventually emerge as an extraordinary man of enormous knowledge and rare depths of practice and experience. He systematized and presented many of the practices that characterize Yoga as it is today. His teachings are one of the pillars of our school at Svastha Yoga.

THE ROOTS OF SVASTHA

The word *svāsthya* literally means "to stay in oneself" or "to be oneself" (*sva* is "self," and the verb root *sthā* means "to stay"). In Ayurveda, *svāsthya* is the definitive word for a state of holistic health and balance (Suśruta Samhitā, Sūtrasthāna 15/41). Ayurveda advocates a personalized approach to treatment, taking into account numerous factors such as the imbalance of the doṣas (groups of biological functions that underlie the paradigm of ayurveda), the body system that is affected, the age, strength, metabolism, constitution, mental state, diet, and lifestyle of the individual, and the environment in which the person lives.

In Yoga, Krishnamacharya's guiding principle was that any teaching had to be modified for the individual to create a state of balanced health. No one among us is entirely like the other. A fit twenty-three-year-old sportswoman with a knee injury, an overweight sixty-eight-year-old retiree with diabetes and low back pain, and a forty-two-year-old stressed executive with allergies are all different from one another, each with his/her distinct needs. If Yoga is to be truly effective for each of them, it has to be taught in a manner suited to their individual requirements.

YOGA AS A THERAPY

Ancient Yoga texts note that ill health is the first and greatest enemy of a calm and focused mind (*Yogasūtras of Patanjali,* 1.30); disease is the principal barrier on the path of Yoga. Fortunately, the practice of Yoga can itself help remove or diminish

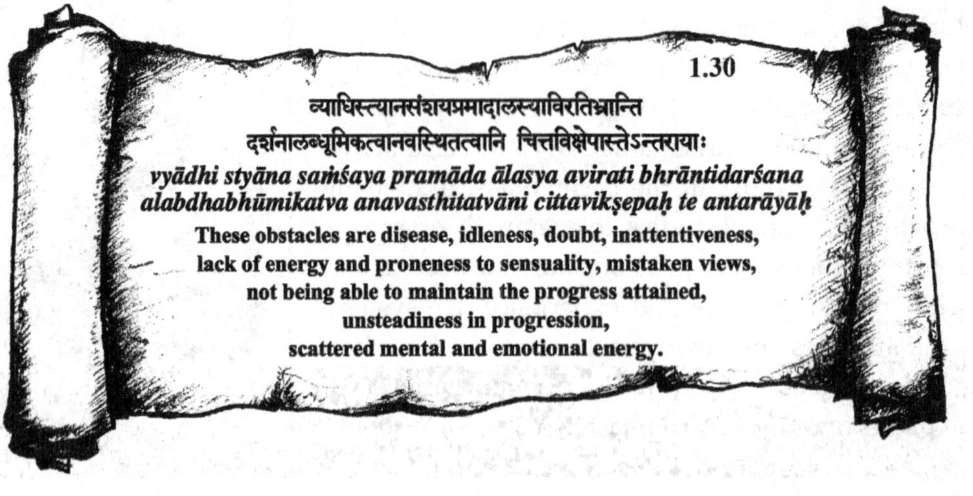
1.30
व्याधिस्त्यानसंशयप्रमादालस्याविरतिभ्रान्ति
दर्शनालब्धभूमिकत्वानवस्थितत्वानि चित्तविक्षेपास्तेऽन्तरायाः
vyādhi styāna saṁśaya pramāda ālasya avirati bhrāntidarśana
alabdhabhūmikatva anavasthitatvāni cittavikṣepaḥ te antarāyāḥ
These obstacles are disease, idleness, doubt, inattentiveness,
lack of energy and proneness to sensuality, mistaken views,
not being able to maintain the progress attained,
unsteadiness in progression,
scattered mental and emotional energy.

ill health. In his commentary on the *Yoga Sūtra*, known as the *Yogavallī* (I.34), Krishnamacharya indicates:

> Just as various medicines and other measures are prescribed by physicians for curing the illnesses of those who are unwell, the revered Patañjali, in his sūtras, has made clear various methods to heal the illnesses of the body through the practice of the limbs of Yoga. Among these many methods, the important are:
>
> 1. Moving the arms, legs, and neck (body parts) with appropriate inhalation and exhalation
> 2. Following appropriate diet
> 3. Avoiding inappropriate travel (disciplined lifestyle)
>
> If Yoga is practiced in the absence of these disciplines, without knowing the correct methods of practice, illnesses will not be healed as said the ancient texts.

The Sanskrit word for "treatment" or "therapy" is *cikitsā*. The root meaning of the word *cikitsā* is "to oppose disease." However, cikitsā is not only about curing disease; Yoga and Ayurveda have the holistic goal of reducing suffering. Curing the disease is a direct pathway to that goal, and Yoga may help in that process. But Yoga also contributes indirectly by helping to tackle related problems and by supporting the principal treatment; sometimes, Yoga Therapy can be about the person rather than the problem.

KEY FEATURES OF YOGA AS THERAPY

The practice of Yoga affects many systems of the body and mind simultaneously. It is, therefore, not advisable to take a reductionist approach to Yoga in clinical practice. We must not only look at the student's spine or their asthma or their blood pressure; we have to view the person as a whole.

The one indispensable requirement for Yoga is the participation of the practitioner. Yoga *requires* that the patient/student *practice*. Yoga Therapy cannot be administered with the teacher doing the work and the student merely being a passive recipient. Hence, Yoga Therapy empowers the patient and depends on the patient empowering him/herself to take an active role in his/her health and to play a major role in the therapeutic process. That, in itself, is a powerful boost to health and awakens support for many positive changes in one's life.

YOGA TRADITION AND MODERN SCIENCE

As we take the field of Yoga forward, one goal lies in combining the knowledge of classical Yoga and Ayurveda with modern science. To achieve health and well-being, we must look not only to tradition but also to science because knowledge is always evolving. Krishnamacharya had great respect for the traditional knowledge he was steeped in, yet he did not hesitate to discard unsound practices or practices that were not effective in modern times. He opined that there is a need to look into the practices of Yoga with a view to revive and revise them.

The database of traditional knowledge is vast. Research can only test some portions of this database as resources, parameters, and possibilities for evidence-based research are always limited. Thus, we have to build our database of tools and practices in Yoga Therapy, not only on modern research, but also on the foundation of effective clinical practices and wise choices made using a sound scientific *approach.*

A scientific approach does not necessarily mean that the traditional methods we use will fit entirely into the paradigm of modern medicine; the paradigm of Yoga and Ayurveda, for example, differs in some ways from that of modern medicine. However, a scientific approach necessarily means that the paradigm and methods we use are open to question. In fact, traditional texts on Ayurveda and Yoga encourage this attitude of exploration.

Theories of modern medicine and traditional systems do not necessarily have to be in complete synchrony for the treatment to work, but each therapist has to be clear of what he/she is doing and why within the chosen paradigm and approach.

A HOLISTIC APPROACH TO YOGA THERAPY

Krishnamacharya's approach to Yoga was characterized by the holistic consideration of the entire person. We can all agree on these factors: We have a body and mind. We breathe, which is an important part of Yoga. We have a lifestyle of activities and various food habits in an environment both animate and inanimate. We can place these factors into a convenient list:

1. Body
2. Breath
3. Mind
4. Diet
5. Lifestyle
6. Environment

We must look into each of these factors to restore or maintain well-being. In Yoga, we have tools to impact the body, breath, and mind directly. And through them, we make changes to the food we eat, the life we lead, and the environment we interact with. Ayurveda speaks substantially to our diet and lifestyle, as well as herbs, through which we may influence our body and mind.

WORKING WITH THE BODY: A FUNCTION-ORIENTED APPROACH

The structure of our body enables its function; function is the goal, and structure is the means. Clinically, wide variations in structure may coexist with normal function. A knee could appear to have significant arthritic changes on an x-ray, but the patient could have good range of movement and a relatively normal gait. Conversely, a person can have low back pain without significant abnormalities on diagnostic imaging. Restoration of "ideal structure" is neither certain nor mandatory. Our aim is restoring function commensurate with the person's requirement.

The figure below outlines our function-oriented approach in Svastha Yoga Therapy in a simple chart.

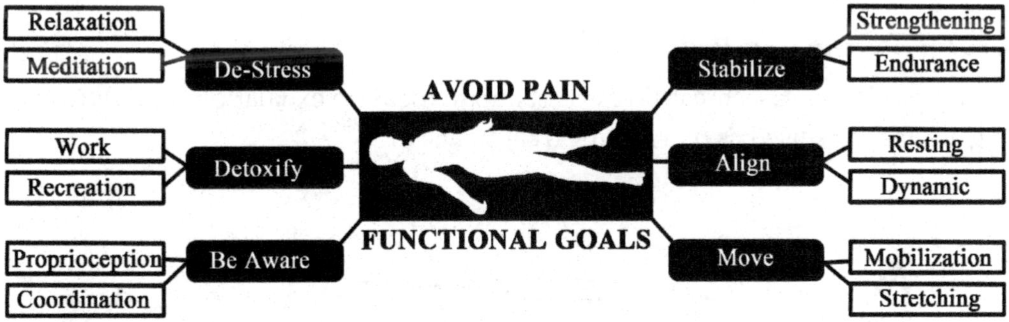

CASE STUDY: LOW BACK PAIN AND SCIATICA

Diana, a forty-three-year-old IT manager, works at a computer and attends meetings on most days. She drives around 45 minutes each way to work five days of the week and does not do any exercise. She is married with two children. Her two episodes of sciatica caused severe pain for about three weeks and occurred five years ago and four months ago, respectively. She still has mild sciatic pain down her left leg with some numbness and tingling sensations. She also has some diffuse low back pain, and, sometimes when the pain in her leg grows better, the pain in her back grows worse (and vice versa).

Diana would like to do Yoga Therapy as an intervention for around 20 minutes in the morning and evening every day. She also wants us to give her some recommendations on how she might strengthen and protect her back when she is at work.

Approach

- Start in a position of minimal pain/discomfort
- Build awareness of posture and move toward the neutral spine
- Strengthen back muscles (extensors) and move into gentle extension
- Engage core stabilization, particularly using exhalation
- Initially avoid flexion, especially flexion-rotation movements
- Over time, transition to a normal Yoga practice, but always have a little attention on neutral spine position and strengthening/stabilization

Useful Āsanas and Prāṇāyāma

In this particular case, breathing was set up to focus on exhalations and the following āsanas were used as therapeutic treatments.

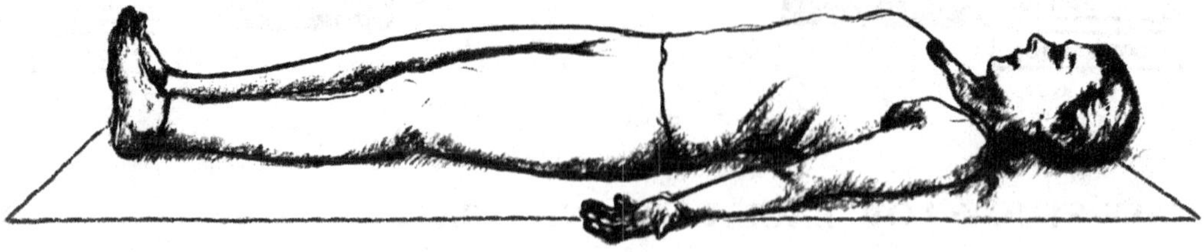

Gentle supine spine extension. Can be done with the knees bent and feet on the mat.

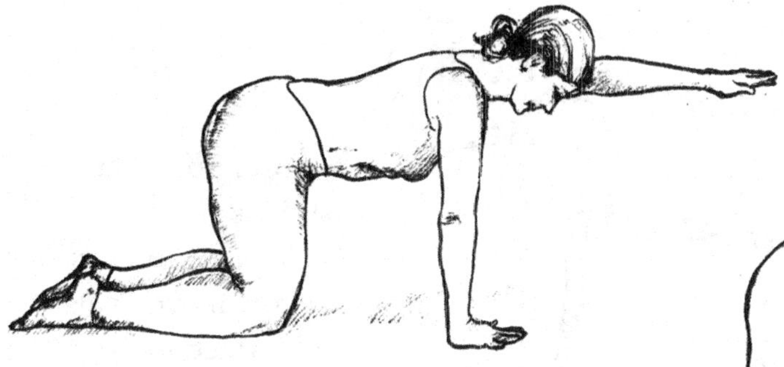

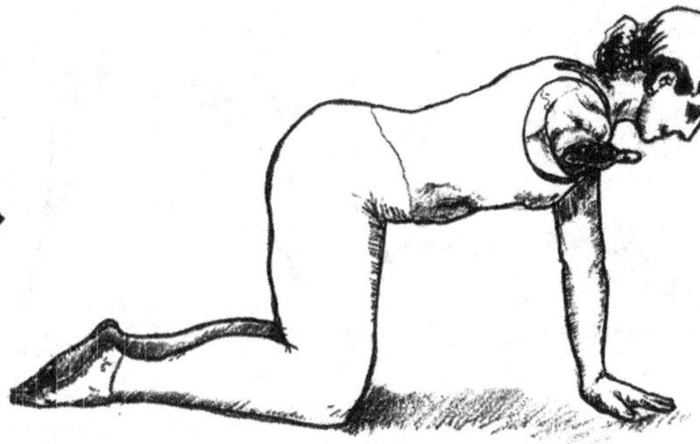

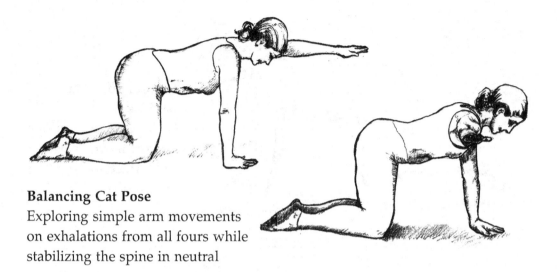

Balancing Cat Pose
Exploring simple arm movements on exhalations from all fours while stabilizing the spine in neutral

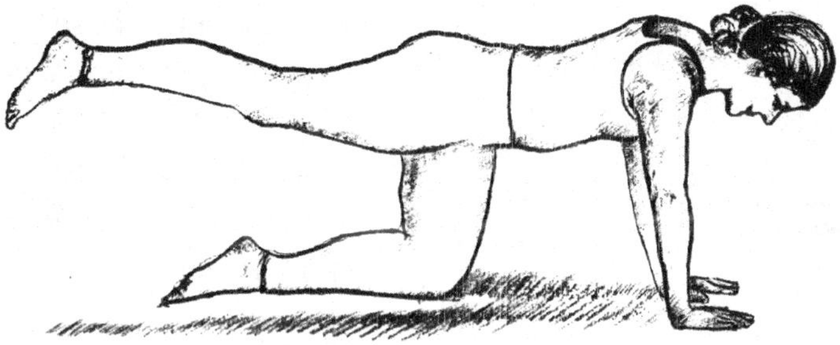

Balancing Cat Pose
Exploring simple leg movements on exhalations from all fours while stabilizing the spine in neutral

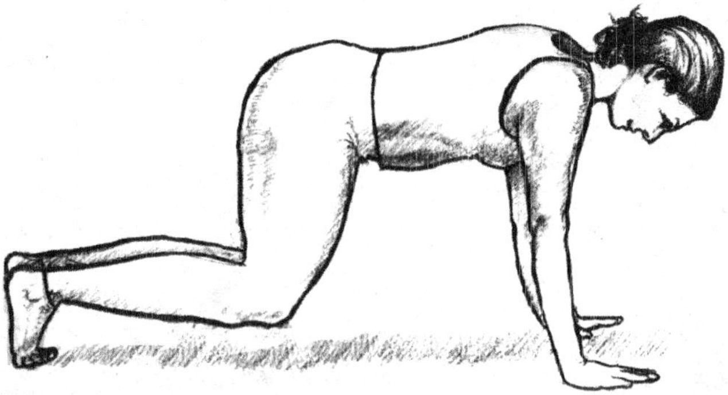

Core Strength
Engaging the abdominal muscles and moving from all fours on exhalations, raise the knees off the floor keeping the spine in neutral

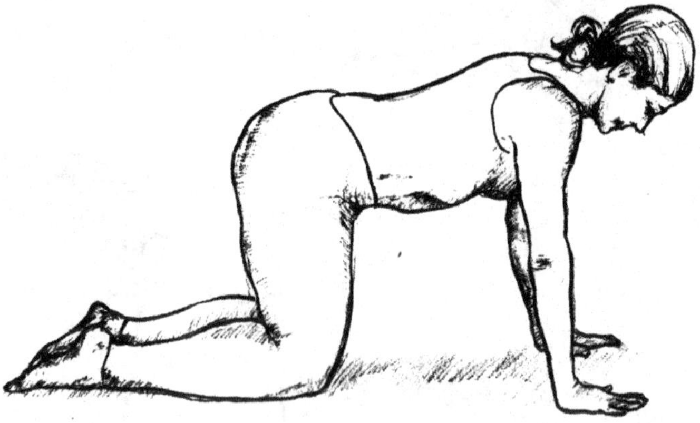

Neutral Spine on All Fours
Gentle flexion-extension cat-cow movements (performed to degree of comfort)

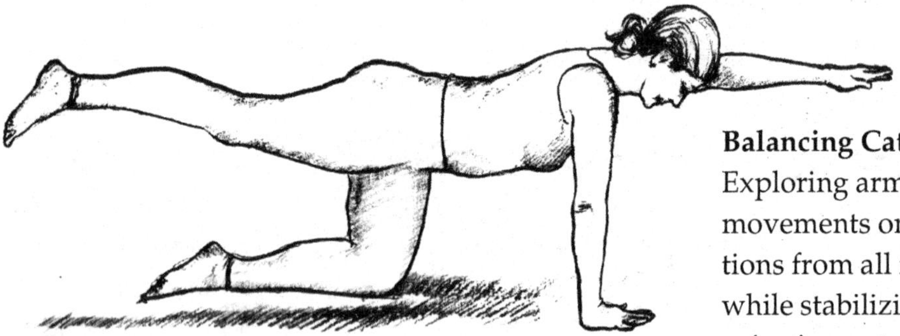

Balancing Cat Pose
Exploring arm and leg movements on exhalations from all fours while stabilizing the spine in neutral

Dolphin Pose
Take the core strengthening exercise into the dolphin pose to challenge overall strength

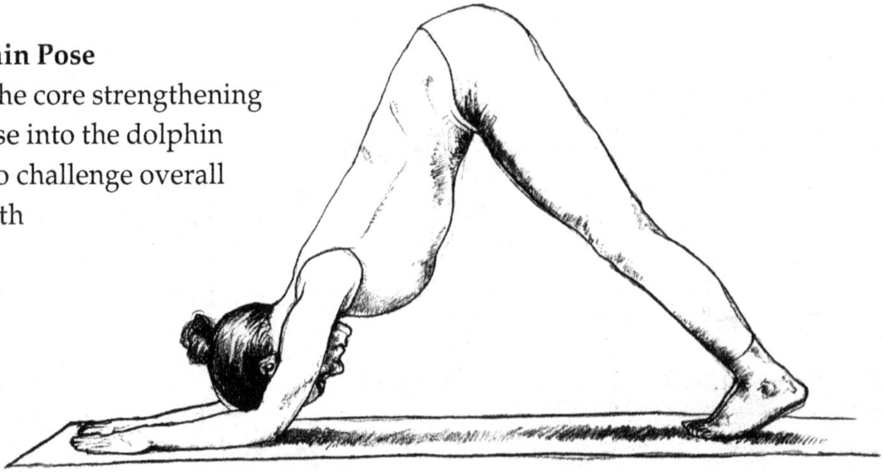

Gentle Cobra Pose
Prone spine extensions done on exhalations to strengthen the back and calm the sciatic nerve

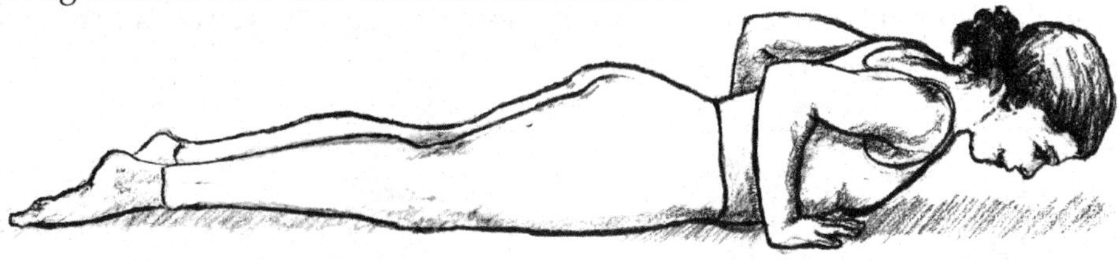

Chair Pose
Strengthening the spine when raising from a chair (half squat or chair pose)

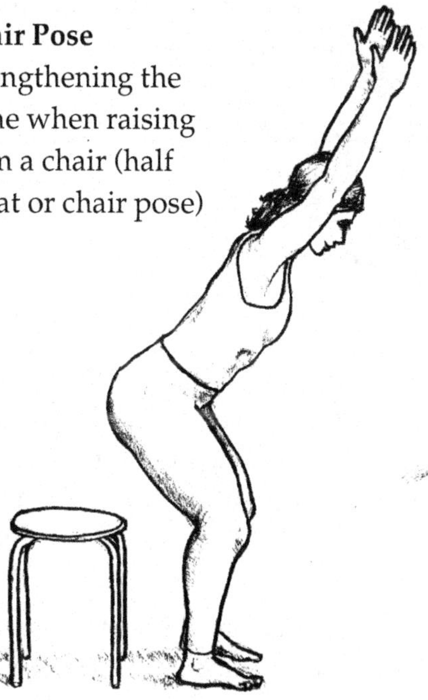

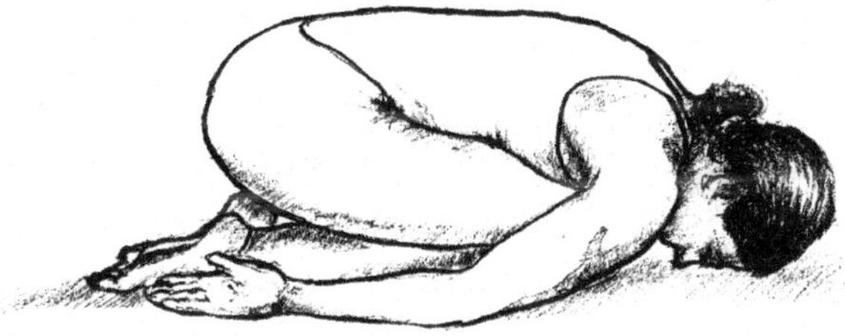

Child's Pose
Once past the initial phase, gentle flexion releases the spinal muscles

Gradually, the intensity of the āsanas was increased to incorporate full dolphin, side plank, standing warrior sequences, and side bends. Forward bends were last to be cautiously incorporated into treatment along with twists after around four months, leading to a mostly normal Yoga practice at around six to eight months.

Lifestyle and Environment

Detoxification requires that we avoid the activities that might create the problem. In this case, the slumped seated position that inevitably takes over when driving or when at the computer has to be combated.

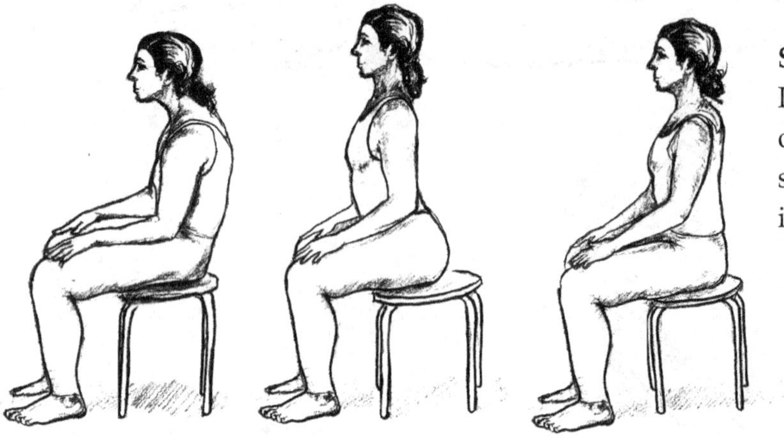

Seated Posture
Raising awareness of one's spine in a seated posture is important.

Incorporating awareness and strengthening of the spine into daily life activities is enormously helpful, providing great reward for little effort and time. From brushing one's teeth to speaking on the phone to getting up from a chair, there are numerous opportunities in daily life to incorporate spine awareness and strengthening.

Mind

Finally, some meditation and relaxation was added to create the mental space to adhere to the physical discipline of āsana practice and daily life spine awareness.

Ayurveda

Ayurvedic suggestions were individualized looking at Diana's doṣa imbalances. Some ayurvedic herbs commonly used in back pain and sciatica are guggulu preparations, rasna preparations, shallaki, ashwagandha for internal use, and mahanarayana oil for external application.

WORKING WITH INTERNAL BODY SYSTEMS

As we look deeper beyond the musculoskeletal system, the role of breathing becomes critical in Yoga Therapy and also plays an important role in Ayurveda. For conciseness and convenience, the chart below is a summary of the many aspects of working with the breath that we focus on in Svastha Yoga Therapy.

Characteristics of the Breath

1. Depth of exhale and inhale.
2. Length of each component (exhale, inhale, holding / pausing).
3. Effort of breathing (muscle work).
4. Pattern of breathing: abdominal / diaphragmatic, chest, combination, etc.

The breath may be influenced by:

1. Direct, conscious modulation.
2. Unconscious modulation (habit patterns).
3. Sound / Chanting.
4. Gravity.
5. Body position.
6. Musculoskeletal restrictions.
7. Overall exertion involved.
8. Imagination / Visualization.
9. Relaxation / Meditation.

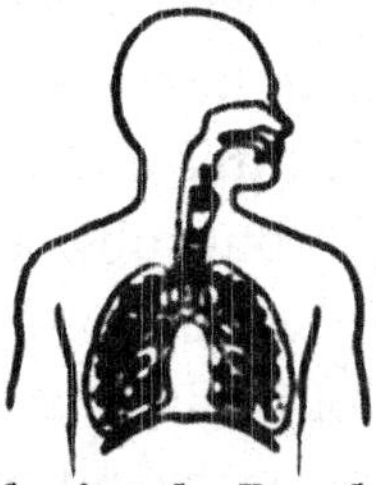

Developing the Breath in Yoga
(in appropriate order of complexity/teaching)

1. Do the breath along with the movement.
2. Develop conscious awareness of breath.
3. Learn to relax and release the breath, focusing on the diaphragm or the abdomen.
4. Deepen the exhale (increase volume, maybe duration). Abdominal muscles are engaged.
5. Deepen the inhale. May come naturally as consequence of emphasizing exhale. Chest expansion is emphasized.
6. Lengthen the exhale (should not be breathless over a couple of cycles).
7. Lengthen the inhale.
8. Develop conscious pause after exhalation.
9. Develop holding after inhalation.
10. Bandhas in asanas.
11. Bandhas in prāṇāyāma.

The breath may be experienced through:

1. Feeling the movement of the air (nostrils, vocal chords).
2. Feeling the proprioception (joints, ligaments, body parts, "hands-on" floor).
3. Energy of the breath.

Goals for the Respiratory System:

1. Symptom relief, to decrease:
   a. Cough and sputum.
   b. Breathlessness.
2. Developing breathing capacity (vital capacity) and easing the work of breathing.
3. Tackling the underlying problem in other ways if possible:
   a. Immune system.
   b. Stress and lifestyle.
   c. Diet, etc.

Working with the breath in Yoga is a layered process, starting from where the person is at and exploring it one step at a time, with patience and wisdom as guides. By modifying the flow and relationship to the breath, we influence the flow of prāṇa (life force) in the body. Classical Yoga texts like the *Haṭha Yoga Pradīpikā* (II, 16–17) and *Yoga Yajñavalkya* (VI, 39–49) emphasize the importance of prāṇāyāma in removing illnesses of the body and mind. The breath is, in turn, related to the doṣas of Ayurveda through heating and cooling practices. Using appropriate āsanas to target the internal systems of the body and combining them with appropriate breathing, we have powerful methods in Yoga to create balance.

CASE STUDY: MENSTRUAL DISORDER

Karen, thirty-two, is an administrative manager at a hospital, and she is under a lot of stress at work. She is in a relationship with a supportive partner, and they have no children. Over the last year, her periods have become more irregular with her menstrual cycle occurring from around twenty-three to thirty-three days. The flow is somewhat heavy on the first day and tapers off from the second day but continues for around five days. She experiences cramping on the first and second day of her periods. Some years ago, in her twenties, her periods were regular, at around twenty-eight days, with only three days of menstrual flow. The cramping was present when she was a teenager but subsided as she reached adulthood and has reappeared only recently in the past year. Her digestion has always been somewhat irregular with episodes of bloating and fullness after meals on two or more days a week. She often delays meals and sometimes skips them because of pressure at work. Karen came to us for Yoga Therapy to increase her energy levels, regularize her periods, and reduce her stress.

Our Approach

The metabolism behind the menstrual cycle is deeply linked to pitta, but the regularity of the cycle and the flow is related to vāta and kapha. In Karen, we see the duration of the cycle becoming irregular and the flow disturbed. Her stress levels are high and her digestion is irregular as well. There is an underlying vāta imbalance with some pitta too because of her lifestyle and stress, which is reflecting in her menstrual cycle.

By working with the breath, in āsana and prāṇāyāma, we can regularize the flow of vāta, particularly the apāna vāyu in the lower abdomen. We may also balance the pitta or heat in the system using prāṇāyāma.

This is a common problem nowadays, which we may use as convenient template to set up a sample practice.

Useful Āsanas and Prāṇāyāma

Helpful āsanas in this case were those that promote exhalation and work on the abdominal region, particularly the lower abdomen where apāna vāyu functions in

Ayurveda. Effortless and pleasant breathing with a sensation of coolness directed to the lower abdominal region along with the following āsanas were used as therapeutic treatment:

- **Apānāsana:** Lying on the back and drawing the knees into the chest on the exhalation, gently compressing the lower abdomen.
- **Bridge:** Lying on the back and raising the hips and spine on the inhalation, breathing into the abdomen and relaxing the lower abdominal region.
- **Lying twist:** Gentle supine twist, stimulating the lower abdominal region and pelvic region, and releasing the rib cage.
- **Legs up on wall:** A pause to focus on the breath.
- **Forward folds:** Child pose, janushirshasana/paschimatanasana (asymmetric or symmetric seated forward bends). This progressively deepens the effect on the lower abdomen and pelvic region.
- **Tadaga mudrā:** Lying stretched out with arms raised and placed on the floor above the head. This position facilitates deepening the exhalation by drawing the lower abdomen upward and the navel toward the spine. If possible and comfortable, waiting for a couple of seconds in the pause after the exhalation is helpful.
- **Mahamudrā:** Modified version of the classical āsana, practicing comfortably long exhalation.
- **Hip openers** and **abdominal release** concluded the practice.
- **Downward dog** and **modified shoulderstand** were options introduced in her practice according to her energy level and time constraints.

Lifestyle and Environment

To create boundaries in the work environment, Karen began to identify particular people or situations that created stress to see if they could be worked around or avoided. She also aimed for more regular hours at work so she could gradually regularize her sleep timings and Yoga practices.

Ayurveda

Our Ayurvedic suggestions focused specifically on her diet. Most important for Karen, she was advised to eat warm cooked foods easy to digest, reduce heavy and raw foods in the diet, avoid spicy or fried foods, and regularize the food items she eats and the timing of her meals altogether. Ayurvedic formulations to normalize function of apāna vāyu were suggested, such as sukumāra rasāyana, and herbs such as shatavari to reduce pitta and for the reproductive system.

WORKING WITH THE MIND

Psychology is the heart of Yoga. The foundational text on Yoga, the *Yoga Sūtras of Patañjali,* is predominantly a text on Yoga psychology. There are numerous far-reaching practices in Yoga that can help us deal with anxiety, stress, depression, anger, trauma, and other psychological issues.

The Cycle of Vṛtti and Saṁskāra

At the center of Yoga psychology is the cycle of vṛtti (activities of the mind in our field of awareness) and saṁskāra (subconscious or stored impressions of the activities of the mind). In our mind, we all see thoughts and emotions. Imperceptible to us, but within our inference, are the latent impressions of these thoughts and

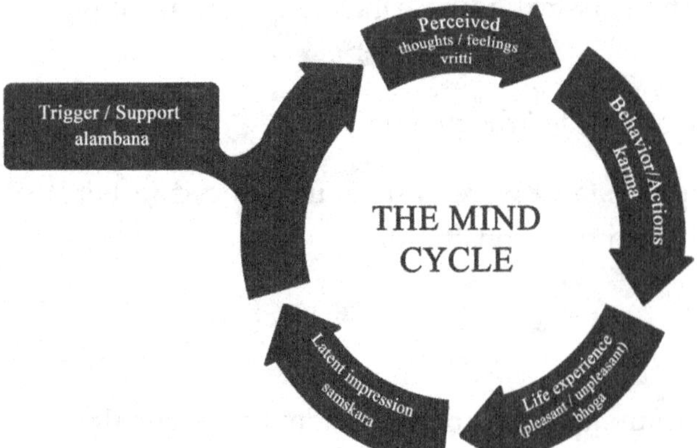

ions. These latent impressions are trigred into thoughts and the thoughts/ emotions leave behind further impressions in our subconscious.

When we act on or express our thoughts and emotions, they become our behavior. Our actions and behavior create our life experience. These life experiences, pleasant and unpleas-t, again impact our mind, leaving d their own separate impressions. Thus, the cycle of the mind incessantly runs our mind and robs us of free will by creating a constant internal dialogue. Through the practice of Yoga as a pathway to mental well-being, we reduce this mental chatter and gradually weaken this automatic cycle, particularly in relation to negative thoughts and emotions, in order to gain greater control over our mind.

Consider, for example, the cycle of how anger develops. Let us hypothetically assume that one day I start a new job in a different city. I do not know my new boss, and, on the first day I meet him, I'm fine with him. Unfortunately, over the first month, I do not get along with him at all. I feel he is dismissive of my work, favoring other colleagues, and standing in the way of my advancement. I feel increasingly angry at every interaction with him. I think angry thoughts about the situation and about him. Soon, over the next few months, the very sight of him is sufficient to bring up a feeling of anger in my mind. At this point, the feeling of anger is the perceived emotion, or vṛtti (thought fluctuation), in my mind. The impression that anger leaves behind in my mind is the saṁskāra. Every time I experience the anger and reinforce the behavior that goes with it, I strengthen the latent impression of anger in my mind. Soon, the trigger just needs to be even hearing my boss's name, and the anger arises in my mind from the storehouse of latent impressions. Conversely, if I were to stop thinking angry thoughts when I interact with my boss and, instead, replace them with a feeling of calmness, then gradually the latent impression of anger would weaken. I would, in time, be able to replace the cycle of anger with a cycle of calmness. This is, of course, not easy but is usually meaningful, both personally and professionally; a practice like this has the capacity to completely transform one's life and pain/disease cycle.

THE PSYCHOLOGICAL TOOLS OF YOGA

Numerous methods and practices in Yoga have a psychological basis. Among them, a few are universal and foremost.

- **Embodiment:** Because our state of mind is continuously reflected in our body and breath, movement and breathing form a strong platform to support any desired psychological change when done with awareness.
- **Minding the mind and mindfulness:** Being watchful of the content of the mind and the thoughts and feelings that pass through it forms the foundation for creating changes in the mind. Meditation and mindfulness are related practices as both are based on directing one's attention.

- **Opposing negative thoughts:** Giving in to negative thinking based on our emotions creates a cycle of support for negative emotions with verbalized thoughts. When we are depressed, we may tell ourselves that we are useless and life does not have anything to offer us. These negative thoughts should be noted and opposed.
- **Creating positive thoughts and emotions:** Emotions such as gratitude, kindness, and friendliness are powerful determinants of our quality of life and our relationships. Nurturing them appropriately can greatly enhance our life experience and remove psychological problems.
- **Mantra meditation and/or chanting:** Found in most meditation traditions across the world, the use of sound and chanting helps cut off the pointless internal dialogue of the mind and serve as an anchor to focus the mind on the desired change.
- **Rituals and sacredness:** Devotion and surrender to a higher power (or if one is not inclined in that direction, the creation of specialness or sacredness around the practice) also has a profound impact on the mind. This may be cultivated consciously in the Yoga practice, or in rituals designed specifically for that purpose, and then that attitude can be transferred into daily life activities.

CASE REVIEW: DEPRESSION

Rachel, thirty-five, works as a part-time web designer at a small company and has had a long history of chronic mild depression with two severe episodes in her twenties. She suffered from postpartum depression after the birth of her two children, who are now seven and ten, respectively. Most of the time, she experiences low mood and low energy, has a reluctance to engage in social activity, and a lack of joy in life. Her husband is supportive, and she has a stable family life, but she is currently on medication because her moods fluctuate so often. She was consulting a psychotherapist some years ago but has discontinued her sessions since then, even though she is aware that her problem persists. A hallmark of depression, she finds herself thinking negative thoughts about her life and herself, even though there is nothing in particular that is problematic. As of now, she is not doing any exercise consistently. Yet, Rachel would like to try Yoga Therapy to see if it could help her remain in a better continued state of mind overall, or, at the very least, she would like to make the effort for the sake of her family.

Our Approach

Rachel's motivation is reasonably good, which is often the first barrier. Exercise has been found to be a good antidepressant. Working from the body, the sense of heaviness and lethargy that accompanies depression can be combated by introducing an āsana practice with a vinyāsa background moving freely with the breath. Moving the body and the breath in this way forms a solid foundation on which the practice of mindfulness can be anchored. While doing the āsana practice, Karen had the possibility to watch the body and breath as well as the mind without getting caught up or carried away by the contents of the mind.

Next, we focused on opposing the negative thoughts in the mind by identifying the common pattern of ruminating on negative thoughts about herself, her life, and others around her. When she found herself engaged in these thoughts, the practice of pratipakṣa bhāvana (cultivating the opposite and reminding herself that these thoughts are neither true nor useful) provided Rachel with a rational basis for her to oppose the thoughts and seek to remove them from the mind.

Another very useful practice for her was meditation with a mantra. Choosing a mantra or affirmation like "I am strong from within," or "I find value and meaning in life," is helpful in retraining the mind.

In addition, we suggested the practice of mindfully appreciating the small things in life, whenever the possibility suggested itself. For instance, she was able to mindfully savor the moments with her children or other family members that she found enjoyable.

Useful Āsanas and Prāṇāyāma

In this case, we used anuloma ujjāyi or nāḍi-śodhana-prāṇāyāma as a seated breathing practice and relaxed ujjāyi breathing during her āsana practice. The following āsanas were also used as therapeutic treatments:

- A few rounds of dynamic, flowing **sun salutations** as a warm up.
- **Warrior sequence** and **chest opening** formed a key part of her practice, as an opposition to the slumped spine posture of depression, and to energize the body and mind by engaging the large muscles of legs, hips, and torso.
- **Inversions** in moderation, one of the days she felt like doing them, to give her a sense of calm.

- A simple **forward bend** and **lying twist** to conclude her practice, not staying for long in either.

Environment

Rachel was told to avoid situations that she finds particularly depressing, particularly periods of rumination where she does not have an activity and tends to sink into a depressive mood. We encouraged her to adopt a change in environment—a new activity or meeting friends or extended family—on a regular basis, at least once a month.

Ayurveda

To support the positive mental changes, Rachel began to make changes in her lifestyle like bringing regularity to waking and sleep times and avoiding overeating and heavy foods. Using gently warming and aromatic herbs such as ginger, long pepper, and holy basil was also recommended along with other more specifically useful herbs such as brahmi, shankhapushpi, and ashvagandha.

CONCLUSION

The aim of Svastha Yoga is holistic health. We do not conceive of Svastha Yoga as a "style" of practicing Yoga; rather, Svastha Yoga is doing Yoga in a way that helps to lead *you,* the individual, toward svāsthya (the state of well-being in body and mind). The foundation for these teachings rests on four pillars. One, the teachings of the great yogī Krishnamacharya. Two, the wisdom of classical Yoga, especially from the *Yoga Sūtras of Patañjali.* Three, the substantial knowledge base and concepts of Ayurveda. And four, integration with modern medicine.

Our vision of Svastha Yoga is dynamic and inclusive, combining clinical pragmatism and traditional depth to provide each individual with what they need most for their health. Nevertheless, in this process, we are always reminded that health is a moving target; Yoga and Ayurveda play a part, but so do many other modalities. Holistic health requires knowing not only strengths but also limitations. Thus, the goal of svāsthya can be met only by working together across boundaries with different practitioners and health specialties, coming together to serve the holistic needs of the individual.

The American Viniyoga Institute

Gary Kraftsow, M.A., and Clare Collins, Ph.D.

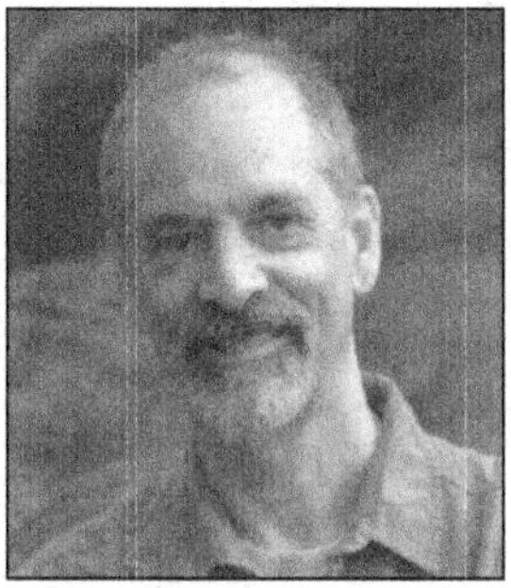

Gary Kraftsow has been a pioneer in the transmission of Yoga for health, healing, and personal transformation for more than thirty years. His journey as a Yoga student, practitioner, teacher, therapist, and teacher of Yoga teachers and therapists began at age nineteen when he traveled to Madras, now Chennai, India, to study Śaiva Siddhānta, the Śaiva Tantra of south India, with the respected mystic/scholar, V. A. Devasenapathi, and Yoga with T. K. V. Desikachar, son and student of T. Krishnamacharya. Gary is the founder of the American Viniyoga Institute (AVI) and author of *Yoga for Wellness* and *Yoga for Transformation.*

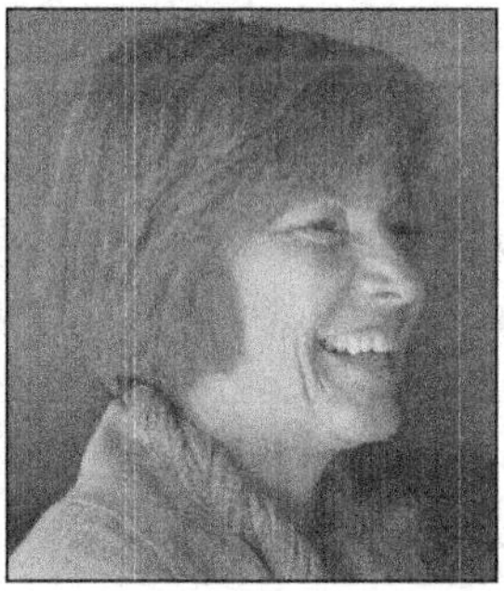

Clare Collins has been practicing and teaching Yoga Therapy since 2003. She is a senior faculty member at the American Viniyoga Institute and a training coordinator of the AVI Yoga Therapist Training Program. She is a Professor Emeritus of Nursing at Michigan State University and a Fellow of the American Academy of Nursing.

OVERVIEW

The American Viniyoga Institute (AVI) is an organization of practitioners and professionals sharing core values, guided by the spirit of Viniyoga, and dedicated to offering quality experiential educational and professional training opportunities in the fields of health and fitness, therapy and self-care, and personal growth and transformation. AVI began as Maui Yoga Therapy in 1983 in Makawao, Hawaii. Several years later, at T. K. V. Desikachar's request, the name was changed to the American Viniyoga Institute to more accurately reflect the intention and scope of its work. AVI currently offers 200-, 300-, and 500-hour certification programs for Yoga teachers, and a 1,000-hour certification program for Yoga Therapists. The AVI Viniyoga Therapist Training Program is a clinical training program that educates experienced Yoga teachers in the theory, principles, adaptation, and application of the tools of Yoga for individuals and groups with health conditions.

In this chapter, we will present the hallmarks of the Viniyoga approach and the philosophical perspective underlying our approach to Yoga and Yoga Therapy. We will discuss the relevance of our approach to Yoga teachers and Yoga Therapists and describe key elements of the Viniyoga Therapist Training Program. Last, we will summarize current research on the Viniyoga approach as well as the future direction of our program.

THE VINIYOGA APPROACH

The Viniyoga approach evolved out of the teachings transmitted by T. Krishnamacharya and T. K. V. Desikachar of Chennai, India. *Viniyoga* is an ancient Sanskrit term that implies differentiation, adaptation, and appropriate application. As a style of practice, Viniyoga refers to an approach to Yoga that adapts the various means and methods of practice to the unique condition, needs, and interests of the individual. As a result, each practitioner is given the tools to individualize and actualize the process of self-discovery and personal transformation. The central features of the Viniyoga approach to Yoga and Yoga Therapy are discussed extensively in books by Kraftsow and in the articles listed in the reference section of this chapter. The specific application of the Viniyoga approach to structural, physiological, and emotional health issues is the focus of the AVI Viniyoga Therapist Training Program.

A TRIBUTE TO T. K. V. DESIKACHAR BY GARY KRAFTSOW

I first became a student of T. K. V. Desikachar in 1974. Desikachar had been a dedicated student of his father, T. Krishnamacharya, since childhood. His formal education was in Western science, and he graduated with a degree in structural engineering. The confluence of his lifelong immersion in Vedic teachings, his education in Western science, and his training as an engineer made Desikachar uniquely qualified to adapt and transmit the ancient science of Yoga Therapy into the modern world.

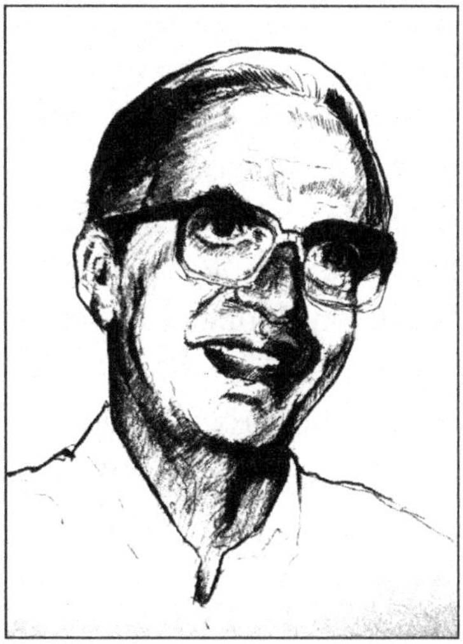

T. K. V. Desikachar

I was an undergraduate student at Colgate University when I began studying with Desikachar. Early on in my studies, Desikachar initiated me in a personal practice that included āsana (posture), prāṇāyāma (breathing practices), mantra japa (mantra repetition), chanting of the *Yoga Sūtras* and sections from the *Upaniṣads,* and meditation. As I went on to graduate school in religious studies at University of California–Santa Barbara, Desikachar encouraged me to study Ayurveda as well as the modern fields of biology and psychology. He had earlier predicted that I would make my career bridging Yoga and Yoga Therapy with modern health care. Toward that end, he taught me vijñāna darśana (the art and science of observation)—how to assess what was happening in my students at the anatomical, physiological, and psychological levels. He also taught me how to understand what I was observing in the context of the student's lifestyle, family life, and social context. He trained me to *see,* to understand what I was seeing, and, on the basis of that understanding, to adapt and apply relevant practices to help an individual reduce his/her suffering, manage symptoms, and achieve his/her goals through personal practice.

Desikachar's ability to observe deeply never ceased to amaze me. His practical perspective on the meaning and purpose of Yoga teachings and practices made his work accessible, relevant, and effective for all who came to learn from him. He initiated me into the *Yoga Vidyā,* the "living body" of yogic knowledge and taught me how to understand and apply its teachings and practices—for myself as well as my students—and taught me the importance of *observation* as well as the skills to observe myself and others. Importantly, he taught me how to access the insight and transformational power of the wisdom of the ancients through inner practice. His teachings are the inspiration for my life work, and I will be forever grateful for his presence in my life.

YOGA THERAPY DEFINED

Yoga Therapy, derived from the Yoga tradition of Patañjali and the Ayurvedic system of health, refers to the adaptation and application of Yoga techniques and practices to help individuals facing health challenges at any level reduce suffering, manage symptoms, improve function, and shift perspective on themselves and their condition. Our approach to Yoga Therapy is to treat the whole person (see the figure below), who is seeking to change attitudes and actions that inhibit the natural healing process, and to cultivate attitudes and actions that support it.

The general long-term goals of Yoga Therapy include:

- Reducing the symptoms of suffering that can be reduced
- Managing the symptoms that cannot be reduced
- Rooting out causes wherever possible
- Improving life function
- Shifting attitude and perspective in relationship to life's challenges

We refer to our approach to Yoga Therapy as Viniyogatherapy™. A central feature of our approach is that we work comprehensively, addressing musculoskeletal, physiological, and emotional conditions though the use of strategies derived from the Yoga tradition. Whereas many Yoga Therapy training programs emphasize only musc loskeletal health, our program contains equivalent focus on physiological and em tional health. Our goal is to train Yoga Th apists who can work in diverse sett including Yoga schools, independent pr healthcare settings, and community-based programs. In the next sections, we will summarize

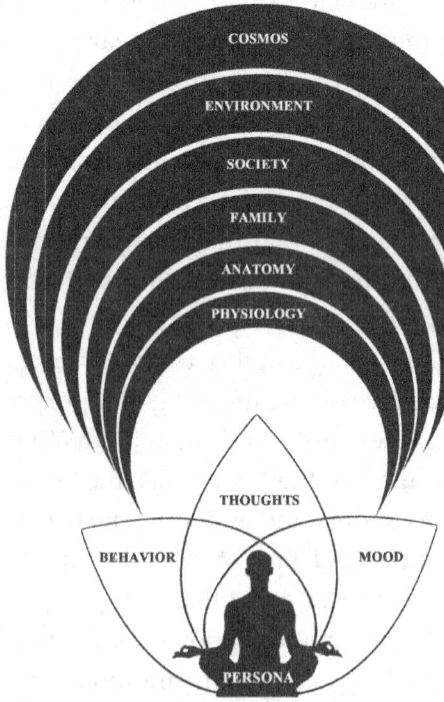

A Multidimensional Approach

the key insights from the Vedic tradition and foundation principles that form the basis of the AVI approach to Yoga and Yoga Therapy.

VEDIC PERSPECTIVES

The foundational insights from the Vedic traditions that inform the perspective of Yoga, Yoga Therapy, and Ayurveda include the ideas of ātman (pure consciousness) and Brahman (absolute reality); the reality of dukha (suffering); the quest for vidyā (knowledge) that would take one beyond suffering; sādhana (the path of practice) through which transformation occurs; and several multidimensional models of the human system including pañca vāyu (five winds) and pañca maya (five dimensions). Patañjali's dualistic model of puruṣa (the seer) and prakṛti (the seen) informs the perspective of a Yoga Therapist. Ultimately, the person (ātman or puruṣa) is not their symptoms or diagnosis (prakṛti).

Building on this foundation, the Yoga tradition affirms that who we are in essence is an unchanging source of pure awareness known as the ātman or puruṣa that dwells within a changing multidimensional universe called prakṛti. *Puruṣa,* translated from Sanskrit as "city dweller," lives within the manifest multidimensional universe and includes aspects that we normally consider to be part of our self, such as our thoughts, feelings, and physical body, as well as those things that we normally consider external to our being, such as our family, social networks, and the natural world. According to this view, the entirety of manifest existence beyond ātman (our essential Self) is composed of ephemeral convergences within a vast field of ongoing change. Fundamentally, Yoga affirms that we are not these changing things and that our suffering comes from our mistaken identification with, and attachment to, them.

On a practical level, Yoga teaches that through the application of intelligence, which is an innate quality of puruṣa (pure undifferentiated awareness), and appropriate methods, we can influence the direction of change in each of these dimensions. As we refine our relationships within each dimension, we begin to see with more and more clarity *who we truly are,* rather than remaining in our misidentification with and attachment to changing internal conditions and external circumstances and thus stay stuck in suffering (Kraftsow, 2002; 2011). These concepts form the basis for the Viniyoga approach to Yoga Therapy.

PHILOSOPHICAL PERSPECTIVE: A MULTIDIMENSIONAL APPROACH TO YOGA THERAPY

A foundational principle for assessment and treatment in the Viniyoga Therapy approach is the recognition of our multidimensional nature. These dimensions of thought, mood, behavior, the body's physiology, the physical body itself, family, society, the physical environment, and the surrounding cosmos can be represented as spheres that overlap and interpenetrate one another (see the figure on page 472). This multidimensional model, used in the AVI Therapist training program, is an extrapolation and synthesis of teachings implicit in Vedic and Western models of the human system. Each sphere carries the potential to affect and be affected by each of the other spheres. The innermost essence of who we are, puruṣa (pure undifferentiated awareness), dwells within and pervades each of these dimensions (Kraftsow, 2011–2012).

THE SPHERES OF THE SELF

The first three overlapping spheres constitute svabhāva (our basic human character) and sense of self. The ancient sages devised methods and a practice-based process called sādhana to help us break our identification with changing experience, see things clearly as they are, and gain the insight that leads to freedom. As our sādhana (practice) advances, svabhāva (self-identity) becomes progressively purified and transparent until it becomes emptied, revealing svarūpa (our true nature, the power of pure awareness). Until then, our svabhāva is formed by three interpenetrating aspects, thought, mood, and behavior, each of which is influenced by our memories and conditioning. When an event triggers a reaction in one dimension, it can drive activity in another.

The thought sphere represents our self-concept, values, priorities, and all of our conceptualization about the world in which we live, including our relationships with those ideas. Our goal in Yoga is to attain clarity of thought, which requires wisdom and discrimination. Traditional yogic methods for cultivating wisdom and the ability to discriminate include vicāra (inquiry), svadhyāya (self-reflection), and various forms of meditation supported by the study of sacred texts.

The mood sphere represents our emotional responses to changing internal conditions and external circumstances. Our moods are profoundly influenced by both our conscious memories and as our unconscious conditioning. This sphere is further influenced by changing thoughts and behaviors and can, in turn, influence each of these spheres. Traditional yogic methods of working within the mood sphere include meditation, chanting, mantra japa with an emphasis on artha (meaning) and bhāva (feeling or attitude), prayer, saṅga (right relationships), and satsaṅga (association with what is ultimately true). These methods help cultivate prema (love) and ānanda (bliss).

The behavior sphere represents our habitual addictive patterns as well as our intentional activity. As with the other spheres, our behavior is profoundly influenced by our conscious memories and unconscious conditioning. It is also influenced by our changing thoughts and moods, which, in turn, influence our experience in each of these spheres. Intention and strength of will underlie behavior. Saṁkalpa (determination) implies the ability to strengthen our will and to set and activate an intention. Saṁkalpa is the foundation of all Yogic practice. Determination is what helps us overcome our habits and develop our capacity for impulse control. Traditional methods of activating intention and strengthening will involve practices that are done consciously through sustained effort with an emphasis on tapas (discipline) and self-restraint. For example, this might include giving something up that we are habituated to, such as a particular type of food. These methods may include mantra japa and ritual activities among other practices.

The three spheres above interpenetrate and influence each other and each is profoundly affected and even driven by our conscious memories and unconscious conditioning. One of the fundamental goals in Yoga and Yoga Therapy is to become free from the twisted journey of our thoughts, feelings, desires, conflicts, distractions, and habitual and dysfunctional behavioral patterns, all of which dissipate our energy.

Toward this end, Yoga places a great deal of importance on purifying our memory and elevating our unconscious conditioning to the level of the conscious mind. Bringing these unconscious impressions and impulses into the conscious realm is the first step toward freeing us from their influence. The integrated practice of linking breath, sound, meaning, and feeling through prāṇāyāma, meditation, and mantra japa helps us harness and powerfully direct the totality of our undissipated energy toward deep transformation.

The dynamic interplay among the three internal spheres influences and is influenced by the next sphere: physiology. The physiological sphere represents the bodily systems, including the sympathetic and parasympathetic function of the autonomic nervous system (ANS), which is of particular importance to Yoga. The ANS, along with the endocrine system, regulates other physiological functions of the body such as digestion, respiration, and cardiovascular rhythms. The sympathetic function is the fight-or-flight response, activated when we perceive danger. The parasympathetic function is the rest-and-repose mode activated when we are at rest. The yogic insight about the mind-body relationship coincides with the modern field of psychoneuroimmunology and shows how our ANS responds profoundly to the inner spheres, including our changing thoughts, emotions, and behavior as well as the outer spheres beyond our physiology.

The most potent traditional methods of working with the physiological sphere are controlled breath in āsana and prāṇāyāma and forms of relaxation including Yoga nidrā. In the dimension of physiology, breath work can help to improve respiratory fitness, balance cardiovascular rhythm, stimulate immune function, and promote sympathetic/parasympathetic regulation (Kraftsow, 1999; 2002; Wolever, 2012), among other benefits. In addition, there are teachings and practices about the conscious use of dietary restrictions, as well as the use of cleansing techniques and herbal preparations.

The next sphere comprises our anatomy and represents our physical structure, encompassing the musculoskeletal and neuromuscular systems. This includes the somatic nervous system (also called the voluntary nervous system), which enables us to react consciously to environmental changes. As with the physiological sphere, the condition of our anatomical sphere is profoundly influenced by all of the inner spheres as well as the outer spheres beyond our anatomy. Āsana is the traditional primary yogic method of working with the anatomical sphere (Kraftsow, 2010). Among other benefits, āsana can help improve structural or skeletal alignment, increase structural stability, release chronic muscular contractions, strengthen what's weak, and develop better functional movement patterns.

The remaining four spheres represent increasingly external dimensions of human experience. These dimensions are described in detail in other writings (Kraftsow, 2011–2012; Dubrovsky, 2009).

RELEVANCE OF YOGA THERAPY IN MODERN TIMES

Although Yoga Therapy is a new and emerging profession in the modern world, its roots reach back thousands of years into Vedic teachings and science. From the depth of their own inner journey, the sages of old brought forth profound insights about the nature of the human condition, as well as extensive teachings and powerful practices about understanding and transforming suffering at every level.

Yoga Therapy has a vital role to play in overcoming some of the challenges in modern Western health care. That role, in part, lies in helping to shift the paradigm from one based on illness and practitioner-oriented care to a paradigm based instead on wellness and holistic self-care. The Yoga community has both a tremendous opportunity and a responsibility to bring forward teachings in a credible and legitimate way (Kraftsow, 2010). Our ability to meet that responsibility is, in part, dependent on our commitment to studying these teachings, reflecting on their insightful implications, and experiencing their transformational potential through practice (Kraftsow, 2011–2012).

RELEVANCE TO YOGA TEACHERS, YOGA THERAPISTS, AND YOGA THERAPY CLIENTS

In AVI Yoga teacher training programs, we educate Yoga teachers about the principles of the Viniyoga approach, the philosophical tradition underlying the approach, and specific tools (asana, prāṇāyāma, meditation, chanting, and ritual) that can be used in both Yoga teaching and the Yoga Therapist role. The prerequisite to enrollment in the AVI Viniyoga Therapist Program is completion of AVI's 300- or 500-hour Yoga teacher training certification program. The AVI Viniyoga Therapist Program helps students deepen their understanding of these tools and teaches skills in clinical assessment, clinical decision making, and appropriate application of Yoga to specific conditions. An important element of both our teacher training and therapist training programs is our emphasis on the personal practice of the Yoga teacher and Yoga Therapist as a tool for self-awareness and personal growth.

A Viniyoga therapist is trained in the process of assessing a client's condition; uncovering the client's goals relative to their condition; development of treatment strategies; empowering their clients to engage in consistent personal practice; and helping their clients build a balanced perspective of themselves in relation to their own conditions.

We educate our therapists that the goal of practice is not about teaching our clients to master the various methods of practice, but rather to master themselves.

With that as a goal, we adapt the Yoga methods to suit the needs of the clients and educate the clients to understand how they can apply the methods to manage their own condition.

For the Yoga Therapy client, Viniyogatherapy empowers them to play a greater role in their own health care. Three critical parts in this process include:

1. **Self-observation** training through which an individual becomes conscious of how his/her actions influence the condition. This self-observation extends from neuromuscular movement patterns to patterns of eating, exercising, and sleeping, patterns of emotional reactivity, and habits of thought and behavior.

2. **Behavioral modification** through which an individual begins the process of transformation. This involves saṁyoga (engaging in beneficial associations, practices, and behaviors) and viyoga (eliminating dysfunctional associations, habits, and activities).

3. **Adaptation of the methods of practice** to keep them interesting and relevant to the individual's changing condition through time.

VINIYOGATHERAPY: ASSESSMENT AND TREATMENT APPROACHES

AVI is committed to educating professionals in the breadth of Yoga teachings and practices, training them to assess their clients at a multidimensional level, develop short- and long-term treatment goals and strategies, creatively adapt and apply appropriate methods, and empower their clients to engage in personal practice. As a baseline, all trainees are competent to work with clients at the structural, physiological, and psychosocial levels. They understand how to adapt and appropriately apply āsana, prāṇāyāma, bandha (specialized psychophysical practices), sound and chanting, relaxation, self-reflection, meditation, mantra (sacred words or syllables to access higher potential), tantra (a system of yogic philosophy, practices, and ritual oriented toward worldly achievement and/or liberation), prayer, and personal ritual. At the same time, we encourage each trainee to specialize in areas of interest or expertise, whether it is system specific, such as anatomy or physiology; condition specific, such as asthma or depression; or demographic specific, such as children or seniors.

To help therapists learn to assess their clients, they are trained in Western models and science, particularly anatomy, pathophysiology, psychology, and treatment approaches. They are also trained thoroughly in Vedic models of science, particularly the guṇas (attributes or qualities of materiality), doṣas (quality of physical body, and cakras (energy centers lying within the subtle body). They are taught methods to assess clients at a multidimensional level through the use of observation, intake, and questioning, and by reading the body through the use of breath and movement diagnosis.

Case study examples of assessment and treatment approaches using Viniyoga principles can be found in numerous publications by AVI founder, Gary Kraftsow, and others. For example, *Yoga for Wellness* (Kraftsow, 1999) includes extensive case studies of Yoga approaches to clients with specific structural, physiological, and emotional conditions. Recent publications include specific applications for clients with allergies (Kelley, 2004), chronic fatigue syndrome (Kraftsow, 2007), depressed mood (Kraftsow, 2011–2012), and life-threatening illness (Dubrovsky, 2009).

CLINICAL RESEARCH FINDINGS

Recent biomedical research supports the efficacy of the Viniyoga approach for the treatment of low back pain, workplace stress, and cancer. We have been honored to participate in the development of the Yoga protocols for these projects, as well as the implementation phases for workplace stress reduction and cancer studies.

In two large-scale, randomized clinical trials on chronic low back pain (Sherman, et al., 2005; Sherman, et al., 2010; Sherman, et al., 2011), a twelve-week standardized Viniyoga program was found to be comparable in effectiveness to a physical therapy–based stretching program of similar intensity. In an editorial following the publication of the Sherman study, Timothy Carey, M.D., M.P.H., recommends that healthcare professionals consider both Yoga and PT-based stretching programs as effective treatment approaches, provided the group-based programs contain similar features as those included in the clinical trial (Carey, 2011).

In a multisite study of workplace stress reduction, a twelve-week Viniyoga intervention was found to be comparable in effectiveness to a mindfulness-based approach to stress reduction. The rationale for the use of the Viniyoga approach and the specific emphasis of the Yoga protocol are detailed in articles by Wolever and Bobinet, et al., 2012; and Kusnick, Kraftsow, and Hilliker, 2012.

In the area of cancer care, Fouladbakhsh conducted a study of the effectiveness of a Viniyoga-based intervention in easing breathing distress among patients with lung cancer (Fouladbakhsh, 2013). The National Cancer Institute (NCI) has recently funded a multisite clinical trial to further test the efficacy of this treatment approach in a large sample of patients with lung cancer (Fouladbakhsh, 2013; personal communication).

CONCLUSION

The Viniyoga approach to Yoga Therapy offers a comprehensive, multidimensional approach deeply rooted in the teachings and practices of traditional Yoga and Ayurveda. Our goal is to prepare Yoga Therapists to practice in diverse settings, whether in private practice or in a hospital or holistic clinic. We train our graduates to work in a complementary fashion with their client's primary caregivers. Our training incorporates biomedical perspectives from contemporary health care, enabling our graduates to understand the conditions, diagnoses, and treatments their clients may bring to them from other healthcare practitioners—and how to shape their treatment strategies while safely respecting that information. At the same time, we are working hard to establish a condition-specific research base, documenting the effectiveness of Viniyogatherapy in a broad range of conditions.

As of October 2013, 120 students have been certified as Yoga Therapists through the AVI and 158 are currently enrolled in various stages of our training program. Our training programs continue to evolve as we incorporate new perspectives, teaching strategies, and mentoring processes to enhance the educational experience of our Yoga Therapy students. We are enthusiastic about the potential of our approach to help clients manage their own conditions, reduce suffering, and improve their quality of life through Yoga.

REFERENCES

Carey, T. "Comparative Effectiveness Studies in Low Back Pain: Progress and Goals." *Archives of Internal Medicine* 171.22 (2011): 2026–2027. Print.

Dubrovsky, A. "Radical Healing: Yoga with Gary Kraftsow." *Yoga Plus Joyful Living* (Spring 2009): 38–43. Print.

Fouladbakhsh, J. M., et al. "Honoring the Spirit of Research Within: The Yoga and More (CAM) Research Interest Group." *Journal of Nursing Education and Practice* 2.3 (2013): 132. Print.

Kraftsow, G. *Yoga for Wellness: Healing with the Timeless Tradition of Viniyoga*. New York: Penguin, 1999. Print.

——. *Yoga for Transformation: Ancient Teachings and Holistic Practices for Healing Body, Mind and Heart.* New York: Penguin Compass, 2002. Print.

——. "Righting the Balance of Emotional Well-Being." *Yoga International* (Winter 2011–2012): 48–56. Print.

——. "Asana as a Tool: A Viniyoga Approach." *Integral Yoga Magazine* (Summer 2010): 22–23. Print.

——. "A Living Healing Tradition." *Yoga International* Winter (2010): 32–37. Print.

——. "Defining Yoga Therapy: A Call to Action." *International Journal of Yoga Therapy* 20 (2010): 12–14. Print.

Kusnick, C., G. Kraftsow, and M. Hilliker. "Building Bridges for Yoga Therapy Research: The Aetna, Inc. Mind-Body Pilot Study on Chronic and High Stress." *International Journal of Yoga Therapy* 22 (2012): 91–92. Print.

——. In "Chronic Fatigue Syndrome" (Chapter 14). *Yoga as Medicine: The Yogic Prescription for Health and Healing*, Timothy McCall. New York: Bantam Dell, 2007, 243–260. Print.

Sherman, K., et al. "Comparison of Yoga Versus Stretching for Chronic Low Back Pain: Protocol for the Yoga Exercise Self-Care (YES)." *Trials* 11 (2010): 36. Print.

Sherman, K., et al. "Comparing Yoga, Exercise, and a Self-Care Book for Chronic Low Back Pain: A Randomized, Controlled Trial." *Annals of Internal Medicine* 143.12 (2005): 849–856. Print.

Sherman, K. J., et al. "A Randomized Trial Comparing Yoga, Stretching, and a Self-Care Book for Chronic Low Back Pain." *Archives of Internal Medicine* 171.22 (2011): 2019–2026. Print.

Wolever, R.Q., et al. "Effective and Viable Mind-Body Stress Reduction in the Workplace: A Randomized Controlled Trial." *Journal of Occupational Health Psychology* 17.2 (2012): 246–258. Print.

The Breathing Project

Leslie Kaminoff

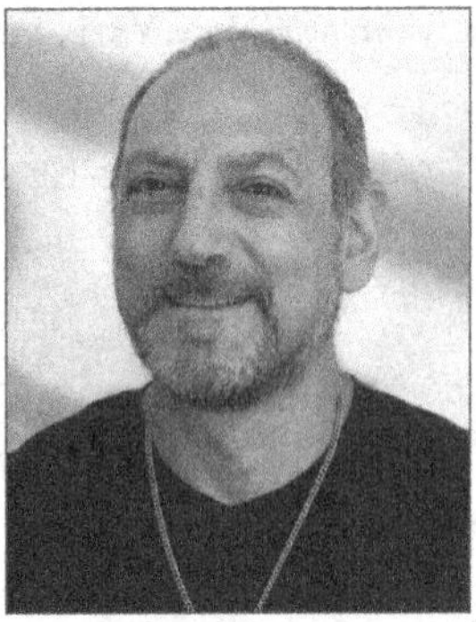

Leslie Kaminoff is a Yoga educator inspired by the tradition of T. K. V. Desikachar. He is recognized internationally as a specialist in the fields of Yoga, breath anatomy, and bodywork. For over three decades he has led workshops and developed specialized education for many leading Yoga associations, schools, and training programs in America and throughout the world. Leslie is the founder of The Breathing Project, a New York City–based educational nonprofit dedicated to teaching individualized, breath-centered Yoga. Leslie created and teaches The Breathing Project's unique yearlong course in Yoga anatomy, also available online at yogaanatomy.net. He is the coauthor, with Amy Matthews, of the bestselling book *Yoga Anatomy*. You can follow him on Twitter (@lkaminoff), Facebook (LeslieKaminoffYogaAnatomy), and on YouTube (YogaAnatomy), and learn more at YogaAnatomy.org.

INTRODUCTION

In December 2001, I founded The Breathing Project, a New York nonprofit educational corporation, after a four-year hiatus from teaching group classes or trainings while focusing primarily on my private Yoga and bodywork. Like many others who were deeply affected that year by the events of September 11, I took stock of my life and priorities and decided that I needed to get back to teaching. By any reasonable standard, it was an insane time to take on such a big commitment scarcely three months since the 9/11 attacks. Most everyone I knew was still in a state of shock, my private practice was down about 50 percent, my close friend Michael Hoffman[1] had just died after a protracted illness, and I was about to begin the task of writing my first book.

On the other hand, it was the perfect time. I was feeling an urgent need to teach, to begin writing about Yoga, the breath, and the body, and to transmit what I'd learned through my studies with my teacher T. K. V. Desikachar. I was also feeling an urgent need to teach and work out of a larger space in order to reach a larger community. As recent events had just proven, life can be unexpectedly short, so whatever risk I faced pursuing my dreams was nothing compared to the risk of putting off that pursuit.

The Breathing Project hosted its first official public event on May 30, 2002, a Vedic chanting concert with Desikachar and his family. The concert was a big success, playing to a full house at the Advent Lutheran Church at 93rd and Broadway. This was followed by a remarkable ten-month discussion with other teachers deeply influenced by our tradition who were likewise eager to create the first New York City studio dedicated to teaching the individualized, breath-centered principles of Yoga in the tradition of Desikachar and Krishnamacharya. Our real estate search resulted in a beautiful, light-filled open space at 15 West 26th Street in Manhattan, which we opened on March 13, 2003 (my forty-fifth birthday!), and this is the space that the Breathing Project still occupies today. At the Breathing Project, it is our mission/intention to create innovative learning opportunities based on experiences of body, breath, and mind. We teach principles of human structure and movement in relationship to the individual nature of every body.

A PROCESS OF REJUVENATION

I can't think of a better way to introduce some of the insights I've gained over the past thirty-five years working as a Yoga educator and bodyworker than by honoring my teacher, T. K. V. Desikachar with great humility and gratitude.

When I teach workshops about the healing potential of Yoga, I play a section of a 1996 documentary I helped to produce in which Desikachar talks about the students who show up at the Krishnamacharya Yoga Mandiram seeking help. His simple words express very beautifully the essence of how Yoga can help:

---

1. Michael Hoffman was the executive director of the Aperture Foundation, the original publishers of *Health Healing and Beyond: Yoga and the Living Tradition of Krishnamacharya*, a remarkable book that came into being when I introduced Michael to Desikachar.

> The most important problem is suffering. When somebody suffers, they cannot meditate, they cannot worship, they cannot pray. When these people suffer, and they go to the usual system of healthcare and it doesn't work, they suffer more. For some reason, the usual system of medical and healthcare is not able to understand the person who is suffering. They know a lot about the problem . . . they know a lot about the disease . . . they know a lot about illness . . . it's amazing how much they know, but the relationship between this illness and the person is not so much emphasized. So, when the person goes to all these people and still they are not better, they become desperate. It's not just illness, it's what I call "the relationship to the illness.
>
> We [at KYM] talk to these people. We say, "You have some resources which are not just medicine. There's something you have: you can still breathe . . . you can still talk . . . you can sit and move. That means you still have the energy that can heal you. Let us direct and use this energy . . . who knows? It may do something good" (Desikachar, 1996).

Desikachar goes on in the video to emphasize the importance of the relationship between the student and the teacher:

> Care, love and attention give the student confidence. With a new positive attitude they can begin to work on their body and their breath, which creates a process of rejuvenation. I don't know how it happens . . . it happens. I can't say it's because of this technique or that technique, but it happens, and they subjectively feel better, which makes them feel more confident, which motivates them to do more Yoga more positively, so the healing begins.
>
> Even if they're sick, they feel better, which makes them more prepared for other aspects, like meditation . . . which can lead them to discover important things about themselves. This is Yoga . . . one thing leading to another." (Desikachar, 1996).

REFLECTIONS ON THE TEACHINGS I RECEIVED FROM T. K. V. DESIKACHAR

In both my private practice and in the clinics I lead at The Breathing Project, people with all manner of suffering show up for help. As I meet these people who are seeking healing through Yoga, my unspoken gut reaction is typically, "I'm just a

Yoga teacher . . . not a doctor! Who am I to address this condition?" I regain focus in those moments by remembering my teacher's simple words in the passage above, when he is clearly referring to prāṇa (life force): "You can still talk . . . you can sit and move . . . that means you still have the energy that can heal you."

In my practice, this principle has evolved into a quick checklist for new students: *Are they breathing? Are they able to focus their attention? Can they move their body voluntarily?* If the answers are even a little bit of "yes," then they can practice Yoga and reap immediate benefits. It is my contention that the most profound healing derived from Yoga practice comes from the simplest things we teach, not the most complex. The first, simplest thing that we ask people to do is also the most powerful: bringing the body and mind together through the medium of the breath.

As soon as a person engages in this act of integration, what immediately becomes apparent are any obstacles that make it difficult to coordinate mind, body, and breath. This principle is what allows āsana practice to become a true tool of Yoga. Breath and postural practices help us identify and resolve obstructions to prāṇa—on whatever dimension we may find them. Therefore, Yoga practice is not about doing the āsanas; it's about undoing what's in the way of the āsanas.

Undoing an obstruction lodged in any layer of our system will have an effect on all of the others because we are multidimensional beings inseparably constituted of body, breath, senses, mind, emotions, intellect, and soul. This is the "process of rejuvenation" Desikachar referred to, and, as he said, it is not "because of this technique or that technique," it is because whenever a person attempts to learn a new way of breathing and moving, by definition, they are unlearning their old way of breathing and moving. The result is our internal spaces become more open to the flow of life force. This is why I question the value of becoming obsessed with the minutiae of posture and breath at the expense of this bigger picture. Of course, there are correct ways to do specific exercises and breathing patterns, but the ultimate goal is to gain freedom from our old patterns, not achieve āsana perfection. I see way too many teachers and practitioners who have become trapped in their Yoga-acquired patterns. As Desikachar also said: "Our Yoga practice always has to be a little more clever than our habits" (notes from live lectures, 1988–1997). Yoga is first and foremost about freedom . . . and that includes freedom from the techniques that previously freed us.

THUNDERSTRUCK BY PRACTICALITY

A hallmark of Desikachar's teachings is their uncompromising practicality. In a modern context, it's important to remember that Desikachar, his teacher Krishnamacharya, and his teacher's teacher Sri Rama Mohana Bramachari were all householders, not swamis. The down-to-earth responsibilities of having a job, wife, and children leaves little room for pie-in-the-sky spirituality that characterizes much of the Yoga germinated within the ashramic culture of Vedantic renunciation.

In a 1992 interview with Desikachar, when one of my questions veered into this territory, I received a stunning corrective takedown. We were discussing the nature of dukha (suffering) and how its recognition is a prerequisite for Yoga. I was having trouble with the idea of suffering being any kind of a foundation for my Yoga, so I asked, "What is underneath it all? Which stuff is the basic nature? In consciousness there is no duḥkha, just ānanda (bliss)!"

Becoming very animated, Desikachar exclaimed, "What do I know about basic nature? If somebody told me there is a pot of gold under my house, but I don't even know where my house is, what good is that? Now I suffer more because before, I didn't even know about the gold, and now somebody comes and tells me, 'You've got a pot of gold . . . go and dig it up!' If I don't even know where my house is, maybe I am suffering more because of this pot of gold."

I was thunderstruck! All I could manage to say was, "That is a brilliant analogy. I can see that is the dilemma of most people who—"

Cutting me off, Desikachar leapt in again, "It is not a dilemma . . . it is a fact! The more I tell you, 'there is something deep inside you that is always happy . . . there is always ānanda . . . you are that ānanda . . . your true nature is ānanda . . . ' it makes you feel much worse!"

Eventually, I managed to get back on track by asking what is beyond this dilemma of sukha (good space) and dukha. He answered, "Well, this is a big question, and I agree that Patañjali uses dukha as the first step toward happiness. This is his strategy: 'There is going to be dukha. Don't feel ashamed of that because that is going to take you to a place where you may have less dukha!' This is the fantastic idea of Patañjali . . . that there is nothing to be ashamed of! It is the best thing that can happen to me . . . the moment I recognize I am in trouble!" (Desikachar, 1992).

In the house analogy above, Desikachar was actually referencing an idea about the dispersion of prāṇa that comes from the *Yoga Yajñavalkya*. There, the sage refers to a person in a state of ill health as having some of his prāṇa scattered outside the limits of his physical body; this is the man who Desikachar described as having lost the location of his house. Preaching to him about the splendor of his bliss body is useless until his basic health is restored. Health cannot be returned without concentrating prāṇa within his physical body through the simple tools of breath and movement (*Yoga Yajñavalkya* VI, 35–38). As Desikachar, himself has said, "The recognition of confusion is a form of clarity" (notes from live lectures, 1988–1997), I add the complementary observation that nonrecognition of confusion is the source of all suffering. This is consistent with Patañjali's great teaching from the second chapter in which avidyā (ignorance) is identified as the root cause of all the kleśas (obstructions).

This takes us back to the basic foundations of a breath-centered Yoga practice. When we reduce dukha (bad space), our prāṇa doesn't get pushed to the outside because we've made more sukha (good space) on the inside. Simple, direct, and profoundly practical.

THE FOUNDATIONS OF BREATH-CENTERED YOGA

How do we begin to reduce dukha? We first must recognize that it exists. This isn't always as easy as it sounds because many of our patterns are so deeply ingrained we have a hard time recognizing them. The practice of breath-centered āsana offers immediate and accessible feedback about our habitual ways of using our bodies, breath, and mind.

As I often remind our students at The Breathing Project, if Yoga isn't about doing the āsanas, but about undoing what's in the way of the āsanas, then the same holds true for breathing practices—we learn new ways to breathe so we can unlearn our old ways of breathing. When we combine breath and āsana, we are employing some of our most powerful tools for transformation.

The breath is a great teacher of Yoga practice, as defined by Patañjali: "Tapas svādhyāya īśvara-praṇidhānāni kriyā-yogaḥ" (YS II.1) can shed some light. The first of the three components of this definition is *tapah,* which means to cook, or purify and is often translated as austerity. In practical terms, it simply means working outside our accustomed patterns of habitual behavior (which does involve a considerable amount of friction—thus heat, or cooking).

When tapah is practiced with an attitude of svadhyāya (self-reflection), we begin to discover behaviors that may be obstructing our prāṇa. When truly attentive, we also notice that not everything needs to be or can be changed. Additionally, there are many things, which—by their nature—are actually unchangeable. Recognition of that which is unchangeable is where the third component of kriyā Yoga, īśvara praṇidhāna, guides our actions. *Īśvara praṇidhāna* is commonly translated as "surrender to the lord," but I favor Desikachar's profoundly practical interpretation: "In the final analysis, we are not the masters of all we do . . . " (Desikachar, 1995).

When encountering something over which we have no direct control, the only rational attitude is one of surrender. There is an anatomical basis for this teaching, and it is rooted in the nature of the breath. The human breathing mechanism operates in a delicate balance between voluntary and autonomic behavior. Anyone who's practiced prāṇāyāma as breath "control" knows how limited that control is! Fortunately, Krishnamacharya (the grammarian) reminds us that the yama (restraint) in prāṇāyāma actually derives from the word *ayama,* which means to lengthen, extend, or unobstruct. I suggest there is an equivalence between tapah, yama, and the voluntary aspect of our breathing, and īśvara praṇidhāna, āyāma, and the involuntary aspect of our breathing. I also see an equivalence between kriyā Yoga and Reinhold Niebhur's famous serenity prayer in which we ask for the strength to change the things we can (tapah), the serenity to accept the things we cannot change (īśvara praṇidhāna), and the wisdom to know the difference (svadhyāya). It's not surprising to me that thinkers as diverse as Patañjali and Niebhur came to the same conclusion: nature built these principles into the way life force courses through our bodies, where I believe the original sūtras can be found.

By placing the breath at the core of āsana, prāṇāyāma, and meditation practice, the Krishnamacharya/Desikachar lineage hands us the ultimate tool for both effecting change and gathering feedback about the deepest levels of our system's function. By honoring the breath as our ultimate teacher and guide, we have the power to balance our anatomy and physiology with our Yoga practice.

THE TEACHING OF BREATH-CENTERED YOGA

Based on the principles outlined above, I have developed statements that underpin my teachings at The Breathing Project. I offer them as inspiration for further investigation:

- If a person is breathing, can move their body, and can focus their attention, they can practice Yoga.
- Yoga practice teaches us how to uncover and resolve obstructions to prāṇa (life force).
- Yoga is not about doing the āsanas; it's about undoing what's in the way of the āsanas.
- The maximum benefits of Yoga practice are derived from the simplest things we teach, not the most complex.
- The simplest thing Yoga students are taught is to coordinate long, slow movements of the body with long, slow movements of the breath.
- When you learn a new way of breathing and moving, by definition you are unlearning your old way of breathing and moving.
- The first task with any student is to help him/her more fully inhabit their physical body by drawing his/her prāṇa inward. If he/she can't feel what's happening inside, he/she needs to recognize that.
- Healthy movement is well-distributed movement—i.e., a little bit of movement from a lot of places.
- Unhealthy movement is too much movement coming from too few places, too many times.
- There are no straight lines in the body. All movement exists as three-dimensional spirals moving through three-dimensional space.
- There are no parts in the body; everything is connected to everything else.
- We can find pathways of connection in an infinite variety of ways.
- Changing breathing by definition changes posture . . . and vice versa.
- To get something unusual to move, you need to get usual movements to be still.
- Support starts from the ground up.
- Breath starts from the top down.
- For every movement in the body, there is an opposing movement that travels in the opposite direction.

- Initiating the action of exhaling from the bottom upward can help to ground the feet, legs, and pelvis.
- Initiating the action of inhaling from the top downward can help to generate lift and support for the upper spine, rib cage, and shoulder girdle.
- As important as the details of technique may be in determining outcomes, far more powerful is the quality of relationship between student and teacher.

THE TEACHING RELATIONSHIP

My teacher said that his father, Tirumalai Krishnamacharya, would permit people to address him only as "Professor." Not only did Krishnamacharya reject all other titles, including "Guru," he went so far as to say: "The moment I say I am a Yogi, I am not a Yogi!" (Desikachar, 1992). I have observed Desikachar do many things over the years to deflate authoritarian situations, both publicly and privately.

One of my strongest early impressions of him occurred at a public event—one of a series of large seminars that had been organized by a group of Desikachar's senior students. Viniyoga America had come together, not just for the purpose of bringing Desikachar to the United States to teach, but to form a certification program. I was very keen on getting involved in that program because I was certain this was the tradition in which I wanted to study and the certification program was the way to do it. We were all very excited to begin the training with Desikachar. The year was 1989, and it was the summer after I met him at Colgate University in upstate New York.

However, at the very first meeting of the inaugural weeklong seminar, Desikachar announced he didn't want to have anything to do with a certification. He explained that certification had become an obstacle to having the sort of individual relationships with his students he had enjoyed up to that point. There was something, he had concluded, that was antithetical to these teachings in offering a standardized curriculum to groups of students.

I clearly remember him saying he was feeling constricted because he was now obliged to deal with this thing called Viniyoga America, whereas before it was just his individual students and friends. In addition to scuttling the certification program, he also said he would appreciate it very much if Viniyoga America would dissolve itself. At this point, just about everyone in the room was going a little crazy. These senior students who had been studying with him for years had put tremendous effort into creating Viniyoga America—the seminars and the certification program—and now their teacher was just blowing it all apart!

Desikachar's courage to say "no" to Viniyoga America becoming a certifying organization was clearly a turning point for the entire future of these teachings in America. It sent a clear message that he would honor the essence of his father's tradition, rooted in the value of individualized one-on-one connections between teacher and student.

From that moment on, I have had nothing but the most intense admiration for my teacher. Whenever I've observed Desikachar having an opportunity to step into the role of a guru or have a large organization under him, he went in the other direction. This was his consistent pattern.

As the new kid on the block, I didn't have anything invested in Viniyoga America, and Desikachar's announcement was easy for me to take. I had only wanted to be in the certification because it was a chance to spend time with him. I was certain he wasn't going to stop teaching and I knew I would keep learning from him whenever and whatever he was presenting, which is just what I did.

Desikachar completed his break from Viniyoga years later, shortly after I started The Breathing Project in New York City. In 2003, he sent a message to all his students saying: "If you want to continue to have a connection with me, I request that you stop having a connection with the word *Viniyoga*." I wasn't any more invested in that word than I had been in Viniyoga America or its certification program. It was clear to me he was simply finishing what he had started fifteen years earlier. We dropped use of the word immediately and replaced it with "Breath-Centered Individualized Yoga."

My teacher has a unique connection to each of his students. What shines through in our relationship is the extraordinarily respectful way he's dealt with me. There were several times I desperately wanted him to just give me an answer. I would be struggling mightily with some really fundamental concepts that simply weren't working for me, and all I wanted was to know "the solution" that would end my confusion. In those times, all he would say is, "What does your experience tell you about this issue?" That really wasn't what I wanted in the moment, but it's definitely what I needed to hear in the long term.

This reserve demonstrates Desikachar's extreme maturity as a teacher. As best I can, I aspire to that example in all my interactions with my students. I try to be conscious of putting aside my answers to their questions and attempt to redirect their inquires into themselves. A famous quote from the martial arts innovator Bruce Lee in the September 1971 issue of *Black Belt Magazine* perfectly sums up my experiences learning from Desikachar:

> A teacher, a really good sensei, is never a "giver" of "truth"; he is a guide, a 'pointer' to the truth that the student must discover for himself. A good teacher, therefore, studies each student individually and encourages the student to explore himself, both internally and externally, until, ultimately, the student is integrated with his being. . . . A good teacher is a catalyst. Besides possessing a deep understanding, he must also have a responsive mind with great flexibility and sensitivity (Lee, 1971).

Whenever I was around Desikachar, what I remember the most is the feeling of being absolutely, completely naked. Naked because he sees everything—particularly all the things I work so hard to keep others from seeing. I have always felt completely vulnerable with him because I've known how completely I was being seen; yet because he is such a true teacher, he has never taken advantage of that vulnerability.

HONORING THE INDIVIDUAL

Desikachar's approach to Yoga is rooted in his insistence that the primary vehicle for transmission of teaching is the personal relationship between teacher and student. The Breathing Project's policies and procedures were created to value and honor that relationship by not overly interfering with it. Students have a direct relationship with their teachers. The Breathing Project isn't the kind of studio where a teacher is an employee who can just "punch the clock" and not be involved in promoting their classes. It takes highly motivated, gifted, and entrepreneurial teachers to thrive in this environment and our core teachers are just that.

In particular, Amy Matthews, who subsequently became my partner in writing, teaching, and managing this unique space, consistently embodies the qualities of a teacher who honors individuals. After Desikachar, Amy is the person who has most influenced my own teaching perspective. Aside from being an endless source of detailed anatomical knowledge, Amy is responsible for pushing me to question and define my teaching philosophy on an ongoing basis, bringing to the table her experience teaching, her degree in philosophy, and her extensive study with the founder of Body-Mind Centering, Bonnie Bainbridge Cohen. Through dynamic dialogue (including differing opinions), we challenge each other to refine our concepts and teaching language.

At The Breathing Project, we strive to teach avoiding floating abstractions that can't be grounded or anchored in students' actual embodied experience. For example, some questions regularly posed in class: *Should the breath move from top to bottom or bottom to top? . . . Should the sacrum counter-nutate (where the top part of the sacrum would move down and forward relative to the pelvis) in backward bends? . . . Should the hamstrings stretch in forward bends?* To us, the problematic word in those questions isn't *should,* it's *the.* These kinds of questions suffer from a problem we call "decontextualization." The context of Yoga practice is always an individual human being: breathing, back-bending, and forward-bending are actions people do with their bodies. Any discussion of these activities must start with the actual person doing them. There is no such thing as *the* breath, sacrum, or hamstrings. Putting *the* in front of these words turns them into floating abstractions—ideas that have no actual referent in reality.

Bringing this to the attention of the questioner requires them to rethink some pretty basic premises, primary among them the desire to have a one-size-fits-all rule that works for everyone. At The Breathing Project, a lot of this rethinking happens.

Similarly, we challenge specific therapeutic claims commonly made for āsana practice such as salamba Sarvaṅgāsana (shoulderstand) helps the thyroid . . . virasana (hero's pose) fixes knee problems . . . sālamba śīrṣāsana (headstand) brings more blood to the brain. Aside from being based on shaky understanding of anatomy and physiology, these statements are devoid of context. Claims such as these ascribe intrinsic properties to āsana that if properly "administered" would have the desired, same effect on everyone—regardless of individual differences. Considering such broad declarations aren't even made about meticulously measured pharmaceuticals, how can it be true of Yoga techniques?

Amy illustrated a corollary of this principle a few years ago while revising her brilliant āsana analysis for the second edition of our book *Yoga Anatomy.* She was very excited about a specific word she had been able to completely eliminate from that section: *stretch*! This took me by surprise, and a very interesting conversation ensued. Amy explained the need to differentiate the concept of "lengthening" (a valid description of what a body structure has to do in order to assume a particular āsana) from "stretch" (a subjective description of a sensation, which may or may not arise as a result of that lengthening). Many people won't feel a stretching sensation in their muscles in certain poses. If those students are told they should feel a stretch, they may push themselves into unsafe ranges of motion.

At The Breathing Project, our primary goal is to question whatever interferes with students' ability to embody their own experience and truth. This is more than just a philosophical problem in Yoga language; it's the state of most educational systems. We've been taught to rely on outside authority to know if something is right and appropriate and good enough. As Yoga educators the challenge we face when teaching is to unhook people from some external authority defining what "should" happen or how to do it "right." In the end, only an individual student can decide what is enough, what feels good, and what to avoid. This is what Amy and I refer to as embodiment in the context of Yoga practice. We regularly ask our students to tune into their inner experience as a source of authority and wisdom. We ask them what they are noticing when they practice, especially when a therapeutic outcome is desired.

THERAPY VERSUS EDUCATION

Personally, I'm opposed to the term *Yoga Therapist*. I feel it would be a betrayal of the trust our students have placed in us to turn Yoga Therapy into another healthcare profession. So, I call myself a Yoga Educator since what I do is education, plain and simple. This process of education frequently has a therapeutic outcome, but that has to do with helping people achieve more independence, more embodiment. Once our students gain more sensitivity to what is going on inside, they become far more empowered to deal with whatever obstacles may arise to their own prāṇa, or life force.

In previous writing, I have advocated for the inclusion of Yoga as a subject for study in University education (Kaminoff, 2008). Subsequently, many of my friends who work in academia have enlightened me about the extreme politics and territoriality of the higher education system. I have come to realize that we do not need to make ourselves any more acceptable to the educational institutions of the world than to the healthcare industry. I say we can do better.

My experience of the past few years putting advanced studies courses online has demonstrated that the future of education is in the open, unregulated, free market of ideas that can be instantly accessed. Through the online education Amy and I offer at YogaAnatomy.net, we create tremendous value, interaction, and accountability with a rapidly growing community of students in over forty countries. This exciting frontier provides a vast opportunity to continue sharing Desikachar's teachings at The Breathing Project.

MY WORDS TO DESIKACHAR

On the tenth anniversary of the start of my student-teacher relationship with Desikachar, I had the opportunity to express my gratitude in a letter. My words remain as true today as they were on July 30, 1998 when I wrote the letter:

> Dear Sir,
> It seems hard to believe, but exactly ten years have gone by since our first meeting. I wanted to take this opportunity to let you know how much our association has meant to me. I know that our actual contact over the past decade has been, at best, intermittent—yet for me, our connection has been constant.
>
> The strength of this connection lies in the example you've set in all our dealings together. As I stated during my last visit to the Mandiram, there is something far more important than all the things you've ever said to me, and that is all the things you could have said, but didn't. I am grateful that you have based all your interactions with me on your faith that the answers I seek reside within me—and I am grateful for the times when that faith had to be stronger than my own.
>
> I will treasure for the rest of my life these last ten years as your student.
>
> Thank you.
> Leslie

Urban Zen Integrative Therapy

Rodney Yee and Colleen Saidman Yee

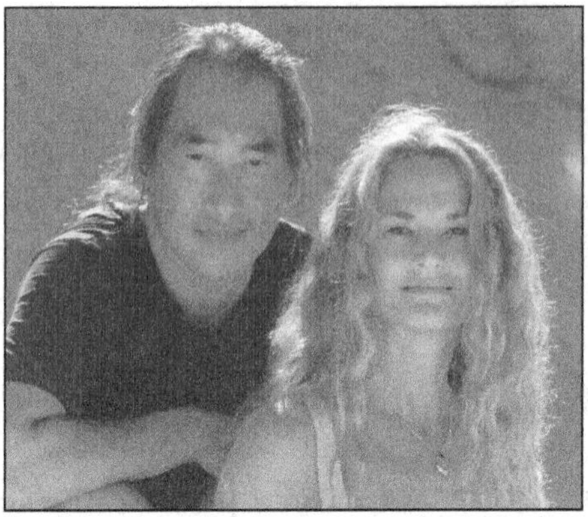

Rodney Yee is the cofounder and former owner of Piedmont Yoga Studio in Oakland, California. He has created dozens of DVDs through the Yoga lifestyle company, Gaiam, and is the author of *Yoga: The Poetry of the Body* and *Moving Toward Balance* (with Nina Zolotow). His wife, **Colleen Saidman Yee**, is a graduate of Jivamukti Yoga's Teacher Training Program and opened Yoga Shanti in Sag Harbor, New York, in 1999. Together, Rodney and Colleen are the coexecutive directors of Donna Karan's Urban Zen Integrative Therapy Program, a 500-hour program that trains therapists to work with patients in hospitals and other settings using five integrative modalities—Yoga Therapy, aromatherapy, Reiki, contemplative end-of-life care, and nutrition. They also helped create and are featured in Gaiam Yoga Studio (www.GaiamYogaStudio.com), an online Yoga club, and they teach workshops, retreats, and teacher trainings worldwide.

INTRODUCTION TO URBAN ZEN INTEGRATIVE THERAPY

There are two major contributions that Yoga can give to the world of medicine: relaxation and mindfulness. In complement to the monumental strides and capabilities of modern medicine, Yoga Therapy can help create the optimum environment for natural healing to take place. Yogic relaxation techniques consist of physically aligned poses and movements, breath exercises, and philosophical shifts of the mind that guide us through complex, convoluted mazes of physical, emotional, and intellectual tensions, which can erect the monoliths of stress and disease. When we evoke and enhance our relaxation response through Yoga, the mind and body work more efficiently toward balance. Similarly, mindfulness techniques focus the power of the mind on the moment-by-moment truth and take away many unnecessary worries. Yogic mindfulness practices consist of meditations that evoke relaxed concentration, broad awareness, and total integration. Collectively, relaxation and mindfulness lead to skill in action and are enhanced by important and accurate observations of oneself and one's world.

On its own, Yoga is a profound mind-body therapy. There are currently a number of pioneers who are setting out to fully integrate Yoga into the health and wellness worlds and are discovering powerful cocktails with revolutionary results in the yogic sciences. Identifying and extracting the Yoga techniques that are relevant to health care and that can be safely utilized by the general public is a daunting task, in and of itself. Alongside that task is the work of understanding and implementing these Yoga techniques into the everyday fabric of the present and future modern healthcare paradigm. This new marriage between conventional medicine and complementary medicine is the future of medicine, and respected in-depth training programs that teach effective, well-tested, and safe techniques that understand how to properly interface with the healthcare industry are invaluable.

After Donna Karan lost her husband to a seven-year battle with lung cancer in 2001, she was inspired to make the complementary health practices that had made the last years of her husband's life more livable and beautiful accessible to all. Donna's life had always been blessed by the best conventional and alternative healthcare professionals and she took this tragedy as an opportunity to rally these experts together in a ten-day Well-Being Conference and to ask them what their vision was for the future of health care. It was from this conference, which housed over a thousand of the best of Western and the best of Eastern healthcare professionals from all over the world, that the foundation of Urban Zen Integrative Therapy was formed.

Urban Zen Integrative Therapy (UZIT), founded in 2007 through the vision of Donna Karan, Colleen Saidman Yee, and Rodney Yee, has developed a methodology that pulls together five different modalities into a comprehensive integrative system that promotes relaxation and mindfulness. These modalities are Yoga Therapy, Reiki, essential oil therapy, nutrition, and contemplative care. The confluence of these therapies exponentially increases the efficacy of each of these amazing care components. Imagine your client in the most precise and supportive restorative pose, inhaling his/her favorite smell, receiving Reiki, and being led through breath-awareness techniques and body-scan meditations. These integrative therapies have been refined, combined, and detailed to be applicable in dealing with pain, anxiety, nausea, insomnia, and constipation (PANIC™)—the common symptoms of so many illnesses.

Through Donna Karan, we have been fortunate to attract the foremost pioneers in their respective fields to participate in the development of this program and the continued education of the trainees. The Senior Yoga faculty are Colleen Saidman Yee, Rodney Yee, Mary Taylor, Richard Freeman, and Richard Rosen. The Senior Contemplative Care faculty is Roshi Joan Halifax, Mary Taylor, Robert "Chodo" Campbell, and Koshin Paley Ellison. The Reiki masters are Lena Falth, Eleonore Koury, and Arleta Soares, with Pamela Miles as a founding Reiki Master. The Nutrition component was compiled by Susan Luck, and we have been fortunate to have been given instruction by Dean Ornish, M.D., Mark Hyman, M.D., Christiane Northrup, M.D., Neal Barnard, M.D., T. Colin Campbell, M.D., among many others. The Essential Oil faculty has been led by Tracy Griffiths and supported by Gary Young, Mae Ming Racer, Marc Schreuder, Doug Corrigan, and Gina Killpack, from Young Living Essential Oils. The medical advisors and contributors have included Mark Hyman, Susan Luck, Barbara Dossey, and Bonnie Shaub. It is through these respected colleagues and many others who are too numerous to name that UZIT has come to life. We are constantly reflecting, observing, and refining our methodology to better serve individuals in all situations and all times throughout their lives.

THE UZIT TRAINING PROGRAM

The UZIT Training Program starts with self-care practices. Our belief is that the health practitioner must embody these practices in their own lives on a daily basis in order to effectively support his/her client(s) with them. Through the coursework, we define the meaning of self-care and demonstrate the integral role that self-care plays in the life and work of the caregiver. Students assess their own self-care needs and how they are, or are not, being met. In addition, students identify an individualized path toward improved self-care that can be practically incorporated into their lives.

For example, after three months of UZIT training, a fifteen-year career nurse from UCLA medical center stood before the door of a patient who she had to take off life support. She stood in taḍāsana (mountain pose) centering herself, drawing in the scent of a peaceful and calming essential oil blend, doing self-Reiki, giving herself a body scan, and observing her own breath. After about a minute, she placed her hand on the doorknob, turned it, and entered the room. The patient's family, who surrounded the bed, looked up. Once they went through their initial introductions, the nurse led everyone in some simple Yoga, gave Reiki, and offered a lavender essential oil. With deep presence from all in the room, she removed the patient from the life support. She said that it was the first time in fifteen years where she felt she had done her job thoroughly.

In UZIT, we feel it is from our trainees' own centering and balance, from their own relaxation and mindfulness practices, that their service emanates to others.

Thus, we encourage the trainees to practice the UZIT therapies below on themselves on a daily basis.

YOGA THERAPY

The UZIT Program begins with Yoga Therapy. The Yoga practices that we have chosen to focus on are in-bed movements, restorative poses, breath awareness techniques, and body scan meditations.

In-Bed Movements

These are movements that articulate the joints of the body and can be done by virtually anyone in almost any situation. A great example is flexing and pointing the feet to articulate the ankle joints and all the joints of the feet. This simple exercise, done in coordination with the breath, immediately gets the practitioner out of his/her head and into their feet; it also promotes circulation and digestion.

Other in-bed movements are those that specifically alleviate the symptoms of PANIC. As an example, when a person is anxious, he/she tends to have a lot of tension in the neck and shoulders, so one might do sun salutation arms in concert with the breath to bring circulation and opening to the tense muscles and restore equilibrium to the emotions. These movements will also focus the mind on the breath and break the cycle of the mind fixating on whatever is causing fear.

Moreover, there are many movements based on Yoga postures that can be replicated in the bed to what we call "any amount" that will enhance circulation, respiration, and digestion. For instance, a patient can do trikoṇāsana (triangle pose) with minimal movement while lying on his/her back in bed. This allows for all of the neurological patterning of this pose to be experienced with very little physical output.

Restorative Poses

These are poses that are completely supported to enhance deep relaxation through optimizing the breath. A supported relaxation pose (below) creates the perfect architecture for the body to enhance easy breathing.

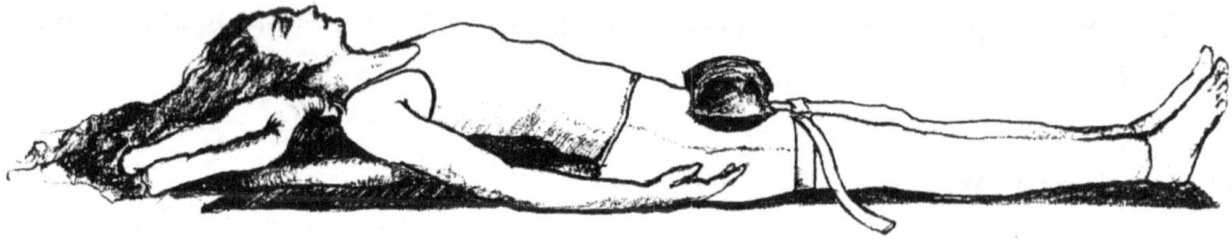

Additionally, restorative poses can be applied to the specific symptom of PANIC that the UZIT Therapist is trying to alleviate or lessen. A good example is child's pose fully supported on one's side (below). This restorative pose is beneficial for nausea and allows access to the back of the body so Reiki can be applied at the same time.

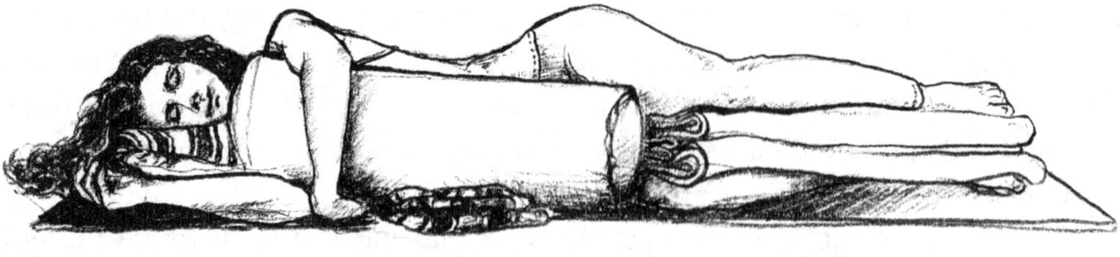

Ultimately, restorative poses are tailored for the individual's specific needs. Even though there are basic restorative poses that we utilize in UZIT sessions, there are many variations for each pose that can make the poses so much more effective in individual circumstances. If someone has lower back problems and is doing a supported reclined supta baddha koṇāsana (cobbler's pose), he/she might adjust the pose by lowering the bolster under the torso while raising his/her feet higher from the floor. These kinds of details make all the difference in the world in Yoga Therapy.

Breath Awareness Techniques

In UZIT, we observe the breath to focus the mind. How does one facilitate easy free breathing? Simple observation of the breath is one of the most effective methods. The main obstacle to this technique is the inability of the participant to train themselves to do something so subtle and elusive. Therefore, we devise breathing exercises to keep the practitioner intrigued. As we mentioned above in the restorative pose section, there are many positions that naturally quiet the mind and illuminate the breath. A great technique is to place one's hands or a prop on the belly or the chest to highlight the movements that are occurring from breathing.

Paying attention to the shifting direction of the breath contributes to quieting the nervous system. When a person gets anxious, their breathing often gets short and restricted. The direction of the breath is usually drawn very quickly up toward the neck and head. If one can change the direction of the inhalation down toward the feet in that situation, the tension and pressure can be released from the neck and head, and the nervous system begins to calm down. When people are given the instruction to take a deep breath, the patient can tend to accentuate the push of the breath upward, which can increase anxiety and disconnectedness. In supported relaxation poses, we sometimes place weights on the thighs to bring mental focus to the breath and to draw the breath down and complete the exhalation. Reiki on the upper thighs can further enhance this breath direction.

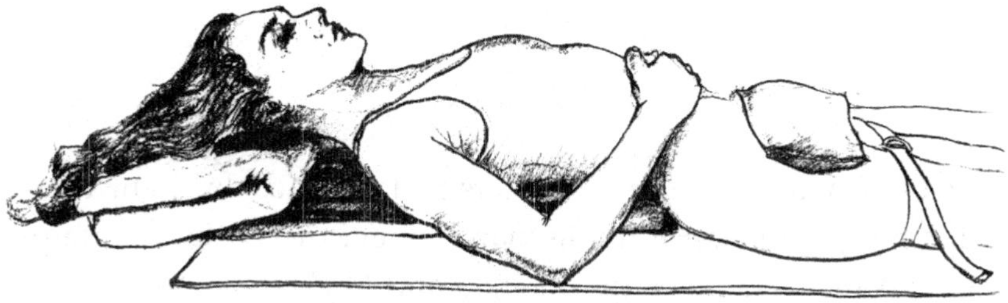

Directing the breath to certain bodily locations helps one observe tension and resistance patterns in the body. Where there is tension in the body, the absorption of the breath is restricted. Changing the patient's posture is an easy way to shift where the breath moves freely and where it is restricted. By consciously breathing into the area that is restricted, or by doing a posture that naturally opens that area, the restriction is observed. The mindfulness that is directed into the restricted area is a significant key in integrating that isolated tension back into the symphony of body-mind confluence.

Body Scan Meditations

Body scan meditations keep the mind focused on the present moment sensations arising in the body. The key to leading a body scan meditation is that the talker should use only verbs that denote noticing or observation. There is nothing for the patient to do except to see things as they are in the present moment without any embellishment or judgment. The scan should be done at a rhythm that flows from one observation to the next.

Furthermore, body scans can follow specific systems to have continuity with the aspect(s) of PANIC one is working on. For example, a digestive body scan (detailed later in this chapter) is done in tandem with the essential oil Di-Gize along with simple in-bed movements and a restorative pose that focus on the natural function of the digestive tract. Combining these therapies in an integrative, scientific approach makes body scan meditations even more effective.

The beauty about body scans is that they can start from different locations, which is obvious when dealing with severe pain. We start the body scan as far from the epicenter of the pain as possible and then move through the entire body. This directs the patient to focus on sensations arising in other parts of the body that are not as extreme as the epicenter so that the process is initially tangible without avoiding the source of difficulty.

REIKI

Reiki is a Japanese vibrational energy therapy facilitated by light touch, on or slightly off the body, to balance the human biofield. It is a technique proven to reduce stress and increase relaxation (Vitale and O'Connor, 2006) and promote healing by channeling the body's healing energy (Miles and True, 2003; Potter, 2003; Brown, 1995). In UZIT, Reiki is an interactive and experiential skill. Students learn what Reiki energy therapy is, how and why it works, and how to give Reiki to themselves and to others. In addition, UZIT practitioners are provided with suggested Reiki protocols to help reduce the PANIC symptoms of pain, anxiety, nausea, insomnia, and constipation, as well as exhaustion.

The Reiki Level One course in UZIT involves the following:

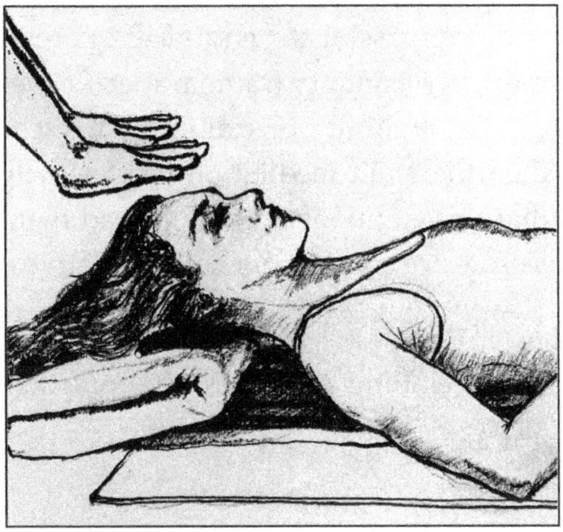

- Overview of Reiki, its history, and how it works
- Introduction of hand positions
- Attunement
- Relationship with Yoga Therapies
- 2nd attunement
- Self-practice
- Medical Reiki and practice on others

AROMATHERAPY

The essential oil therapy component in UZIT training is intended to provide a comprehensive understanding of what essential oils are, why they are used, how they work, and where they pertain to PANIC. We focus on nine basic oils and the simple and efficacious application of these oils in both private and clinical settings for practitioners whose patients wish to integrate essential oils into their medical treatment. An ideal way to supplement allopathic medical care and enhance complementary healing practices such as Reiki, therapeutic-grade essential oils can be used to calm, energize, balance, purify, and rejuvenate the mind and body.

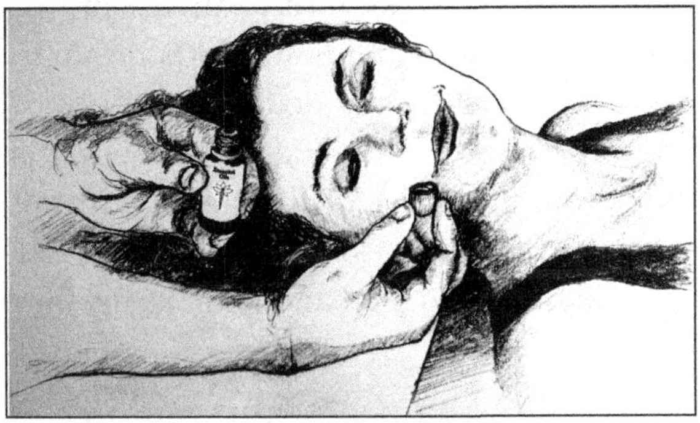

CONTEMPLATIVE CARE

The Urban Zen Integrative Therapy Program trains caregivers in a contemplative approach to psychosocial, spiritual, and ethical aspects of care of the sick. Our main focus is the cultivation of mindful awareness, emotional balance, equanimity, and compassion around issues of illness. These mental qualities and the practices that open the pathways to their mastery are needed if caregivers are to provide mindful and compassionate end-of-life care for the patient and effective self-care that reduces secondary trauma; specifically, caregiver burn-out, and moral distress.

Throughout our trainings, we teach components of contemplative care, and then the main meditation teacher will come to present. We find more and more that this component is the thread that ties the whole program together. The main lessons we share about contemplative care include:

- Philosophy
- Developing a formal sitting practice
- Observing oneself
- Bearing witness
- Creating a community support system

NUTRITION

At Urban Zen Integrative Therapy, we understand that nutrition is an integral part of self-care and a necessary component of wellness promotion and disease prevention. Our training presents practical information on food and nutrition grounded in current research and clinical advances. Students are provided with the foundations of nutrition education for everyday application in an effort to enhance personal balance and well-being. By learning the principles of functional nutrition, nutrition guidelines, and basic information on food and its effect on the body, individuals are able to assess their personal relationship to food and to make healthier choices for themselves in the future.

SELF-CARE AND INTEGRATION OF MODALITIES

As students practice these therapies daily, they hone their observation skills and connect more deeply with their "center." Much of the quietness and depth they develop inside themselves is transferred nonverbally through their presence and touch. It is through their own self-practice that they are able to deliver these skills safely and effectively to others at home, with friends and clients, and in clinical settings.

UZIT CLINICAL ROTATIONS

UZIT Therapists' first clinical rotations were at Beth Israel Hospital. For about six months, we prepared the groundwork at the medical oncology floor, a twenty-four-bed unit where about 70 percent of the patients have throat and neck cancer. Donna Karan gave a generous donation to remodel an existing meeting room into a sanctuary where patients could find peace and quiet and where nurses and doctors could be given UZIT sessions in between their rounds. Donna's donation also supported an Urban Zen Day that educated the staff on the UZIT sessions and allowed them to personally experience the same treatments their patients would receive. We sent two of our very best therapists to work on the floor, to organize and pave the way for the upcoming clinical rotations. Concurrently, we set up a medical study to surmise the efficacy of the program, which was to later show a million dollars' worth of savings in one year in pain and sleep medications (Kligler, 2011).

To date, there have now been more than 15,000 UZIT sessions given and received at Beth Israel Hospital. There are also countless stories of how UZIT has become integral to the health and wellness of the entire hospital (Kligler, et al., 2011), from the patient and their families, to the administration, to the volunteer staff, and to the nurses and doctors. We envision this as a model that could be duplicated at hospitals all around the nation.

Our practitioners are trained to enter a situation empty of ideas and empty of an agenda. It is this blank slate that is the foundation for keen listening and profound observations. Before entering a patient's room, there is an entire protocol to follow to get the proper information. UZIT practitioners are expected to gather information such as:

- What is the patient's diagnosis?
- When was the patient diagnosed?
- How long has the patient been in the hospital?
- Do the nurses have any specific concerns about the patient?
- Who is there supporting the patient? Staff, family, friends?

They are trained to make mental notes about the room and the patient. For example, some questions they may ask themselves as they enter the room include:

- Does the patient have any visitors or a healthcare practitioner with them?
- Are they in a single room or do they have a suite mate?
- Are there flowers or cards present that signify someone is caring for them?
- What is the general environment of the room? How is the temperature? The lighting? The smell? The auditory environment?

Observations directly about the patient come from questions like:

- Are they asleep? Did they just finish a meal?
- How is their breathing? Short? Ragged? Held? Labored? Smooth? Easy?
- What body position are they in?
- What is the color of their skin?
- How coherent are they?

Through the UZIT Therapist's conversation with the patient and other observations and information gathered, the therapist assesses which symptom or symptoms of PANIC their session will address. Throughout the session, it is the therapist's constant observations and skillful listening that lead the way. Training oneself to be constantly centered, empty, and receptive is where each therapist's self-practice comes into play.

As UZIT became an integral player at Beth Israel Hospital, nurses and doctors utilized the UZIT Therapists constantly. Nurses would tell a UZIT to go into a room to calm a patient down. UZIT Therapists would give a Yoga class to the staff in the UZ Sanctuary. A family member would help with a session so that they could bring the practices and lessons home with them. Sessions were given presurgery and postsurgery with incredible results at Beth Israel Hospital. And the word is spreading! The chief cardiologist at UCLA medical center is now prescribing UZIT sessions for his patients and has plans to do further research on our techniques and study our approach in the near future.

SO WHAT IS A UZIT SESSION?

Once a patient has been assessed, a standard UZIT session starts with in-bed movements. Take a patient experiencing constipation for example. The UZIT session could involve prescribed movements that replicate walking to help with the peristaltic movements of the intestinal tract. After the movement portion of the session, the UZIT Therapist might set the patient up in a digestive restorative pose such as reclined cobblers pose (below) with the pelvis in an anterior tilt and the head higher than the chest, the chest higher than the pelvis, and the legs fully supported and folded as deeply as comfortable. This pose would help facilitate the digestive flow and would be a perfect physical set up for a digestive body scan, where the practitioner talks the patient through noticing the present moment state of different aspects of the digestive tract. As the UZIT Therapist gets the patient to observe the areas of the body that are named, there is an opportunity for a spontaneous release of tension and a return toward an unimpeded flow of

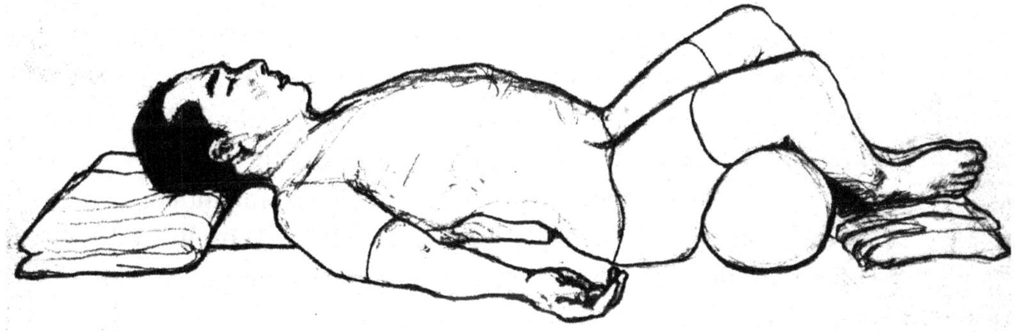

absorption and movement in the digestive tract. The following is a sample of a digestive body scan and what the UZIT Therapist might say to the patient:

- Notice your lips. Observe the placement of your lips. Feel the moisture of your lips.
- No need to make any changes. No judgment, just simple observation of what is.
- Feel your teeth and the shape of the cavity of your mouth.
- Sense the placement of your tongue.
- Feel your throat down through your esophagus, the tube that connects your mouth to your stomach.
- Observe any sensations and movements in your stomach. Feel how the rhythm of the breath is in concert with the movements of the stomach.
- Sense the beginning of your intestinal tract. Know that you have twenty to thirty feet of intestinal tract. Feel any sensations that are arising in that area.
- Notice the movement of your lower belly rising and falling with the breath.
- Observe how this long coiled tube finishes at the anus. Just sensing the digestive tract and observing the sensations that are arising in this specific pathway will help free the tensions that are adding to the constipation.

Simultaneously, the practitioner can use Di-Gize, an essential oil blend that assists in unlocking constipation, while performing the body scan. Of course, the patient is always asked whether or not the essential oil that is being utilized is pleasing and desired, and there are always several options of different essential oils for specific symptoms if a particular oil is not appealing. We have enjoyed wonderful and invaluable success in including these oils with our UZIT sessions, and the results and patient satisfaction level have often been miraculous.

After the practitioner informs and educates the patient about Reiki and is given permission to use it, Reiki is commonly applied throughout the session. Depending on the symptoms and one's educated intuition, the Reiki practitioner may begin the session at different parts of the body but, because it can be delivered with the hands either lightly touching or hovering above, Reiki is a perfect modality in all settings to help relax and restore balance to the patient.

Since the symptoms of PANIC cause restrictions and contortions to the breath, we can restore calmness to the mind and relaxation to the body by moving toward free and easy breathing. The most efficient route to free and easy breathing starts in a good restorative posture and then introduces *breath observation—not breath control*. The trick is to keep bringing the patient's attention back to watching his/her breath with as little judgment as possible. We call this "open-minded focused observation." Throughout the session, breath awareness is encouraged through simple techniques like putting a folded blanket on the patient's belly and having him/her feel the weight of the blanket rise and fall as previously mentioned. The UZIT Therapist can help the patient's observation return to the breath by calling out the breaths as they occur. This breath awareness can be utilized in the Yoga Therapy movement practices as well as in the restorative poses.

During the in-bed movements, the UZIT guides the patient to coordinate his/her movements with the breath. For instance, a typical movement for constipation is to bend the legs toward the chest. Bringing the legs into the chest is coordinated with the exhale, and lowering the leg back down is coordinated with the inhale. When the breath leads the movement, the physical exercises transcend the physical realm and become important components to train the mind to stay steady in the present moment. As many Yoga masters have stated, the breath is the ruler of the mind and the body (Haṭha Yoga Pradipika 4.29), and it is the bridge that links the mind to the body (Haṭha Tatva Kaumudi 37.11, 37.13). The moment the mind, breath, and body are yoked together, there is an optimal environment for natural healing and balance.

At Urban Zen we have charted the symptoms of PANIC and have created, sequenced, and layered specific courses of action to take with each healing art. It is common for a patient to have more than one symptom of PANIC and the UZIT session has to morph into a hybrid of practices, finding the intricate balance to a whole solution. It is when the UZIT Therapist learns how to integrate the modalities together within a single session that the true potential of this integrative therapy is realized. The layering of multiple oils, a variety of movements, multiple restorative poses, a combination of body scans, and a mixture of breath awareness exercises might all be used in a single session to address the symptoms at hand.

CURRENT IMPLEMENTATIONS

As of 2014, UZIT sessions are now being offered at Beth Israel Medical Center, NYU Medical Center, and Montefiore Medical Center in New York City; Southampton Hospital in Long Island, NY; UCLA Health System in Los Angeles, CA; Wexner Medical Center at the Ohio State University and Wexner Heritage Village in Columbus, Kent State Nursing school in Kent, Ohio; as well as many other venues. They have also been used in crisis situations such as in relief efforts in Haiti and for the victims of Hurricane Katrina. UZIT Therapists are deployed in public schools in the Oakland Unified School District (California) for the administration, teachers, parents, and students. UZIT classes are also being taught in Yoga studios, and we have come to realize that there are endless numbers of people and places in need of this service.

CONCLUSION

One of the best aspects of the UZIT practices is that the practitioner can so easily integrate them into his/her everyday life. Simple meditations, easy-to-remember body movements, breath awareness exercises, self-Reiki, restorative poses, essential oil aromatherapy, and good nutrition practices can be incorporated on a daily basis at home, at work, and in the hospital setting. The Urban Zen Integrative Therapist offers patients and students suggestions of vital practices that they can do at home alone or with their families.

Relaxation and mindfulness are practices that facilitate our ability to get the most out of the arising moment, no matter what the moment entails. If individuals can integrate these practices into their everyday lives, then when a crisis takes place the therapies will be readily available, extremely beneficial, and so much more effective. So much of health care is about everyday care and even moment-by-moment care. Living life is about being present. Thus, in times of trouble as well as in ordinary life, the confluence of Urban Zen Integrative Therapies is an amazing methodology to promote relaxed, mindful, and awakened living.

REFERENCES

Brown, C. "Alternative Medicine Comes to the OR." *Medical Economics* 2.17 (1995): 207–219. Print.

Kligler, B., et al. "Impact of the Urban Zen Initiative on Patient's Experience of Admission to an Inpatient Oncology Floor: A Mixed--Methods Analysis." *The Journal of Alternative and Complementary Medicine* 17.8 (2011): 729–734. Print.

Kligler, B., et al. "Cost Savings in Inpatient Oncology Through an Integrative Medicine Approach." *The American Journal of Managed Care* 17.2 (2011): 779–784. Print.

Miles P., and G. True. "Reiki: Review of Biofield Therapy, History, Theory, Practice, and Research." *Alternative Therapies* 9.2 (2003): 62–71. Print.

Potter, P. "What Are the Distinctions Between Reiki and Therapeutic Touch?" *Clinical Journal of Oncology Nursing* 7.1 (2003): 89–91. Print.

Sundara Deva. "Hatha Tattva Kaumudi (Moonlight on the Principles of Hatha Yoga)." 18th Century.

Svatmarama Yogendra. "Hatha Yoga Pradipika (Light on the Forceful Yoga)." Mid-14th century.

Vitale, A. T., and P. C. O'Connor. "The Effect of Reiki on Pain and Anxiety in Women with Abdominal Hysterectomies: A Quasi-Experimental Pilot Study." *Holistic Nursing Practice* 20.7 (2006): 263–272. Print.

The Yoga Therapy Rx Program at Loyola Marymount University Where Yoga Meets Modern Medicine

Larry Payne, Ph.D.

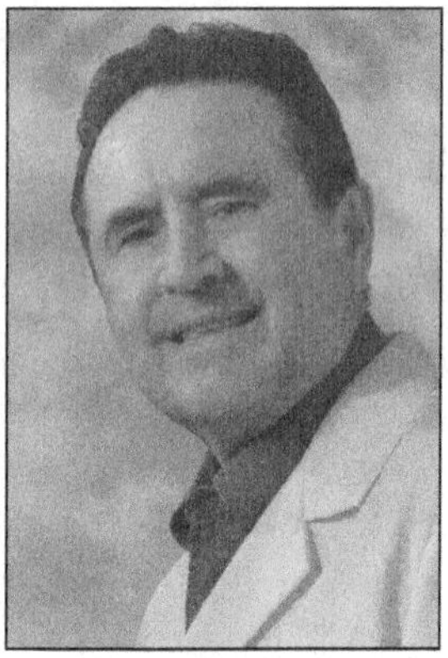

Larry Payne is the founding director of the Yoga Therapy Rx and Prime of Life Yoga Training Programs at Loyola Marymount University. His own Yoga journey began in a quest for relief from chronic back pain, which led him to India, where he studied with many of the great Yoga masters, including his teacher, T. K. V. Desikachar. He is the cofounder of the International Association of Yoga Therapists and the founding director of Samata International Yoga & Health Center in Los Angeles, California. Additionally, Larry is the coauthor of *Yoga for Dummies* with Georg Feuerstein, Ph.D., and *Yoga Rx* with Richard Usatine, M.D.

OUR ROOTS AND OUR PHILOSOPHY

The seeds of the Yoga Therapy Rx Program at Loyola Marymount University (LMU) in Los Angeles, California, were sown when I experienced a life-changing wave of relief from chronic back pain after taking my first Yoga class in 1976. The profundity of this experience led me on a global quest to learn everything I could about health and healing. Twelve years of high stress had taken their toll on me as the West Coast Sales Representative of *McCall's* magazine, and I was ready for a new direction. I immediately got hooked on Yoga and quickly found my way to India.

In India, I met with many of the great modern Yoga masters: Professor Sri T.

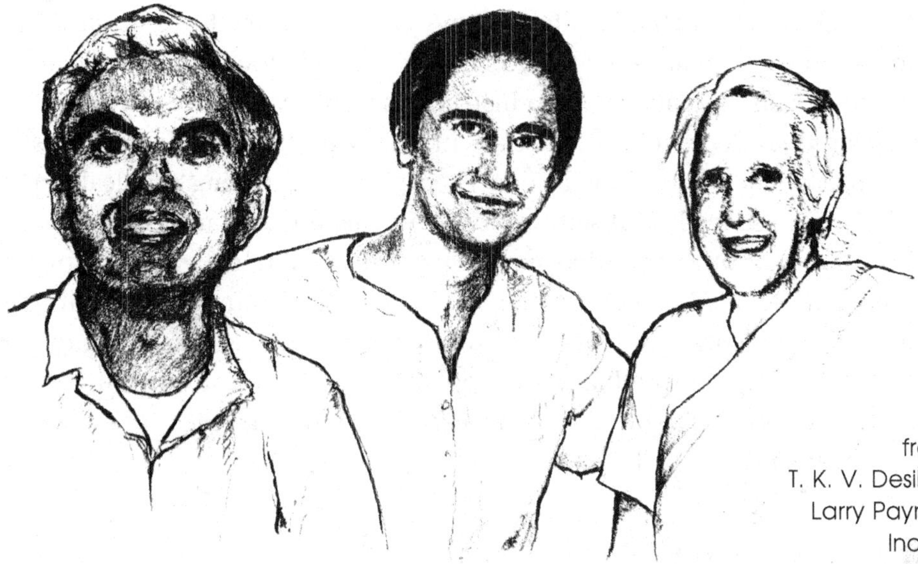

from left:
T. K. V. Desikachar,
Larry Payne, and
Indra Devi

Krishnamacharya, B. K. S. Iyengar, Yogi Bhajan of Kundalini Yoga, Satya Sai Baba, Bhagwan Shree Rajneesh (now known as Osho), Indra Devi (Krishnamacharya's first female student and a dear friend of mine), and Swami Vishnudevananda of Sivananda Yoga. But it was T. K. V. Desikachar, the son and student of Sri T. Krishnamacharya, who became my teacher and mentor. His lineage has guided my career path, and I owe a debt of gratitude to him for my lasting pain relief and personal growth.

After coming back from India, I collaborated with LeRoy Perry, D.C., in founding the first Yoga Therapy center in Los Angeles at the International Sports Medicine Institute in 1984. Then, in 1989, Richard Miller, Ph.D., and I brought together an ecumenical group of Yoga traditions to found the International Association of Yoga Therapists (IAYT). And today, more than one hundred Yoga Therapy training programs have memberships in IAYT.

Inspired by T. K. V. Desikachar, the Yoga Therapy Rx Training Program at LMU is a marriage between Yoga Therapy and modern integrative medicine. Our eclectic faculty has more than thirty highly renowned professionals in their respective fields presenting an array of perspectives and applications of Yoga to offer students an enriching experience not limited to a single point of view. Students are encouraged to explore their areas of interest and eventually find their own respective niches. Among the faculty are physicians, chiropractors, physical therapists, doctors of traditional Chinese medicine (TCM) and Oriental medicine, mental health professionals, and master Yoga instructors from a variety of lineages.

We opened our doors to our first class in 2005 with the intention to transform certified Yoga teachers into skilled Yoga Therapists by applying classical applications of Yoga for use in clinical settings to help treat common ailments and conditions. Our four-year program offers a rigorous didactic and experiential course of study, and our teaching philosophy encourages critical thinking as well as the acquisition of knowledge. Students draw upon the emerging and growing research literature on Yoga Therapy and its many applications. Further, students are encouraged to consider conducting their own research to expand the base of evidence as part of their careers in Yoga Therapy.

WHAT IS YOGA THERAPY?

Yoga is a practice that optimizes the health of the body and quiets the mind. Yoga Therapy has been described and defined in a myriad of ways. What the many modern interpretations of Yoga Therapy have in common is an understanding of the vital integration of mind, body, and spirit to heal the whole person. Yoga Therapy, as practiced in the West, is a synthesis of the ageless wisdom of the East with the most recent knowledge in complementary health care from the West.

The teachers who have developed Yoga Therapy as a field come to it from their areas of practice and expertise, and, accordingly, their definitions vary from one another. According to the late Yoga scholar, Georg Feuerstein, Ph.D., "Yoga Therapy is of modern coinage and represents a first effort to integrate traditional yogic concepts and techniques with Western medical and psychological knowledge" (Taylor, 2007). From the medical perspective, Art Brownstein, M.D., defines *Yoga Therapy* as "consisting of the application of yogic principles, methods, and techniques to specific human ailments. In its ideal application, Yoga Therapy is preventive in nature, as is Yoga itself, but it is also restorative in many instances, palliative in others, and curative in many others" (Brownstein, 2013). Judith Lasater, Ph.D., P.T., defines *Yoga Therapy* as "the use of the techniques of Yoga to create, stimulate, and maintain an optimum state of physical, emotional, mental, and spiritual health" (Lasater, n.d.). From the psychological perspective, Richard Miller, Ph.D., says *Yoga Therapy* is "the application of yogic principles to a particular person with the objective of achieving a particular spiritual, psychological, or physiological goal" (Miller, n.d.). And Michael Lee describes *Yoga Therapy* as "a holistic healing art . . . that invites presence and awareness. Using age-old yogic approaches to deeper presence and awareness, we are able to know ourselves more fully. Out of that knowing, we are more easily moved to embrace the opportunity for change, growth, and enhanced well-being in body, feelings, thought, and spirit" (Lee, n.d.).

Simply put, we can think of Yoga Therapy as a replacement therapy that is replacing old bad habits with new and better ones. Yoga Therapy views the mind, body, and spirit as interconnected and advocates changes in lifestyle. It can be a means to manage illness or facilitate healing. It encompasses not only the body and the movements we do on the Yoga mat but how we live and treat others and ourselves off the mat. Different from group Yoga classes, Yoga Therapy adapts the practice of Yoga to the needs of individuals with specific or persistent health problems that are not usually addressed in a group format.

A BRIEF HISTORY OF YOGA THERAPY

Yoga Therapy originated in ancient India and was initially practiced in combination with Ayurveda (also known as Siddha medicine in Southern India). Yoga and Ayurveda have common roots in Sāṁkhya, the oldest of Indian philosophies, the goal of which is to find freedom from pain and suffering. Within the Sāṁkhya philosophical system, which is systematic, clear, concrete, and specific, Yoga and Ayurveda are considered techniques by which the root causes of pain can be removed (Samkhya Philosophy, n.d.).

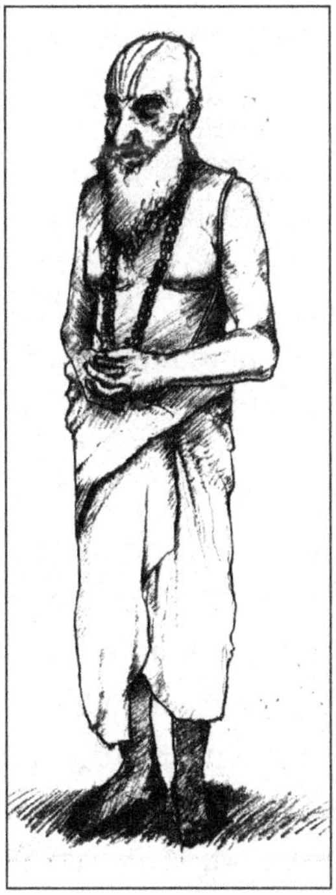
Sri T. Krishnamacharya

Indian Yoga Therapy in its present form can be traced back to Sri T. Krishnamacharya in the 1920s and 1930s and two other prominent Yoga Therapy centers still in existence today. Kaivalyadhama Yoga Hospital, founded by Swami Kuvalayananda in 1930 in Lonavala, near Pune, India, and the Yoga Institute of Santa Cruz near Mumbai, founded in 1918 by Shri Yogendraji, were the first to combine Yoga Therapy with Western medicine. They also championed scientific research, which was mainly published in Indian journals. Krishnamacharya, on the other hand, used his own blend of Yoga and Ayurveda encompassing ritual, chanting, food choices, herbs, advanced breathing, relaxation, and āsana. He also produced students who became the West's most influential teachers of Indian therapeutic Yoga, including his son, T. K. V. Desikachar, and his nephew, B. K. S. Iyengar, among others.

THE GROWING BASE OF EVIDENCE SUPPORTING YOGA THERAPY

There is a growing body of research demonstrating positive results with the therapeutic use of Yoga in a wide range of clinical situations. The website for the National Institute for Complementary and Alternative Medicine (NCCAM) of the National Institutes of Health (NIH) even spotlights a journal article discussing not just whether Yoga practice is effective for back pain relief, but whether or not the frequency of group classes made a difference in the study population (Boah, et al., 2013). Search for "Yoga Therapy" on the NCCAM website, and you will get scores and scores of hits on recent and current studies. The specificity and validity of the research analyzing Yoga Therapy is growing!
According to the NCCAM:

> Recent studies in people with chronic low-back pain suggest that a carefully adapted set of Yoga poses may help reduce pain and improve function (the ability to walk and move). Studies also suggest that practicing Yoga (as well as other forms of regular exercise) might have other health benefits such as reducing heart rate and blood pressure, and may also help relieve anxiety and depression (Yoga for Health, 2013).

A scan of the S-VYASA website lists over 200 research publications reporting on Yoga and its impact on a vast array of physical, medical, and mental conditions and situations, including memory, empathy, diabetes, and polycystic ovarian syndrome, to name a few (List of Research Publications on Yoga, 2013).

Yoga is fast becoming the treatment modality of choice for veterans suffering from posttraumatic stress disorder (PTSD), some of them having suffered for decades without noted improvement prior to practicing Yoga. As reported by Public Radio International (PRI), Yoga has become a standard treatment for vets with PTSD (Kaplan, 2013). According to Stanford University researcher Emma Seppala,

Ph.D., Yoga-based breathing, in particular, rhythmic breathing techniques from the Sudarshan Kriyā Yoga tradition, and exercises dramatically decreased PTSD in veterans, and the positive effects achieved in her study lasted a full year after the study period (Brandt, 2013). Harvard University investigator Sat Bir S. Khalsa, Ph.D., attributes Yoga's power of addressing symptoms of PTSD to the changes in the brain that result from the combination of the physicality of the postures and the regulation of the breath that direct the focus to the present moment while quieting down the hormone-related stress cycle (Zimmerman, 2010).

The efficacy of Yoga as a complementary treatment modality with breast cancer patients and survivors is also an area of active investigation. Researchers from the University of Calgary found decreases in depression, fatigue, anxiety, tension, diarrhea, confusion, anger, and emotional irritability among the Yoga practitioners as compared to their control group (Carlson, et al., 2006). A 2002 study by the Swami Vivekananda Yoga Research Foundation (S-VYASA), conducted in conjunction with the Bangalore Institute of Oncology, reported the surprising outcome that study participants assigned to the Yoga practice group experienced a decrease in the toxicity of treatments. This is a very important finding because when patients are unable to tolerate the treatment's side effects, physicians may need to reduce the dose and possibly compromise their effectiveness of the treatment.

For those seeking to utilize Yoga as a therapeutic modality, the NIH urges the careful selection of an instructor who is experienced with, and attentive to, the needs of the individual and the medical issues involved. Because everyone's body is different, Yoga postures should be modified based on individual abilities (Yoga for Health, 2013).

THE YOGA THERAPY RX PROGRAM AT LOYOLA MARYMOUNT UNIVERSITY

Yoga Therapy includes a variety of activities, including āsanas (postures), prāṇāyāma (breathing techniques), dhyāna (meditation), and lifestyle practices, and, accordingly, a therapist's training needs to be multidimensional. The concepts and framework of the Yoga Therapy Rx Program at LMU, inspired by T. K. V. Desikachar, were designed to incorporate licensed health professionals into an integrative approach. For each topic, the medical view and etiology are presented as well as the therapeutic applications of Yoga to the condition, thus grooming the Yoga Therapist in training to participate as an active member of the client's health-care team.

The full course of training at the LMU Yoga Therapy Rx Program offers four levels:

The Basic Program, Level I: Level I begins the course of study by building a firm understanding of the musculoskeletal system. I have observed, and other experienced Yoga Therapists will likely agree, that musculoskeletal pain comprises the most common reasons for which people seek out Yoga Therapy. LMU-trained Yoga Therapists are taught to be discerning and to recognize when a presenting problem may be masking a more serious medical condition and thus fall outside the Yoga Therapist's scope of practice. The first year curriculum includes the principles of practice, anatomy, and the origin and treatment of common lower back, upper back, knee, and hip problems.

In the first level, our Yoga Therapy students learn to communicate effectively with the medical profession and clients alike. They conduct systematic assessments and document their findings utilizing SOAP notes, a convention common to all areas of health and medical care. SOAP notes include noting the client's subjective complaints (what the client experiences); the therapist's objective evaluations (what the therapist observes and measures); the therapist's assessment of the problem (based on the array observations); and a plan of treatment. Prescriptive Yoga routines are drawn out in simple stick figures to give the client a take-home plan that is customized to meet his/her specific needs according to the assessment. This method of approach facilitates revising routines as often as necessary to match the client's changing needs. Higher technological methods such as digital recordings may also be utilized in certain clinical situations.

The Advanced Program, Level II: Level II provides background and tools to work with conditions related to the body's internal systems: circulatory, respiratory, digestive, nervous, reproductive, and endocrine. Faculty includes various medical and mental healthcare specialists. Although Yoga Therapists don't "treat" medical conditions in our philosophy, Yoga Therapy can be a powerful adjunct to medical treatment, supporting healing and improving quality of life. This level incorporates a general understanding of the relationship between Yoga Therapy and Ayurveda and connects the therapeutic practices with Yoga's philosophical foundation in the *Yoga Sūtras of Patañjali.*

The Clinical Program, Level III: Level III consists of practicum experience in a clinical setting covering the topic areas presented in didactic fashion in Levels I and II. Level III is an immersive clinical experience where clinical instructors work with patients and the Yoga Therapy students observe the application of Yoga tools and principles to particular situations and conditions. They also get to study the clinical interaction between the Yoga Therapist and the patients, and they have opportunities to ask questions of both the instructor and the patient during the course of the session. Additional case studies and lectures presented by the faculty further expand the Yoga Therapy student's ability to analyze presenting situations and devise treatment strategies.

The Integrative Medicine Program, Level IV: Level IV moves the Yoga Therapist student to Yoga Therapy intern status. During this culminating year of training, Yoga Therapist interns immerse themselves in all aspects of the clinical process and patient care in a community clinic treating underserved populations. They work directly alongside treating physicians as part of the integrative team approach to patient care. The setting of this practice year reinforces the Yoga principle of selfless service, or karma Yoga. The year also includes weekend sessions in the classroom where the Yoga Therapist interns present their cases to one another and the instructors.

YOGA THERAPY IS AN EMERGING SPECIALTY

Yoga, as it was traditionally taught, was a personal, one-on-one transmission of knowledge from teacher to student. By its very nature, Yoga is therapeutic and has long served that function, even if not specifically spelled out. Yoga Therapy as a field is now coming of age, as evidenced by conversations at organizational levels concerning ensuring high standards of training and assurances to the public that go beyond the reputation of a particular teacher or lineage. An objective of IAYT is to ensure that Yoga Therapists are highly qualified, and the organization set forth a recognized registration standard of 800 hours of study in 2013 (Kepner, 2013). To meet these new standards, graduates of the four-year Yoga Therapy Rx Program have access to additional programs and coursework through Loyola Marymount University and the program's instructors. An independent credentialing program is also available through Samata International Yoga and Health Center.

LEARNING FOR LIFE

"If you are going to teach, you need a teacher."

—SRI T. KRISHNAMACHARYA

Yoga Therapy students at LMU are encouraged to explore the large and varied list of recommended resources and develop a personal reference library. Continuing education workshops are offered to enable graduates to maintain current knowledge in their areas of interest. The adjunct Mentor's Program provides current students and alumni opportunities to study with any of the program's faculty members in greater depth. A teachers' blog provides a way for all who are interested in Yoga Therapy to keep current with developments in the field.

THE YOGA THERAPY RX MODEL OF CARE

A core and unifying concept in Yoga Therapy is to approach the whole person. The Yoga Therapy Rx Program at LMU provides its students with a variety of tools to assess clients in this fashion. The Morris-Payne Standard Evaluation, developed by Rick Morris, D.C., associate director of Level I and me, guides the Yoga Therapist in conducting a thorough assessment. This assessment includes detailed observations of the client's movements and posture, measuring the range of motion in a number of areas, assessing quality of life issues, and measuring breath capacity. To further capture the client's subjective experience of pain and its impact on his/her daily life, the conventional visual analog scale of pain is used where patients rate the severity of their discomfort from 0–10 and describe the quality of pain they are experiencing. In addition, we utilize the Patient-Specific Functional Scale (PSFS) to grade disabilities with daily activities and measure functional outcomes for orthopedic conditions.

The art of offering Yoga Therapy to clients is two-fold. First is the mastery of the interview and assessment process, which involves active listening, relating to the client as an individual, and interpreting the various data to get an understanding of that individual's experience and needs. Second, and perhaps even more critical, is knowing *what to give to whom and when,* based on the thoroughness of the therapist's evaluation.

The development of an individual treatment program in our Yoga Therapy model at LMU follows an eight-step wellness plan and is customized to meet the needs of each person. In summary, the eight steps are outlined in the following table:

TABLE 1. EIGHT-STEP WELLNESS PLAN

STEP	EXAMPLES
Mind-Set	Practices and habits to encourage a positive frame of mind are recommended. This includes bhāvana (visualization, affirmation), laughter, spending time in nature, social support, meditation, and goal setting.
Biomechanical Re-Education	Ergonomic improvements based on biomechanics are considered. This includes looking at a person's workstation and work habits; sitting and walking styles; and sleep environment and habits, including one's mattress, pillow, and sleeping positions.
Personalized Āsana Routine	A short, sustainable Yoga āsana program (10 to 20 minutes) to be practiced once or twice daily is designed and modified as progress is achieved. Teaching tools and techniques such as illustrating the routine with stick figures and having the client teach it back to the Yoga Therapist allows him/her to check the client's understanding and encourages compliance.
Journaling	A daily log is kept to record the client's recommended practices and to help him/her stay on track. The client is encouraged to note his/her feelings and *ah ha* moments as they arise, which can be elucidating and reinforcing.
Food Choices	A healthful diet that is varied, close to nature, and respectful of the planet is recommended. Healthful intakes may be achieved in many ways and should take into account the preferences and economics of the individual.

STEP	EXAMPLES
Adequate Hydration	Staying hydrated is especially helpful when healing the musculoskeletal system. Six to eight glasses of water daily, or the equivalent in other healthful beverages, is recommended.
Breathing Breaks	Incorporating short prāṇāyāma routines into the daily routine targeted to the client's needs is an integral part of the Yoga prescription.
Adequate Rest	Sleep deprivation and inadequate rest have wide-ranging negative physical, emotional, and mental consequences. Sleep hygiene is discussed to encourage sufficient sleep on a regular basis.

CONCLUSION

As a Yoga Therapist, I have seen the power a short, well-designed, individualized daily Yoga practice has in transforming lives. People who might never think of themselves as yogis or yoginis can benefit from incorporating the wisdom and carefully selected practices of Yoga into their daily routines. Through the practice, they find relief from their discomforts and pain, while others with serious chronic medical conditions and/or stress cultivate resources to better cope with their situations.

Now, some thirty-five years after my own fortunate and life-changing acquaintance with Yoga, I am wholeheartedly dedicated to the continued evolution of the field of Yoga Therapy. As it takes its place as a complementary therapeutic modality in modern integrative medicine, my goal is to continue to develop and refine a comprehensive academic Yoga Therapy training model that sits comfortably in the college setting. The body of research supporting the efficacy of Yoga Therapy is growing and the number of trained Yoga Therapists serving the public is equally expanding. These dedicated, hardworking, educated individuals therapeutically apply the tools of Yoga in well informed and discerning ways to benefit patients and clients.

REFERENCES

Boah, A. R., et al. "Weekly and Twice-Weekly Yoga Classes Offer Similar Low-Back Pain Relief in Low-Income Minority Populations." National Center for Complementary and Alternative Medicine, 1 July 2013. Web. Retrieved 5 Sept. 2013. http://nccam.nih.gov/research/results/spotlight/072013.

Brandt, M. "The Promise of Yoga-Based Treatments to Help Veterans with PTSD." ScopeBlog, Stanford Medicine, 23 May 2013. Web. Retrieved 5 Sept. 2013. http://scopeblog.stanford.edu/2013/05/23/the-promise-of-yoga-based-treatments-to-help-veterans-with-ptsd/.

Brownstein, A. "Contemporary Definitions of Yoga Therapy." IAYT, n.d. Web. Retrieved 5 Sept. 2013. http://www.iayt.org/?page=ContemporaryDefiniti.

Carlson, L. E., et al. "A Pilot Study of Yoga for Breast Cancer Survivors: Physical and Psychological Benefits." *Psycho-Oncology* 15.10 (2006): 891–897. Wiley Interscience, 2005. DOI: 10.1002/pon.1021. Web. Retrieved 5 Sept. 2013. PDF available at http://people.ucalgary.ca/~lcarlso/Yoga%20PON%20Culos-Reed.pdf.

Kaplan, S. "Yoga Now Standard Treatment for Vets with PTSD." Public Radio International, PRI's The World, 21 March 2013. Web. Retrieved 5 Sept. 2013. http://pri.org/stories/2013-03-21/yoga-now-standard-treatment-vets-ptsd.

Kepner, J. President, IAYT. Personal interview. June 2013.

Lasater, J. "Contemporary Definitions of Yoga Therapy." IAYT, n.d. Web. Retrieved 5 Sept. 2013. http://www.iayt.org/?page=ContemporaryDefiniti.

Lee, M. "Contemporary Definitions of Yoga Therapy." IAYT, n.d. Web. Retrieved 5 Sept. 2013. http://www.iayt.org/?page=ContemporaryDefiniti.

List of Research Publications on Yoga. S-Vyasa University, Aug. 2013. Web. Retrieved 5 Sept. 2013. http://svyasa.org/research/research-publications/.

Miller, R. "Contemporary Definitions of Yoga Therapy." IAYT, n.d. Web. Retrieved 5 Sept. 2013. http://www.iayt.org/?page=ContemporaryDefiniti.

Samkhya Philosophy: Foundation for Yoga and Ayurveda. Yoga International, n.d. Web. Retrieved 5 Sept. 2013. http://yogainternational.com/assets/content/ecourses/Samkhya-Philosophy-Lecture-Notes.pdf.

Taylor, M. J. "What Is Yoga Therapy? An IAYT Definition." Yoga Therapy in Practice, IATY. Dec. 2007. Web, Retrieved 5 Sept. 2013. http://www.ihttp://www.matthewjtaylor.com/whatisYRx.pdf.

Yoga for Health. National Center for Complementary and Alternative Medicine, 25 July 2013. Web. Retrieved 5 Sept. 2013. http://nccam.nih.gov/health/yoga/introduction.htm.

Zimmerman, Rachel. "Harvard, Brigham Study: Yoga Eases Veterans PTSD Symptoms." WBUR's CommonHealth, 8 Dec. 2010. Web. Retrieved 5 Sept. 2013. http://commonhealth.wbur.org/2010/12/harvard-brigham-medical-study-yoga-veterans-ptsd.

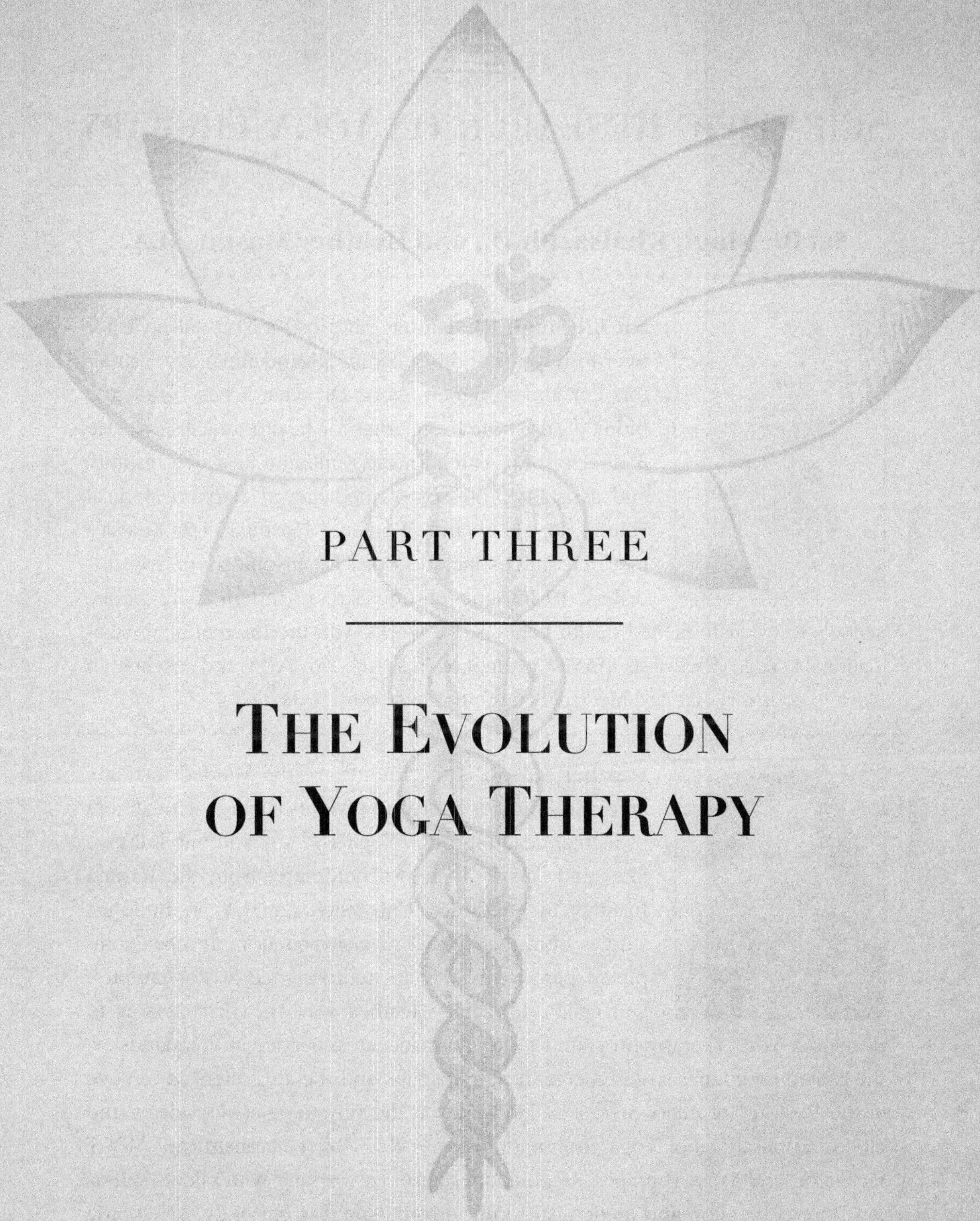

PART THREE

THE EVOLUTION OF YOGA THERAPY

Scientific Research on Yoga Therapy

Sat Bir Singh Khalsa, Ph.D., and Heather Mason, M.A.

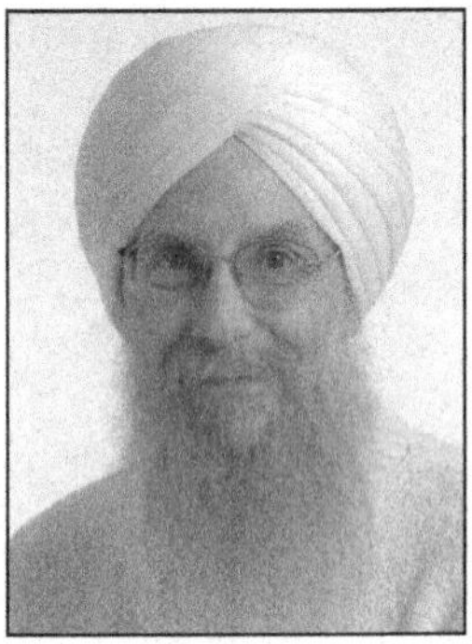

Sat Bir Singh Khalsa has practiced a Yoga lifestyle for over forty years and is a certified Kundalini Yoga instructor. For almost fifteen years, Dr. Khalsa has conducted biomedical research on Yoga for health and disease. He is director of research for the Kundalini Research Institute and assistant professor of medicine at Harvard Medical School, Brigham and Women's Hospital. Dr. Khalsa's research studies include Yoga for insomnia, anxiety disorders, PTSD, and chronic stress, and in K–12 public schools to evaluate mental health benefits. He works with the International Association of Yoga Therapists (IAYT) promoting research on Yoga and teaches an elective course at Harvard Medical School in mind-body medicine.

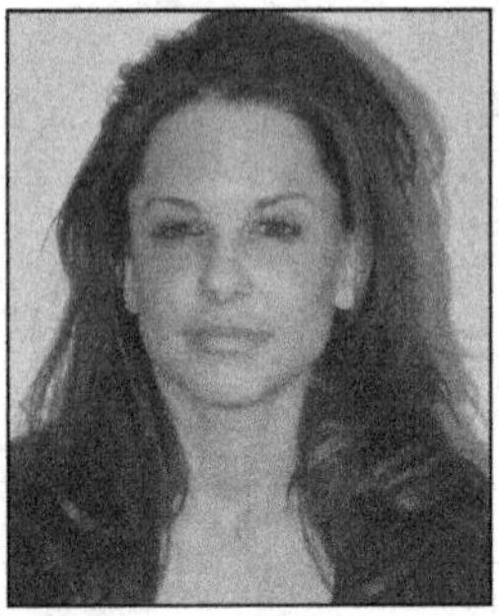

Heather Mason is the founder of the Minded Institute, an organization dedicated to revolutionizing the treatment of mental health through Yoga Therapy and mindfulness. She holds an M.A. in psychotherapy from the Karuna Institute at Middlesex University, an M.A. in Buddhist studies from the SOAS University London, and has completed part of an M.S. in neuroscience at Roehampton University. In 2008, Heather was the first person to develop a Yoga Therapy program for the traumatic stress service at the Maudsley, the United Kingdom's largest mental health hospital, and she also offers an elective at the Boston University School of Medicine on the physiological correlates and clinical applications of Yoga and mindfulness. A RYT 500 Yoga instructor, MBCT facilitator, and Yoga Therapist, Heather specializes in working with clients suffering from depression and anxiety spectrum disorders and is currently developing mind-body programs for the United Kingdom's largest mental health charity, Mind.

THE RATIONALE FOR SCIENTIFIC RESEARCH ON YOGA THERAPY

Yoga Therapy is a holistic practice that respects and addresses the entire individual —mind, body, and spirit. Scientific biomedical research, on the other hand, is largely reductionistic and seeks to verify treatment efficacy and elucidate underlying therapeutic mechanisms by evaluating therapies in rigorous experimental design settings that are often very different from the actual clinical application of the therapy. Furthermore, full-time research on Yoga or Yoga Therapy involves substantial resources both in labor and in costs. Even a small preliminary Yoga Therapy clinical trial grant can cost the taxpayer over a half-million dollars, funds that perhaps could be more rightfully applied in providing Yoga and Yoga Therapy to underserved populations. Therefore, the rationale for why we should conduct research on Yoga Therapy deserves consideration (Khalsa, 2007; Khalsa and Gould, 2012).

One rationale for Yoga research is that it can be used to boost the prestige, profile, and ultimately the popularity of Yoga Therapy through resulting media coverage, a strategy actively employed by a number of Yoga organizations and individuals. Yet, Yoga appears to be prospering without this particularly expensive form of marketing strategy. The current popularity of Yoga is unprecedented. A 2012 *Yoga Journal* survey revealed that 20 million Americans are practicing Yoga. Yoga is widely revered as a practice associated with health and well-being and is even being widely used by the advertising industry to sell consumer products.

Perhaps a stronger rationale for Yoga research is about safety from the perspective of the Public Health Service, the watchdog agency responsible for public health. In the face of the burgeoning use of complementary and alternative medicine (CAM) and Yoga Therapy, the National Center for Complementary and Alternative Medicine (NCCAM) has succinctly stated this rationale: "Despite their potential, untested CAM therapies may have unintended negative consequences. They may interfere with or displace effective treatments . . . and they may absorb resources that might be better invested in more appropriate treatment. Thus, it is critical to evaluate widely used CAM treatments for both safety and efficacy" (NCCAM 5-year strategic plan 2001–2005).

However, there is a much stronger rationale for researching Yoga that is based on availability and is more appealing to those of us committed to the promotion of Yoga. Despite its popularity, Yoga has been largely restricted to narrow segments of the population. Demographic analyses from U.S. Yoga surveys have shown a clear skewing in favor of higher incomes, higher education, white-collar occupations, and middle-aged or young adults. There is also a strong gender imbalance favoring women (about 3:1) and an uneven geographical distribution in the United States (Birdee, et al., 2008). While examples of initiatives to provide Yoga to underserved populations exist, it is unlikely that these initiatives will fully penetrate the demographics of the population sufficiently to ultimately result in a truly widespread use of Yoga.

A viable solution to this problem is to embed Yoga into societal systems that already penetrate the entire population: the education and the healthcare systems. Unfortunately, the popularity of Yoga and anecdotal evidence of its benefits are insufficient to justify the incorporation of Yoga into these systems. Carefully designed and executed research studies that convincingly validate its physical and psychological benefits will be required before it can be broadly applied to a large number of populations (children, the elderly, patients, etc.) and institutions (hospitals, schools, offices, etc.). A CAM study confirmed that "the primary obstacles to incorporating CAM into mainstream healthcare were the following: lack of research on efficacy [and] uncertainty that offering CAM is profitable or that research demonstrates cost-effectiveness" (Pelletier, 2002). Although some research exists for Yoga, much more is needed.

It is indeed possible to imbed a health/wellness behavior into our society as a widespread practice. A classical historical example of this is the incorporation of dental hygiene education into the public schools in the United States at the beginning of the twentieth century in response to the high burden of oral health problems and the knowledge of the benefits of proper dental hygiene. The result has been the full incorporation of dental hygiene into our education and healthcare systems to the point where it is now a widespread cultural norm. It is necessary to compare and contrast this to Yoga, which is essentially a "mind-body hygiene."

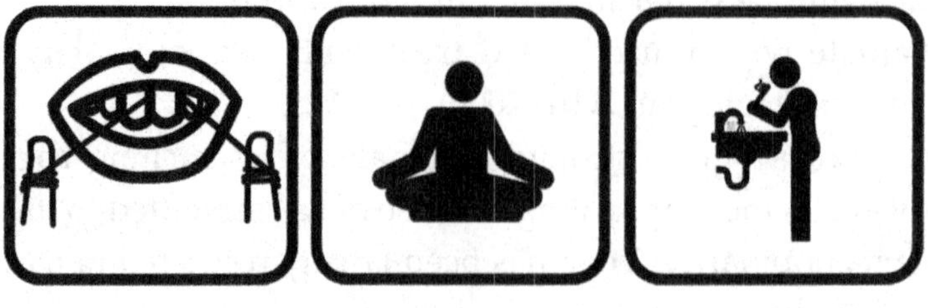

Mind-body practices such as Yoga and meditation are not taught routinely in school systems or prescribed by doctors. Current physical education promotes competitive sports and focuses on exercise only to develop muscle strength and cardiorespiratory endurance. Education in skills for maintaining socio-emotional and psychological health are even less apparent, if present at all. We are a society raised without effective self-care/preventive techniques necessary to deal with stress, emotion, attachment, grief, tension, and the wide array of associated physical symptoms. Consequently, we are burdened with relatively high levels of dysfunctional attitudes, maladaptive behaviors, distress, and mood disturbances, as well as a lower sense of well-being and impaired quality of life—all of which can lead to or exacerbate medical and psychiatric conditions.

Those of us actively involved in a personal Yoga practice, instruction, and Yoga Therapy believe that widespread practice would have a deep positive and transforming impact on the physical and psychological health of society as a whole and reduce the high economic burden of our healthcare system. As an adjunct/complementary self-care medical treatment, Yoga Therapy has enormous potential to cost-effectively treat disorders that are often treated superficially, symptomatically, and ineffectively with drugs and surgery. But Yoga research will ultimately provide the basis and support for incorporating Yoga-based practices into our healthcare system. This will, of course, take time as we await the necessary critical mass of Yoga research studies and replications of these studies by different investigators in different institutions on different populations in different settings.

BASIC RESEARCH ON THE PSYCHOPHYSIOLOGY OF YOGA

Research on the psychophysiological effects of Yoga practice began with Swami Kuvalayananda's efforts in the 1920s to apply modern research methods to elucidate the psychophysiology of Yoga practices. This work and a number of additional classic studies set the stage for future work showing the capability of individuals to self-regulate internal psychological and physiological states with Yoga practice (Funderburk, 1977; Pratap, 1971). Bagchi and Wenger (Bagchi and Wenger, 1957), in their early seminal Yoga research study of master practitioners in India, concluded that "physiologically yogic meditation represents deep relaxation of the autonomic nervous system without drowsiness or sleep and a type of cerebral activity without highly accelerated electrophysiological manifestation but probably with more or less insensibility to some outside stimuli for a short or long time." Subsequently, Herbert Benson, M.D., at Harvard Medical School demonstrated that meditation could induce what he termed the *relaxation response.* This is a self-regulatory, coordinated psychophysiological downregulation of the stress system with a generalized reduction in both cognitive and somatic arousal as observed in hypothalamic pituitary axis and the autonomic nervous system that is the opposite of the well-known stress or fight-or-flight response (Benson, 1975). Later Yoga research studies examining its component techniques of postures/exercises, breathing techniques, and meditation/mindfulness practices both in isolation and in combination have further confirmed these early results that Yoga is an excellent stress-management and emotion-regulation practice (Arpita, 1990; Gharote, 1991; Li and Goldsmith, 2012; Streeter, et al., 2012; Dunn, 2008; Ospina, et al., 2007). From recent research, there are now very compelling brain-imaging and genomic-expression studies on Yoga and meditation showing positive changes in psychophysiological functioning, and even anatomical structure, in the systems involved in stress, resilience, and emotion regulation (Streeter, et al., 2012; Saatcioglu, 2013). Given that many disease states are caused or exacerbated by unmanaged stress and mood, this represents a significant underlying mechanism by which Yoga Therapy exerts its benefit.

Other research has demonstrated the ability of Yoga practices to enhance mind/body awareness or mindfulness (Mehling, et al., 2011). This is an important characteristic that can be of great importance in facilitating behavior change in patients with lifestyle diseases such as obesity and type 2 diabetes, which are occurring in near epidemic proportions and constitute the greatest burden on healthcare costs. Āsana (posture) and prāṇāyāma (breathing) practices have been shown to provide direct improvements in musculoskeletal and respiratory functioning (Abel, et al., 2013; Raub, 2002), which are also likely of benefit in improving symptom management in a variety of disease states. Finally, Yoga is also a contemplative, transpersonal, and transformative practice that can lead to dramatic changes in spirituality and self-concept, which are also invaluable assets in contributing to the potential therapeutic benefit of Yoga in patient populations (Luskin, 2004).

HISTORY AND BREADTH OF RESEARCH ON YOGA THERAPY

Research on therapeutic applications of Yoga and meditation began more recently than that of basic research (Gharote, 1991), and, although there are reviews of this literature, many of these are restricted to specific disorders (Bussing, et al., 2012). The past few decades have seen a dramatic increase in the quantity and quality of research in academic journals on Yoga as a therapeutic intervention. A 2004 bibliometric analysis of Yoga Therapy research publications revealed 181 studies in eighty-one journals in fifteen countries. The majority of research focused on mental health conditions, cardiovascular disorders, and pulmonary disease (Khalsa, 2004). In the subsequent eight years, research has more than doubled, with a remarkable surge in cancer trials and increased frequency in studies exploring conditions not previously tested. A large number of Yoga Therapy research review papers have been published (Bussing, et al., 2012).

All of the reviews on Yoga Therapy research literature highlight the weaknesses in the quality of research by citing small sample size, the low percentage of randomized controlled trials, and/or the lack of trials with active controls, and/or the heterogeneity of Yoga interventions, including the frequency/duration of practice. Such limitations in this body of research is not surprising, though, given that Yoga Therapy research is a new field and is likely to improve in quality over time. Reviews are generally optimistic that further research will yield positive outcomes and that enough evidence exists to recommend therapeutic Yoga to treat conditions directly and/or as a supportive or adjunct treatment to increase self-competence, physical fitness, and well-being.

MENTAL HEALTH DISORDERS

The volume of research published on Yoga Therapy for mental health exceeds that of any other health condition, which is consistent with a 2008 U.S. survey report that the primary therapeutic use of Yoga in the public was for mental health problems (Birdee, 2008). Historically, Yoga research in this area has focused on the two major disorders of depression and anxiety; however, recent studies have begun to expand the scope of conditions evaluated. A heavily publicized review that analyzed the use of Yoga for a variety of psychiatric conditions (excluding anxiety disorders) revealed preliminary evidence for Yoga as an adjunct treatment in schizophrenia, attention deficit hyperactivity disorder (ADHD), and sleep complaints (Balasubramaniam, et al., 2013). Reviews have also noted that more evidence exists for the efficacy of Yoga in depression than for any other psychiatric problem (Bussing, et al., 2012; Balasubramaniam, et al., 2013). Other publications and reviews have reiterated Yoga's utility for depression, including its benefit for major depressive disorder, dysthymia, and elevated depressive symptoms (Pilkington, et al., 2005; da Silva, et al., 2009; Uebelacker, et al., 2010; Cramer, et al., 2013). In describing the rationale of Yoga for depression, Uebelacker has hypothesized that Yoga offers unique therapeutic benefit because it integrates techniques of mindfulness, movement, and breathwork, all of which are effective in the management of depression (Uebelacker, et al., 2010).

Evidence revealing the therapeutic use of Yoga for anxiety is mixed. Most of the research on anxiety has not focused directly on anxiety spectrum disorder populations but rather on anxiety itself as an outcome measure (Li and Goldsmith, 2012; da Silva, et al., 2009). Exceptions include a trial for obsessive compulsive disorder (Shannahoff-Khalsa, et al., 1999), the first trial on generalized anxiety disorder published in 2012 (Katzman, et al., 2012), and a number of trials of Yoga for posttraumatic stress disorder (van der Kolk, 2006; Staples, et al. 2013; Descilo, et al., 2010; Telles, et al., 2010) for which there is growing interest. Notably, in 2006, Bessel van der Kolk, a leader in trauma research, first articulated a proposed neuroscientific basis for body-based therapies such as Yoga for trauma (van der Kolk, 2006). Subsequent review papers on research studies of Yoga for trauma have also discussed the scientific rationale and underlying mechanisms that may be involved (Streeter, et al., 2012; Cabral, et al., 2011; Telles, et al., 2012).

B. N. Gangadhar, M.D., at the National Institute of Mental Health and Neurosciences in India has recently become a prominent researcher in the field of Yoga research for psychiatric conditions and has conducted trials on autonomic, neurological, and psychological changes that occur through Yoga practice. A recent issue of the *Indian Journal of Psychiatry* highlighted a dozen papers from his group on Yoga for mental health conditions, including schizophrenia, depression, and the first trial of Yoga for psychosis (Khalsa, 2013). Such findings have expanded the conception of the potential of Yoga Therapy for all mental health disorders.

MUSCULOSKELETAL CONDITIONS

The use of Yoga for musculoskeletal conditions is increasingly popular as evidenced by a U.S. survey, which revealed that relief of musculoskeletal problems was a primary incentive for practice (Birdee, et al., 2008). The benefit of Yoga for musculoskeletal problems is also supported by research reviews, which have concluded that

Yoga may lead to improvements in pain and functional outcome and is one of the more promising mind-body therapies (Chou and Huffman, 2007; Cramer, et al., 2013).

The predominant research area on therapeutic Yoga practices is for lower back pain (LBP), although clinical trials of other back pain conditions like kyphosis and neck pain are also revealing Yoga's benefit. Reviews report that Yoga is mildly better than exercise in reducing disability and pain symptoms in LBP and moderately preferable to self-care and education (Cramer, et al., 2007; Hill, 2013). However, the field is riddled with debate over preferred style of Yoga and duration of intervention to achieve the best results. Additionally, different studies have examined a variety of differing levels of LBP severity, thereby complicating clear conclusions about Yoga's benefit (Tilbrook, et al., 2011).

The research of Karen Sherman, Ph.D., M.P.H., offers a prime example of this complication. In a 2011 study, Sherman reported Yoga was equal to stretching on all measures of LPB, thereby challenging Yoga's potentially unique benefit, even in relationship to perceived stress (Sherman, et al., 2013). However, in a subsequent paper Sherman elaborated on these findings revealing that the study excluded moderate and acute back pain and that participants exhibited low levels of stress prior to the intervention. Sherman hypothesized that Yoga might offer greater benefit in more acute LBP populations than stretching would, specifically in stress reduction (Sherman, et al., 2013). Evidence for the efficacy of Yoga for other musculoskeletal conditions is mixed. A few trials were published showing that Yoga was superior to exercise in reducing pain and disability and improving quality of life. Cramer and colleagues examined Yoga versus exercise for neck pain. After a nine-week Yoga intervention and a twelve-month follow-up, both revealed the same level improvement, in function, pain intensity, and mental quality of life (Cramer, et al., 2013; Cramer, Dobos, et al. 2013).

Reviewers analyzing published evidence on joint issues suggest that Yoga may have less efficacy than for other musculoskeletal conditions. In a review paper evaluating eight trials on osteoarthritis, Haaz concluded that Yoga is equal to or better than exercise in reducing swollen joints and pain, while a rigorous analysis by Cramer that ultimately only examined two studies was skeptical about the evidence for both osteoarthritis and rheumatoid arthritis (Haaz and Bartlett, 2011; Cramer, et al., 2013). Furthermore, two studies on carpal tunnel syndrome found Yoga was superior to a splint in increasing grip strength and decreasing pain (Garfinkel, 1998; Garfinkel and Schumacher, 2000).

CARDIOVASCULAR CONDITIONS

The first trial published on Yoga Therapy was conducted in 1973 by British cardiologist Patel, revealing Yoga's potential for decreasing hypertension (Patel, 1973). Since this initial study, the field of Yoga Therapy research for cardiovascular conditions has blossomed into one of the more prolific areas, and evidence supports Yoga's role in reducing risk of cardiovascular disease and its utility in treatment and rehabilitation. The beneficial properties of Yoga were explored in a 2004 review (Jayasinghe, 2004), which described thirteen studies and a 2005 review identifying seventy studies, of which sixteen were analyzed (Innes, et al., 2005). These reviews have suggested that Yoga reduces cardiovascular risk factors including high levels of cholesterol and triglycerides, improves anthropometric characteristics, reduces sympathetic tone, increases heart-rate-variability, and decreases hypertension.

This positive evidence has stimulated a growth in trials evaluating Yoga's benefit for specific cardiovascular pathologies and outcomes. Findings have included improved lipid profiles in postmyocardial infarction, increased baroreflex sensitivity (BRS) in ischemia heart disease and chronic heart failure, and improvement of symptoms in atrial fibrillation and ventricular arrhythmia (Khare and Rai, 2002; Howie-Esquivel, et al., 2010; Lakkireddy, et al., 2013; Dabhade, et al., 2012). The evaluation of Yoga for hypertension has undergone consistent research ever since Patel's early research. A 2013 review of Yoga for hypertension found that traditional Yoga interventions produce significant reductions in diastolic and systolic blood pressure even in comparison to exercise (Hagins, et al., 2013).

A notable effort in this area has been the study of discrete Yoga practices on cardiovascular health. For example, Italian cardiologist and Yoga researcher Luciano Bernardi, M.D., has conducted extensive research on slow breathing demonstrating its efficacy in improving baroreflex sensitivity, decreasing the respiratory chemoreflex, and improving oxygen saturation, all of which are important in cardiovascular conditions (Bernardi, et al., 2001; Bernardi, et al., 2001; Joseph, et al., 2005).

In his landmark 1990 study, Dean Ornish, M.D., revealed the efficacy of a full yogic lifestyle program in cardiac rehabilitation (Ornish, et al., 1990). In a rigorous research trial that included diet, relaxation, and lifestyle management, Dr. Ornish found participants could reverse coronary heart disease; an outcome that has never before been demonstrated with any intervention. His yearlong trial reduced stenosis in participants while a usual care group had increased blockage. This evidence has been seminal in demonstrating the potential impact of behavioral and mind-body medicine and has directly contributed to the decision by Medicare to reimburse participation in Dr. Ornish's lifestyle program for heart disease.

PULMONARY CONDITIONS

As breathing practices are an inherent part of Yoga practice, it should not be surprising that research on Yoga for respiratory complaints has been and continues to be a large area of research. In fact, according to the 2004 bibliometric analysis, there were more publications in non-Yoga journals on asthma than on any other discrete disorder (Khalsa, 2004). Additionally, the largest trial in Yoga Therapy research was a noncontrolled study of asthmatics by Nagendra in 1986 in which 570 participants were followed for three to fifty-four months. Evidence in that study revealed a positive correlation between amount of practice and significant positive outcomes such as reduced cortisone and increased peak respiratory flow (Nagendra and Nagarathna, 1986). Various other Indian studies before 2000 have measured reductions in medication, better exercise tolerance, and improvement in overall lung functioning following a Yoga intervention. However, in the only review devoted to research on Yoga Therapy for asthma, the author noted the weaknesses in poor study design and suggested that findings were generally insignificant especially in comparison to control conditions (Posadzki and Ernst, 2011). His negative conclusion is supported by a rigorous study that reported only moderate gains even in absence of a control condition and a study of complete lifestyle intervention versus usual care. In the latter study, although the quality of life improved, no changes in pulmonary functioning were expressed (Singh, et al., 1990; Kligler, et al., 2011).

In a review of complementary alternative medicine (CAM) therapy trials for asthma, Burgess included review of Yoga studies and found some evidence of benefit. He also noted that review of this literature was particularly problematic due to the high level of interventions used across studies and poor characterization of breath practices (Burgess, et al., 2011). Consequently, reviewers often compare "yogic breathing" against another breathing technique, unaware that the other technique is also a style of yogic breathing, leading to confusion about what Yoga can actually offer.

Reviewers have experienced similar challenges in examining studies of Yoga programs for chronic obstructive pulmonary disease (COPD) in respect to the variety of interventions used with twenty-four weeks being the most popular. Even still, reviewers are generally agreed that evidence supports the conclusion that Yoga practice may reduce dyspnea and increase exercise tolerance in COPD (Holland, et al., 2012; Donesky, et al., 2012).

METABOLIC CONDITIONS

Metabolic disorders are on the rise worldwide with type 2 diabetes reaching epidemic levels particularly in low- and middle-income countries. Since the 1990s, a growing need for cost-effective treatments has stimulated substantial research interest in Yoga's role in the treatment of diabetes. Three reviews have investigated the influence of Yoga on metabolic disease (Aljasir, Bryson, and Al-Shehri, 2010; Yang, 2007; Innes and Vincent, 2007). Yang's review described Yoga's overall benefit in reducing risk factors for chronic disease in general while the other two reviews focused solely on type 2 diabetes. Aljasir's review was particularly critical, stating that the current trials are virtually inconclusive, yet Innes was more optimistic in reporting that "Yoga may improve indices of risk in adults with type 2 diabetes." Her analysis suggested a multidimensional role for Yoga in the treatment and prevention of diabetes, including decreasing fasting plasma blood glucose and reducing insulin resistance, as well as improving lipid and anthropometric profiles.

Evidence also indicates that Yoga may reduce obesity in both adults and children. A 2013 review by Rioux confirmed the link between Yoga and weight reduction, noting the fact that greater frequency and length of practice, coupled with a complete yogic program and diet, were most effective in reducing weight. Even so, in Rioux's review, there were very few studies suggesting that Yoga was superior to exercise (Rioux and Ritenbaugh, 2013).

CANCER

Cancer is by far the fastest growing area of Yoga Therapy research over the past decade. In fact, the research has been so prolific that it has prompted over a dozen review papers, eight of which were published in 2012 alone (Bower, et al., 2005; Smith and Pukall, 2009; Cramer, et al., 2012; Cote and Daneault, 2012; Zhang, et al., 2013; Cramer, et al., 2012; Harder, Parlour, and Jenkins, 2012; Levine and Balk,

2012; Buffart, et al., 2012). The most robust area of research on cancer has been conducted on women with breast cancer currently undergoing radiation or chemotherapy, followed by rapid growth in trials on breast cancer survivors. Comparably little evidence exists for the effects on men with cancer or on other types of cancer. In general, these research trials have not focused on reducing biometric markers of cancer or tumor reduction but rather were directed at evaluating changes in psychological characteristics, including mood, quality of life, and well-being measures. Two studies have reported reductions in cortisol levels in cancer patients and many more have investigated sleep and physical functioning (Vadiraja, et al., 2009; Banasik, et al., 2011; Saper, et al., 2009). Notably, one study revealed that participation in a Yoga intervention reduced immune suppression postsurgery in breast cancer (Rao, et al., 2008).

It has been suggested that, due to ethical concerns that have placed priority on patient preference over that of research design issues, most Yoga cancer studies have not incorporated randomized controlled trials in which participants cannot choose their intervention. Although this bias must be considered in evaluating the outcomes, the overwhelming majority of clinical trials have reported decreased distress, anxiety, depression, and improved quality of life (QOL). Although not surprising given the overwhelming existing research evidence for such psychological benefits of Yoga practice, this is of great significance in the cancer patient population given that emotional well-being is correlated with better prognosis. Research on Yoga Therapy for cancer has also focused on improving daily functioning, such as reduction in cancer-related fatigue and enhanced physical functioning, but findings have differed among trials. Mild improvements in sleep have also been reported, but there are mixed results in the literature.

One of the leaders in the field of Yoga research for cancer is Lorenzo Cohen, M.D., at M.D. Anderson Cancer Center, who has investigated QOL for breast cancer patients undergoing radiation and sleep quality in lymphoma patients (Cohen, et al., 2004; Chandwani, et al., 2010). His laboratory is currently conducting a large-scale clinical trial funded by the National Cancer Institute at the NIH investigating the efficacy and cost benefit of including Yoga in the treatment of women with breast cancer as part of usual care (the largest grant to date ever awarded for Yoga Therapy research). As this institution is considered one of the world's premiere cancer hospitals, positive results from this study may favorably impact the medical community's perception of Yoga as an adjunct treatment for cancer patients.

NEUROLOGICAL AND IMMUNE DISORDERS

Yoga Therapy for neurological, immune, and pain disorders is a relatively new area of research with only a handful of publications. A review of Yoga research in neurological disorders by Mishra offered limited, but promising, evidence for the therapeutic application of Yoga in epilepsy for reducing seizures and improving quality of life; a couple of trials on multiple sclerosis found Yoga superior to exercise in improving mood and physical symptoms (Mishra, et al., 2012). Additionally, there is one very preliminary study on Yoga and traumatic brain injury reporting enhanced physical and respiratory functioning (Silverthorne, et al., 2012) and a few studies on Yoga for neurodegenerative disorders such as Alzheimer's disease that express psychological benefit, but, to date, no significant changes in cognitive functioning (Gallego, et al., 2011; Litchke, et al., 2012). Clinical trials for Yoga and fibromyalgia, a pain disorder with a strong neurological component, which influences perception of pain and experience of pain, suggest that Yoga may improve psychological and physical symptoms as compared to usual care (Cramer, et al., 2013).

Some studies have provided evidence that Yoga supports immunological resiliency, specifically in populations with higher levels of stress who are more prone to disease (Gopal, 2011; Black, et al., 2013). Two earlier studies using Yoga-based practices reported significant improvement in immune indices (Cruess, et al., 2000; Antoni, et al., 2000) while the only study on Yoga and HIV found significant positive changes in cardiovascular disease risk factors, but no change in immunological markers (Cade, et al., 2010).

SPECIAL POPULATIONS

Yoga has also been evaluated for special populations and conditions that are not actual disease states such as pregnancy, menopause, children/adolescents, and the elderly. Yoga for pregnancy has become quite popular in the general public and research has confirmed that prenatal Yoga has significant benefit; it may reduce pain and discomfort, perceived stress, and improve quality of life and labor parameters (Curtis, Weinrib, and Katz, 2012; Babbar, Parks-Savage, and Chauhan, 2012). Notably, one review of prenatal Yoga also found that the regular practice of Yoga improved birth weight and reduced preterm labor (Babbar, Parks-Savage, and

Chauhan, 2012). On the other hand, the evidence for the efficacy of Yoga on menopausal symptoms is mixed. Reviewers agree that there is no significant evidence to support Yoga's role in reducing physical complaints; however, one review revealed that the practice of Yoga enhanced quality of life and psychological well-being in menopausal women (Lee, et al., 2009; Cramer, et al., 2012).

For the elderly, Yoga may be a significant practice in maintaining and even improving well-being. A 2012 review that focused on Yoga's physical benefits verified that Yoga improved fitness, strength, and perceived health and that Yoga may be superior to exercise (Patel, Newstead, and Ferrer, 2012). On trials devoted to mood measures of geriatric populations, Yoga has been reported to successfully reduce stress, anxiety, and depressive symptoms (Chong, et al., 2011).

Positive benefits have been reported for Yoga in children and adolescents for a variety of conditions including stress, mood, self-concept, and weight management, as well as for both cognitive and physical performance (Galantino, Galbavy, and Quinn, 2008; Birdee, et al., 2009). There is currently a popular and growing movement promoting the incorporation of Yoga practices within public school settings. Research on these interventions in school settings is just beginning, although a review has been published citing twelve studies with apparent benefit but that lack rigor in research design characteristics (Serwacki and Cook-Cottone, 2012). Lastly, a few randomized controlled trials have been published, showing improvements in adolescents in mood and resilience (Khalsa, et al., 2012).

PREVENTION AND WELLNESS

Although Yoga Therapy is usually defined as the use of Yoga in the treatment of disease, it is equally relevant and perhaps even more important as a form of preventive medicine. As a complete lifestyle, Yoga affords practitioners a range of positive habits and practices that cultivate and maintain well-being. Evidence revealing Yoga's role as a preventive strategy is supported by both surveys of long-term practitioners and prospective studies. In 2008, a U.S. survey reported 58 percent of practitioners believed that Yoga maintained well-being (Birdee, et al., 2008) while a 2012 survey observed a significant correlation between practice hours, well-being, and resilience (Ross, et al., 2012). Long-term Yoga practice was a predictor of psychological wellness in women over age forty-five, was correlated with improved quality of life and sleep in the elderly, improved hormonal modulation and sleep quality in the elderly, and reduced weight, blood pressure, and glucose levels in long-term practitioners (Moliver, et al., 2013; Bankar, Chaudhari, and Chaudhari, 2013; Vera, et al., 2009; Yang, 2007).

It is likely that these health measures reflect the benefits of actual Yoga practice and the lifestyles changes that naturally emerge from regular practice. A recent U.S. survey study compared health outcomes for practitioners and nonpractitioners, finding positive health outcomes for practitioners in comparison to non-practitioners, and that superior health outcomes were associated behaviors that were correlated with long-term practice (Ross, et al., 2013). Practitioners not only stretched their bodies and meditated but also smoked less, exercised more, and ate healthier, thus contributing to their overall long-term health.

CONCLUSION

The current explosion in the popularity of research in Yoga Therapy and meditation is likely to continue as more of the general public experiences their benefits. There are numerous young scientists and investigators interested in adopting this field of research, and more and more academic and clinical institutions are adopting integrative medicine practices such as Yoga. The application of modern scientific methodologies such as molecular biological assays and brain-imaging techniques is growing rapidly in Yoga research and will not only help elucidate the full range of improvements but will also provide valuable information on the mechanisms of action of these contemplative practices. The current medical and scientific research paradigm still prevails and is held by many conventional biomedical researchers who are still focused on treating disease symptoms with pharmaceuticals or surgical procedures. This continues to some degree to impede Yoga research, as grant review panels mostly consist of conventional allopathic medicine researchers. Furthermore, federal funding limitations also add to the challenge of acquiring Yoga research grants. Because of this, private philanthropic funding of Yoga research as a potential for stable support would be welcome. Ultimately, the publication of rigorously conducted Yoga research trials will justify continued and expanded funding and the continuation of the recent dramatic growth in Yoga research.

REFERENCES

Abel, A. N., L. K. Lloyd, and J. S. Williams. "The Effects of Regular Yoga Practice on Pulmonary Function in Healthy Individuals: A Literature Review." *Journal of Alternative and Complementary Medicine* 19.3 (2013): 185–90. Print.

Aljasir, B., Bryson, M., and B. Al-Shehri. "Yoga Practice for the Management of Type II Diabetes Mellitus in Adults: A Systematic Review." *Evidence Based Complementary and Alternative Medicine* 7.4 (2010): 399–408. Print.

Antoni, M. H., et al. "Cognitive–Behavioral Stress Management Intervention Effects on Anxiety, 24-Hour Urinary Norepinephrine Output, and T-Cytotoxic/Suppressor Cells over Time Among Symptomatic HIV-Infected Gay Men." *Journal of Consulting and Clinical Psychology* 68.1 (2000): 31–45. Print.

Arpita, J. "Physiological and Psychological Effects of Hatha Yoga: A Review of the Literature." *Journal of the International Association of Yoga Therapists* 1.I-II (1990): 1–28. Print.

Babbar, S., A. C. Parks-Savage, and S. P. Chauhan. "Yoga During Pregnancy: A Review." *American Journal of Perinatology* 29.6 (2012): 459–464. Print.

Bagchi, B. K., and M. A. Wenger. "Electro-Physiological Correlates of Some Yogi Exercises." *Electroencephalography and Clinical Neurophysiology* 7 Supplement (1957): 132–149. Print.

Balasubramaniam, M., S. Telles, and P. M. Doraiswamy. "Yoga on Our Minds: A Systematic Review of Yoga for Neuropsychiatric Disorders." *Frontiers in Psychiatry,* 25 January 2013, 3:117. Web. doi: 10.3389/fpsyt.2012.00117.

Banasik, J., et al. "Effect of Iyengar Yoga Practice on Fatigue and Diurnal Salivary Cortisol Concentration in Breast Cancer Survivors." *Journal of the American Academy of Nurse Practitioners* 23.3 (2011): 135–142. Print.

Bankar, M. A., S. K. Chaudhari, and K. D. Chaudhari. "Impact of Long-Term Yoga Practice on Sleep Quality and Quality of Life in the Elderly." *Journal of Ayurveda and Integrative Medicine* 4.1 (2013): 28–32. Print.

Benson, H. *The Relaxation Response.* New York: William Morrow/Harper Collins, 1975; 2000. Print.

Bernardi, L., et al. "Slow Breathing Reduces Chemoreflex Response to Hypoxia and Hypercapnia, and Increases Baroreflex Sensitivity." *Journal of Hypertension* 19.12 (2001): 2221–2229. Print.

Bernardi, L., et al. "Effect of Rosary Prayer and Yoga Mantras on Autonomic Cardiovascular Rhythms: Comparative Study." *British Medical Journal* 323.7327 (2001): 1446–1449. Print.

Birdee, G. S., et al. "Characteristics of Yoga Users: Results of a National Survey." *Journal of General International Medicine* 23.10 (2008): 1653–1658. Print.

Birdee, G. S., et al. "Clinical Applications of Yoga for the Pediatric Population: A Systematic Review." *Academic Pediatrics* 9.4 (2009): 212–220.e1–9. Print.

Black, D. S., et al. "Yogic Meditation Reverses NF-kappaB and IRF-Related Transcriptome Dynamics in Leukocytes of Family Dementia Caregivers in a Randomized Controlled Trial." *Psychoneuroendocrinology* 38.3 (2013): 348–355. Print.

Bower, J. E., et al. "Yoga for Cancer Patients and Survivors." *Cancer Control* 12.3 (2005): 165–171. Print.

Buffart, L. M., et al. "Physical and Psychosocial Benefits of Yoga in Cancer Patients and Survivors: A Systematic Review and Meta-Analysis of Randomized Controlled Trials." BioMedCentral.com, 27 Nov. 2012. 12:559. Web. doi:10.1186/1471-2407-12-559.

Burgess, J., et al. "Systematic Review of the Effectiveness of Breathing Retraining in Asthma Management." *Expert Review of Respiratory Medicine* 5.6 (2011): 789–807. Print.

Bussing, A., et al. "Effects of Yoga on Mental and Physical Health: A Short Summary of Reviews." *Evidence-Based Complementary and Alternative Medicine* 2012: Article ID 165410. 18 July 2012. Web. http://www.hindawi.com/journals/ecam/2012/165410/.

Cabral, P., H. B. Meyer, and D. Ames. "Effectiveness of Yoga Therapy as a Complementary Treatment for Major Psychiatric Disorders: A Meta-Analysis. Primary Care Companion for CNS Disorders." 13.4 (2011): n.p. Print.

Cade, W. T., et al. "Yoga Lifestyle Intervention Reduces Blood Pressure in HIV-Infected Adults with Cardiovascular Disease Risk Factors." *HIV Medicine* 11.6 (2010): 379–388. Print.

Chandwani, K. D., et al. "Yoga Improves Quality of Life and Benefit Finding in Women Undergoing Radiotherapy for Breast Cancer." *Journal of the Society for Integrative Oncology* 8.2 (2010): 43–55. Print.

Chong, C. S., et al. "Effects of Yoga on Stress Management in Healthy Adults: A Systematic Review." *Alternative Therapies in Health and Medicine* 17.1 (2011): 32–38. Print.

Chou, R., and L. H. Huffman. "Nonpharmacologic Therapies for Acute and Chronic Low Back Pain: A Review of the Evidence for an American Pain Society/American College of Physicians Clinical Practice Guideline." *Annals of Internal Medicine* 147.7 (2007): 492–504. Print.

Cohen, L., et al. "Psychological Adjustment and Sleep Quality in a Randomized Trial of the Effects of a Tibetan Yoga Intervention in Patients with Lymphoma." *Cancer* 100 (2004): 2253–2260. Print.

Cramer, H., et al."Effectiveness of Yoga for Menopausal Symptoms: A Systematic Review and Meta-Analysis of Randomized Controlled Trials." *Evidence-Based Complementary and Alternative Medicine* 2012: Article ID 863905. 1 June 2012. Web. http://www.hindawi.com/journals/ecam/2012/863905/.

Cramer, H., et al. "Yoga for Breast Cancer Patients and Survivors: A Systematic Review and Meta-analysis." BioMedCentral.com, 18 Sept. 2012. 12:412. Web. doi: 10.1186/1471-2407-12-412.

Cramer, H., et al. "Can Yoga Improve Fatigue in Breast Cancer Patients? A Systematic Review." *Acta Oncologica* 51.4 (2012): 559–560. Print.

Cramer, H., et al. "Yoga for Chronic Neck Pain: A 12-Month Follow-Up." *Pain Medicine Journal* 14.4 (2013):541–548. Print.

Cramer, H., et al. "A Systematic Review and Meta-Analysis of Yoga for Low Back Pain." *Clinical Journal of Pain* 29.5 (2013): 450–460. Print.

Cramer, H., et al. "Yoga for Rheumatic Diseases: A Systematic Review." *Rheumatology* (Oxford) 52.11 (2013): 2025–2030. Print.

Cramer, H., et al. "Yoga for Depression: A Systematic Review and Meta-Analysis." *Depression and Anxiety* 30.11 (2013): 1068–1093. Print.

Cramer, H., et al. "Randomized-Controlled Trial Comparing Yoga and Home-Based Exercise for Chronic Neck Pain." *Clinical Journal of Pain* 29.3 (2013): 216–223. Print.

Cote, A., and S. Daneault. "Effect of Yoga on Patients with Cancer: Our Current Understanding. *Canadian Family Physician* 58.9 (2012): e475–479. Print.

Cruess, S., et al. "Reductions in Herpes Simplex Virus Type 2 Antibody Titers After Cognitive Behavioral Stress Management and Relationships with Neuroendocrine Function, Relaxation Skills, and Social Support in HIV-Positive Men." *Psychosomatic Medicine* 62.6 (2000): 828–837. Print.

Curtis, K., A. Weinrib, and J. Katz "Systematic Review of Yoga for Pregnant Women: Current Status and Future Directions." *Evidence-Based Complementary and Alternative Medicine* 2012: Article ID 715942. 14 Aug. 2012. Web. http://www.ncbi.nlm.nih.gov/pmc/articles/ PMC3424788/.

Dabhade, A. M., et al. "Effect of Pranayama (Breathing Exercise) on Arrhythmias in the Human Heart." *Explore (NY)* 8.1 (2012): 12–15. Print.

da Silva, T. L., L. N. Ravindran, and A. V. Ravindran. "Yoga in the Treatment of Mood and Anxiety Disorders: A Review." *Asian Journal of Psychiatry* 2.1 (2009): 6–16. Print.

Descilo, T., et al. "Effects of a Yoga Breath Intervention Alone and in Combination with an Exposure Therapy for Post-Traumatic Stress Disorder and Depression in Survivors of the 2004 South-East Asia Tsunami." *Acta Psychiatrica Scandinavica* 121.14 (2010): 289–300. Print.

Donesky, D., et al. "A Responder Analysis of the Effects of Yoga for Individuals with COPD: Who Benefits and How?" *International Journal of Yoga Therapy* 22 (2012): 23–36. Print.

Dunn, K. D. "A Review of the Literature Examining the Physiological Processes Underlying the Therapeutic Benefits of Hatha Yoga." *Advances in Mind-Body Medicine* 23.10 (2008): 10–18. Print.

Funderburk, J. *Science Studies Yoga: A Review of Physiological Data*. Glenview, IL: Himalayan Institute Press, 1977. Print.

Galantino, M. L., R. Galbavy, and L. Quinn. (2008). "Therapeutic Effects of Yoga for Children: A Systematic Review of the Literature. *Pediatric Physical Therapy* 20.1 (2008): 66–80. Print.

Gallego, Q., et al. "Effects of Hatha-Yoga Program on a Small Group with Alzheimer's Disease." *Journal of Yoga and Physical Therapy* 3 (2011): n.p. Print.

Garfinkel, M. S. "Yoga-Based Intervention for Carpal Tunnel Syndrome: A Randomized Trial." *Journal of the American Medical Association* 280.18 (1998): 1601–1603. Print.

Garfinkel, M., and H. R. Schumacher. "Yoga." *Rheumatic Disease Clinics of North America* 26.1 (2000): 125–132. Print.

Gharote, M. L. "Analytical Survey of Researches in Yoga." *Yoga Mimamsa* 29.4 (1991): 53–68. Print.

Gopal, A. "Effect of Integrated Yoga Practices on Immune Responses in Examination Stress: A Preliminary Study." *International Journal of Yoga* 4.1 (2011): 26–32. Print.

Haaz, S., and S. J. Bartlett. "Yoga for Arthritis: A Scoping Review." *Rheumatic Disease Clinics of North America* 37.1 (2011): 33–46. Print.

Hagins, M., et al. "Effectiveness of Yoga for Hypertension: Systematic Review and Meta-Analysis." *Evidence-Based Complementary and Alternative Medicine* 2013: Article ID 649836. 28 May 2013. Web. doi: 10.1155/2013/649836.

Harder, H., L. Parlour, and V. Jenkins. "Randomised Controlled Trials of Yoga Interventions for Women with Breast Cancer: A Systematic Literature Review." *Support Care Cancer* 20.12 (2012): 3055–3064. Print.

Hill, C. "Is Yoga an Effective Treatment in the Management of Patients with Chronic Low Back Pain Compared with Other Care Modalities—A Systematic Review." *Journal of Complementary & Integrative Medicine* 10.1 (2013): 211–219. Print.

Holland, A. E., et al. "Breathing Exercises for Chronic Obstructive Pulmonary Disease." *Cochrane Database System Review* 10:CD008250. 17 Oct. 2012. Web. doi: 10.1002/14651858.

Howie-Esquivel, J., et al. "Yoga in Heart Failure Patients: A Pilot Study." *Journal of Cardiac Failure* 16.9 (2010): 742–749. Print.

Innes, K. E., C. Bourguignon, and A. G. Taylor. "Risk Indices Associated with the Insulin Resistance Syndrome, Cardiovascular Disease, and Possible Protection with Yoga: A Systematic Review." *Journal of the American Board of Family Medicine* 18.6 (2005): 491–519. Print.

Innes, K. E., and H. K. Vincent. "The Influence of Yoga-Based Programs on Risk Profiles in Adults with Type 2 Diabetes Mellitus: A Systematic Review." *Evidence-Based Complementary and Alternative Medicine* 4.4 (2007): 469–486. Print.

Jayasinghe, S. R. "Yoga in Cardiac Health (A Review)." *European Journal of Cardiovascular Prevention and Rehabilitation* 11.5 (2004): 369–375. Print.

Joseph, C. N., et al. "Slow Breathing Improves Arterial Baroreflex Sensitivity and Decreases Blood Pressure in Essential Hypertension." *Hypertension* 46.4 (2005): 714–718. Print.

Katzman, M. A., et al. "A Multicomponent Yoga-Based, Breath Intervention Program as an Adjunctive Treatment in Patients Suffering from Generalized Anxiety Disorder with or Without Comorbidities." *International Journal of Yoga* 5.1 (2012): 57–65. Print.

Khalsa, S. B. S. "Yoga as a Therapeutic Intervention: A Bibliometric Analysis of Published Research Studies." *Indian Journal of Physiology and Pharmacology* 48.3 (2004): 269–285. Print.

——. "Why Do Yoga Research: Who Cares and What Good Is It?" *International Journal of Yoga Therapy* 17 (2007): 19–20. Print.

——. "Yoga for Psychiatry and Mental Health: An Ancient Practice with Modern Relevance." *Indian Journal of Psychiatry* 55. Supplement 3 (2013): S334–S336. Print.

Khalsa, S. B. S., and J. Gould. *Your Brain on Yoga* (A Harvard Medical School Guide). New York: RosettaBooks, 2012, p. 52. Print.

Khalsa S. B. S., et al. "Evaluation of the Mental Health Benefits of Yoga in a Secondary School: A Preliminary Randomized Controlled Trial." *Journal of Behavioral Health Services* 39.1 (2012): 80–90. Print.

Khare, K. C., and S. Rai. "Study of Lipid Profile in Post–Myocardial Infarction Subjects Following Yogic Lifestyle Intervention." *Indian Practices* 55.6 (2002): 369–373. Print.

Kligler, B., et al. "Randomized Trial of the Effect of an Integrative Medicine Approach to the Management of Asthma in Adults on Disease-Related Quality of Life and Pulmonary Function." *Alternative Therapies in Health and Medicine* 17.1 (2011): 10–15. Print.

Lakkireddy, D., et al. "Effect of Yoga on Arrhythmia Burden, Anxiety, Depression, and Quality of Life in Paroxysmal Atrial Fibrillation: The YOGA My Heart Study." *Journal of the American College of Cardiology* 61.11 (2013): 1177–1182. Print.

Lee, M. S., et al. "Yoga for Menopausal Symptoms: A Systematic Review." *Menopause* 16.3 (2009): 602–608. Print.

Levine, A. S., and J. L. Balk. "Yoga and Quality-of-Life Improvement in Patients with Breast Cancer: A Literature Review." *International Journal of Yoga* 22 (2012): 5–9. Print.

Li, A.W., and C. A. Goldsmith. "The Effects of Yoga on Anxiety and Stress." *Alternative Medicine Review* 17.1 (2012): 21–35. Print.

Litchke, L. G., J. S. Hodges, and R. F. "Benefits of Chair Yoga for Persons with Mild to Severe Alzheimer's Disease." *Activities, Adaptation & Aging* 36.4 (2012): 317–328. Print.

Luskin, F. "Transformative Practices for Integrating Mind-Body-Spirit." *Journal of Alternative and Complementary Medicine* 10 Supplement 1 (2004): S15–S23. Print.

Mehling, W. E., et al. "Body Awareness: A Phenomenological Inquiry into the Common Ground of Mind-Body Therapies." *Philosophy, Ethics, and Humanities in Medicine* 6.1 (2011): 6. Print.

Mishra, S. K., et al. "The Therapeutic Value of Yoga in Neurological Disorders." *Annals of Indian Academy of Neurology* 15.4 (2012): 247–254. Print.

Moliver, N., et al. "Yoga Experience as a Predictor of Psychological Wellness in Women over 45 Years." *International Journal of Yoga* 6.1 (2013): 11–19. Print.

Nagendra, H. R., and R. Nagarathna. "An Integrated Approach of Yoga Therapy for Bronchial Asthma: A 3–54-Month Prospective Study." *Journal of Asthma* 23.3 (1986): 123–137. Print.

Noggle, J. J., et al. "Benefits of Yoga for Psychosocial Well-Being in a US High School Curriculum: A Preliminary Randomized Controlled Trial." *Journal of Developmental and Behavioral Pediatrics* 33.3 (2012): 193–201. Print.

Ornish, D., et al. "Can Lifestyle Changes Reverse Coronary Heart Disease? The Lifestyle Heart Trial." *Lancet* 336.8708 (1990): 129–133. Print.

Ospina, M. B., et al. "Meditation Practices for Health: State of the Research." *Evidence Report Technology Assessment* (Full Report) 155 (2007): 1–263. Print.

Patel, C. H. "Yoga and Biofeedback in the Management of Hypertension." *Lancet* 2.7837 (1973): 1053–1055. Print.

Patel, N. K., A. H. Newstead, and R. I. Ferrer. "The Effects of Yoga on Physical Functioning and Health-Related Quality of Life in Older Adults: A Systematic Review and Meta-Analysis." *Journal of Alternative and Complementary Medicine* 18.10 (2012): 902–917. Print.

Pelletier, K. R. "MindBody Medicine." Interview with Kenneth R. Pelletier by B. Horrigan. *Alternative Therapies in Health and Medicine* 8.6 (2002): 90–99. Print.

Pilkington, K., et al. "Yoga for Depression: The Research Evidence." *Journal of Affective Disorders* 89.1–3 (2005): 13–24. Print.

Posadzki, P., and E. Ernst. "Yoga for Asthma? A Systematic Review of Randomized Clinical Trials." *Journal of Asthma* 48.6 (2011): 632–639. Print.

Pratap V. "Scientific Studies on Yoga—A Review." *Yoga Mimamsa* 13.4 (1971): 1–18. Print.

Rao, R. M., et al. "Influence of Yoga on Mood States, Distress, Quality of Life and Immune Outcomes in Early Stage Breast Cancer Patients Undergoing Surgery." *International Journal of Yoga* 1.1 (2008): 11–20. Print.

Raub, J. A. "Psychophysiologic Effects of Hatha Yoga on Musculoskeletal and Cardiopulmonary Function: A Literature Review." *Journal of Alternative and Complementary Medicine* 8.6 (2002): 797–812. Print.

Rioux, J. G., and C. Ritenbaugh. "Narrative Review of Yoga Intervention Clinical Trials Including Weight-Related Outcomes." *Alternative Therapies in Health and Medicine* 19.3 (2013): 32–46. Print.

Ross, A., et al. "Frequency of Yoga Practice Predicts Health: Results of a National Survey of Yoga Practitioners." *Evidence-Based Complementary and Alternative Medicine* 2012: Article ID 983258. 20 June 2012. Web. http://www.hindawi.com/journals/ecam/2012/983258/.

Ross, A., et al. "National Survey of Yoga Practitioners: Mental and Physical Health Benefits." *Complementary Therapies in Medicine* 21.3 (2013): 313–323. Print.

Saatcioglu, F. "Regulation of Gene Expression by Yoga, Meditation and Related Practices: A Review of Recent Studies." *Asian Journal of Psychiatry* 6.1 (2013): 74–77. Print.

Saper, R. B., et al. "Yoga for Chronic Low Back Pain in a Predominantly Minority Population: A Pilot Randomized Controlled Trial." *Alternative Therapies in Health and Medicine* 15.6 (2009): 18–27. Print.

Serwacki, M. L., and C. Cook-Cottone. "Yoga in the Schools: A Systematic Review of the Literature." *International Journal of Yoga Therapy* 22 (2012): 101–109. Print.

Shannahoff-Khalsa, D. S., et al. "Randomized Controlled Trial of Yogic Meditation Techniques for Patients with Obsessive-Compulsive Disorders." *CNS Spectrums* 4.12 (1999): 34–46. Print.

Sherman, K. J., et al. "A Randomized Trial Comparing Yoga, Stretching, and a Self-Care Book for Chronic Low Back Pain." *Archives of Internal Medicine* 171.22 (2011): 2019–2026. Print.

Sherman, K. J., et al. "Mediators of Yoga and Stretching for Chronic Low Back Pain." *Evidence-Based Complementary and Alternative Medicine* 2013: Article ID 130818. 14 March 2013. Web. http://www.hindawi.com/journals/ecam/2013/130818/.

Silverthorne, C., et al. "Respiratory, Physical, and Psychological Benefits of Breath-Focused Yoga for Adults with Severe Traumatic Brain Injury (TBI): A Brief Pilot Study Report." *International Journal of Yoga* 22 (2012): 47–51. Print.

Singh, V., et al. "Effect of Yoga Breathing Exercises (Pranayama) on Airway Reactivity in Subjects with Asthma." *Lancet* 335.8702 (1990): 1381–1383. Print.

Smith, K. B., and C. F. Pukall. "An Evidence-Based Review of Yoga as a Complementary Intervention for Patients with Cancer." *Psycho-oncology* 18.5 (2009): 465–475. Print.

Staples, J. K., M. F. Hamilton, and M. Uddo. "A Yoga Program for the Symptoms of Post-Traumatic Stress Disorder in Veterans." *Military Medicine* 178.8 (2013): 854–860. Print.

Streeter, C. C., et al. "Effects of Yoga on the Autonomic Nervous System, Gamma-Aminobutyric-Acid, and Allostasis in Epilepsy, Depression, and Post-Traumatic Stress Disorder." *Medical Hypotheses* 78.5 (2012): 571–579. Print.

Telles, S., et al. "Post-Traumatic Stress Symptoms and Heart Rate Variability in Bihar Flood Survivors Following Yoga: A Randomized Controlled Study." *BMC Psychiatry,* 2 Mar. 2010, 10:18. Web. 10:18. doi: 10.1186/1471-244X-10-18.

Telles, S., N. Singh, and A. Balkrishna. "Managing Mental Health Disorders Resulting from Trauma Through Yoga: A Review." *Depression Research and Treatment,* 19 June 2012. Web. doi: 10.1155/2012/401513.

Tilbrook, H. E., et al. "Yoga for Chronic Low Back Pain: A Randomized Trial." *Annals of Internal Medicine* 155.9 (2011): 569–578. Print.

Uebelacker, L. A. "Hatha Yoga for Depression: Critical Review of the Evidence for Efficacy, Plausible Mechanisms of Action, and Directions for Future Research." *Journal of Psychiatric Practice* 16.1 (2010): 22–33. Print.

Vadiraja, H. S., et al. "Effects of a Yoga Program on Cortisol Rhythm and Mood States in Early Breast Cancer Patients Undergoing Adjuvant Radiotherapy: A Randomized Controlled Trial." *Integrative Cancer Therapies* 8.1 (2009): 37–46. Print.

van der Kolk, B. A. "Clinical Implications of Neuroscience Research in PTSD." *Annals of NewYork Academy of Science* 1071 (2006): 277–293. Print.

Vera, F. M., et al. "Subjective Sleep Quality and Hormonal Modulation in Long-Term Yoga Practitioners." *Biological Psychology* 81.3 (2009): 164–168. Print.

Yang, K. "A Review of Yoga Programs for Four Leading Risk Factors of Chronic Diseases." *Journal of Evidence-Based Complementary & Alternative Medicine* 4.4 (2007): 487–491. Print.

Zhang, J., et al. "Effects of Yoga on Psychologic Function and Quality of Life in Women with Breast Cancer: A Meta-Analysis of Randomized Controlled Trials." *Journal of Alternative and Complementary Medicine* 18.11 (2013): 994–1002. Print.

IAYT AND THE FUTURE OF YOGA THERAPY

John Kepner, M.A., M.B.A.

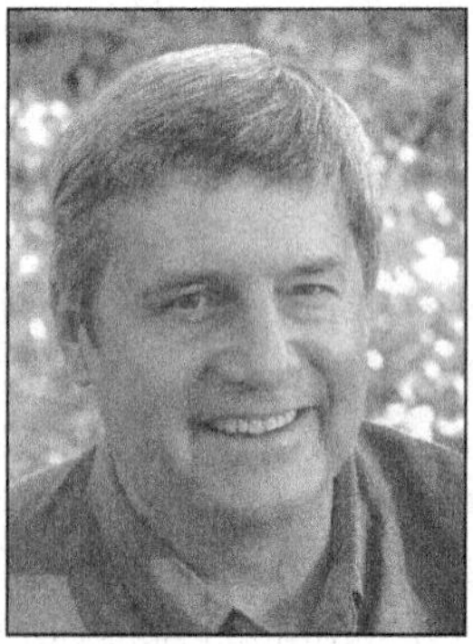

John Kepner has served as the executive director of the International Association of Yoga Therapists (IAYT) since 2003 when IAYT once again established itself as an independent nonprofit organization. He is a practicing Yoga teacher and therapist with a professional background in economics, finance, and nonprofit management. John holds both Yoga teacher and therapist certifications from the American Viniyoga Institute and a teaching certification from A. G. Mohan in Chennai, India. His work for IAYT and his writings often share an economic and public policy perspective.

INTRODUCTION

"Where your talents and the needs of the world cross, therein lies your vocation."

—ARISTOTLE

In my view, much of the future of the professional field of Yoga Therapy is actually being determined *now,* as the field is defining itself through standards. This is so important, yet often not recognized by those not experienced in this fundamental aspect of emerging healthcare fields. Hence, much of this chapter will initially focus on what has been done in the last ten years to actually bring us to a point where we can indeed begin to define the field and thus shape its future. At the end, however, I will share a few thoughts about the future of the field and the work that still needs to be done to bring this precious Indian gift to a much fuller, and much needed, flowering in Western health care.

ABOUT IAYT

The International Association of Yoga Therapists (IAYT) is a professional organization serving Yoga teachers and Yoga Therapists worldwide. Our mission is to establish Yoga as a recognized and respected therapy. Professional interest in the field of Yoga Therapy has soared in the past ten years and IAYT's membership has grown almost five-fold (from less than 700 to over 3,400 members) in almost fifty countries at the beginning of 2014. Perhaps even more illustrative is the growth in professional training. IAYT listed just five schools with Yoga Therapy training programs on our website in 2003. Now, in 2014, we list over 120 member schools. Yoga Therapy, with its comprehensive set of practices and teachings for body, breath, and mind, is one of the answers to a much-needed transformation of our contemporary approach to health *care*. Indeed, "Bridging Yoga and Healthcare" is our tagline at IAYT. Given our mission, though, we are sometimes thought to focus on "medicalizing" Yoga in order to service the healthcare market, hence the importance of our organization's dual slogan, which is, in fact, central to our work, "Keep the Yoga in Yoga Therapy."

The future of Yoga Therapy fundamentally depends on how well the practices and teachings of Yoga serve the needs of people seeking improved health, healing, and spiritual support. Nevertheless, these people are reached through two very different "markets": the classic Yoga student-teacher relationship and the conventional healthcare system. The Yoga market primarily depends upon relationships, local reputations, an expansive notion of health and healing, highly customized individual practices, small group classes, and saṅgha (spiritual community), in addition to the skills of the Yoga Therapist. The conventional system requires all of the auxiliary supports in place for modern health care, including professional journals, continuing education, a conventional-evidence base, clinically proven protocols, credibly accredited training programs, and credentialing. As John Weeks notes, this system is driven, even defined, by "the insurance, research, and even accreditation practices of the larger medical industrial complex" (Weeks, 2006). While the student-teacher relationship and the conventional healthcare systems are commonly uneasy bedfellows and are sometimes at odds with one another, since 1989 the IAYT has been a bridge between the two.

This chapter outlines some of the landmarks to date in creating the future of Yoga Therapy by focusing on credibility, community, and stories about some of the individuals who have been most responsible for establishing the field. The chapter also details some thoughts on the current and future challenges faced by the field to develop Yoga Therapy as both a standalone practice with the classical student-teacher relationship *and* as a complementary therapy that can be part of an integrated approach to health in our Western healthcare system.

A LITTLE PERSPECTIVE

At our first IAYT conference in 2007, Pamela Snider, N.D., one of the leaders of the professional development of naturopathic medicine and the Academic Consortium for Complementary and Alternative Healthcare (ACCAHC) was asked to share some advice and experience with us as a newly emerging field (Weeks, 2007). Dr. Snider gave a moving lecture titled "Accountability and Soul" and led with a classic story that has guided me for years while I've wrestled with the day-to-day aspects of our work at IAYT—the story of the three bricklayers.

> *An old priest was out walking one day and came upon three bricklayers. "What are you doing?" he asked the first bricklayer. "I'm laying bricks," he replied. The second bricklayer was asked the same question and answered, "I'm building a wall." When the third bricklayer was asked the same question, however, he looked up and into the distance, and said, "I'm building a cathedral."*

So, in a real sense, one could view our association as a team of bricklayers, coming together to do our part to serve our field. But instead of walls, I see us as building pillars of credibility, community, standards, research, accreditation, and credentialing, marketing and branding, economic viability, and governance to support the professional association to define and shape the emerging field.

CREDIBILITY: *THE INTERNATIONAL JOURNAL OF YOGA THERAPY*

In professional fields, a credible professional journal is needed to showcase the best practices and contemporary research in the field and to provide a forum to discuss and debate contemporary issues. Professional journals are peer reviewed, indexed in the right databases, such as PubMed, and hosted on scholarly journal websites so the articles can be found by scholars around the world and libraries can subscribe to the publication.

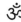

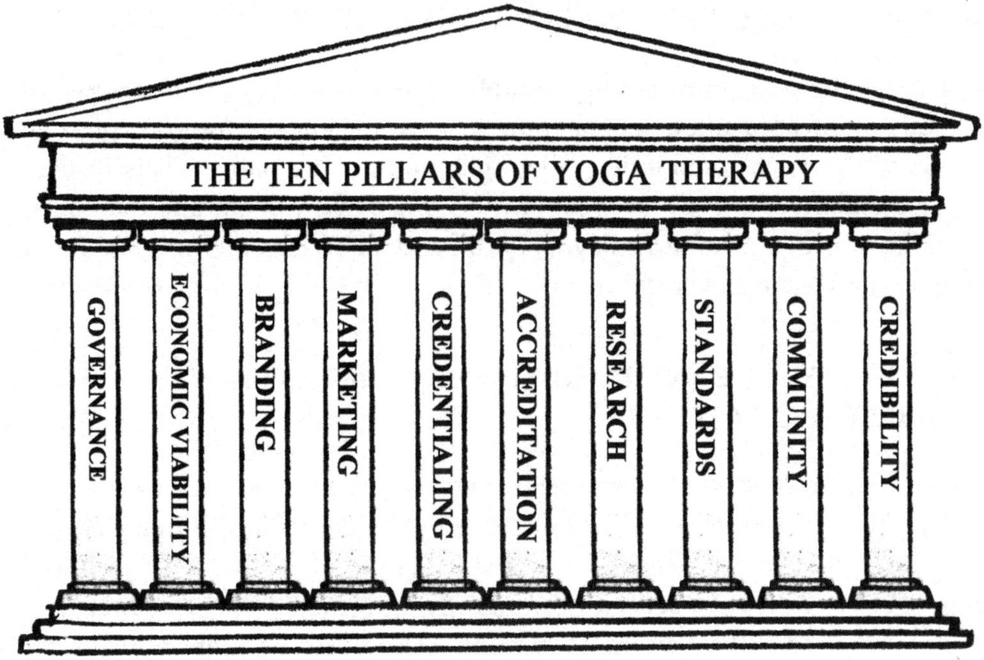

The *International Journal of Yoga Therapy* was started by one of IAYT's founders, Richard Miller, Ph.D., in 1990. At the time of our renewal as an independent organization in 2003, however, we still had few of the necessary scholarly attributes, so our first goal was to establish the professional credibility of the Journal. We were most fortunate to find an extraordinary editor, Kelly McGonigal, Ph.D., who knew how to do this and could do much of it singlehandedly. Much to my surprise, she was able to assemble a well-qualified set of reviewers and immediately took the *Journal* to peer review in 2005 during her first year as editor. Then, after years of hard work by authors, reviewers, copy editors, proofreaders, and graphic designers under her leadership, the *Journal* was finally accepted for indexing in PubMed in 2011.

This may be no feat for established fields, well supported by university departments, NIH research grants, and foundations, but, for an emerging field like Yoga Therapy, this is a landmark accomplishment. Our challenge now is to support the *Journal* better in a more professional way, such as publishing at least two issues a year and providing much additional support for the entire process.

COMMUNITY: RESPECT FOR OUR DIVERSE YOGA TRADITION

A fundamental part of developing community is a genuine sense of respect for the diversity of lineages and personal approaches to the ancient tradition of Yoga. As we say in the Yoga community, "One mountain, many paths." This respect has been a hallmark and a key strength of IAYT since in the beginning due to IAYT's founding president, Dr. Larry Payne, Ph.D., and all of our other original founding members and leaders over the years.

COMMUNITY: THE SYMPOSIUM ON YOGA THERAPY AND RESEARCH (SYTAR)

Professional fields need professional conferences. A professional conference is an annual gathering to bring the members of a field together for continuing education, an opportunity to discuss the issues of the day, to reconnect with old friends, and, most of all, to develop a sense of community and identity. When I first saw this type of gathering at the National Ayurvedic Medical Association (NAMA) conference, which is a sister field and emerging profession in the West as diverse as Yoga, and deeply united by love of their discipline, our thinking at IAYT completely shifted from "Should we have a conference?" to "How can we do this as soon as possible?"

While conferences help to bring people together in a field, they are a tremendous amount of work and involve a great deal of time and financial risk, especially for small organizations without experience, a track record, or even a significant credit history. Fortunately, Veronica Zador (IAYT's first president after the 2003 renewal), and her husband, Ivan Zador, Ph.D., were experienced conference organizers who stepped up to produce our first three conferences. The first conference in 2007 was supported by many of the leaders of the field, who were taking a chance and committing to present at an untested event. We hoped for 400 participants. I still remember the last day of the *early*, early bird registration. Our phones didn't stop ringing! We had 400 registrations before the normal early bird registration even started, and we finally sold out at over 800 participants. So many individuals were working alone, feeling isolated in their town and state, and were thrilled to finally meet their peers from around the United States and the other thirty attending counties. In hindsight, I now see that perhaps the most important result of establishing a professional conference was creating a sense of professional identity and community for Yoga Therapy and Yoga Therapists. To that end of identity and community, I also should note the efforts of Matthew Taylor, Ph.D., P.T., another IAYT president, who later developed the Common Interest Community sessions for IAYT conferences starting in 2009. These are special-interest groups with short presentations, like TED talks, all primarily designed to support networking for people with common interests, such as structural Yoga Therapy, Yoga Therapy and mental health, etc.

STANDARDS

The development of standards is one of the most challenging aspects of becoming a professional field and it is a transformative and often painstaking event. Under the leadership of John Weeks, the Academic Consortium for Complementary and Alternative Healthcare (ACCAHC) was instrumental in guiding IAYT to standards and in providing advice and counsel. Indeed, a commitment to establish standards was a prerequisite to joining the organization and Yoga, via IAYT, was the first nonlicensed field ever represented in the ACCAHC. John led the first two Meetings of Schools at SYTAR, where our community of Yoga Therapy training program directors first gathered and began to address their aspirations and fears for establishing standards. The third meeting had an influential presentation by Dan Seitz, J.D., Ed.D., an experienced leader in emerging complementary alternative medicine (CAM) fields, on regulatory issues for Yoga Therapy that included the necessary characteristics of a standards setting process. He advised, *"Practitioners and educators within emerging fields should engage in inclusive, representational, and transparent decision-making processes to build support for any self-regulatory measures being considered"* (Seitz, 2010). And so, we did, and our community endorsed the standards setting process as long as we followed those guidelines.

Later that year, the board of directors at IAYT established a representative committee of leading educators in our field to set entry-level standards for the training programs for Yoga Therapists. The initial focus was on training and the accreditation of training programs because training establishes the future for the field. Sound training is, of course, a necessary but not sufficient foundation for a good Yoga Therapist. Before the IAYT standards, most of the training programs were simply 300-hour programs after a 200-hour basic teacher training program to fulfill Yoga Alliance's 500-hour registry requirements—and without any real standards for content or competencies. Every program director I talked to said that 300 hours was far from sufficient for the required training to be a Yoga Therapist, but, without higher standards from a recognized leader in the field like IAYT, few schools could increase the length of their training programs.

Setting standards is a prime example of the lengthy, tedious, and sometimes painstaking work by dedicated volunteers required to establish a field. After over two years of steady hard work, in 2011 the committee unanimously recommended, and the IAYT Board adopted, a set of competency-based standards, including a definition of *Yoga Therapy* and a set of training requirements (IAYT, 2012). The standards that were set are essentially at the professional master's level and were above most schools' training programs. Furthermore, the new standards' committee defined *Yoga Therapy* as "The practice of empowering individuals to move towards improved health and well-being through the teachings and practice of Yoga."

RESEARCH: THE SYMPOSIUM ON YOGA RESEARCH (SYR)

Yoga is classified as a "mind-body" medicine by the National Institutes of Health (NIH) and the National Center for Complementary and Alternative Medicine (NCCAM), which funds much of today's conventional research. Healthcare systems, insurance systems, and educational systems all want therapies to be well researched and to have the appropriate base of evidence supporting applied therapies. Such research is slowly emerging in Yoga Therapy, as conventional research is very expensive. Thus funds for Yoga, as well as all CAM practices that cannot be patented, are severely limited.

At IAYT, we recognize that research will help take our field forward and have acted accordingly. After our first three SYTAR conferences, Sat Bir Khalsa, Ph.D., one of the world's leading Yoga researchers and an influential supporter of other researchers, was instrumental in helping us set up the Symposium on Yoga Research (SYR). We supported Dr. Khalsa's vision that it is best to have a standalone research conference for the field, not just a track at a larger Yoga conference where it is hard to identify the researchers, so, in 2010, we launched the first widely publicized academic Yoga research conference in the West at the Himalayan Institute, where Swami Rama became one of the pioneers of Yoga research thirty years prior, and we appointed Sat Bir to the chair of the scientific program committee. We wondered how many people would come to an out-of-the-way ashram for an academic Yoga research conference and assumed around fifty participants based on the attendance of our research tracks at our earlier conferences. We applied for a NCCAM scientific conference grant the first year but were turned down in part because the reviewers thought people wouldn't attend a conference in such a remote location. But when four times the amount of participants came and over 200 people showed up, due to the success of the first conference, NCCAM awarded IAYT a grant for the second year, which was a major recognition for our emerging field!

ACCREDITATION AND CREDENTIALING

Creating credible accreditation and credentialing systems with a solid foundation in IAYT's standards requires more sets of dedicated volunteers, well supported by experienced expertise, especially in an emerging field such as Yoga Therapy. In 2013, the IAYT board established the IAYT Accreditation Committee as a semi-independent committee to accredit Yoga Therapist training programs that meet the new IAYT standards. Again, this requires lengthy, tedious, and painstaking work to develop an actual application, as well as a complete set of policies and procedures for the accreditation process before actual reviewing programs can begin. As of spring 2014, IAYT has thirty-five programs under review, about twice as many as expected.

Yet one more agency is required, one for actual credentialing. My expectation is that this will be established in the 2015–2016 time frame.

Our initial standards for an "IAYT Certified Yoga Therapist (CYTh)" will be graduation from an accredited program or via one of the grandparenting avenues. However, in my view, which aligns with the views of many licensed professionals in our field, Yoga Therapy will not have a credible credentialing system until we also have some form of independent third party testing like other professional fields. Despite the inevitable initial resistance this will bring out from other members of the Yoga community, it's not impossible to do, providing we focus on skills and knowledge that all approaches to Yoga have in common, such as safety, professional therapeutic relationships, and education. One of the most important considerations for referrals from physicians and other healthcare providers is confidence their patients will not be harmed by practitioners of this new discipline, thus some common tests or other quality controls, for safety and ahiṁsa (nonviolence), will help advance the field of Yoga Therapy.

MARKETING AND BRANDING

Accredited programs and credentialed practitioners must be branded and marketed to be recognized by those outside our own field. Credible research and education in the field, as well as accreditation and credentialing are necessary, but not sufficient conditions to establish a viable profession. Judi Barr, the manager of the Yoga Therapy programs at Cleveland Clinic, one of the pioneering hospitals integrating Yoga into their lifestyle medicine program, has said, "The future of Yoga Therapy rests in the rigorous empirical testing of Yoga protocols for specific conditions and symptoms" (Barr, 2013), as clinically proven protocols are demanded by our current healthcare system. Therefore, well-branded protocols, such as Dr. Richard Miller's iRest Yoga Nidrā program, Dr. Dean Ornish's Program for Reversing Heart Disease, and Dr. Jon Kabat-Zinn's Mindfulness Based Stress Reduction are fundamental to the growth and practice of Yoga Therapy in the future. The reductionist nature of protocols is anathema to many Yoga Therapists because working with individuals as a whole, with all their multiple dimensions and aspirations, is fundamental to the classical practice of Yoga Therapy. Richard Miller, who may have done more than anyone else in our field to develop a well-branded protocol in Yoga Therapy, agrees with this line of thinking but also stresses the four steps required to develop accepted protocols: conventional clinical evidence, credentialed practitioners, replicable results, and a manual for the practice (Miller, 2014). Ultimately, the field of Yoga Therapy will have to learn to develop these steps, market the results, and yet still retain the skills and perspectives to work with people as individuals at all times. IAYT has already modestly begun the marketing and branding process for Yoga Therapy, but much more work needs to be done.

ECONOMIC VIABILITY: LICENSING AND INSURANCE COVERAGE

A fundamental requirement for any professional field is economic viability. Most healthcare fields keep fees up by limiting entry through licensing and are sustained by public and private insurance systems. Neither of these is yet directly available for Yoga Therapy. Licensing and Yoga are not very compatible and licensing has been generally resisted by the field to date. Moreover, it can be difficult to distinguish teaching Yoga from Yoga Therapy in a legal realm. As Michael Cohen noted however, title licensure is possibly the best path for regulatory recognition of Yoga Therapy (Cohen, 2008).

Insurance coverage generally requires licensing and can be a trap because insurance coverage may define the field. An oft-quoted observation of Dean Ornish, M.D., is "The practice of medicine is defined by the reimbursement system." The same thing has arguably happened to the chiropractic field once the practice came to be covered by insurance. In some jurisdictions, chiropractors essentially became "just" back doctors, since insurance coverage is so often limited to back care in their field (Weeks, 2006). Insurance coverage is generally limited to addressing disorders and fixing "problems." Yoga Therapy can often do that, but the power and the appeal of Yoga as a practice and/or therapy often lies in the many other dimensions of self-care and spiritual evolution that it provides. Hence, the classic student-teacher relationship, which is outside the constraints of our modern insurance system, and the inherent freedom for personal growth this allows, is the bedrock of the field. This is a fundamental challenge for our field of Yoga Therapy and CAM fields, in general, since the economic structure supporting our system has been so mismanaged and insurance companies, not doctors and therapists, have too much power in patients' care and doctors' decision-making process.

GOVERNANCE

Association governance may appear to be an unusual necessity for the future of a field, but my experience with IAYT and other nonprofits has taught me that it is essential. The missions and programs of associations don't just happen; they are governed and managed by people with widely different backgrounds and often limited experience with governance and management. With many nonprofit organizations, confusion regarding the respective roles of governance and management is all too common and potentially disastrous.

As a result of having our own challenges with governance over the years at IAYT, we adopted the policy governance model of John Carver in 2011 (Carver, 2013). A key virtue of this model is that it clearly distinguishes the roles and responsibilities of governance and management. IAYT is also indebted to our President Emeritus, Eleanor Criswell, Ed.D., for her vision in championing the adoption of this governance model, as well as IAYT's long-term consultant and advocate of this model, Dan Seitz., J.D., Ph.D.

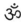

CONCLUSION

So this brings me back to the original quote by Aristotle. Serving the needs of the world with our talents is fundamental, but, in our world today, it takes so much more to cultivate and grow a field, even one as ancient as Yoga, into a recognized and respected therapy. That is what a professional association, when well governed, and well managed, is able to provide.

The Future of Yoga Therapy as a Discipline

I would like to end by outlining the three major future streams of the practice as I see it.

- The classic individual sessions and small classes taught in homes and personal studios, and paid for privately. These sessions, based upon the Yoga Therapist's skill, personal relationships and transmission, are still the heart of Yoga Therapy. I expect to see demand for these to grow as students increasingly recognize and cherish the breadth and depth of the benefits and relationships inherent in this practice, *and* the supply of skilled therapists grows as the new higher standards begin to take effect, all unfettered by insurance and other third party payers. Another factor spurring demand will be the increasing dissatisfaction with the quality, impersonality, and narrow focus of health care provided by third party financing.

- Yoga Therapy as part of what are called integrated lifestyle medicine programs, such as the Dean Ornish Program for Reversing Heart Disease and a variety of similar programs now practiced in the Cleveland Clinic's Center for Lifestyle Medicine. These programs typically encompass diet, exercise, group counseling, and yoga for stress reduction.

  The reason is simple and compelling. As Dean Ornish testified before Congress:

  > Heart disease, diabetes, prostate cancer, breast cancer, and obesity account for 75% of these healthcare costs, and yet these are largely preventable and even reversible by changing diet and lifestyle. Our research, and the work of others, has shown that our bodies have a remarkable capacity to begin healing, and much more quickly than we had once realized, if we address the lifestyle factors that often cause these chronic diseases. (Ornish, 2009)

Getting our healthcare financing system to recognize and support such efforts, however, is the challenge. Only in 2010 was the Dean Ornish program finally accepted for reimbursement by Medicare, after decades of developing the evidence base.

- Branded yoga therapy programs provided privately or as part of corporate, governmental, or other organization treatment and wellness programs. These will be based upon clinically tested protocols with a strong evidence base, such as the iRest program, the Mindfulness Based Stress Reduction program, the Viniyoga Therapy program for Anxiety and Depression, and others as the evidence base develops. Financing the research, of course, will be one of the major limitations. It is encouraging that some of the research is financed by health insurance companies. Branding and marketing programs like these, however, are not something most of the field is used to, much less skilled at—yet.
- At their best, these protocol-based programs will be taught be skilled Yoga Therapists able to adapt the programs to the actual needs of the individuals in the program and not just with blind adherence to the tested protocols. Whether or not our healthcare systems will support such programs and creativity in delivery remains to be seen. Part of this depends on how well these programs are "branded," publicized, and demanded by consumers. Demand by consumers for both branded and unbranded Yoga Therapy programs will be a driving force for Yoga Therapy in the future, since consumer demand has been the key driving force for the acceptance of complementary and alternative medicine in general.

REFERENCES

ACCAHC (Academic Consortium for Complementary and Alternative Health Care). ACCAHC's core membership is those organizations related to complementary and alternative healthcare disciplines that have an accrediting agency recognized by the U.S. Department of Education, have a recognized certification or testing organization, and are licensed for professional practice in at least one state. Full membership is limited to three categories of organizations: Councils of Colleges or Schools, Accrediting Agencies, and Certification and Testing Organizations. In addition, through a separate membership category, ACCAHC includes those Traditional World Medicines or Emerging Professions organizations that show a commitment to exploring public health–related standard-setting, and self-regulatory activities and believe their organizations will benefit from ACCAHC participation. ACCAHC.org. 2014. Web. http://accahc.org/.

Barr, Judi. "Bringing Yoga Therapy into the Mainstream: Lessons from Cleveland Clinic." *International Journal of Yoga Therapy* 23. 2 (2013): 67. Print.

Carver, John. The Policy Governance Model. PolicyGovernance.com. 25 February 2013. Web. 2014. http://www.carvergovernance.com/model.htm.

Cohen, Michael. "The Search for Regulatory Recognition for Yoga Therapy: Legal and Policy Considerations." *International Journal of Yoga Therapy* 18 (2008): 43–50. Print.

IAYT (International Association of Yoga Therapists). "Educational Standards for the Training of Yoga Therapists." 1 July 2012. Web. 2014. http://www.iayt.org/.

Miller, Richard. Private conversations. 2014.

Ornish, Dean. U.S. Senate Health Reform Testimony on Integrative Care: A Pathway to a Healthier Nation. Reprinted in the *International Journal of Yoga Therapy* 19 (2009): 43–46. Print.

Seitz, Dan. "Regulatory Issues for Yoga, Yoga Therapy and Ayurveda." *International Journal of Yoga Therapy* 20 (2010): 34–40. Print. (I am pleased to say that financial support for this paper was provided by our sister organizations, the National Ayurvedic Medical Association (NAMA) and the Yoga Alliance (YA) as well as IAYT. This cooperation makes a statement.)

Weeks, John. "Integrator Blog News and Reports Series on the Future of Yoga Therapy." *Yoga Therapy in Practice* 2.4 (2006): 17. Print.

Weeks, John. "Accountability and Soul: An Interview with Pamela Snider, ND." *Yoga Therapy and Practice* 3.2 (2007): 5–7. Print.

Writing and Reading of Sanskrit Words

Sanskrit words in this book have been written using a form of "Romanized Sanskrit" technically known as IAST or International Alphabet of Sanskrit Transcription, developed in 1894 for the precise transcription of Sanskrit and other Indic languages into common Euro-American or "Roman" letters. IAST has become the most basic academic and literary standard. With the addition of a few "diacritical marks," the usable letters of the "Roman" alphabet of twenty-six letters used in writing standard English may be extended to uniquely represent all forty-eight sounds of classical Sanskrit. To provide immediate initial access to the sound system, the IAST scheme is presented below in a traditional, systematic grammatical format, with sample English words appended as an initial (but not always definitive) guide to pronunciation. A few clarifying details are included in the notes that follow. For alternate spellings, note the "commonly encountered substitutions" cited on the following page.

A SIMPLE PHONETIC GUIDELINE

13 Vowels

a	America	ā	father				
i	mint	ī	ski	e	beta	ai	aisle
ṛ	leader	ṝ	curb				
ḷ	able	—					
u	put	ū	rule	o	note	au	flautist

25 Consonant "Stops"

k	baker	kh	inkhorn	g	glory	gh	peghole	ṅ	sing
c	cello	ch	Churchhill	j	jet	jh	hedghog	ñ	canyon
ṭ	curtain	ṭh	arthouse	ḍ	harder	ḍh	birdhouse	ṇ	turn
t	true	th	hothead	d	dollar	dh	adhere	n	pin
p	vapor	ph	uphill	b	labor	bh	abhore	m	most

4 Semi-vowels, 3 Sibilants, 'h,' *anusvāra* & *visarga*

—	—	h	hello		
y	yellow	ś	shift		
r	radiant	ṣ	lush	ṁ	(*anusvāra*) open nasal, like the "n" in French "bon"
l	letter	s	simple	ḥ	(*visarga*) light echo of preceding vowel
v	vibrant	—			

Commonly Encountered Substitutions *(especially when diacritical marks are unavailable)*

ā = aa	**ī** = ee	**ū** = oo	**ṛ** = ri	**ṝ** = ree	**ḷ** = lri	**ṁ** = m	**ḥ** = h
c = ch	**ch** = chh	**ṅ/ñ/ṇ** = n	**ṭ/ṭh/ḍ/ḍh** = t/th/d/dh	**ś/ṣ** = sh			

SANSKRIT SOUNDS AND THE ENGLISH TONGUE—SOME BASIC NOTES

OṀ NAMAḤ PĀṆINAYE

"Oṁ! Homage to Pāṇini!" This presentation of Sanskrit phonemes is patterned on the analytic description articulated by Pāṇini, the most eminent of the ancient native grammarians of Sanskrit (c. fourth century BCE).

1. Each written character uniquely represents one, and only one, sound or "phoneme."
2. There are no silent or ambiguous letters in written Sanskrit. Sanskrit writing is phonetically literal.
3. Several sounds quite common in the English language simply *do not occur* in classical Sanskrit: the **'a'** in 'act,' the **'e'** in 'bet,' the **'f'** in 'fast,' the **'th'** in 'thorn' or 'that,' and the **'z'** in'zest.'
4. Variant pronunciations of Sanskrit sounds and words by contemporary speakers, Indic and Western, public and private, can become normative within certain populations, even when diction is imprecise from the perspective of classical Sanskrit grammar. Some frequently heard variations include:

ai sometimes pronounced like the 'a' in "date" (e.g., *Jain*).

ṛ is most often written and mispronounced 'ri,' often with a trilled 'r' (e.g., *Krishna* for *Kṛṣṇa*).

ṝ is most often written and mispronounced 'ree,' often with a trilled 'r.'

ḷ is most often written and mispronounced 'lri,' frequently with a trilled 'r' (e.g., *klrip* for *kḷp*).

th is always an aspirated **'t'** and should never be pronounced as in "this" or "path." (see note 5)

ṭh is always an aspirated **'ṭ'** and is also a "retroflex" sound. (see notes 5 & 6)

ph is always an aspirated **'p'** but often mispronounced 'f,' like the 'ph' in "physics." (see notes 3 & 5)

jñ is often variantly pronounced, and sometimes even re-spelled, "gn" or "dn."

v is often written and pronounced **'w,'** especially when immediately preceded by another consonant (e.g., *swāmi* and *Saraswati*); however, Pāṇini describes the sound as a voiced labio-dental (**'v'**).

ṁ is very commonly reduced to a simple nasal stop, usually **'m'** but sometimes **'ṅ'** (ng). (see note 8)

ḥ is frequently underpronounced, as if it were a simple aspiration (**'h'**) without echo. (see note 9)

5. Sanskrit consonants appended with **'h'** are "aspirated" consonants, that is, each of these consonants is sounded with a distinctive puff of air following the consonantal sound. In spoken English, consonants are sometimes aspirated and sometimes unaspirated, but the phonetic nuance is not denoted in the English writing system as it is in the Sanskrit. To illustrate: the **'k'** in 'kind' is a bit aspirated, while the **'k'** in 'lakeside' is not. If these were Sanskrit words, in IAST they would be spelled *"khaind"* and *"leksaid."*

6. The consonants with a dot beneath (**ṭ** - **ṭh** - **ḍ** - **ḍh** - **ṇ** - **ṣ**) are "retroflex" sounds, which are made with the tongue curled up and back towards the roof of the mouth. While these phonemes feel a bit odd at first to some native English speakers, they are of ubiquitous presence in Sanskrit, Hindi, and other Indic languages. They are a distinctive ingredient of the "Indian accent." In English words, when a **'t,'** **'d,'** or **'n'** is preceded by an **'r,'** the tongue is naturally pulled upward into a mildly retroflex position, hence the choice of sample words in the chart above. However, *the sample words offered here should be understosod as imperfect approximations.* To make a genuine retroflex sound, the tongue is curled up and back in a manner more extended than normal for the English tongue. These sounds may require conscious practice to fully master.

7. The "dental" consonants (**t** - **th** - **d** - **dh** - **n**) are pretty close to the English phonemes represented by the same letters. To be precise, however, the tip of the tongue should ideally touch the top of the upper front teeth, rather than squarely on the hard gumline above those teeth. While the natural English pronunciation of these consonants is perhaps closer to Sanskrit "dentals" than to Sanskrit "retroflex" sounds, the English sounds are not precisely identical with either. Given the middling position of the English speaker's tongue, an English **'t,'** **'d,'** or **'n'** is frequently *heard* as a "retroflex" sound by the native Indic speaker's ear.

8. **'ṁ'** (also written with the dot *beneath* the 'm') is called *anusvāra* or "after-sound" and is an open nasalization of the vowel sound that precedes it. "Open" means that the oral cavity is not entirely closed by tongue or lips. This resonant nasalization is quite common in Sanskrit. In Devanāgarī it is written with a mere dot, and this dot is often used as a scribe's shorthand for any one of the five nasal stops: **ṅ** - **ñ** - **ṇ** - **n** - **m**. The genuine *anusvāra* (**ṁ**) often gets reduced to the simple nasal stop **'m'** or sometimes **'ṅ'** (ng).

9. **'ḥ' is called *visarga* or "emission" of breath.** 'ḥ' resolves the preceding vowel sound with a light, puffy echo *of its simplest related vowel.* In the chart, this *short simple vowel* is in the first ***column*** of each ***row*** of related vowels. The subtle, bump-like echo of *visarga* is thus one of four sounds: **a** - **i** - **ṛ** - **u**.

10. From a classical perspective, *anusvāra* (**ṁ**) and *visarga* (**ḥ**) are phonetic *grace notes* to be neither overplayed nor ignored. Two ways to complement a vowel. Despite similarities in IAST transliteration, **'ṁ'** and **'ḥ'** are phonetically distinguishable from the simple consonants **'m'** and **'h.'**

JOHN THOMAS CASEY, PH.D.

John Thomas Casey is a fellow without abiding rank and, at this juncture, about four decades a scholar-yogin, working and studying by the sea in Southern California and Hawai'i, with an inclination to travel.

Following doctoral studies in Asian and Comparative Philosophy at the University of Hawai'i, Dr. Casey has taught courses in Sanskrit, Yoga Studies, Buddhism, World Religions, and related subjects at several Southland schools, including UCLA, UCI, and, most especially, Loyola Marymount University (LMU).

Others endeavors include specialized instruction for Yoga Teaching Teachings and weekend seminars, sacred calligraphy, photography, astrology, Jin Shin Do acupressure, and sound meditations and healing work using Tibetan Singing Bowls.

OṀ

All Sanskrit in this text was translated and interpreted by John Thomas Casey, Ph.D.

Glossary of Sanskrit and English Terms

Countless texts and encyclopedias, both online and offline, were referenced in the compilation of this glossary, as well as respectable websites, the authors' own knowledge (including the consultation of renowned Sanskrit scholar John Casey, Ph.D.), and the source chapters from *Yoga Therapy & Integrative Medicine: Where Ancient Science Meets Modern Medicine.* While none of the sources have been cited or referenced in the glossary, it is acknowledged that this was not intended plagiarism but is simply intended to be an unreferenced resource and guide to assist the reader in understanding unfamiliar terms, names, words, topics, and concepts that he/she may encounter in the general book.

Sanskrit words in this glossary are typically presented in *italics.* The exception is when a Sanskrit word is being used as a proper noun, as in the name of an individual, an institution, a type of *Yoga,* a school of thought, or a genre of literature. It should be duly noted that many of these terms admit of other possible meanings beyond the ones offered here. Also, since there are variations in the way in which different teachers understand and present the proper execution of various yogic practices, so any such descriptions presented here, while legitimate, may admit of other interpretations. Since the dating of ancient Indic texts and persons are typically not known with great precision, most dates provided are educated approximations, some of them continuing to be subject to scholarly debate. The designations "BCE" and "CE" mean "Before Common Era" and "Common Era," and correspond to "BC" and "AD," respectively, while "c." stands for "circa" (approximately).

A. G. Mohan A direct student of Professor Tirumalai Krishnamacharya and founder of Svastha Yoga Therapy, A.G. Mohan is the author of *Yoga for Body, Breath, and Mind* and co-author of *Yoga Therapy* with Indra Mohan (his wife), Ganesh Mohan (his son), and Nitya Mohan (his daughter) as well as *Krishnamacharya: His Life and His Teachings* with his son, Ganesh.

abhiniveśa* or *abhinivesha Defined as "tenacity" or "the will to go on," this is one of the five *kleśas* or subjective afflictions cited in the *Yoga Sūtra,* wherein it is often translated as the "fear of death," "clinging to life," or "fear of impermanence."

Academic Consortium for Complementary and Alternative Healthcare (ACCAHC) An organization dedicated to enhancing the health of individuals and communities by creating and sustaining a network of global educational organizations and agencies, which promote mutual respect, understanding, competence, collaborative activities, and interdisciplinary healthcare education.

accident reconstruction (certification) Designed for law enforcement and private collision investigation professionals, this certification program includes courses in intermediate collision investigation, advanced collision investigation, and collision reconstruction, pedestrian collision investigation, and forensic photography.

acupuncture A system of complementary medicine originating in ancient China that involves placing needles in the skin or tissues at various structural and energetic points to alleviate pain and treat various physical, mental, and emotional conditions.

acupuncturist One who engages in the practice of acupuncture utilizing techniques of electroacupuncture, oriental massage, acupressure, moxibustion, cupping, breathing techniques, exercise, heat, cold, magnets, nutrition, diet, herbs, dietary supplements, and/or plant, animal, and mineral products to promote, maintain, and restore health.

ādi mantra Ong Namo Guru Dev Namo *ādi* = original, beginning, primordial, commencement

1. A primary or commencing *mantra* (prayer, chant, or spell).
2. The syllable *oṁ*. (see *mantra* and *bīja mantra*)
3. A mantra traditionally recited in Kundalini Yoga classes and Kundalini Yoga Therapy.

Advaita Vedānta *advaita* = nondual

vedānta = "end of the Vedas" or "limit of knowledge"

One of the principal subsects of the Vedānta *darśana,* advocating a radically monistic interpretation of the *Upaniṣads,* wherein the whole of Reality is understood as only the One Being, Brahman. All diverse phenomena, the multiplicity of beings, and the *ātman* (soul) in this nondual philosophy are seen as the projective illusions (*māyā*) of Brahman, the Divine Ground of Being or Absolute Reality, where the goal is to "become One" with Brahman. The most influential advocate and systematizer of the Advaita Vedānta perspective was the philosopher, Śaṅkara (c. eighth century CE).

advanced Iyengar teaching certificate Iyengar Yoga teacher certification levels include introductory, intermediate junior, intermediate senior, advanced junior, and advanced senior, most of which have three levels in each category and all advanced Iyengar teaching certificates require the Iyengar family granting their direct approval.

agni 1. Fire, as a physical phenomenon.
2. Fire as one of the five elemental principles. (see *mahābhūta*)
3. The Hindu deity of fire.
4. Sacred ritual fire employed in Vedic *pujas* or worship ceremonies.
5. Biological heat animating all living processes.
6. The body's digestive or internal fire.

agnisāra 1. Literally meaning "fire essence," *Agnisāra kriyā* (or *vahnisāra kriyā*) is a pranayama technique involving emptying the lungs while leaning over and pumping the diaphragm and lower abdomen. This yogic practice is said to stimulate digestive fire, vitalize the energy of the abdomen, strengthen the abdominal muscles, massage and tone the internal organs while restoring them with fresh blood, and to improve digestion, constipation, motility, and elimination.
2. A medicine for the eyes.

ahaṁkāra Lit. "I-making," "individuation," Self-consciousness, sense of ego, or egotism. In the Sāṁkhya metaphysical system, *ahaṁkāra* is the second *tattva* or elemental evolute of *prakṛti* (material Nature) and is joined with *buddhi* (intelligence) and *manas* (mind) to form the *antaḥkaraṇa* or "internal instrument" which constitutes the individual subjective personality.

ahiṁsa One of the five *yamas* or ethical restraints cited in the *Yoga Sūtra*, this is the practice of not harming or injuring other beings in word, deed, thought, and/or action.

Air One of the five elements in each of the systems of Ayurveda and Yoga. Ayurveda lists the other four elements as water, earth, fire, and space and Yoga lists the other four elements as water, earth, fire, and ether. In Yoga philosophy, air is represented by Vayu, the god of the Wind and the father of Hanuman, and symbolizes breathing, expansiveness, vital spirit, lightness, knowledge, inspiration, sound, and, when out of balance, confusion and a lack of groundedness.

Air Medal A military award from the United States Air Force recognizing an act of merit, heroism, or commendable service while participating in an aerial flight.

Albert Schweitzer A Nobel Prize winning philosopher, theologian, musician, author, and physician whose reverence for life helped identify many "diseases of modern civilization."

allopathy A system of medicine that combats disease by using evidence-based remedies and treatments such as drugs and/or surgery.

ālocaka pitta A sub-***doṣa*** specific to the eyes, enabling vision, visual impressions, and color perception.

āma Lit. "uncooked, undigested." Incomplete digestion of food or constipation, resulting in unhealthy accumulation of impurities and toxins within the body, viewed in Ayurveda as being one of the principal causes of disease.

American Viniyoga Institute (AVI) Founded by Gary Kraftsow, AVI is an approach to Yoga Therapy that adapts the various means and methods of practice to the unique condition, needs, and interests of each individual—giving each practitioner the tools to individualize and actualize the process of self-discovery and personal transformation. It is a comprehensive system that implies differentiation, adaptation, and appropriate application of Yoga and includes āsana, pranayama, bandha, sound, chanting, meditation, personal ritual, and study of texts.

anāhatāsana Heart chakra pose or heart opening pose.

ānanda Bliss, joy, esp. the innate bliss of Being.

ānanda-maya-kośa According to the *Taittirīya Upaniṣad,* this is the "sheath made of bliss" or the subtle, innermost shell covering the *ātman* (individual self).

aṇima A yogic *siddhi* or supranormal power of making the physical body subtle in mass or density, or making it as small as an atom. Eternal smallness, minuteness, and fineness.

añjaneyāsana Crescent pose.

anna-maya-kośa According to the *Taittirīya Upaniṣad,* this is the "sheath made of food" or the outermost shell covering the *ātman* or individual self.

antar yoga Lit. "internal yoga." Deep thought, abstraction, or meditation, in contrast with external physical ***yoga*** practices.

anthroposophical medicine Founded by Rudolph Steiner, in association with Ita Wegman, this is a form of alternative medicine that is occasionally at odds with mainstream medicine and draws on a variety of treatment techniques including massage, exercise, counselling, Steiner's spiritual philosophy, and the use of anthroposophic drugs that are similar to those used in homeopathy.

anti-aging medicine A clinical medical specialty focusing on the early detection, prevention, treatment, and reversal of age-related dysfunctions, disorders, and diseases to assist in prolonging a healthy life span in human beings.

anuloma ujjāyi A basic pranayama technique emphasizing the effortlessness and natural ease of the breath. It is performed by breathing through alternative nostrils and uses ***ujjāyi*** breathing on the inhalation breath and a calm, natural, long, and smooth exhalation breath to help relax the nervous system.

anuloma viloma *anuloma* = "with the hair," with the grain, regular
viloma = "against the hair," other than ordinary

Commonly referred to as "alternate nostril breathing," this is a pranayama technique that traditionally involves inhaling through one nostril, retaining the breath, and exhaling through the other nostril in a ratio of 2:8:4 (inhale:retention:exhale), though other variations of the breathing ratio are often applied for various purposes. With respect to yogic breathing, *anuloma* refers to inhalation through both nostrils and exhalation alternately through either nostril that is affected with pauses, rather than with a single smooth movement. The technique is said to restore, equalize, and balance the flow of prana (energy) in the body and sometimes includes skipping the kumbhaka (retention of breath) and breathing with a balanced 1:1 or a parasympathetic-inducing 1:2 inhale to exhale ratio when used in therapeutic situations to decrease potential stress.

apānāsana Downward air/abdominal breath pose or supine knees to chest pose.

apāna vata A foundational aspect of the vata dosha typically located in the lower abdomen that governs the elimination of wastes, sexual function, and the menstrual cycle and manifests as intestinal cramps, menstrual problems, lower back pain, irregularity, diarrhea, prostate issues, constipation, and gas when it is out of balance.

apāna vāyu One of the five vayus (winds or energy channels) in Yoga and originating in the navel and pelvic floor, apāna vāyu governs the outward and downward flow of energy and the exhalation breath. It balances the muladhara chakra and nourishes the organs of digestion, reproduction, and elimination.

aparigraha One of the five ***yamas*** or ethical restraints cited in the *Yoga Sūtra*, this is the practice of nonpossessiveness, nonacceptance, renunciation, being satisfied, and not coveting.

ardha-añjaneyāsana Half crescent pose or kneeling crescent pose.

Army Medical Specialist A distinctive branch of the United States Army, the Army Medical Specialist Corps provides agile healthcare leaders and uniquely trained specialists, who transform health, facilitate collaborative partnerships, foster innovation, improve resiliency, and provide ways of maximizing wellness.

Art of Living's Sahaj Samadhi Meditation Similar to transcendental meditation and Deepak Chopra's Primordial Sound Meditation, this technique of mantra-based meditation is taught by Śrī Śrī Ravi Shankar and The Art of Living Foundation. Sahaj Samadhi literally means "natural enlightenment" and the meditation technique is designed to improve energy, clarity, creativity, and one's inner peace through mantra recitation.

ārtava 1. Conforming to seasons or periods of time.

2. Relating to a woman's menstrual period or menstrual discharge.

artha Aim, purpose, advantage, ambition, meaning, wealth, material prosperity, or monetary success. One of the four *puruṣārthas* or basic human values recognized in Hindu culture.

āsana Classically listed as the third component or limb of Patañjali's *rāja* or *aṣṭāṅga-yoga*, this refers to a stable, comfortable seat for meditation practice. In later Haṭha Yoga, it referred to any formal physical posture, movement, or pose. The practice of physical postures is designed to improve flexibility, strength, energetic flow, endurance, focus, vitality, conditioning, organ health, and overall healing response, as well as reduce stress, strain, and discomfort in the body in Yoga and Yoga Therapy.

Ashtanga See Ashtanga Vinyasa Yoga.

ashwini mudra Literally meaning "horse gesture," this technique rhythmically contracts the anal sphincter to pump energy into the manipura chakra and is often used in pregnancy, uterine problems, and to strengthen the pelvic floor in conjunction with mula bandha (the root lock).

asmitā One of Patañjali's five kleshas (afflictions) Egotism, conceit. One of the five *kleśas* or subjective afflictions cited in Patañjali's *Yoga Sūtra,* this is the material aspect of being that is concerned with one's ego, conceit, or false identity in the world, and one's "I-am-ness" – as in "I am a woman," "I am a father," "I am a lawyer," etc.

assistant professor of medicine This is a scholar, teacher, doctor, and/or academic, who has been awarded a doctoral or professional degree and participates in university affairs at least at the department level for a probationary period before he/she is either offered tenure or terminated.

associate director An associate director of an academic program typically works in association with a program director and under administrative direction, plans, organizes, develops, and/or directs day-to-day department operations, workshops, trainings, and long term objectives.

Ashtanga Vinyasa Yoga Colloquially referred to as Ashtanga Yoga, this dynamic and vigorous style of Haṭha Yoga was founded and popularized by Śrī K. Pattabhi Jois in Mysore, India as a modern-day form of classical Indian Yoga. It employs the use of bandhas, ujjayi pranayama, and specific dṛṣṭis within the context of six vigorous set sequences and series of āsanas that progressively increase in their degree of difficulty. Several popular forms of modern Haṭha Yoga are derived from Ashtanga Vinyasa Yoga including Power Yoga, Vinyasa Yoga, Jivamukti Yoga, and Rocket Yoga. (see *vinyāsa yoga*)

aṣṭāṅga yoga Patañjali's "eight-limbed" path to Yoga outlined in chapter two of the *Yoga Sūtra,* helps develop all aspects of a human being. The eight-component contemplative strategy includes ***yama*** (ethical restraints or moral codes), ***niyama*** (observances and self-purification methods), ***āsana*** (stable seat or postures), ***prāṇāyāma*** (extension and expansion of breath), ***pratyāhāra*** (withdrawal), ***dhāraṇā*** (concentration), ***dhyāna*** (meditation), and ***samādhi*** (absorption). It is also a shortened name for "Ashtanga Vinyasa Yoga."

aṣṭa-sthāna-parikṣa Lit. "eight areas of investigation." Subject material of the eight chapters of the *Carakasaṁhitā,* namely: *sūtra* (general principles of health and healing), *nidāna* (pathology of eight major diseases), *vimāna* (pathology and diagnostics), *śārīra* (anatomy and embryology), *indriya* (diagnosis and prognosis based on perceptible signs), *cikitsā* (specific therapies), *kalpa* (pharmaceutics and toxicology), and *siddhi* (effecive treatment and principles of *pañcakarma*).

asteya One of the five *yamas* or ethical restraints cited in the *Yoga Sūtra,* this is the practice of not stealing and being generous.

asthi In Ayurvedic medicine, this is one of the seven *dhātus* (fundamental tissues of the body) consisting of bone and cartilage.

Atharva Veda The fourth book of the Vedas representing "ancient rishi knowledge" and great antiquity developed independently of the other three (*Ṛg Veda, Sāma Veda,* and *Yajur Veda*). The *Atharva Veda* is not much utilized in formal Vedic rituals but rather consists largely of *mantras,* spells, poetic hymns, and incantations utilized for purposes of both white and black magic that deal with the practical and philosophic aspects of human existence. The *Atharva* is celebrated for its *Pṛthivī Sūkta* (Hymn to Goddess Earth) and its germinal expression of pantheism through its description of the *hiraṇyagarbha* or "golden embryo" out of which Brahmā, the Creator, emerged. It is also the earliest extant Indic text dealing with medical subjects, with a pre-Ayurvedic germ-based theory of disease and advice on the treatment and prevention of disease through the use of *mantras* and medicinal plants.

ātma-jñāna Lit. "self-knowledge," knowledge of soul, or knowledge of the Supreme Spirit.

ātman Lit. "self." In Vedānta philosophy, the individual spiritual soul that transmigrates from life to life. In the nondual Advaita Vedānta, *ātman* is ultimately equated with Brahman, the impersonal Divine Ground of Being, the latter being often referred to as *paramātman,* the transcendental Self or pure consciousness. From the monistic perspective of Advaita, the perceived differentiation of a plurality of selves is seen as a fundamental illusion (*māyā*) brought about by the creative sport (*līlā*) of the One. The *dvaita* (dualistic) interpretation of Vedānta regards the *ātman* as being eternal, indestructible, truly individual, and ontologically distinct from Brahman.

Autobiography of a Yogi A spiritual classic written by Indian guru, Paramahansa Yogananda, this book has introduced millions of practitioners and teachers to Kriya Yoga, Indian spirituality, and Eastern mysticism. It follows Yogananda's autobiographical spiritual adventures in India and the United States and was named as one of the "100 Most Important Spiritual Books of the 20th Century" by HarperCollins Publishers.

avidyā The first of the five ***kleśas*** or subjective afflictions cited in Patañjali's *Yoga Sūtra,* this is viewed as the field from which the other *kleśas* arise and the underlying cause of individual suffering. It is "not knowing" or one's ignorance concerning the true nature of existence and can also refer to the ignorance that develops from one's misidentification of what is real, especially in terms of the ultimate status of one's own self.

āyāma Stretching, lengthening, extending, unobstructed expansion. Compounded with *prāṇa* in the generic term for yogic breathing practices, namely, *prāṇāyāma.*

Ayurveda *āyus* = life, vitality, health, longevity; *veda* = knowledge. Translated as "the science of life" and considered the most traditional and ancient system of medicine in India, this is a specialized field within holistic alternative medicine that observes the doshas, koshas, and gunas and seeks to bring an individual into greater overall balance, harmony, and equilibrium through treatments like pañca karma and diet and lifestyle modification techniques.

Ayurvedic health science practitioner An introductory or semi-introductory level training for Ayurvedic practitioners in the United States consisting of a minimum of 500–1000 hours of course work. The term is sometimes used synonymously with the term ayurvedic wellness counselor (AWC) and often designates an additional training following the completion of an AWC program.

Ayurvedic medicine and surgery (et al.) A $5\frac{1}{2}$ year bachelor's degree in India that requires a Statutory Board exam for entrance.

Ayurvedic Wellness Counselor (AWC) The initial 500-hour introductory level training program for Ayurvedic practitioners in the United States, which typically focuses on the first goal of Ayurveda: to preserve the health of the healthy. It can include topics of, but not limited to, the philosophy of Ayurvedic health, physiology, psychology, nutrition and herbology, Yoga, body work, pathology, assessments, and introductions to disease and clinical management.

Ayurvedic Yoga Therapy Founded by Mukunda and Chinnamasta Stiles, Ayurvedic Yoga Therapy is an approach to Yoga Therapy and Ayurveda that focuses on bringing equilibrium to the doshas and finding the root causes of dis-ease, including but not limited to stress, inflammation, tumor, and congestion to bring the body-mind-heart back to balance.

azidothymidine (AZT) A type of antiretroviral drug used in the treatment of HIV/AIDS.

B. K. S. Iyengar Named as "one of the 100 most influential people in the world" by *Time Magazine*, B.K.S. Iyengar was an innovative Yoga master and guru who founded the Ramamani Iyengar Memorial Yoga Institute in Pune, India. A student of Professor Tirumalai Krishnamacharya, he created and developed the style of Haṭha Yoga known as Iyengar Yoga, which highlights six main features: alignment, breathing, timing, props, women's adaptations, and therapeutics. He wrote several books on Yoga including *Light on Yoga, Light on Pranayama, Light on Life,* and *Light on the Yoga Sutras of Patanjali.*

baddha-koṇāsana Bound angle pose or butterfly pose.

bālāsana Child's pose.

bandha Translated as "lock," "hold," or "tighten," these are psycho-muscular contractions or energetic practices in Haṭha Yoga that involve internally controlling, closing, and locking valves in the spine and energetic body to influence the flow of *prāṇa* (energy). There are three main bandhas: ***mūla*** *bandha* (the root lock or perineal/cervical lock), *uḍḍiyāna bandha* (the abdominal or belly lock), and *jalandhāra bandha* (the throat lock) and when all three are engaged together it is known as maha bandha (the great lock).

Bangalore Institute of Oncology A specialty care oncology center and hospital in Sampangiramnagar, Bangalore, India.

basti One of the six shat karmas (cleansing techniques) mentioned in the *Haṭha Yoga Pradīpikā* and one of the *pañca karma* treatments of Ayurveda, this is the Indian version of an enema for cleaning the lower abdomen and colon and is performed by sucking air or water into the anus using a catheter tube.

Beatles, The See The Beatles.

Bele Noci Sanitarium A special facility in Russia where the KGB would train their agents in the 1970s that had special chamber rooms where light, sound, and temperature were all controlled.

Bernard Osher Foundation Founded in 1977 by Bernard Osher, the Osher Foundation seeks to improve quality of life through support for higher education and the arts by providing post-secondary scholarship funding to colleges and universities across the nation. It also benefits programs in integrative medicine in the United States and Sweden, including centers at the University of California, San Francisco, Harvard Medical School and Brigham and Women's Hospital in Boston, and the Karolinska Institute in Stockholm.

Bhagavad Gītā Written by the sage Vyasa and literally translated as "The Song of The Lord," this 700-verse work is the sixth book in the Mahabharata and is largely considered as the Hindu Bible. One of the longest epic poems in the world, it highlights the ethical and moral struggles of human life in the allegorical tale of Krishna, Arjuna, and the Pandava brothers on the battefield with their cousins, the Kauravas, during the Kurukshetra War. Among other things, Kṛṣṇa, an *avatāra* (incarnation) of the god Viṣṇu, instructs Arjuna, a virtuous prince, on the various ways of being spiritual, including *jñāna-yoga* (*yoga* of knowledge), *bhakti-yoga* (*yoga* of religious devotion), and *karma yoga* (*yoga* of selfless action).

Bhakti Yoga One of the four main paths to Yoga, this is the path of worship, devotion, and love and typically includes practices like chanting, mantra japa and recitation, ceremonial offerings, faith in one's istha devata (chosen form of The Divine), and surrendering to God, as the Beloved.

bhastrikā Defined as "bellows breath," this pranayama technique combines anuloma viloma (alternate nostril breathing) with kapalabhati (skull shining breathing) and is performed by breathing forcible through the nostrils aiming toward equal intensity and time for both inhalations and exhalations like the pumping of a blacksmith's bellows. It is good for sluggishness, depression, a slow metabolism, and digestive issues.

bhāva 1. Being, becoming; existing, occurring; appearance, feeling, attitude.

2. That which exists; thing or substance; a being or living creature.

3. Nature, condition, state of being, character, temperament.

4. Any state of mind or body, way of thinking or feeling, sentiment.

bhāvana 1. Causing to be, effecting, producing, displaying, manifesting, affirming.

2. Forming in the mind, conception, imagination, visualization, guided imagery, meditation.

3. In Buddhism, mental cultivation or mood developed through meditation practice.

4. In Ayurveda, the process of levigation in the preparation of medicinal agents, wherein an ingredient is ground into a fine powder or paste, increasing its effectiveness upon ingestion.

bhramarī Translated as "bee breathing," this pranayama technique resembles the soft humming sound of a bee and is produced by closing the tragus (cartilaginous flap of the external ear) while making a prolonged *M* sound or the sound of a buzzing bee. It is said to be good for anger issues, insomnia, sinus problems, anxiety, and stress.

bhū mudrā Earth ***mudrā***. A gesture signifying one's connection with Mother Earth, this hand position is performed by extending the index and middle fingers in the shape of a "peace sign" and placing them in direct contact with the ground. It is said to evoke feelings of trust, support, and being rooted to the Earth.

bhujaṅgāsana Cobra pose or serpent pose.

bīja mantra The "seed syllables" of mantras, these one-syllable sounds have inherent connections to spiritual principles, the invocation of deities or the energies and qualities they represent, the focusing of awareness on specific points or chakras (energy centers) in the body, or the starting point for more elaborate mantras, though typically they do not have meaning on their own. The most well-known and ubiquitous *bīja mantra* is the *praṇava* or sacred syllable ***oṁ***.

bitilāsana Cow pose.

board certified A classification within medical and alternative health professions like osteopathy, general medicine, chiropractic, and acupuncture, distinguishing that a governing body of professionals and peers has tested and approved that particular practitioner's skills, knowledge, and application of therapeutic interventions.

brahmacarya* or *brahmacharya Lit. "holy conduct," this is one of the five *yamas* or ethical restraints cited in Patañjali's *Yoga Sūtra* and is the practice of self-restraint, continence, moderation, proper behavior and lifestyle, and preserving one's energy. The term *brahmacarya* has often been translated as celibacy, reflecting an imprecise and overly reductive understanding of the term.

Brahman In Hinduism, the Divine Ground of Being from which all existence arises. In order to preserve the relevance of convention religion, a distinction is made between *nirguṇa brahman* or *brahman* beyond characteristic, referring to the transpersonal and transcendental nature of the one Being, and *sāguṇa brahman* or Brahman with characteristics, referring to the personified creative agency of the initial individuation of the Divine in the form of Brahmā, the Creator of this world order. Many followers of Hindu religious traditions centered around Śiva, Viṣṇu, or the Goddess regard their principal deity as the supreme personality of Brahman.

Breathing Project, The A New York City–based educational nonprofit organization founded by Leslie Kaminoff dedicated to teaching individualized, breath-centered Yoga and creating innovative learning opportunities based on experiences of body, breath, and mind.

breathwork Of, or relating to, a variety of breathing and pranayama practices found in Yoga and Yoga therapy that teach an individual to harness, balance, expand, and/or control one's breath, mental state, and energy.

Brūgger relief position An exercise invented by Swiss neurologist Dr. Alois Brūgger to reduce physical muscle tension and stress on the spine in a poor, rounded, and/or slumping posture. This technique is performed by externally rotating the arms, turning the palms forward/up, lightly engaging the abdominal muscles, and bringing the chin in slightly toward the neck.

buddhi Intelligence, the faculty of discrimination and reason, or the highest state of mind. In the Sāṁkhya metaphysical system, *buddhi* is the first *tattva* or elemental evolute of *prakṛti* or material Nature and is joined with *ahaṁkāra* (self-consciousness) and *manas* (mind) to form the *antaḥkaraṇa* or "internal instrument" that constitutes the individual subjective personality.

cakra* or *chakras Lit. "disk, circle, wheel." In Yoga subtle anatomy, an energy center in the body. There are seven major chakras aligned along the central energy channel, *suṣumna,* from the pelvic floor to the crown of the head. Each is associated with an elemental energy and is generative of certain psycho-spiritual functions, potentials, and referred to as a "lotus," with the petals representing major energy channels or ***nāḍis*** that converge at that place.

cakrāsana* or *chakrāsana Wheel pose. (Also *ūrdva dhanurāsana* or upward-facing bow pose.)

candra bhedana* or *chandra bhedana Lit. "moon piercing." A *prāṇāyāma* breathing technique of inhaling through the left nostril and exhaling through the right nostril, thus amplifying the cool "lunar" energy conducted through the *iḍā nāḍī,* clearing and purifying the major energy channel on the left side of the body.

Caraka Samhita This "compendium of Caraka" is one of two foundational Indic texts in the Ayurvedic medicine system along with the *Sushruta Samhita.* Although the surviving edition has been dated to its reputed compiler, the physician Caraka, around the fourth or fifth century CE, it may be based on an original work written a few centuries before. Caraka received his medical training at the renowned academy of Takṣaśilā (Taxila), ancient capital of Gandhāra, near present-day Islamabad, Pakistan. It is said that Buddha's physician, Jīvaka also studied there, which suggests a formal medical tradition that dates back to at least the sixth century BCE. The *Carakasaṁhitā* is structured around "eight areas of investigation." (see *aṣṭa-sthāna-parikṣa* and *Suśrutasaṁhitā*)

Caraka Samhita—Sutrastanam A specific section of the *Caraka Samhita* that focuses on the body, mind, and primal qualities of Nature and their role in disease, discernment, well-being, and happiness.

Centers for Disease Control and Prevention (CDC) The health protection agency of the United States, the CDC works to protect Americans from health, safety, and security threats, both foreign and domestic, from mostly an allopathic model of care. It collaborates with other organizations and responds publicly with information and tools that people and communities use to protect their health through health promotion, prevention of disease, injury and disability, and preparedness.

Certified Yoga Therapist A credential designation within the field of Yoga Therapy implying that a therapist, healthcare provider, or a Yoga instructor has completed all exams and coursework necessary to graduate from a particular school's Yoga Therapist certification program. This title does not necessarily distinguish the program's accreditation status with the International Association of Yoga Therapists and/or the practitioner's competency, acumen, and skill level in working with patients.

check-in Time and space created in a Yoga Therapy session that assists practitioners in reflecting on their own physical, mental, and/or emotional situation. It can also be used for community sharing and to review any mudras, affirmations, āsanas, meditations, and/or breathing techniques previously given to the Yoga practitioner(s).

Chi Gong See qi gong.

Chinese herbs Various herbs, herbal concoctions, and herbal combinations originating in China that are used to treat illness, disease, and imbalance in Chinese Medicine and acupuncture.

Chinese Medicine A system of complementary medicine originating in ancient China that involves utilizing techniques of acupuncture, oriental massage, acupressure, moxibustion, cupping, breathing techniques, exercise, heat, cold, magnets, nutrition, diet, herbs, dietary supplements, and/or plant, animal, and mineral products to promote, maintain, and restore health, alleviate pain, and treat various physical, mental, and emotional conditions.

cikitsā Lit. "treatment" or "therapy."

cin mudrā* or *chin mudrā (Read "*cin*" as "*cit*," as in "*citta*.") "Consciousness gesture." A meditative hand gesture where the thumb and forefinger are joined together and the remaining fingers are extended. It may be distinguished from the *jñāna mudrā* or "knowledge *mudrā*" in that the hand is opened upward, thus opening out consciousness to awareness of All. Sitting in full lotus posture with hands extended over the knees in *cin mudrā* is the quintessential image of meditation in the Yoga tradition.

citta or ***chitta*** Lit. "noticed," thinking, reflecting, imagining; thought; the mind and its activities in the broadest sense.

citta mudrā* or *chitta mudrā Translated as "gesture of witness consciousness," this hand gesture supports the awakening of witness consciousness in which thoughts, feelings, and limiting beliefs are seen more clearly, without identifying with them. It directs breath, awareness, and energy into the throat and head and is for balancing the vijnanamaya kosha. It is performed by touching the pads of the index fingers to the tips of thumbs on the same hand and extending the other fingers straight out as the hands are brought together in front of the chest with the pads of the middle, ring, and little fingers touching the same fingers on the opposite hand. The thumbs touch along their length and the tips of the index fingers also touch so that they form a line parallel to the earth.

citta-vṛtti-nirodha Patañjali's definition of *Yoga* in the second aphorism of the *Yoga Sūtra,* "[*Yoga* is] the arresting of the movements of the mind" or "[Yoga is] the cessation of the movements and modifications of the 'mind-stuff.'"

Classical Yoga An indistinct system (or systems) of Yoga found in ancient texts like *The Vedas,* Patañjali's Yoga Sūtra, *The Bhagavad Gītā, The Ramayana,* and *The Upaniṣads.* Often, this term is used when specifically referring to Rāja Yoga or Patanjali and his eight-limbed path known classically as *aṣṭāṅga yoga.*

clinical hypnotherapist A practitioner who uses hypnosis in a clinical setting for stress management, personal growth, stopping smoking, losing weight, health maintenance, alleviating or eliminating phobias, and/or coping with pain.

complementary and alternative medicine (CAM) A group of diverse medical and healthcare systems, practices, and products that are not presently considered to be part of conventional medicine and/or accepted standards of care that consist of medical doctors, doctors of osteopathy, and allied health professionals, such as nurses and physical therapists.

core quality A facet of healing in Integrative Yoga Therapy that is awakened through the introduction and use of an educational theme such as the importance of body awareness, posture, or breathing.

Cyrex Laboratories A clinical immunology laboratory in Arizona specializing in functional immunology, multitissue antibody testing, and autoimmunity.

cytochrome p450 system Located predominantly in the liver, cytochrome p450 enzymes are essential for the systemic production of cholesterol, steroids, and prostacyclins, the detoxification of foreign chemicals, and the metabolism of drugs.

darśana 1. Seeing, observing, looking, noticing, observation, perception.

2. Inspection, examination.

3. Audience, meeting.

4. View, doctrine, philosophical system.

5. A generic term for any one of the six orthodox Hindu "perspectives" or philosophical schools of thought. The six are typically presented in three related pairs: **Nyāya** and **Vaiṣeśikā, Pūrva Mīmāṁsa** and **Uttara Mīmāṁsa (Vedānta), Sāṁkhya** and **Yoga.**

Dartmouth-Coop Test An outcome measure used in clinical practice and developed by a collaborative research network of 233 primary care clinicians in conjunction with Dartmouth Medical School, the dimensions of health status measured by the test include physical endurance, emotional health, daily activities, social activities, social support, level of pain, change in health, overall health, and one's quality of life.

Dean Ornish, M.D. A Clinical Professor of Medicine at the University of San Francisco School of Medicine and the founder of the Preventive Medicine Research Institute in Sausalito, California, Dr. Dean Ornish is a student of the late Indian guru, Swami Satchidananda, and is the first person in the Western world to scientifically prove that heart disease could be reversed without drugs or surgery. His methods relied primarily on Yoga and a low fat, plant-based diet, which was considered the traditional diet of yogis in India, and his program for heart disease has been approved by Medicare, the gold standard for mainstream medicine in America.

Deepak Chopra's Primordial Sound Meditation Similar to transcendental meditation and The Art of Living's Sahaj Samadhi meditation, this mantra-based technique is rooted in the Vedic tradition of India and promotes "restful awareness," deep physical relaxation, inner calm, and an alert yet quiet mind through mantra recitation.

deha The body; form, shape; mass, appearance, bulk.

Department of Family and Community Medicine (at University Hospital) A specific health division at the University of Texas Health Science Center in San Antonio that focuses on Family Practice and Community Medicine.

dev* or *deva 1. A god or deity. (Feminine: *devī*.)

2. Heavenly, divine; a terrestial thing of high excellence.

3. Transparent or nonphysical.

dhanurāsana Bow pose.

dhāraṇā Classically listed as the sixth component or limb of Patañjali's *rāja* or *aṣṭāṅga-yoga*, this is the starting point for meditation practice. According to the *Yoga Sūtra*, *Dhāraṇā* is "the mind's locking onto a point," harnessing and steadying one's concentration, and retaining a single-pointed focus.

dharma 1. In Hinduism, duty, sacred duty, righteous duty, social ethics, propriety, law. One of the four *puruṣārthas* or basic human values.

2. In Buddhism, teachings and practices conducive to awakening.

3. In philosophy, a classifiable phenomena, true purpose, vocation, or essential principle.

***dhātus* (foundational tissues of the body)** Lit. "layer, stratum." A constituent part or ingredient.

1. The five *mahābhūtas* (great elements).

2. The three *doṣas* (bodily humors).

3. The seven tissues of the body in Ayurveda and Yoga consisting of ***rasa*** (plasma), ***rakta*** (blood), ***maṁsa*** (muscle), ***meda*** (adipose), ***asthi*** (bone and cartilage), ***majja*** (marrow and nerves), ***śukra/artava*** (male/female reproductive fluids).

dhautī Lit. "washing, cleansing." One of the six shat karmas (cleansing techniques) mentioned in the *Haṭha Yoga Pradīpikā,* this involves swallowing a moistened piece of thin muslin cloth into the stomach to cleanse the digestive tract. The cloth in presoaked in salt water, then about 12 feet of it is swallowed, and, finally, it is slowly and carefully pulled back up and out of the mouth. It takes a great deal of guidance and discipline to perform this cleansing technique and should only be done by a healthy person under supervision by a teacher.

dhyāna Classically listed as the seventh component or limb of Patañjali's *rāja* or *aṣṭāṅga-yoga,* this is where *dhāraṇā* (concentration) evolves and becomes meditation. In this limb, which commonly involves an object of meditation that is divine, godly, and holy, or more practically involves just an activity or a practice, the individual and the experience of the act of meditating dissolves and what emerges is the awareness, being-ness, or evenness of consciousness toward the object of meditation.

diploma [as in diploma in Yoga] Offered at the Institute of Medical Sciences at Banaras Hindu University in India, the diploma in Yoga is part of a $5^1/_2$ year course in Yoga and Ayurveda.

***dīrga* breathing** Also called "*dīrgha prāṇāyāma,*" this basic breathing technique employs a three-part complete breath that completely fills the thorax beginning in the abdomen, then continuing to the diaphragm/rib cage, and lastly filling the chest on a long, slow, and smooth inhalation breath (and the exhalation breath simply reverses the flow of the inhale) utilizing the full capacity of the lungs.

dīrga prāṇāyāma *See dīrga* breathing.

Divine Farmer (Shen Nong) Known as the "Emperor of the Five Grains," Shen Nong, literally meaning "The Divine Farmer," lived about 5,000 years ago and is credited with introducing the Chinese culture to agriculture and the use of herbal medicine. He is regarded as one of the two "legendary founders" of Chinese Medicine along with The Yellow Emperor.

doctorate in chiropractic A four-year doctorate level postgraduate degree that consists of about 5,000 contact hours in anatomy, spinal biomechanics, physiology, biochemistry, pathology, microbiology, pharmatoxicology, psychology, dietetics and nutrition, public health, history-taking skills, general physical examination, laboratory diagnosis, differential diagnosis, radiology, sports science and physical therapeutics, rehabilitation, neurology, orthopedics, massage, and adjustment technique, including a minimum 1,000 hours of supervised clinical training.

doṣas or ***doshas*** The doshas, *vata, pitta,* and *kapha,* are known as the "three bodily humors," "qualities of life," or "constitutions" that represent the combinations, permutations, and interplay of the five basic elements of creation (ether/space, air/wind, fire, earth, and water) in Ayurveda and Yoga Therapy. All people are said to have the qualities of vata (wind, gas), pitta (file, bile), and kapha (phlegm, mucus), but one (or two) are usually more primary and dominant, which has/have great influence on an individual's body type, personality, and general constitution. The cause of dysfunction and disease in Ayurveda is viewed as a lack of proper cellular function due to an excess or deficiency of vata, pitta, or kapha at the cellular level. (see ***prakṛti***)

doṣa gati **(movement of dosha)** Referencing the cyclic movement of each ***doṣa*** from the hollow structures of the gastrointenstinal tract to the denser *dhātus* or bodily tissues and back, as well as from the GI tract to the places of elimination. The ***doṣas*** alternate in dominance during these movements, which run through two complete cycles daily. Understanding of the *doṣa gatis* is important in choosing the optimal timing for various Ayurvedic *cikitsās* or therapeutic treatments.

Dr. Ram Murthy An Indian medical doctor who taught Yoga as a therapy in the New York area in the 1950s.

dṛṣṭi or dṛṣṭi 1. Seeing, viewing, beholding.

2. Sight, the faculty of seeing; the pupil of the eye.

3. The mind's eye, wisdom, intelligence.

4. View, notion, theory, doctrine, system.

5. Where one focuses the eyes during meditation or āsana practice.

duḥkha Lit. "a bad space." Suffering, pain, uneasiness, trouble, or difficulty physically, mentally, emotionally, and/or spiritually. In Buddhism, *duḥkha* is embodied in the first of the Four Noble Truths, i.e., that life, as ordinarily experienced, is permeated with sorrows.

Du Mai One of the "Eight Extraordinary Vessels" in Chinese meridian theory, this vessel, known as the governing vessel, controls the Yang channels, the Guardian Qi, and the Yang Qi, or "fire" of the body. It originates deep in the dantien near the perineum and travels posteriorly along the spine, up over the head, down past the third eye, and concluding at the junction between the upper lip and the gums. It is used to treat brain issues, spinal cord pain, heaviness, stroke, psychological issues, headache, migraines, dizziness, tinnitus, pain/swelling in the face/head, and stiffness in the shoulders, neck, and back.

dveṣa One of the five *kleśas* or subjective afflictions cited in Patañjali's *Yoga Sūtra,* this is the aversion, aggression, repugnancy, enmity, hatred, and anger that develops when an individual doesn't get what he/she desires.

Earth One of the five elements in each of the systems of Chinese Medicine, Ayurveda, and Yoga. Chinese Medicine lists the other four elements as water, fire, metal, and wood; Ayurveda lists the other four elements as water, fire, wind/air, and space; and, Yoga lists the other four elements as water, fire, ether, and air. In Yoga philosophy, earth is represented by Prithvi, the goddess of earth, and symbolizes nature, foundation, structure, rootedness, and when out of balance, instability and dryness.

editor-in-chief The person who heads all departments at a publication or press organization that is ultimately responsible for delegating and managing tasks to staff, general operations, overseeing projects, and making final editorial decisions on content, facts, grammar, style, design, and photos.

ego-I This is the identification with the belief of being separate or a "separate self," which creates inner and outer division in people and feelings of separation, disharmony, and constriction. This belief in separation generates a feeling that "something's missing," "wrong," or "off" in people's lives.

Eight Extraordinary Channels Consisting of the ren mai, yin qiao mai, du mai, yang qiao mai, chong mai, yin wei mai, dai mai, and yang wei mai, these channels are paired with the twelve primary energy channels as the main parts of the channel system in Chinese Medicine and are intended to "act like reservoirs of energy" to the primary channels, which are referred to as "rivers" of energy and regulate the change of life cycles.

Eight Extraordinary Meridians See Eight Extraordinary Channels.

extended exhalation breath practice A breathing practice focusing on gradually extending the exhalation breath beginning with an exhalation to inhalation ratio that is slightly greater than than a 1:1 ratio and works toward an exhalation breath that is twice-as-long as the inhalation breath. It has been seen that lengthening the exhalation breath stimulates the parasympathetic (rest and restore) nervous system and produces favorable psychological and physiologic effects.

family medicine A form of primary care medicine providing comprehensive general health care that is not limited to a certain age, gender, and/or disease and does not specialize in any specific part of the body. It is also sometimes referred to as family practice medicine or general practice medicine.

felt-sense A psychotherapy term that refers to a method of establishing more inner awareness that is not consciously thought or verbalized but is experienced in the body. An aspect of focusing, it is that deeper sense in people that accepts, feels, engages in, or holistically, what someone is "working on."

fight-or-flight response The stress response delivered by the sympathetic nervous system, this is activated when there is impending harm, a perceived threat to survival, and/or stress. Effects include increased heart and lung actions, inhibited salivation, slowing/stopping of digestion, constriction of blood vessels, and suppression of the immune system.

Fire One of the five elements in each of the systems of Chinese Medicine, Ayurveda, and Yoga. Chinese Medicine lists the other four elements as water, earth, metal, and wood; Ayurveda lists the other four elements as water, earth, wind/air, and space; and, Yoga lists the other four elements as water, earth, ether, and air. In Yoga philosophy, fire is represented by Agni, the god of fire, and symbolizes purity, burning karma, activity, the sun, transformation, and, when out of balance, agitation and anger.

follow-up A subsequent session with a client following an initial examination or treatment.

foundation of life In Ayurvedic medicine, this is the "holy trinity," otherwise referred to as sharira (body), sattva (mind), and atma (consciousness).

four pillars of life: dharma, artha, kama, and moksha In Ayurveda, Vedic astrology, Jyotish astrology, and Yoga philosophy these are the four aims, goals, or pillars of life. They include dharma (righteous duty), artha (monetary success), kama (love or fulfillment of positive desire), and moksha (enlightenment, self-realization, or liberation).

Ganesh Mohan A doctor, trained in both modern medicine and Ayurveda, and a scholar of Vedic chanting, Patañjali's *Yoga Sūtra,* and Svastha Yoga Therapy, Ganesh Mohan is coauthor of *Yoga Therapy* with A. G. Mohan (his father), Indra Mohan (his wife), and Nitya Mohan (his sister) as well as *Krishnamacharya: His Life and His Teachings* with his father, A. G. Mohan.

garuḍāsana Garuda pose or eagle pose. A pose in Yoga Therapy that can be used as a passive proprioceptive neuromuscular facilitation (PNF) stretch to assist in the treatment of frozen shoulder and other orthopedically-based range of motion deficiencies.

Golgi tendon organ Also called the GTO, this is the proprioceptive receptor in the nervous system that is sensitive to changes in the tension of a muscle or tendon.

gomukhāsana Cow face pose. A pose in Yoga Therapy that can be used as a passive proprioceptive neuromuscular facilitation (PNF) stretch to assist in the treatment of frozen shoulder, lengthening of the external rotator muscles (infraspinatus and teres minor muscles), and other orthopedically-based range of motion deficiencies.

gu One-half of the Indian and Sanskrit term, *guru,* meaning "teacher" or "master," the word, *gu,* itself, means "darkness" or "shadows."

guṇas The process by which evolution is created and carried out in Sāṁkhya philosophy, the *guṇas* are properties, strings, threads, attributes, or tendencies of behavorial and natural phenomena and consist of an ever-changing balance of the qualities of materiality and ***prakṛti*** (nature): ***rājas*** (activity, energy, passion, action, movement, or pain), ***tamas*** (heaviness, density, inertia, ignorance, or dullness), and ***sattva*** (purity, light, rhythm, beauty, joy, or balance).

gurmukhī **or** ***gurumukhi*** **language** The customary script of the Punjabi language in India and literally meaning "from the mouth of the Guru," gurumukhi (also written as ***gurmukhī***) is a writing system (rather than a language) developed in northwest India during the sixteenth century CE, from the pre-existing Lahnda script, by Guru Angad, the second patriarch of the Sikh religion. It is the most often used language in the mantras of Kundalini Yoga and Kundalini Yoga Therapy as taught by Yogi Bhajan.

guru Made up of two Indian and Sanskrit words, gu (darkness or shadows) and ru (light or dispel), this is a "teacher," "master," and/or principle, which "removes or dispels the darkness," "brings light to the shadows," and/or "awakens the light within." Other meanings include heavy, great, large, important, serious, venerable, respectable, and a venerable or respectable person, especially a teacher, family member, or spiritual preceptor.

Guru Krishnamacharya See *Krishnamacharya.*

Guru Ram Das Center for Medicine and Humanology Founded as a nonprofit organization by Yogi Bhajan and currently directed by Shanti Shanti Kaur Khalsa, the mission of the center is to bring the techniques of Kundalini Yoga and Meditation into the healthcare field as a treatment modality for those with life-threatening or chronic illness such as asthma, diabetes, HIV disease, cancer, heart disease, chronic pain, and depression.

gyan mudra Translated as the "seal of knowledge," this hand gesture is for expanding breath, awareness and energy, honoring the Divine order within all of creation, balancing the *ānanda-maya-kośa,* opening the ajna chakra, and cultivating silence in the mind. It is performed by touching the tip of the index finger with the tip of the thumb while leaving the other fingers straight out. It may be distinquished from *cin mudra* or "consciousness *mudrā*" in that the hand is turned downward, thus drawing awareness inward to the seat of understanding. It has been practiced for thousands of years by yogis for peace, calmness, wisdom, and spiritual progress and it is the hand position of Kundalini Yoga Therapy's Healthy, Happy, Holy Breathing technique as well as countless other yogic techniques. In Vajrayāna Buddhism, a "wisdom seal" or visualized consort is utilized in visualization practices involved in the arousing and channeling of internal subtle energies within the central *nāḍi.*

Gyana Yoga Also referred to as *Jnana Yoga* and known as one of the four main paths to Yoga, this is the path of philosophic insight, mastering avidya (ignorance), and enlightening the mind. It typically includes practices like contemplation, satsang, viveka (discernment), and self-inquiry.

halāsana Plow pose.

haṁsi mudrā* or *hansi mudra Known as the "gesture of the inner smile," this hand gesture is for lightness, ease, and balancing the anandamaya kosha. It is performed by touching the tips of the index, middle, and ring fingers to the tips of the thumbs on the same hand while extending the little fingers straight out and resting the backs of the hands on the thighs.

Haṭha Yoga Lit. "***yoga*** of a forceful kind," Haṭha Yoga is a subsystem of Rāja Yoga (the classical or royal path) that was systematized circa ninth century CE. Derived from the two words ha (sun) and tha (moon), Haṭha Yoga places emphasis on the vigorous physical practices of *āsana, prāṇāyāma, mudrā,* and *bandha* to create balance in the body and transform the psychophysical organism of the *yogin* into a superior instrument for contemplative practice, intended to bring about the experience of divine union, and the attainment of spiritual realization or freedom. From a therapeutic perspective, the Haṭha Yoga system believes that physical illness impedes the practice of *samādhi* (absorption with the Divine) and must be addressed within the context of the practice.

Haṭhapradīpikā* or *Haṭha Yoga Pradīpikā Authored by Swami Svatmarama, a disciple of Gorakhnath, around the fourteenth to fifteenth century CE, this is the most widely used manual on Haṭha Yoga and one of the three classical texts of Haṭha Yoga along with the *Gheranda*

Samhita and the *Shiva Samhita*. The *Haṭha Yoga Pradīpikā* is a prominent summary text of four chapters and 395 verses and has received many Sanskrit translations and commentaries over the years to try to clarify its meanings and uses. All in all, it has been considered as a possible starting point for the entire system of Yoga Therapy.

health care A system, organization, clinic, or health-oriented professional that assists others in maintaining, preserving, and restoring health by the treatment and/or prevention of disease.

heart-rate-variability The variation in the beat-to-beat interval in between heartbeats, heart-rate variability is a cardiovascular risk factor that has been scientifically shown to positively improve with the practice of Yoga and Yoga Therapy.

Himalayan Institute An international nonprofit organization founded by the Indian guru, Swami Rama, and currently led by Pandit Rajmani Tigunait, that promotes Yoga and holistic health through Yoga retreats, online courses and classes, residential ashram programs and trainings, health products and services, and humanitarian projects.

holy trinity In Ayurvedic medicine, this is "the foundation of life," otherwise referred to as sharira (body), sattva (mind), and atma (consciousness).

homeopathy Also known as "homeopathic medicine" and based on the principle that "like cures like," this system of alternative medicine believes that engaging in natural techniques and healthy lifestyle practices reestablishes homeostasis when out of balance and that, if a substance causes symptoms in a healthy person, giving the person a very small amount of the same substance may actually cure the illness.

hou-tian-zhi-jing (or Postnatal Essence) A source of Jing in Taoist Yoga and Chinese Medicine, this type of acquired constitution, literally defined as "After Heaven Essence" or "Postnatal Essence," is derived from the refined parts of the ingested food, continuous exercise, and emotional and mental stimulation from a person's environment.

***Huang-di Nei-Jing* (Inner Classic of the Yellow Emperor)** Dating back to at least 300 to 100 BCE and likely much farther as an oral tradition, this work was written by the legendary Yellow Emperor and is the earliest written source and the most important foundational and fundamental text in Chinese medicine and Chinese medical theory.

I Ching See *Yijing*.

IAYT Accreditation Committee A group of expert Yoga Therapists and educators appointed by the IAYT Board that helped develop competency-based educational standards that define the foundation of knowledge, key terms, skills, requirements, necessary hours of training, and abilities for the safe and effective practice of Yoga Therapy and the training of Yoga Therapists.

IAYT Certified Yoga Therapist (CYTh) The title and credential associated with a Yoga Therapist, who has graduated from an IAYT accredited program or received the designation via one of IAYT's grand parenting avenues.

iḍā In *Yoga* subtle anatomy, one of the three main *nāḍīs* (channels of energy) running the length of the body and intersecting at the major *chakras,* or energy plexuses, distributed along the central axis. *Iḍā* is the energy channel of the left side, beginning at the base of the spine and terminating at the left nostril. Along with the *piṅgalā nāḍi* (right channel) and the *suṣumṇa nāḍi* (central channel), the *iḍā nāḍi* (left channel) represents the *chandra nāḍi,* the moon, comfort, introverted activities, mental processes, the Ganges River, the color white, femininity, the parasympathetic nervous system, and the left side of the spine/body.

Indra Devi Born as Eugenie V. Peterson and known as "The First Lady of Yoga," Indra Devi became the first female student of Professor Tirumalai Krishnamacharya after he was convinced to accept her as a student by the Maharāja of Mysore. She met every challenge her teacher, Krishnamacharya, set out for her and was so successful that he asked her to spread the teachings of Yoga all over the world, which she did in Argentina, Mexico, and the United States where her clients included Hollywood socialites, dignitaries, and thousands of people seeking to change their lifestyle and/or heal their injuries through the practices of Yoga.

Indra Mohan One of only a few people who received a postgraduate diploma in Yoga from Professor Krishnamacharya, Indra Mohan has been practicing and teaching yoga for more than three decades and is coauthor of *Yoga Therapy* with A. G. Mohan (her husband), Ganesh Mohan (her son), and Nitya Mohan (her daughter).

integrative medicine This system of medicine highlights the importance of a supportive and effective doctor-patient relationship and combines conventional Western medicine with alternative or complementary treatments and CAM approaches, such as herbal medicine, acupuncture, massage, chiropractic, biofeedback, naturopathy, Yoga Therapy, and stress reduction techniques to achieve optimal health and healing of the whole person in body, mind, and spirit (known in conventional medicine as a bio-psycho-social-spiritual approach).

integrative medicine specialist A doctor or therapist who specializes in integrative medicine and/or provides individualized treatment plans focused on the underlying cause of disease in the "whole person" by addressing his/her physical, emotional, mental, dietary, genetic, environmental, and lifestyle issues, as well as other risk factors and prevention-based health strategies.

Integrative Yoga Therapy (IYT) Founded by Joseph LePage, IYT's approach to Yoga Therapy is based on the model of the five koshas from the *Taittiriya Upanishad.* It is an experiential approach to learning and a complete healing program that allows students to integrate in-depth information through the creative process using a wide variety of Yoga tools that are grounded in a unique ten-step therapeutic process, which is successfully being used in a variety of healing environments, including hospitals and clinical settings.

International Association of Yoga Therapists (IAYT) Founded in 1989 by Larry Payne, Ph.D., and Richard Miller, Ph.D., the IAYT supports research and education in Yoga and serves as a professional organization for Yoga teachers and Yoga Therapists worldwide.

IAYT's mission is to establish Yoga as a recognized and respected therapy, a healing art, and a science for its approximately 3,400 members and 120 member schools spanning over 50 countries worldwide.

iRest Yoga Nidra Founded by Richard Miller, Ph.D., iRest Yoga Nidra is a modern-day secular rendition of Yoga nidra and a transformative practice derived from the nondual tantric (*tan* "to extend" and *tra* "to liberate") teachings of meditation. It supports psychological, physical, and spiritual healing and has been scientifically validated by the Surgeon General's Pain Management Task Force as a Tier-1 approach for pain management and the Defense Centers of Excellence as a complementary medicine for the treatment of PTSD. It has been used at military and veteran hospitals, homeless shelters, chemical dependency units, and in university settings and is comprised of a series of inquiries designed to extend one's understanding of and to liberate the mind's penchant to divide what's whole into separate parts. Ultimately, the iRest protocol is *integrative* as it supports the healing of unresolved physical and psychological issues and is *restorative* as it restores the body-mind to its inherent felt-sense of peace and equanimity that is present no matter our ever-changing circumstances.

īśvara praṇidhāna One of the five *niyamas* or observances listed in Patañjali's ***Yoga Sūtra,*** this is literally "placing the Lord in front" and keeps one's highest spiritual ideal in the foreground of one's attention. From a theistic perspective, it involves the practice of total devotion, surrender, and absolute love for one's chosen concept of God, Divinity, and/or Spirit, in form or within. From a nontheistic perspective, it involves one's devotion to a ***guru,*** saint, preceptor, or an alternative image or concept of a spiritually perfected being.

Iyengar Yoga Created and developed by Yoga master, B. K. S. Iyengar, Iyengar Yoga is a style of Haṭha Yoga and Yoga Therapy that focuses on reducing discomfort, keeping the body attentive, and settling the mind with an emphasis on detail, precision, and alignment in the practice and performance of āsanas (postures) and pranayama (breathing techniques). The style highlights six main features: alignment, breathing, timing, props, women's adaptations, and therapeutics. It is a scientifically-proven complementary treatment methodology for modulating the cardiac parasympathetic system, carpal tunnel syndrome, osteoarthritis, and a host of other ailments.

Iyengar/Kolar wall lean This exercise was originally designed by Yoga master, B. K. S. Iyengar, as a preparatory pose for headstands and was later developed as a thoracic spine mobilization exercise by famed Czechoslovakian physiotherapy specialist, Pavel Kolar, P.T., Ph.D., of the Prague Rehabilitation School. It is performed by sitting in a chair that is facing the wall and placing the elbows directly in front of the shoulders with the fingers interlaced. The chest is then dropped forward in the direction of the wall and the thoracic spine is mobilized in a posterior to anterior translation (from back to front) between the scapulas to improve cervical and thoracic range of motion and reduce intervertebral restrictions.

jala neti See *neti.*

jalāśaya mudrā Translated as the "peaceful lake," this hand gesture is for instilling relaxation and serenity of the mind, decreasing feelings of judgment and anger, and balancing the ***mano-maya-kośa***. It is performed by interlacing the first three fingers together while pointing and extending the ring and pinky fingers outward and pointing away from the abdomen.

Jing Literally translated as "essence," this is one of the "three treasures" that fuels and nourishes human beings along with Qi (energy) and Shen (spirit). It is the body's most dense physical matter and the material basis for the physical body. It is stored in the kidney region and is often referred to as the "kidney essence."

jing luo In Chinese Medicine, these are the subtle channels, or meridians, where Qi (energy) flows and is distributed and additionally are the main channels of communication in the body.

jivān sañjīvāni Living *sañjīvāni* or life-promoting. (see *sañjīvāni*)

jñāna Literally "knowing" or "becoming acquainted with," this is knowledge, especially higher knowledge, derived from scriptural study, self-study, and/or meditative experience.

jñāna mudrā See *gyan mudra*.

kaivalya The ultimate goal posited by the Sāṁkhya and Yoga *darśanas*, this is spiritual autonomy, isolation, aloneness, the absolute state, or that source of certain knowledge in wellness of being.

Kaivalyadhama Yoga Hospital Located in Lonavala, India, (also spelled Lonalva) and founded in 1930 by Swami Kuvalayananda, this was one of the first hospitals in the world dedicated to the study of Yoga Therapy and Western medicine. Still in existence today, the hospital's approach combines Yoga Therapy with naturopathic therapies and Ayurveda and has pioneered scientific research on Yoga and its evidence-based benefits for health.

Kaivalyadhama Yoga Institute Located in Lonavala, India, (also spelled Lonalva) and founded in 1924 by Swami Kuvalayananda, the institute is one of the foremost Yoga research institutes in the world and one of the oldest and most traditional schools offering Yoga in its original form. Kaivalyadhama's specific aim is to bring together traditional Yoga with modern science, as neither is thought to be complete without the other. A leader in the field of scientific research on Yoga, their work falls primarily in two quantitative directions: 1) creating, designing, and administering cutting-edge studies into the effects of Yoga practices, such as āsanas, kriyas, and pranayama, on diverse subjects like school children or police officers and 2) creating, designing, and administering studies into the benefits of Yoga on various afflictions, such as obesity, diabetes, stress, and blindness.

kāki mudrā Literally meaning "crow's gesture" and also classified as a form of *prāṇāyāma*, *kāki mūdra* is performed by rolling the tongue and placing it just behind the lips (like in sitali prāṇāyāma) in a U-shape to make it look like a "crow's beak." The inhalation breath is drawn or sipped in via a tube-like or straw-like opening where the lips are pursed like a crow's lips and it is cooling by nature, then the lips are retracted for the exhale, which is completed through the nose. It is said that this technique is helpful for people with high blood pressure, anger issues (by drawing attention inward toward the heart center), constipation, skin diseases, overheating, weakness in the facial muscles, and liver problems.

kāma One of the four *puruṣārthas* or basic human values, this consists of the sensual pleasures like desire, love, enjoyment, and sensuality.

kapālabhāti One of the six shat karmas (cleansing techniques) mentioned in the Haṭha Yoga Pradīpikā and literally meaning "skull shining," this is a joy-inducing diaphragmatic breathing technique that is performed with forceful exhalations followed by passive inhalations. Essentially, the lower belly near the umbilicus is quickly contracted or pumped as air is pushed out of the lungs and the passive release of the contraction allows the belly to rebound and suck air into the lungs. This technique has been shown to be effective in gastroparesis, sluggishness, head fogginess, depression, stress, and to cleanse the sinuses of the head.

kapha One of the three *doshas,* along with *pitta* and *vata,* kapha is located primarily in the chest, thorax, and upper stomach and represents the building block materials, or "glue" that holds the cells together, the energy that forms the body's structure (bones, muscles, and tendons), and is characterized as cool, moist, and stable. Made up elementally of earth and water, it receives nourishment through the elements of water and earth and is said to lubricate joints, moisturize the skin, maintain immunity, and heal irritation, inflammation, and ulceration by replacing them with scar tissue. In balance, kapha is expressed as love, calmness, and forgiveness. Out of balance, it leads to attachment, greed, mucus, phlegm, and envy.

Karma Yoga One of the four main paths to Yoga and classically promoted by Kṛṣṇa in the *Bhagavad Gītā,* this is the path of work, selfless service, giving without expecting results, consistent and impeccable behavior , and doing one's duty, ***dharma*** (duty, responsibility), remaining ever unattached to the fruits of one's actions. Called "The Yoga of Action," it typically includes practices like volunteering, serving others cheerfully and willingly, following the ***yamas*** (ethical restraints or moral codes) and *niyamas* (observances and self-purification methods), and as Mother Theresa said, performing "love in action."

khecarī mudrā Called the "most important mudra in all of Yoga" by Swami Lahiri Mahasaya, the "best of all mudras" by Swami Sivananda, and highly recommended in the *Haṭha Yoga Pradīpikā,* this gesture denoting "the bliss and expansion of consciousness" is performed by touching the tip of the tongue to the rear of the palate and placing it as far back as possible toward the nasal cavity without straining. It is said to quiet hunger, dispel disease, conquer death, and awaken the spiritual energies of the body by drawing the prana (energy) from the spine and chakras up toward the head, brain, and the Vaishvanara (Universal Spirit).

kledaka kapha One of the "subdoshas" of *kapha,* kledaka kapha governs the mucosal lining of the stomach and is intricately related to the digestive system, phlegm in the stomach, and excessive saliva. When it is balanced, it leads to steady, smooth, and stable digestion. When imbalanced, it can lead to nausea, constipation, and/or digestion becoming slow and sluggish.

kleśas* or *kleshas The five obstacles, afflictions, or obstructions of the mind outlined by Patanjali in Sutra II.3 of the ***Yoga Sūtra***. The five kleshas include *avidyā* (ignorance, mistaking the Real), *asmitā* (ego, self-importance, or self-involvement), *rāga* (attachment or passion), *dveśa* (aversion), *abhiniveśa* (fear of impermanence and death or the tenacity of mundane existence).

kośas* or *koshas Translated as "sheaths" or "casings," these are commonly referred to in Indian philosophy as the *pañca maya kosha* model, or the five bodies or coverings of the atman (self). They are also a reference to the phenomena of the material world as being composed of the five *mahābhūtas* or fundamental elements of earth, water, fire, wind, and space and come from the *Taittirīya Upaniṣad* where "the pure light of the transcendental Self" or one's spiritual soul essence is described as being covered or enveloped by five successive sheaths: *anna-maya-kośa* (the sheath composed of food), *prāṇāmāyāma-maya-kośa* (sheath composed of life force energy), *mano-maya-kośa* (sheath composed of mind), *vijñāna-maya-kośa* (sheath composed of awareness), and *ānanda-maya-kośa* (sheath composed of bliss). In modern health care, the *kosha* model of body integration extolls the value of understanding that, not only is physical regional interdependence important in optimizing health, so too are all of the other aspects of the human experience, including social, emotional, psychological, and spiritual influences.

Krishnamacharya The founder of the Yogashala at the Jaganmohan Palace in Mysore, India, and regarded as the "Father of Modern Yoga," Professor Tirumalai Krishnamacharya was a scholar, philosopher, grammarian, and guru who taught many of modern Yoga's master teachers, including B. K. S. Iyengar, K. Pattabhi Jois, Indra Devi, and T. K. V. Desikachar. Author of *Yoga Makaranda*, *Yogaasangalu*, *Yoga Rahasya*, and *Yogavalli*, he is largely responsible for Haṭha Yoga's revival and expansion to the West and for its evolution as a therapeutic practice that can be specifically adapted to an individual.

Krishnamacharya Written in 2010 by A. G. and Ganesh Mohan, this book is a personal tribute to Professor Tirumalai Krishnamacharya that draws on the Mohans' memories of the great guru, as well as Krishnamacharya's own diaries and recorded materials, to present a fascinating view of the master and his teachings.

Krishnamacharya Yoga Mandiram (KYM) Founded in Chennai, India, in 1976 by T. K. V. Desikachar, the son and student of Professor Tirumalai Krishnamacharya, KYM focuses on quality Yoga teachings that respect the needs, interests, abilities, and secular faiths of its students. It is largely considered as one of the premier Yoga centers in the world and is recognized as a Public Charitable Trust, by the Government of India.

kriyā Literally defined as "completed action," this refers to a practice or technique in Yoga intended to create a specific result. It may refer to: 1) the six shat karma kriyas, or cleansing practices, listed in the *Haṭha Yoga Pradīpikā;* 2) Kundalini Yoga sets, series, practices, and/or breathing exercises combining breath, āsana, *bandha*, *mudrā*, mantra, and dṛṣṭi that have a desired purpose to affect various nerves, glands, or organs; 3) spinal energy *prāṇāyāma* exercises from the system of *Kriyā Yoga* that teach Yoga practitioners to move energy through their *chakras* and spines around the six spinal centers of the medullary, cervical, dorsal, lumbar, sacral, and coccygeal plexuses; 4) A religious rite or ceremony, sacrifice; or, 5) A medical treatment or practice applying a remedy, cure.

Kriyā Yoga 1. In the *Yoga Sūtra,* the preliminary yogic practices of *tapas* (austerity), *svādhyāya* (personal study), and *īśvara-praṇidhāna* (spiritual devotion), which, together, also constitute three of the five *niyamas* or observances in Patañjali's *aṣṭāṅga-yoga.*

2. A system of Yoga revived in the modern era by the great Himalayan guru, Mahavatar Babaji, Kriyā Yoga promotes the practice of *kriyas,* or simple, psychological methods by which human blood can be decarbonated, recharged with oxygen, and transmuted into life current to rejuvenate the brain and spinal centers and prevent the decay of tissues. The Kriyā Yoga path is intended to rapidly accelerate spiritual development and God-communion and employs various practical methods for expanding awareness in contrast to the effort of radically stilling the mind through sitting practice alone. Kriyā Yoga utilizes the methods found in *haṭha* and *kuṇḍalinī yoga,* including *āsana* (physical postures), *prāṇāyāma* (breathing techniques), *bandha* and *mudrā* (energy locks and seals), along with visualization practices to rotate subtle energies through *nāḍis* and *chakras* (psychic passageways and energy centers).

kriyās See ***kriyā***.

Kṣurikā Upaniṣad* or *Kshurika-Upanishad Literally meaning, "to sit down near the knife," this ancient text refers to the sharp mind of wisdom informed by *yoga and* sketches out the yogic concept of subtle anatomy, referring to the 72,000 *nāḍis* of the body, with a special emphasis on the central and side channels of ***suṣumna, iḍā,*** and ***piṅgala***. This brief and minor *Upaniṣad* explores ways to cut through one's attachments to the material world and refers to the focus, the wisdom, and the freeing of tension and energy in the marma points that one creates through the practices of meditation and pranayama.

kubera mudrā Dedicated to Kubera, the god of wealth and regent of the north in Indian cosmology, this hand gesture is for self-confidence, courage, drawing money to oneself, wealth, self-esteem, and balancing the *mano-maya-kośa.* It is performed by touching the tips of the thumb, index finger, and middle finger together while the ring finger and little finger are drawn into the palm as if making a fist.

Kum Nye Translated as "massage of the subtle body," and similar to qigong from Taoist Yoga and Chinese Medicine, these Tibetan Yoga and medical body movement practices are slow, massage-like, semireligious, and healing in nature. They are used in Integrative Yoga Therapy to heal the *prāṇāmāyāma-maya-kośa* (energy body) and are an aspect of pranic healing designed to cultivate and channel healing energy to specific areas of the body.

kumbhakāsana Plank pose, retention pose, urn-like pose, or upper push-up position.

kuṇḍalinī śakti Literally defined as "circular or coiled energy," this is the indwelling dormant spiritual and corporeal energy that lies coiled up in the *mūladhāra cakra* at the base of the spine.

When it is "awakened" through the various practices of Yoga, it moves up the spine like a serpent toward the brain and the *sahasrāra cakra* (the thousand-petaled lotus of the mind), ultimately leading the Yoga practitioner to higher states of consciousness and realization.

Kundalini Yoga Introduced to the United States in 1968 by Yogi Bhajan, who founded the Happy, Healthy, Holy Organization (3HO), Kundalini Yoga is often referred to as the "Yoga of Awareness." A universal and sacred science of the mind and body that elevates the spirit, it is founded on the principles of Sikh Dharma as a householder path to Yoga that teaches practitioners how to live fully engaged in the world, yet detached from it. It is rooted in the practices of discipline, self-awareness, and self-dedication and combines various yogic technologies like kriyas, pranayama, mudras, mantras, bandhas, and āsanas to balance and improve the performance of the glandular, digestive, respiratory, cardiovascular, and nervous systems.

Kundalini Yoga Therapy (KYT) The process of empowering individuals toward improved health and well-being through the application of the philosophy and practice of Kundalini Yoga, KYT is an approach that teaches Yoga therapeutically to the unique individual who has the condition, rather than address the condition itself. It includes Yoga and meditation practices, yogic psychology, self-reflection, and yogic recommendations on lifestyle and diet and has been scientifically applied to individuals being treated for and/or recovering from all forms of cancer, chronic fatigue, fibromyalgia, stroke, heart disease, diabetes, arthritis, psychological conditions, such as depression and anxiety, and life transitions.

Leslie Kaminoff A Yoga educator inspired by the tradition of his teacher, T. K. V. Desikachar, and founder of the Breathing Project in New York City, Leslie Kaminoff is the coauthor of the bestselling book *Yoga Anatomy* with Amy Matthews and for over three decades has led workshops, trainings, and developed specialized education for many leading Yoga associations, schools, and training programs in America and throughout the world.

licensed marriage and family therapist Licensed relationship specialists trained to assess, diagnose, and treat individuals, couples, families, and groups to achieve more adequate, satisfying, and productive marriages, family dynamics, personal relationships, and social adjustments. Requirements for licensure include a related doctoral or two-year master's degree, passage of a comprehensive written and oral examination, and at least 3,000 hours of supervised experience.

licensed professional clinical counselor Licensed counseling specialists providing treatment for individuals, couples, and groups experiencing social, relationship, emotional, and/or vocational difficulties, as well as crisis intervention counseling. Requirements for licensure include a related doctoral or two year master's degree, passage of a comprehensive written and oral examination, and at least 3,000 hours of supervised experience.

life-song Vedantic in nature, this is the individual contribution that a person makes to the "sung tune" of life and life's *melodia,* which emerges, conjointly, from all beings as one melody.

life-threatening Fear or anxiety felt in a grave and possibly dangerous situation of potential illness, extreme harm, crisis, and/or threat to one's life.

mahābhūta The five "great elements," of Indian cosmology, which are *ākāśa* (space/ether), *vāyu* (wind/air), *agni* (fire), *apas* (water), and *pṛthivī* (earth). These appear formally as five *tattvas* or elementary principles in the Sāṁkhya metaphysical system.

Mahānirvāṇa One of the classical source texts addressing the practice of Yoga nidra along with the *Trika-Shāsana* (as found in the *Shiva Sutras*), the *Māṇḍūkya and Taittirīya Upaniṣads*, the *Tripura Rahasya*, the *Yogatārāvalī*, and Patañjali's ***Yoga Sūtra***. The *Mahānirvāṇa Tantra* was the first Indian tantric text translated into English (1913) and is a dialogue between Śiva and Pārvatī, filled with complex tantric *pujas* or ritual performances, visualizations, and *mantras*, complemented by teachings concerning the oneness of *brahman* and instructions on the means of achieving the self-realization that confers ultimate freedom.

Maharishi Mahesh Yogi Founder of the popular style of meditation known as TM, or Transcendental meditation, he is "the meditation teacher of The Beatles," whose fame helped introduce and popularize The Maharishi and Yoga culture in the West. Maharishi's ancient, mantra-based TM technique was the inspiration for research conducted by Dr. Herbert Benson at Harvard University in the 1970s that, for the first time in the Western world, scientifically proved that meditation could lower blood pressure, relax the heart and blood vessels, and initiate "the relaxation response," the neurophysiological antithesis of the fight-or-flight reaction.

mahāsamādhi Lit. "great absorption," this is the final liberation or final conscious exit from the body made by an accomplished ***yogin*** or an enlightened person at the time of physical death when the spirit leaves the body.

mahima A yogic *siddhi* or supranormal power obtained through the practice of Yoga, this is the ability to expand one's body to a great or infinitely large size.

majjas In Ayurvedic medicine, this is one of the seven *dhātus* (fundamental tissues of the body) consisting of nerve, bone marrow, and connective tissue.

makarāsana Crocodile pose.

māṁsa In Ayurvedic medicine, this is one of the seven *dhātus* (fundamental tissues of the body) consisting of muscle, flesh, and meat.

maṇḍala Translated as circular, round, disk, sun, moon, or a halo around them, this is a spiritual and ritualistic symbol representing beauty, balance, dedication, and the Universe in both Hindu and Buddhist culture. Typically, mandalas are drawn featuring a square with four gates containing a circle with a center point. In Yoga Therapy, the concept is used metaphorically to symbolize the entry points for care that a therapist may choose while working with a patient. In Vajrayāna Buddhism, this is a complex psycho-cosmic diagram used in visualization practices and seen as a symbolic residence of the meditation deity (Tib. *yidam* or "mind bond") and as a symbolic outline of the spiritual worldview and the path of attainment.

Māṇḍūkya and Taittirīya Upaniṣads Two of the classical source texts addressing the practice of Yoga nidra along with the *Trika-Shāsana* (as found in the *Shiva Sutras*), the *Mahānirvāṇa*, the *Tripura Rahasya*, the *Yogatārāvalī*, and Patañjali's *Yoga Sūtra.*

mano-maya-kośa According to the *Taittirīya Upaniṣad,* this is the "sheath made of mind" or, one of the intermediate shells covering the *ātman* or individual self. *Manas* here means the thinking or instrumental mind, as distinguished from the faculty of discrimination (*vijñāna*), upon which it depends.

mantra 1. Mental instrument or device.

2. Prayer, sacred words, or a song of praise, esp. those found in the Vedas.

3. A sacred verbal formula or chant addrssed to an individual deity.

4. A mystical verse or magical formula, incantation, charm, or spell.

5. A yogic science based on the knowledge that sound is a form of energy having structure, power, and a definite predictable effect on the body, the chakras, and the human psyche.

mantra japa Literally meaning "to repeat internally," this is a spiritual practice from Bhakti Yoga, the path of devotion, which is often performed on a japa mala (string of beads) and involves the meditative repetition or whispering of mantras, sacred syllables, a devotional prayer, and/or affirmations that invoke the name of a divine power, energy, or guru.

mārga A concept from Svastha Yoga Therapy, this is one's "path, route, way, method, or passage" through life that helps a Yoga Therapist decide whether a practice is appropriate for a particular individual. The other two aspects that factor into the decision of what is appropriate include the individual's deha (body, shape, appearance, mass) and vrttibheda (differences in mental modifications).

marīcyāsana Spinal twist pose named for Marīci, one of the Seven Sages.

mārjāryāsana Cat pose.

master of arts degree A two to three year postgraduate degree in English, history, geography, communications, Chinese Medicine, or any of the humanities like philosophy, social sciences, fine arts, and/or theology.

master's degree in holistic health education An interdisciplinary two to three year master's degree that integrates Eastern and Western approaches to health including the philosophy of the interconnectedness of all nature and principles, strategies, and concepts related to treating the whole person and optimizing one's quality of life through mind-body-spirit integration.

Matra Majmundar An occupational therapist, perinatal educator, Yoga Therapist, and consultant at Stanford University's Rehabilitation Stroke Research Centre, Matra Majmundar trained at the internationally renowned Kaivalyadhama Yoga Institute and has worked as a stroke research therapist at the R&D department of Veteran Hospital in Palo Alto, CA.

matyāsana Fish pose.

Mawangdui Currently considered "the most important collection of ancient [Chinese] texts, medical or otherwise," these were discovered in 1973 and include illustrations of the Chinese Medicine practices of Daoyin (Guiding [the Qi] and Stretching [the muscles and joints]). The texts cover "therapeutic exercises comparable to the exercises practiced by Taoists of later times," illustrating that the author, Hua Tuo, likely described physical health practices that were "extant before his time."

mayurāsana Peacock pose.

McKenzie extension exercises Rehabilitation exercises developed by world renowned physical therapist and spinal specialist, Robin McKenzie, C.N.Z.M., O.B.E., F.C.S.P. (Hon), F.N.Z.S.P. (Hon), founder of The McKenzie Method of Mechanical Diagnostics and Therapy. The exercises are Yoga-like movements that focus on the extension of the spine and include, but are not limited to, bhujangāsana (cobra pose), belly sphinxes, standing back bends, gluteal bridges, and salabāsana (locust pose) variations, which decrease the pressure on the discs and nerves when properly and appropriately applied.

meda In Ayurvedic medicine, this is one of the seven *dhātus* (fundamental tissues of the body) consisting of fat and adipose tissue. *Medā*, as the root of *Asparagus racemosus, is* an ingredient sometimes used in Ayurvedic medicinal preparations.

medical director A doctor or physician who provides leadership, guidance, oversight, and quality assurance to a group of doctors or physicians, a medical or healthcare practice, and/or a hospital.

Meetings of Schools at SYTAR An annual meeting held at the Symposium on Yoga Therapy and Research where member schools of the International Association of Yoga Therapists have the opportunity to review, discuss, and collaborate on the issues and challenges facing the field of Yoga Therapy.

Menninger Institute Originally founded in 1925 in Topeka, Kansas, this is one of the leading in-patient psychiatric hospitals in the United States and it was the site of pivotal Yoga research involving Swami Rama in the 1970s. Their work has assisted in the development of innovative approaches for treating mentally ill patients, training psychiatrists, and helping veterans hospitals and law enforcement agencies incorporate information about mental illness into their staff training.

Michael Lerner, Ph.D. A student of the late Indian guru, Swami Satchidananda, Dr. Lerner is the author of *Choices in Healing: Integrating the Best of Conventional and Complementary Approaches to Cancer* and founder of Commonweal Cancer Treatment Center in Northern California.

micro-skills The finer, more advanced points and details of a particular skill or technique that one learns through repetitive practice.

Mīmāṁsa (Pūrvamīmāṁsa) One of the six darshans, or systems of Indian Vedic philosophy, this is a philosophy that teaches that truth is not accessible to reason and observation and that the nature of dharma must be inferred from the supreme authority of the revelations in the Vedas, which are considered "eternal, authorless, and infallible."

mind-body An experiential science that studies the connection between our thoughts, perceptions, behaviors, and insights and how we feel, understand, and experience ourselves physically, energetically, emotionally, and spiritually.

mind-body medicine A system of medicine that focuses on the interactions between the brain, the body, the mind, and one's behavior and the ways in which emotional, mental, social, spiritual, experiential, and behavioral factors can directly affect health.

mind-body therapy A mind-body medicine approach that uses one's mental capacity to affect bodily function and symptoms. It typically includes practices like Yoga and Yoga Therapy, Reiki, meditation, aromatherapy, mindful eating, hypnosis, prayer, tai chi/qigong, and other alternative therapies that incorporate the senses, the mind, and/or the body into an appropriate treatment methodology.

Mira Alfassa (The Mother) A French-born woman, artist, and spiritual teacher known to her followers as "The Mother" or "The Mother" of Śrī Aurobindo ashram, she was a spiritual collaborator and student of the great Indian guru, Śrī Aurobindo. Her writings, prayers, reflections, essays, sayings, letters, and personal notes were all well-preserved and are featured in the 17-volume text, *Collective Works of the Mother.*

mokṣa* or *moksha One of the four *puruṣārthas* or basic human values, this is freedom, liberation, self-liberation, or the ultimate spiritual release.

Morris-Payne Standard Evaluation A methodology for beginning Yoga Therapists to measure and document the body, breath, and mind of their clients, tools for this evaluation consist of an instructional DVD, color manual, goniometer, The Dartmouth Coop quality of life test, and the use of sound for breath measurement.

Morris-Payne Yoga Therapy Exam See Morris-Payne Standard Evaluation.

MTHFR The abbreviation for an enzyme known as methylenetetrahydrofolate reductase (NAD(P)H) that plays a role in processing amino acids, building proteins, and activating folic acid, which itself has many uses like serotonin production, detoxification, creating red and white blood cells, and making DNA. It is tested in preventive medicine when a person has elevated homocysteine levels, which may indicate an increased risk of developing premature cardiovascular disease (CVD) and/or thrombosis, and for those prone to depression, immune dysfunction, and low energy.

mudrās Literally defined as "seal" or "gesture," these are symbolic, energetic, meditative, expressive, ritualistic, and/or healing positions made with the body or any of its parts in the Hindu and Buddhist traditions, yet most commonly appearing as gestures, movements, or postures of the hands and fingers in Yoga and Yoga Therapy. They are often used therapeutically and psycho-energetically in conjunction with *prāṇāyāma* (breathing techniques), *āsana* (postures), and meditation to stimulate different parts of the brain, body, prana (energy), and/or character of an individual.

mūla bandha Translated as "the root lock," this is an energetic and psycho-physical practice in Haṭha Yoga that involves engaging, closing, and locking the perenium muscle and the floor of the pelvis to influence the flow of prana (energy). It creates an internal compression and upward pull from the pelvic floor to draw *apāna* upward into the central energy channel, *suṣumna,* and to awaken the dormant *kuṇḍalinī* energy at the root *chakra* of the body. This is one of the three main *bandhas,* along with *uddīyāna bandha* (the abdominal or belly lock) and *jalandhāra bandha* (the neck lock), that together make up *maha bandha* (the great lock) when all three are engaged together.

mūladhāra cakra Lit. the "Root Support," this is one of the seven primary chakras in traditional Yoga systems and the root chakra at the base of the pelvis near the coccygeal plexus, which is commonly associated with the color red, the seed mantra syllable "lam," and the element of Earth.

nāḍī* or *nāḍīs An aspect of the physical, subtle, and/or energetic bodies in the *pranamaya knosha,* these are energy pathways or conduits of energy in Yoga that are similar to meridians or channels of energy in Chinese Medicine. There are said to be over 72,000 *nāḍīs* in each person and three main nāḍīs: *iḍā* nāḍī (left channel), *piṅgalā nāḍī* (right channel) and ***suṣumṇa*** *nāḍī* (central channel), which lie in a criss-crossing pattern along and parallel to the spine. These *nāḍīs* are not necessarily identifiable as gross physical structures but can refer to any vein or artery in the body.

nāḍī-śodhana* or *nāḍī shodhana See nāḍī shodhana pranayama.

nāḍī-śodhana-prāṇāyāma Literally defined as "nerve cleansing," "channel purification," or "channel clearing breathing" and commonly referred to as "alternate nostril breathing," this is a pranayama technique that is said "to balance the sun and moon" and restore, equalize, and balance the flow of prana (energy) in the body and *the iḍā* and *piṅgalā nāḍī,* which begin at the *mūladhāra chakra* and terminate at the left and right nostrils, respectively. It involves inhaling through one nostril and exhaling through the other nostril with the breath being natural and effortless. While the *Gheranda Samhita* says that traditionally nāḍī shodhana includes breath retention, fixed ratio breathing, and the repetition of *bīja* (seed) mantras, beginners usually skip the *kumbhaka* (breath retention) and the fixed ratios to help make the technique more accessible and further calm the nerves, decrease anxiety and stress, and harmonize the mind. Eventually, in the advanced technique, breath retentions and fixed ratios are added back in like in *samavṛtti* (equal breathing) *nāḍī-śodhana-prāṇāyāma* at a classical 1:1:1:1 inhale to retention to exhale to retention ratio.

namas (namaḥ, namo) Lit. "a bend or bow," this is a gesture of honor, respect, or homage. Often found in devotional *mantras* and forming part of the customary Indian greeting *namaste* (bow to you).

nasya One of the five classic purification methods of *pañca karma* and an Ayurvedic parallel to the therapeutic practice of *neti,* which cleanses the nasal passageway, this is a dosha cleansing exercise for the air channel that is said to clear and lubricate the sinus passageways, strengthen the mind and concentration, and relieve acute and chronic sinus problems such as allergies, mucous congestion, dry nasal passage, and snoring. It is performed with a person lying on his/her back with a pillow under the scapula whereby five drops of sesame oil, ghee, vacha medicated oil, or any other medicated ghee is put into each nostril, which passes through the nose, sinuses, and pharynx. After lying down for a minute or two and the nasal passageway is cleansed, the person sits up and has the upper back and neck gently massaged.

naṭarājāsana Dancer's pose, Lord of the dance pose, or king dancer pose.

National Center for Complementary and Alternative Medicine (NCCAM) A division of the National Institutes of Health (NIH), this a United States government agency that investigates complementary and alternative medicine (CAM) healing practices in the context of scientific and clinical methodology. Its four areas of focus include research, research training and career development, outreach, and integration.

National Institutes of Health (NIH) One of the world's foremost medical research centers and a division of the United States Department of Health and Human Services, this is the primary government agency responsible for biomedical and health-related research. It funds intramural, in-house research and extramural, non-NIH research grants in the fields of clinical research, genetics-related research, prevention research, cancer research, and biotechnological research, and also disseminates authoritative information on health-related topics to the public and healthcare professionals.

naturopathic doctor A doctor who specializes in natural therapies and assists patients in creating an internal and external healing environment that facilitates the body's inherent ability to identify, restore, maintain, and remove barriers to optimal health.

naturopathic medicine An alternative holistic medical system that provides a framework for approaching the treatment of illness, proactive prevention, and the promotion of health in a comprehensive, diagnostic, and natural way. Naturopathic medicine serves as an umbrella for a full spectrum of natural therapies including dietary nutrition and nutritional supplements, intravenous (IV) nutrients, lifestyle counseling, botanical medicine, homeopathy, hydrotherapy, naturopathic manipulation therapy (musculoskeletal bodywork techniques), and therapeutic exercise for the optimal healing of each individual.

naturopathy Literally, the "nature of disease," this alternative holistic system of medicine teaches that optimal health is achieved and illness is best remedied by identifying and treating the underlying causes of disease and by strengthening the inherent homeostatic mechanisms of the body using naturopathic medicine and natural therapies.

nauli One of the six shat karmas (cleansing techniques) mentioned in the *Haṭha Yoga Pradīpikā*, this practice is performed by contracting the rectus abdominus on an exhale breath while leaning forward with the knees slightly bent in an upright position. The hands are placed on each thigh for support, and after a full exhalation, the abdomen is drawn in and contracted so that a center, vertical pillar of abdominal muscle is formed. Pressing back and forth—left to right and right to left—causes a circular "churning" of the whole gastrointestinal (GI) tract, improves digestion of food, decreases constipation, awakens kundalini shakti, and performs cleansing of the subdoshas of kledaka kapha, samana vayu, pachaka pitta, and apana vayu.

Nei-Jing See *Huang-di Nei-Jing*.

neti One of the six *ṣaṭkarma* (cleansing techniques) mentioned in the *Haṭha Yoga Pradīpikā*, this practice involves cleansing of the nasal passage as well as the throat. It can be done with *jala neti* (water neti) or with *sutra neti* (a big wick, thread, or string dipped into salty water) and is a practice used by many traditions for colds and coughs, sinusitis, tonsillitis, adenoid inflammation, and eye, nose, and throat problems. *Jala neti* is performed using sterilized and lukewarm saltwater, which is poured into one nostril, so that it leaves through the other nostril, and the procedure is then repeated on the other side. *Sutra neti* is performed by putting the wick, thread, or string in one nostril, moving it back and down to the throat, then swallowing it into the mouth. Once in the mouth, the wick, thread, or string is grasped with the fingers and brought out of the mouth. Then, the cleansing commences by drawing the thread back and forth, pulling it forward through the nose and then downward through the mouth as if the nasal passage is being flossed. This is a quite powerful cleansing process and can be intense. This kind of *neti* usually requires guidance from a teacher.

netra basti One of the five classic purification methods of *pañca karma* and an Ayurvedic parallel to the therapeutic practice of *trāṭaka,* which cleanses and strengthens the eyes, this is a cleansing practice that benefits alochaka pitta, improves vision, and decreases straining and tension in the eye muscles. It is performed by placing a whole-wheat doughnut of wheat flour and water around the orbit of the eye and sealing it with a little water on the inside and outside of the dough. This creates a little pool around the eye. Lukewarm ghee in liquid form is then poured into this pool over the eye. With the ghee covering the eye, it is opened and closed repeatedly until tears occur in the other eye just like in the practice of *trāṭaka.*

neuroscience The scientific study of the brain and nervous system.

nirodha Literally defined as "restraint, stopping, arresting, inhibition, cessation." In Yoga, this is the arresting of the movements of the mind through meditation practice. In Buddhism, this is the elimination of suffering through bringing the mechanism of desire and craving to a halt.

nirvāṇa A term often used in Buddhism, Hinduism, Jainism, and Sikhism, and known in Yoga as samadhi (total absorption), this is the complete release of suffering, desire, and delusion, which leads one to spiritual peace and enlightenment. In a practical, microcosmic, and more worldly application in Yoga Therapy and sports science, this is a steady stillness of the mind, a meditative ability, and/or an internal yogic trance state known as "The Zone" that athletes can train, reinforce, and self-initiate when they work out, when they practice Yoga, when they study, when they are running, when they are jumping and throwing, when they prepare for competition, and when they are on the field of play actually competing.

Nitya Mohan An expert in Vedic chanting with a degree in music, Nitya Mohan is coauthor of *Yoga Therapy* with A. G. Mohan (her father), Indra Mohan (her mother), and Ganesh Mohan (her brother).

niyamas Classically listed as the second component or limb of Patañjali's *rāja* or *aṣṭāṅga-yoga*, these are social adherences, self-purification methods, observances, or qualities to nourish that lead an individual to a healthier, more *sattvic* lifestyle and include *tapas* (austerity), *svādhyāya* (personal or self-study), *īśvara-praṇidhāna* (devotion), *saucha* (purity), and *saṁtoṣa* (contentment).

Nyāya One of the six *darśanas*, or systems of Indian Vedic philosophy and often paired with *Vaiśeṣika*, this is a philosophy that uses analytic and syllogistic logic and the Vedas to prove existence of God, and that epistemologically validates the sources of knowledge so one can obtain release from suffering. The four sources of knowledge in this philosophy include perception, inference, comparison, and testimony.

Ohm Test A Yoga Therapy outcome measure and part of the Morris-Payne Standard Evaluation, this is a simple yogic tool and exercise to measure lung capacity changes before and after a series of treatments. The test is performed by instructing the Yoga practitioner to take in as deep a breath as possible and make the longest, continuous sound possible, vocalizing *Aum, Ah, Ma,* or *Sa* during the exhalation. A pitch tool can be used (when available) to replicate and standardize the exact level of sound and the best time of three attempts is recorded with a watch.

ojas Literally translated as "vigor" and primarily located in the region of the heart, this is a refined form of *kapha dosha,* which is said to be the "purest substance in the universe" or the "subtle essence" and is the ultimate end result of digestion, metabolism, absorption, and assimilation. When it is in balance, it provides a healthy foundation for the immune system and vitality, contains nurturing and nourishing qualities like breast milk and the placenta, and contributes to higher states of consciousness, purity of thought, optimal health, positive feelings, creativity, and bliss. When it is deficient, it results in weakness, fatigue, and disease.

oṁ The *ādi mantra* and most celebrated *bīja mantra* or seed syllable of Indic religious culture. Frequently intoned at the beginning of a *mantra,* prayer, or religious text, *oṁ* is highly praised in many of the *Upaniṣads* and is succinctly analyzed as the essence of all existence in the *Māṇḍūkya Upaniṣad.*

oṁ māṇi padme hūṁ Lit. "oṁ, the jewel in the lotus, hūṁ," this is a popular *mantra* of Mahāyāna Buddhism and is especially ubiquitous in Tibetan Buddhism as the *mantra* of Avalokiteśvara, the Bodhisattva or Compassion.

oncology and elder services departments A special department in a hospital or medical center dedicated to cancer treatment, research, and/or care for older individuals.

One Minute Breath A breath-based meditation technique from Kundalini Yoga Therapy and Kriya Yoga, this technique is a three-part breath consisting of a 20-20-20 (or 1-1-1) inhale to retention to exhalation ratio. It is performed by inhaling to the count of 20 or by repeating the mantra *Sa Ta Na Ma* five times at a pace of one second per syllable, retaining the breath for a count of 20, and finally, slowly exhaling to a count of 20, which makes the total time for each cycle of breath one minute. Often, beginners are advised to begin the technique by counting to 5-5-5 or 10-10-10 and progressing up to 20-20-20 as their body's ability to stay relaxed and take in deeper, more balanced breaths without straining improves. The technique calms anxiety and fear, develops intuition and concentration, and optimizes coordination between the two hemispheres of the brain.

Ong The sound representing the infinite within the finite or the creator within creation.

Oriental medicine See Chinese medicine.

pacaka pitta or pachaka pitta One of the "subdoshas" of *pitta,* pachaka pitta is the first seat of pitta in the body located in the small intestine and stomach. It governs the biological heat of digestion and is often referred to as the "digestive fire." When unbalanced, it leads to foul smelling breath and stool, acid indigestion, and ulcers.

padmāsana Lotus pose.

pain-free The condition of being without pain or discomfort during an exercise, Yoga practice, treatment, and/or life experience.

pañca karma The chief purification and detoxification method in Ayurvedic medicine, this system teaches that the doshas are "at home" in the gastrointestinal (GI) tract and, because of changes in the season, changes in diet, changes in emotions, and changes in the internal and external environment, the doshas move out of the GI tract and into the tissues of the body where they are *not* at home and cause pathological changes and disease. The "five actions" or "five purification practices" of pañca karma are designed to help the doshas flow back to the GI tract to restore health and include *vamana* (therapeutic vomiting), *virechana* (purgation), *nasya* (nasal cleansing), *niroha/basti* (enema), and *anuvāsana/snehana* (oleation massage).

pañca maya or pancha maya See *kośa.*

pañca vāyu Literally translated as the five "winds," energy channels, or movements of energy, these are the vital forces or channels of energy that describe the movement, location, and/or flow of prāṇa (life force energy) in the body. The five vayus include : *prāṇa vāyu* (vitalizing breath, centered in the chest), *apāna vāyu* (the downward-voiding wind, centered in the organs of elimination and reproduction), *udāna vāyu* (upward-moving wind, centered in the throat, face, and extremities), *samāna vāyu* (digestive energy, centered in the abdomen), and *vyāna vāyu* (circulation throughout the entire body of energy and nutrients derived from breath and food).

Paramahansa Yogananda Founder of Self-Realization Fellowship and one of the main proponents of modern Kriyā Yoga, Paramahansa Yogananda was an Indian guru, who introduced millions of practitioners and teachers to Kriyā Yoga, Indian spirituality, and Eastern mysticism through his book, *Autobiography of a Yogi.*

parāvṛtta-trikoṇāsana Revolved triangle pose.

Parliament of World Religions An organization created to cultivate harmony among the world's religious and spiritual communities and to bring about a more just, peaceful, and sustainable world, the Parliament of World Religions was the forum where Swami Vivekananda introduced Yoga to the Western world in 1893.

pārśva-bakāsana Side crow pose or side crane pose.

paścimottanāsana Seated back stretch pose or seated forward bend pose.

past president Not the current, but the former, president, leader, or head of a corporation, professional organization, club, or group of people.

Patañjali 1. The legendary author of the *Yoga Sūtra,* about whom very little is known with any real certainty. The dating of his career is subject to considerable debate, although numerous contemporary scholars place the writing of the *Yoga Sūtra* circa second or third century CE.

2. Another Patañjali, circa second century BCE, is credited with authorship of the *Mahābhāṣya,* an advanced treatise on Sanskrit grammar and linguistics.

3. Yet another Patañjali, whose dates are not well documented, is credited with authoring redactions of the *Caraka Saṁhitā* and the *Suśruta Saṁhitā,* two of the earliest medical treatises of the Ayurveda tradition, although neither of these redacted versions is extant today.

Patañjali's *Yoga Sūtra* The foundational text for classical Yoga, *aṣṭāṅga yoga,* Rāja Yoga, and the *darśana* of Yoga, this compilation was written down by the great sage, Patanjali, around 200–400 B.C.E, and contains 195 *sūtra* or "aphorisms," which describe the evolution of the yogic path. It is divided into 4 *padās* or chapters, where each chapter consists of a different aspect of the Yoga practice, including but not limited to the traditional eight limbs of Yoga and Kriyā Yoga (the Yoga of action).

Patient-Specific Functional Scale (PSFS) A questionnaire used in rehabilitative medicine and Yoga Therapy to quantify activity limitations with daily activities, grade disabilities, and measure functional outcomes for patients with orthopedic conditions.

Pattabhi Jois Officially, Śrī K. Pattabhi Jois and commonly referred to as "Guruji," he was a direct student of Professor Tirumalai Krishnamacharya and the founder of the modern style of Haṭha Yoga known as Ashtanga Vinyasa Yoga as well as the founder of the Ashtanga Yoga Research Institute in Mysore, India.

pauri kriyā A *prāṇāyāma*-based meditation technique from Kundalini Yoga combining controlled breathing, syllable visualization and recitation, and coordinated finger movements that has been clinically proven to benefit self-efficacy beliefs and the therapeutic application of meditation. To perform the technique, inhale and divide the breath into eight equal, separate parts, like sniffs, while sitting comfortably with the eyes closed. On the first segment of the eight parts, silently repeat the sound of *Sa* and press the tips of the index finger and thumb firmly together, on the second *Ta* press the middle finger and thumb tips, on the third *Na* press the ring finger and thumb tips, and on the fourth *Ma* press the little finger and thumb tips together. Silently repeat *Sa* on the fifth, *Ta* on the sixth, *Na* on the seventh, and *Ma* on the eighth part of the eight-part inhalation with the finger positions for the fifth through eighth parts of the breath coordinating to the sounds listed above. To exhale the breath, recite aloud, *Sa Ta Na Ma, Sa Ta Na Ma,* in a monotone. Coordinate the pressing of the thumb tips to the fingers with the corresponding sounds, just as was done during the silent eight-part inhalation. If the mind wanders, simply return the attention to the breath, sound, and finger sequence of the meditation.

pedorthist A professional who has specialized training in the art of designing, making, and/or use of corrective footwear, foot orthotics, pedorthic devices, and the assessment of lower limb anatomy and biomechanics.

phenotype A person's observable physical traits and characteristics, how he/she appears to the world, and what is expressed in his/her body and mind.

Phoenix Rising Yoga Therapy Founded by Michael Lee, this is a reflective and experiential approach to Yoga Therapy that supports people in their quest for greater authenticity and wholeness by providing the opportunity to unfold in accordance with one's "true nature." It is a healing technique designed for the myriad of "lifestyle disorders" and psychoemotional issues and is composed of meditations, process-based practices that facilitate presence, and focused relaxed awareness on the breath, the body in āsana (posture) held at a point of therapeutic tolerable discomfort, the subsequent layers of emotions that arise, and the thoughts sparked by the experience.

Phoenix Rising Yoga Therapy Training Program A Yoga Therapy training program combining ancient yogic wisdom with cutting edge techniques from contemporary psychological dialogue that guides a client safely and with awareness to the edge of deep physical sensations where the body and mind not only meet but engage each other. Trainees are taught ways to assist clients in listening to their body's wisdom and are guided to listen to clients without judgment to help them experience the empowerment they need to let go of the "need to change" feeling, which opens up the space for deep acceptance and the release of underlying charged emotions or beliefs that have often manifested into chronic aches and pains.

piṅgalā In *Yoga* subtle anatomy, one of the three main *nāḍīs* (channels of energy) running the length of the body and intersecting at the major *chakras*, or energy plexuses, distributed along the central axis. *Piṅgalā* is the energy channel of the right side, beginning at the base of the spine and terminating at the right nostril. Along with the *iḍā nāḍī* (left channel) and the *suṣumṇa nāḍī* (central channel), the *piṅgalā nāḍī* (right channel) represents the *sūrya nāḍi, the* solar channel, the sun, activity, extroverted activities, vital processes, the Yamuna River, the sympathetic nervous system, masculinity, and the right side of the spine/body.

pitta One of the three *doṣas*, along with *kapha* and *vāta*, *pitta* is located primarily in the chest, thorax, and upper stomach and represents the heat and energy of digestion, absorption, assimilation, nutrition, metabolism, body temperature, and the transformation of food into ahar rasa (digested food). It is characterized as hot, sharp, penetrating, volatile, and oily and is associated with the metabolic functions of the body. Made up elementally of fire and water, it is responsible for color and complexion of the skin, luster of the eyes, and absorption of sensory information into cognitive knowledge. In balance, *pitta* promotes understanding and intelligence. Out of balance, *pitta* arouses anger, bile, hatred, and jealousy.

Polarity Therapy This is an alternative health therapy that works with the human energy field and involves energy-based bodywork, exercise, verbal and psychological coaching, dietary modification, and self-awareness techniques. It focuses on experiencing health through the easeful flow of energy in the human body and assisting energy to return to its natural state of balance by removing energy that is blocked or fixed due to stress, pain, disease, and/or other lifestyle factors.

Positive and Negative Syndrome Scale (PANSS) An outcome measure used in the mental health fields that is designed to assess and track the severity of symptoms in patients with schizophrenia.

postgraduate A program, degree, or certification of advanced study that is typically completed after a traditional four year bachelor's degree, a master's degree, and/or a professional degree.

Postnatal Essence Known in Chinese Medicine as *hou-tian-zhi-jing*, this is one of the two main sources of Jing, which is responsible for growth, development, reproduction and helps distinguish organic life from inorganic material. This type of essence is derived from the refined parts of "ingested food and continuous exercise, emotional, and mental stimulation from a person's environment."

Power Yoga Founded by Beryl Bender Birch and Bryan Kest independently of one another, this is a flowing, vigorous, and fitness-like style of Haṭha Yoga derived from Ashtanga Vinyasa Yoga that employs physically challenging ***āsanas*** (postures), breath-oriented *vinyāsa* movements, and the use of *ujjāyi* prāṇāyāma.

prabhāva Might, power, majesty, dignity, strength, splendor, beauty. In Ayurveda, the specific effects or actions of a medicinal compound or substance above and beyond the properties of the individual components.

prakopa 1. Effervescence, excitement, provocation.

2. In Ayurveda, aggravation or inflamation—the second phase of the disease process. (see *saṁcaya*)

prakṛti 1. Cause, original source, or substance; nature, character, or constitution.

2. In Sāṁkhya philosophy, "the seen," nature, or the material world, as distinguished from *puruṣa* or spirit, and consisting of three constituent qualities or *guṇas*: *sattva*, *rājas*, and *tamas.*

3. In Ayurveda, an individual's basic or original psycho-physical constitution, resulting from karmic influences from prior lives, perinatal conditions, etc. Seven types are recognized and are labeled on the basis of *doṣa* dominance: *vāta*, *pitta*, *kapha*, *vāta-pitta*, *vāta-kapha*, *pitta-kapha*, and, more rarely, an evenly balanced *vāta-pitta-kapha.*

prakṛuti See *prakṛti.*

prāṇa Defined as "life force energy" since the time of the Vedas, this is the principle creative energy that is responsible for the body's life, maintenance, vigor, vitality, power, energy, breath, respiration, and health. At its essence, it is the energy that manifests and flows through nature, creation, and all things throughout the universe. In Sāṁkhya philosophy, it is *puruṣa* (spirit) and in Ayurveda it is one or all of five vital energies of the body. (see *pañca vāyu*)

prāṇa-apāṇa The two main energy channels or currents in the body, prāṇa represents the upward and inward flow of energy, expansion, and the inhalation breath while apāṇa represents the downward and outward flow of energy, contraction, and the exhalation breath. Together, like positive charges and negative charges, both forces are thought to be needed in Yoga to create balance and harmony in a well-coordinated energy system. (see *pañca vāyu*)

prāṇa-kośa See *prāṇa-maya-kośa.*

prāṇa-maya-kośa According to the *Taittirīya Upaniṣad,* this is the "sheath made of breath and life force" or an intermediate shell covering the *ātman* (individual self) and supporting the *anna-maya-koṣa* or "sheath made of food."

prāṇa-vaha-srota This is the air channel in Ayurvedic Medicine and Yoga Therapy that is responsible for taking *prāṇa* (energy) into the body. It governs the respiratory and circulatory systems and is in charge of charge of oxygen and blood flow, gas exchange, kindling the digestive fire, and maintaining body temperature.

prāṇa-vāyu One of the five vāyus (winds or energy currents, qualities, and channels) in Yoga and originating in the diaphragm, heart, and throat, prāṇa vāyu governs the inward and upward flow of energy and the inhalation breath. It balances the anahata chakra, governs sensory perceptions and mental experiences, nourishes the vital organs, and is the driving force for all the other vāyus. (see *pañca vāyu*)

prāṇāyāma Classically listed as the fourth component or limb of Patañjali's ***rāja*** or ***aṣṭāṅga-yoga,*** these are a variety of breathing practices found in Yoga that lead an individual to mastery over breath and life force, and ultimately to render the breath long and subtle, as an aid to achieving deep meditative states and a healthier, more *sattvic* lifestyle. Commonly translated as "extension of breath," "energy expansion," or "energy control," the techniques as a collective group are considered the "ultimate medicine" within the field of Yoga Therapy and have a wide range of clinically-proven psychophysical benefits including decreased stress, increased vitality, mental calmness, concentrative acuity, improved energetic flow, emotional balance, organ cleansing, and, as a goal, the experience of *samādhi* (absorption). In the later ***Haṭha Yoga*** traditions, intensive *prāṇāyāma* practices are employed to help arouse and amplify latent *kuṇḍalinī* energies.

***prāṇi* or pranee** Lit. breathing, living, alive. In Yoga, this is the actual person, human being, living creature, animal, or sentient being who moves prāṇa (life force energy) through his/her physical and energetic body and awakens the cells with life by bringing energy into action.

prasāra Spreading or stretching out, extension; opening the mouth.

pratipakṣa bhāvana Literally meaning "moving to the other side of being," this concept is found in Chapter 2 of Patañjali's *Yoga Sūtra* and is a replacement therapy technique, which cultivates the opposite thought that one is suffering from and/or acts as if a new, more harmonizing thought is already being experienced and expressed. For example, replacing feelings of anger, violence, stress, and hate with feelings of compassion, peacefulness, relaxation, and love.

pratipakṣa-bhāvana See *pratipakṣa bhāvana.*

pratyāhāra Classically listed as the fifth component or limb of Patañjali's *rāja* or *aṣṭāṅga-yoga,* this is translated as "withdrawing the attention from the physical senses" and the process of inner and outer alignment or synchronization. It relates to a variety of techniques that shift one from an externalized practice to an internalized practice, which leads to the restoration of the senses to their natural functioning and guides one into deeper practices of concentration, meditation, and absorption.

prema Love, affection, kindness, tender regard, fondness.

Prenatal Essence Known in Chinese Medicine as *xian-tian-zhi-jing,* this is one of the two main sources of Jing, which is responsible for growth, development, reproduction, and helps distinguish organic life from inorganic material. This type of essence is what we genetically inherit and is "fixed at birth and, together with Original Qi, determines an individual's basic makeup and constitution."

president The current leader or head of a corporation, professional organization, club, or group of people.

professor This is an accomplished and recognized scholar, teacher, academic, and/or an expert in the arts or sciences, who has been awarded an educational position of influence, tenure, and/or a department chair at a university.

professor of neurology A professor specializing in the study of the brain and nervous system.

Professor Tirumalai Krishnamacharya See Krishnamacharya.

pṛthivī mudrā Translated as the "gesture of the earth," this hand gesture is for balancing the annamaya kosha, cultivating the energy of the earth element, and instilling groundedness, self-assurance, and stability, especially in the creation of endurance or strength in muscles. It is performed by joining the thumbs of each hand to the tips of the ring fingers while extending the remaining fingers with the hands resting on the thighs with the palms facing upward.

psycho-emotional Any type of psychological interaction with the emotions and/or one's ability to embrace thoughts and feelings. In Yoga Therapy, this typically relates to the *mano-maya-kośa,* or the dimension of oneself that is made up of the thoughts and feelings that compose his/her personality.

psychology An academic and applied science involving the study of one's mental function, mental processing, behavior, perception, cognition, attention, motivation, personality, interpersonal relationships, and/or unconscious and conscious observations of the world.

psychophysiological Traditionally known in alternative medicine as the "mind-body connection," this is any type of psychological interaction or mental process that creates a physical, physiological, and/or molecular change in a person. In Yoga Therapy, this approach uses the mind as a functioning device and through affirmation, mantra, meditation, and/or a thought-based technique for administering change, rather than simply manipulating the person's physical structure, mental and neurological processes are enlisted to aid in the fight against pain, disease, and/or illness.

psychosocial Any type of psychological interaction with and/or within a social environment. In Yoga Therapy, this typically relates to one's sangha (community) and the environment of social support one creates when dealing with pain, disease, and/or illness.

psychotherapy A psychologically-based therapeutic interaction or treatment between a trained professional and a client, patient, family, couple, or group that involves the exploration of thoughts, feelings, and behaviors for the purpose of increasing one's sense of well-being and improving one's functionality in the world and quality of life.

Ptah, Egyptian Creator God The creator God in Egyptian cosmology, who existed before all things, and whose thoughts and word brought the world into existence. He generally is depicted as a green man with a divine beard carrying a scepter (for power), an ankh (for life), and a djed (for stability), which are the three symbols of the creative power of a God in Egyptian culture.

purāṇas Sometimes referred to as "the fifth Veda" and "belonging to an olden or ancient time," this text introduces the creation of the universe, its destruction and renovation, the genealogy of the gods and sages, the reigns of the kings, the beginning of the human race, deity worship, and the "trimurti of the three *gunas*" known as *sattva, tamas,* and *rājas.*

Purna Yoga Translated as "Integral Yoga" and founded by Aadil and Savitri Palkhivala, this is a holistic style of Yoga that maintains the core belief that all parts of the human being need to be addressed for healing to happen. In the therapeutic application of Purna Yoga, a wide variety of tools are synthesized from various methodologies, including āsana and prāṇāyāma techniques from the Iyengar Yoga tradition, meditation techniques from the lineage of Śrī Aurobindo, philosophic study from the teachings of the *Vedas,* the four purusharthas, the *Bhagavad Gītā,* Patanjali, and Śrī Aurobindo, and nutrition and lifestyle practices from Ayurveda, Chinese nutritional herbology, and naturopathy.

puruṣa 1. Man, male, person, human being.

2. Soul, spirit, pure undifferentiated awareness, or the personal and animating principle in humans and other living beings.

3. In Sāṁkhya, "the seer," or the individual, immaterial spirit as a passive spectator of *prakṛti* (the phenomenal world).

4. Supreme Being or Soul of the universe, esp. when prefixed with *para, parama,* or *uttama,* thence identifiable with Brahmā, Viṣṇu, Śiva, or the Goddess.

puruṣamṛgāsana Sphinx pose or kneeling sphinx pose.

puruṣārtha *puruṣa* = person *artha* = aim or purpose

Traditional Hindu culture recognizes four fundamental existential human values: *kāma* (love, sensual enjoyment), *artha* (wealth, power, worldly ambition), *dharma* (sacred duty, social ethics), and *mokṣa* (freedom, spiritual liberation).

Pūrva-Mimāṁsā *mīmāṁsa* = examination *pūrva* = before, in front, previous, former

One of the six *darśanas* or schools of orthodox Hindu philosophy, paired with *Uttara Mīmāṁsā.* Philosophical analysis of the Vedas, providing rules for their interpretation, along with rational justifications for the observance of Vedic rituals.

Qi (or Chi) Known as prāṇa (life force energy) in Yoga and Ayurveda, this is one of the "three treasures" in Chinese Medicine, along with Jing (essence) and Shen (spirit), and represents the fundamental quality of being and becoming that has no beginning and no end. It is the "vital substance," which links mind, body, and spirit and is the energy that makes up all things in the universe, organic and inorganic.

Qi Gong Translated as "life energy" and also commonly referred to as Chi Gung or Chi Gong, this Taoist Yoga and Chinese medicine practice is designed to improve health, cultivate awareness, and balance the chi/qi (energy) of the body through highly specific movements, breathing techniques, and movement meditations.

qualified medical examiner Primary, secondary, and alternative healthcare physicians who are certified by a workers' compensation department to examine injured workers to evaluate disability and write medical-legal reports, which are used to determine an injured worker's eligibility for workers' compensation benefits

rāga One of the five *kleśas* or subjective afflictions cited in Patañjali's ***Yoga Sūtra,*** this is the attachment and desire for pleasurable, passionate, and attractive things, which create mindless actions and bring only temporary happiness. In Yoga Therapy, this manifests as redness and inflammation. In classical Indian music, this is a musical note, harmony, formula, or melody.

Rāja Yoga One of the four main paths to Yoga, this is the path of psychic control or "the royal path" and typically includes practices found within Patañjali's *Yoga Sūtra,* including his eight-limbed path to Yoga, classically referred to as *aṣṭāṅga yoga.* It includes practices that help develop all aspects of a human being like the *yama* (ethical restraints), *niyama* (observances), *āsana* (stable seat), *prāṇāyāma* (extension of breath), *pratyāhāra* (withdrawal), *dhāraṇā* (concentration), *dhyāna* (meditation), and *samādhi* (absorption).

rājas Part of the balance of the "trimurti of the three *gunas,*"and the three constituents of *prakṛti* (nature) along with *tamas* and *sattva,* this represents the qualities of movement, heat, energy, motility, and transformation. In a psycho-spiritual context, when *rājas* is out of balance it is associated with passion, restlessness, greed, activity, and pain.

rakta In Ayurvedic medicine, this is one of the seven *dhātus* (fundamental tissues of the body) consisting of blood, which is the primary vehicle for prana (energy).

rakta mokṣa The Ayurvedic practice of bloodletting.

rasa In Ayurvedic medicine, this is one of the seven *dhātus* (fundamental tissues of the body) consisting of plasma and noncellular portions of the blood like lymph and interstitial fluids. It is also considered to be one of six tastes: *madhura* (sweet), *amla* (sour), *lavana* (salty), *katu* (pungent), *tikta* (bitter), and *kaśaya* (astringent). The effects of these flavors on the *doṣas* is taken into account when prescribing therapeutic treatments.

rasāyana 1. A drug used as a vermifuge or an antiparasitic in Ayurveda.

2. An elixir vitae intended to prolong life or prevent old age.

relaxation response Outlined in studies on meditation performed by Harvard researcher, Herbert Benson, M.D., in the 1970s, this is a self-regulatory, coordinated psychophysiological down regulation of the sympathetic nervous system with a generalized reduction in both cognitive and somatic arousal. It is the neurophysiological antithesis, or mirror opposite, of the well-known fight-or-flight stress response and instead activates the parasympathetic, "rest and digest," system as natural and instinctive as the stress response, which can be measured through such parameters as a slower heart rate, lower blood pressure, decreased oxygen consumption, and improved metabolic function.

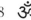

Ren Mai One of the "Eight Extraordinary Vessels" in Chinese meridian theory, this vessel, known as the conception vessel, controls the Yin channels and circulates the Yin Qi, including blood, essence, and body fluids, to nourish and lubricate all of the abdominal and thoracic organs and channels. It originates deep in the abdomen, near the uterus in females, and travels along the central axis of the front side of the body concluding at the cheeks and the infraorbital region just below the eyes. It is used to treat menstruation issues, reproductive problems, impotence, hernia, and gastrointestinal and digestive dysfunctions.

resveratrol A substance found in red wine that is one of the chief activating factors of the Sirt 1 gene (which is said to cause the breakdown of fat cells), increases DNA repair, suppresses bad or disruptive genes, and actively contributes to the longevity effect in genetic medicine.

Richard Usatine, M.D. A Columbia University–trained doctor and full professor in the Department of Family and Community Medicine at the University of Texas Health Science Center, he cofounded the first Yoga in Medicine course at a U.S. medical school while on faculty at UCLA and also coauthored the book, *Yoga Rx,* with Larry Payne, Ph.D.

Ru One-half of the Indian and Sanskrit term, *guru,* meaning "teacher" or "master," the word, *ru,* itself, means "light," "brightness," or "to dispel."

sādhana Lit. "means of achievement," this is a daily Yoga or spiritual practice that can involve one or more of various activities, such as meditation, chanting, religious devotion, visualizations, and the physical practices of Haṭha Yoga, undertaken in pursuit of various attainments, the supreme of which is *mokṣa* (spiritual freedom or liberation).

Sahaja Yoga *Sahaja* = congenital, innate, original, natural. This is a system of Yoga and meditation founded in the 1970s by Indian guru, Śrī Mataji Mirmala, that aims to produce the experience of self-realization through Kundalini awakening and an inner transformation, which results in one becoming more moral, united, integrated, and balanced. The teachings of Sahaja Yoga make explicit assertions that various diseases are causally connected with problems in specific *chakras* and key *nāḍis* in the body and can be effectively corrected through implementation of the methods that they teach.

sahasrāra cakra* or *sahasrāra chakra One of the seven primary *chakras* in the body in traditional Yoga systems, this is the crown chakra at the top of the head or above the head and is said to be the "thousand petal lotus of the mind," which opens up in samadhi (absorption). It is commonly thought of as the linking point of the individual soul with the transcendental Spirit and is associated with the color violet or white, the seed mantra syllable ***oṁ*** or having no sound, and the element of Light.

Śaiva Siddhānta A traditional, "settled," or normative branch from the Śaivite Tantra sect of the Tamil region of south India, it promotes a dualistic and nondualistic philosophy that focuses on the tantric worship of Śiva, devotional rites, cosmology and theological concepts, ritual initiation, bhakti poetry, and, ultimately, liberation.

Śaiva Tantra A general term referring to several Indic religious traditions, such as *Śaiva Siddānta, Kapālika, Tantric Śaivism,* and *Kashmir Śaivism,* this philosophy describes how the formless supreme principle manifests throughout the universe. It centers around Śiva as the as the creator, preserver, destroyer, revealer, and concealer of all that exists and employs concepts, rituals, and yogic practices of *tantra* (like Shakti existing within Shiva), the union of Shiva and Shakti, guru worship, asceticism and self-purification practices.

śakti* or *shakti 1. Power, strength, might, energy, capability.

2. The active, manifesting power of the Divine, often personified as the Goddess in her various forms.

3. Any *devī*, especially the consort of a male *deva.*

śalabhāsana Locust pose.

sālamba bhujaṅgāsana Supported cobra or serpent pose.

sālamba sarvaṅgāsana Shoulderstand or all limbs standing on the shoulders pose.

sālamba śīrṣāsana Headstand or all limbs standing on the head pose.

samādhi Classically listed as the eighth component or limb of Patañjali's *rāja* or *aṣṭāṅga-yoga,* this is the state of deep contemplative absorption in Yoga that is experienced by an individual once he/she merges with the object of his/her meditation. It is said to be the ultimate state of pure consciousness that transcends the realms of body, logic, time, analytical ability, intellect, and mind. While Patañjali identifies four increasingly subtle levels of *samādhi,* culminating in a fifth state called *nirbīja* (seedless) *samādhi,* which transcends phenomenal experience altogether and constitutes *kaivalya* (radical autonomy of the Seer), additional forms and manifestations of *samādhi* can be found in many other texts and traditions.

śamana cikitsā or shamana chikitsa Also called "pacifying therapy," these Ayurvedic treatments are performed for the alleviation of the symptoms of a disease when a person is not strong enough to bear the strain of *pañca karma.* Complemented with *śodhana cikitsā* or purification treatment, *śamana cikitsā* leads to palliation, pacification, or neutralization but usually does not get all the way to the root cause of the disease.

samāna vāyu One of the five *vāyus* (winds or energy channels) in Yoga and originating in the center of the navel in the solar plexus, *samāna vāyu* governs the balance between *apāna vāyu* (downward and outward forces) and *prāṇa-vāyu* (upward and inward forces). It is responsible for processing and assimilating breath and nutrients from food, enhancing cell production and cell repair, stimulating the *manipura* chakra, and balancing the organs of digestion and elimination.

samatā 1. Equality, sameness, identity with.

2. Equableness, normal condition.

3. Equanimity, balance; benevolence.

Samata International Yoga & Health Center Established in 1980 by Larry Payne, Ph.D., and inspired by the teachings of T. K. V. Desikachar, son of the late Professor Śrī T. Krishnamacharya of Mysore, India, the style of Yoga taught at Samata features Yoga postures (āsanas) and breathing techniques (prāṇāyāma) therapeutically adapted with respect to individual differences in age, physical and mental health, culture, religion, philosophy, and occupation.

samavṛtti Defined as "equal breathing," this prāṇāyāma technique is performed by balancing the breath in length, depth, and speed with respect to puraka (inhalation), rechaka (exhalation), and kumbhaka (holding or retaining the breath). The most common samavṛitti practices include a 1:1 inhalation to exhalation ratio as well as a more advanced 1:1:1:1 inhalation to retention to exhalation to retention ratio. It is said to be good for balancing one's mind, calming one's mood and temper, releasing stress, teaching concentration and moderation, and preparing one for higher states of meditation.

saṁhitā Translated as "compendium," "compilation," or "collection," this is gathering of knowledge or wisdom that is generally associated with the Vedas and other ancient yogic and/or Ayurvedic texts, which include a collection of mantras, authors, techniques, hymns, or systemic-based approaches to health.

saṁkalpa or sankalpa Definite intention, determination, or decision; will, volition, purpose.

sāṁkhya One of the six *darśanas,* or systems of Indian Vedic philosophy, *sāṁkhya* seeks to explicate the relationship between *puruṣa* (transcendental individual spirit/pure consciousness/witness) and *prakṛti* (matter or material Nature) with *viveka* (clear discernment). *Puruṣa* is unknowable and beyond the senses, words, and the mind while *prakṛti* is the cause of the manifest physical universe—of everything except *prakṛti*—and is composed of the three *gunas.* There is no creator god in *sāṁkhya,* like Brahman or Shiva, because in this philosophy each jiva (individual soul) is bound to experience human suffering as a synergy of *puruṣa* (soul) and *prakṛti* (physical form/body) and, just like the *darśana* of Yoga, the goal is to achieve *mokṣa* (liberation).

saṁskāra 1. Memories; mental impressions or imprints left on the subconscious mind from past and present experiences.

2. Conditioned dispositions and volitions that are the product of psychic formations accumulated in this or prior lifetimes.

3. A sacred or sanctifying ceremony performed as a Vedic purification rite of passage for persons of the first three castes.

4. In Ayurveda, the processing of a medication to increase its natural properties, add additional properties, and/or to delete undesirable properties, such as the toxic characteristic of a metallic ingredient.

saṁtoṣa or santosha One of the five *niyamas* or observances cited in the *Yoga Sūtra,* this is the practice of contentment and feeling satisfied.

saṁyoga The practice of combining, associating, or connecting two (or more) behaviors, concepts, medicines, or practices to create a more powerful and potent effect or outcome. Union or synthesis. In Ayurveda, this is combining healthy foods based on general principles and individual constitutions with respect to the *doṣas* and body type. Sometimes, *saṁyoga* can result from *avidyā* (ignorance) as the tendency to confuse the character and/or value of two objects, which are similar in nature or close in proximity like *puruṣa* and *prakṛti.*

Sanātana Dharma Lit. "everlasting *dharma.*" The eternal set of duties performed on the path to Eternal Truth that usually has Yoga, Ayurveda, and/or Hindu orthodox origins, Sanātana Dharma consists of cultivating virtues such as honesty, refraining from injuring living beings, purity, goodwill, mercy, patience, self-restraint, generosity, and asceticism.

sañjīvani Lit. "life-giving." In Hindu mythology, a magical herb that could cure any disease and even bring the dead back to life. Identified by some today with the lythophytic plant of south India, *Selaginella bryoteris,* which affords therapeutic protection from heat stroke and cellular damage due to ultraviolet exposure and oxidative stress.

sangha Spiritual community or right relationships.

sarvaṅgāsana Shoulderstand or whole body pose.

ṣaṭkarma See *shat karmas.*

satsaṅga Association with the good and the true and literally meaning "to be in the company of truth," this is an assembly of people who gather with a guru or teacher to listen to, talk about, meditate and reflect on, discuss, and assimilate the truth.

sattva Part of the balance of the "trimurti of the three *gunas,*" along with *rājas* and *tamas,* this represents a state of purity, harmony, joy, goodness, balance, health, and contentment that is free from sickness when the doshas are brought into equilibrium. In the yogic and Ayurvedic traditions, an overabundance of *rājas* and/or *tamas* causes suffering as it leads one away from *sattva. Sattva* is also being, existence, entity, spirit, nature, and true essence. As a material constituent, it is the component of light, radiance, vibration, and illumination.

sattva guṇa See *sattva.*

satya One of the five *niyamas* or observances cited in the *Yoga Sūtra,* this is the practice of honoring one's word, telling the truth, and being honest..

Satyananda Saraswati One of the twentieth century's chief proponents of the practice of Yoga nidra, Satyananda Saraswati was a disciple of Swami Sivananda and founder of the Bihar School of Yoga.

Śavāsana* or *shavāsana Corpse pose.

Science of Life, The Known most commonly in Sanskrit as *Ayurveda,* this is the scientific study of the ancient healing arts of Ayurveda and the ways in which an individual can live a life of wholeness, balance, and good health.

Self See True Self.

self at essence See True Self.

self-realization In Yoga philosophy, this is the realization of the unification of *jivatma* (the living self) and *paramatma* (the supreme self) on all levels of one's being. It is the knowledge of the True Self beyond delusion and identification with the material phenomena or the world and ego. In a practical sense, it is the fulfillment, embodiment, and unification of one's human potential with one's divine potential. It is said to be possible through any of the four main paths to Yoga: *Rāja* , *Jñāna*, *Karma*, and *Bhakti*.

Selvarajan Yesudian An Indian-born Yoga teacher, who authored a book called *Yoga and Health* with Elisabeth Haisch in the 1950s and went on to found the first school of Yoga in Switzerland.

serratus punches An exercise from rehabilitative medicine and Yoga Therapy that can isolate, engage, and re-educate the serratus anterior muscle of the scapula, which is one of the chief stabilizers of the shoulder and has the tendency toward hypotonicity, weakness, and/or inhibition. The exercise is performed by lying supine on the floor with one arm directly in front of the shoulder holding a weight with the elbow straight. The arm is repetitively moved to push the weight away from the body in a small punching motion to initiate activity in the serratus anterior muscle.

setu bandha sarvāṅgāsana Bridge pose.

setu bandhāsana See *setu bandha sarvāṅgāsana*.

seven *dhātus* See *dhātus*.

Shabad Kriya A technique from Kundalini Yoga that has been used as a therapeutic insomnia treatment for thousands of years, the effectiveness of this meditation technique is the 22-beat cycle. To perform the kriya, the practitioner is to inhale in four equal parts, mentally vibrating the mantra, *Sa Ta Na Ma,* with one syllable for each part of the inhalation. The breath is then gently retained without strain while mentally vibrating the sound of the mantra for four cycles holding the breath for a total of 16 beats. Finally, the exhale is done completely in two equal strokes with the mental sound *Wahe Guru*. The technique is for chronic insomnia as well as for balancing the natural rhythms in brain, neural, and endocrine function.

sharira, sattva,* and *atma In Ayurvedic medicine, this is the "foundation of life" or the "holy trinity" otherwise referred to as sharira (body), sattva (mind), and atma (consciousness).

shat karmas* or *ṣaṭkarma Lit. "six procedures" or "six actions," these are extraordinary purification or cleansing practices performed in the Haṭha Yoga tradition to cleanse the body and heal internal disorders. They include *dhauti* (cleansing), *basti* (yogic enema), *neti* (nasal cleansing), *trāṭaka* (focused gazing), *nauli* (abdominal massage), and *kapālabhātī* (skull shining).

shavāsana See *savāsana*.

sheetali See *śītalī.*

Shen Literally translated as "spirit," this is one of the "three treasures" that fuels and nourishes human beings along with Qi (energy) and Jing (essence). It is one's awareness, the vitality and stability of the mind, the human spirit, and the soul. It is stored in the upper dantien and is often associated with the heart.

shitkari prāṇāyāma or sītkārī prāṇāyāma Literally meaning "hissing" or "that which cools," this *prāṇāyāma* technique is performed by opening the lips slightly with the teeth pressed together and the tongue just behind the lower palate. While taking in the inhalation breath a soft hissing or "ssss" sound is made while the exhalation breath follows through both nostrils of the nose. It is said to cool the body and calm thirst and hunger.

Shiva Sūtras* or *Śiva Sūtras Written by Vasugupta, this is one of the central texts of *Kashmir Śaivism,* which discusses nondualism, and is a classical source text addressing the practice of *Yoga nidrā.*

Shri Yogendraji Born as Mani Haribhai Desai and known as the "Father of Modern Yoga Renaissance," he founded The Yoga Institute of Santa Cruz in Mumbai, India, in 1918 and is credited with creating a medically-based form of Haṭha Yoga and research that would later lead to the development of Yoga Therapy. He is responsible for simplifying Yoga āsanas and bringing yogic technologies to the common householder and is the author of several books on Yoga as well as the journal, *Yoga and Total Health,* which he first published in 1933.

shukra/artava* or *śukra In Ayurvedic medicine, this is one of the seven *dhātus* (fundamental tissues of the body) consisting of male and female reproductive tissues and fluids. In essence, it is any clear, pure, bright, or resplendent liquid (water, *soma,* juice, etc.).

shushumna* or *suṣumṇa In *Yoga* subtle anatomy, one of the three main *nāḍīs* (channels of energy) running the length of the body and intersecting at the major *chakras,* or energy plexuses, from the base of the spine (*mūladhara chakra*) to the crown of the head (*sahasrāra chakra*). Along with the ida nāḍī (left channel) and the pingala nāḍī (right channel), the *suṣumṇa* nāḍī (central channel) runs directly along the spinal cord in the center energy channel and represents inner attentiveness, illumination, self-realization, awakened kundalini, the Saraswati River, and the union of duality. Considered to be empty most of the time, the techniques of Haṭha Yoga are intended to awaken the typically dormant *kuṇḍalinī* energy concentrated at the *mūladhāra cakra,* drawing it into *suṣumṇa* and thence upward to the *sahasrāra cakra,* thereby bringing about cosmic consciousness and spiritual liberation.

Siddha medicine (Ayurveda in Southern India) One of the oldest medical systems known to mankind, this approach developed in southern India and is part of the trio Indian medicines: Ayurveda, Siddha, and Unani. It is based on balancing the three humors in equilibrium as well as the elements and claims to revitalize and rejuvenate dysfunctional organs that cause the disease through a variety of cleansing treatments, prāṇāyāma exercises, and herbal and mineral medicines.

siddhi **(supernatural powers, skills)** Lit. "accomplishment, attainment, fulfillment, success" and discussed in Patañjali's *Yoga Sūtra,* these are spiritual, magical, psychic, and/or supernatural powers that can be obtained through sadhana (spiritual practice), tapas (austerity), ritual, special plants, magic, and/or the practice of Yoga and meditation. Traditionally, there are eight powers that can be acquired, which include *aṇima* (reducing one's body to the size of an atom), *mahima* (expanding one's body to an infinitely large size), *garima* (infinite heaviness), *laghima* (weightlessness), *prapti* (ability to acquire anything anywhere), *prakamya* (realizing all desires), *istva* (absolute lordship over all of creation), and *vastva* (control over everything including the five elements). In Ayurveda, *siddhis* can also refer to a cure or the healing of a disease.

siṁhāsana Lion pose.

śīrṣāsana See *sālamba śīrṣāsana.*

śītalī **or** ***sheetali prāṇāyāma*** Lit. "cooling" and also known as the "whistle breath" in Kundalini Yoga Therapy, this *prāṇāyāma* technique is performed by curling the tongue (if possible) and placing it just behind pursed lips. In a method similar to whistling, the inhale is taken in through the pursed mouth and the exhale is calmly released through the nose. It is said to cool the body, calm the mind, remove excess heat, lower blood pressure, reduce stress, and depress the sympathetic nervous system.

Sivananda Yoga Vedanta Center Founded by Swami Vishnudevananda, author of *The Complete Illustrated Book of Yoga* and one of the top authorities on Haṭha Yoga and Rāja Yoga in the twentieth century, this a worldwide nonprofit organization dedicated to the teachings of Vishnudevananda's guru, Swami Sivananda. The teachings of Sivananda Yoga Vedanta Center are traditional Haṭha Yoga and classical Vedanta intended to bring physical, mental, and spiritual well-being and are best summarized in the six words: Serve, Love, Give, Purify, Meditate, Realize.

snehana One of the five classic purification methods of *pañca karma* and an Ayurvedic parallel to the therapeutic practice of *anuvāsana,* this is the application of oils to lubricate the body as a prepatory technique for deeper cleansing practices in *pañca karma.* Quite literally, *snehana* is "lubricating, rubbing, or smearing with oil or unguents."

socio-emotional Any type of social interaction that effects the emotions, stress, mood, attitude, well-being, behavior, and/or one's ability to embrace thoughts and feelings.

sociology The scientific study of the origins, development, and organization of human social behavior.

Source See Spirit.

Space One of the five elements in each of the systems of Ayurveda and Yoga, which list the other four elements as water, earth, fire, and air/wind. In Yoga philosophy, space, often referred to as *akasha,* or ether, is the subtle material that fills the universe, the space in which everything exists/happens, and the source of all matter. It symbolizes emptiness, presence, infinity, vibration, and the space that the other elements fill, and, when out of balance, the loss of one's hearing or voice and the destruction of tissues that are replaced by space.

Spirit A common name in Yoga and other systems of Eastern mysticism for the God, Soul, Supreme Being, Source, Consciousness, Intelligence, and/or Great and Holy Spirit that lives in each being, animate and inanimate, and forms the natural order of the universe.

Sport + Yoga See Yoga and Health.

sports medicine A branch of medicine that deals with the treatment and prevention of injuries related to sports, athletic performance, exercise, or physical fitness using medications, injections, training, and/or surgery. This is contrasted to the application of science to sports, known as *sports science,* as the word *medicine* is usually related to drugs and/or surgery. Sports science describes the physics of the body and the application of motion, i.e., the kinetics of the body, while sports medicine falls under the larger umbrella of sports science.

Sports Science and Medical Advisory Board for America's Schools Program A nonprofit group that shares information and advice about sports science with the general public and raises money for education programs for children from kindergarten to twelfth grade.

Śrī Aurobindo Born Aurobindo Ghose and founder of a method of spiritual practice called "Integral Yoga," he was an Indian guru, a spiritual master, a philosopher, and a poet. The central theme of his vision was the evolution and transformation of human life into a life divine through the scientific application of Yoga and meditation, which was taken up by his spiritual collaborator, Mira Alfassa (The Mother), after his *mahāsamādhi* in Pondicherry, India. His main literary contributions include *The Life Divine, Synthesis of Yoga, Savitri,* and several commentaries on the *Vedas, Upaniṣads,* and *Bhagavad Gītā.*

Śrī Brahmananda Saraswati Formally "Swami Shankaracharya Brahmananda of the Saraswati branch of the ancient Swami Order" and the teacher of Mahirishi Mahesh Yogi, founder of Transcendental Meditation, Śrī Brahmananda Saraswati was a spiritual master in the Radhaswami School of Surat Shabd Yoga tradition and one of the twentieth century's chief proponents of the practice of Yoga nidrā.

Śrī Rama Mohana Bramachari An Indian guru, Yoga master, and householder, who was the teacher of Professor Tirumalai Krishnamacharya, Śrī Rama Mohana Bramachari lived in a cave in the mountains of Tibet and taught Krishnamacharya over 3,000 āsanas, Patañjali's *Yoga Sūtra,* the therapeutic uses of Yoga, āsana, and pranayama, and how to stop his heart from beating.

srotas 1. Bodily channels.

2. Currents or beds of a river or stream; torrent.

3. Courses or currents of food and nutriment in the body.

4. Apertures in the body (eyes, ears, nose, mouth, etc.).

Stress Reduction Cognitive Behavioral Treatment (SR-CBT) A psychotherapeutic treatment program that reduces stress by addressing dysfunctional emotions, maladaptive behaviors, and cognitive processes using meditation and other Yoga and lifestyle modification techniques.

Structural Yoga Therapy Founded by Mukunda and Chinnamasta Stiles, this is a systematic approach to Yoga Therapy that adapts Yoga to an individual's unique body and seeks to reduce pain, reestablish muscle tone, and free up normal ranges of mobility and motion (ROM). It is designed as a physically-based system but has far reaching implications into work with the subtle body, and, through the study of postural language and body reading, the system posits that a wealth of information is expressed through the physical form that can be used to gauge the efficiency of the various systems of the body and treat an assortment of physical, visceral, and mental health issues.

sūcī randhrāsana Eye of the needle pose.

Sudarshan Kriya Yoga Translated as "proper vision by purifying action," this is a *prāṇāyāma* technique taught by The Art of Living Foundation that incorporates ujjayi prāṇāyāma, bhastrika prāṇāyāma, and an advanced form of rhythmic, cyclical breathing with slow, medium, and fast cycles. It has been clinically found to alleviate anxiety, reduce depression, and decrease PTSD and stress in various scientific studies.

sudarśana kriyā See Sudarshan Kriya Yoga.

sukha Lit. "good space" or "having a good axle hole," this is one of the descriptive terms used to define āsana in Patañjali's *Yoga Sūtra*. It has a variety of definitions including pleasant, agreeable, gentle, comfortable, happy; happiness, joy, prosperity, ease.

sukhāsana Easy pose.

sukumāra rasāyana Lit. "fair youth elixir," this is a complex Ayurvedic formulation and treatment made using a variety of Indian herbs. It is said to be good for bloating, digestive problems, women's issues, piles, constipation, rheumatic disorders, vaginal complaints, and normalizing the function of *apāna vata*.

śūnyatā Similar to *Brahman* in Hinduism, the *Tao* in Taoism, *Qi* in Chinese Medicine, and *Prāṇa* in Yoga, this Buddhist term represents emptiness and openness. *śūnyatā* is said to be the infinite expansiveness of the unseen universal life force energy that exists without a beginning or an end and is the point from which all energy and action in life manifests. In Buddhism, the assertion that all selves and objects are ultimately empty of permanence or truly substantial self-nature. All phenomena are thus viewed as transient and radically interdependent.

supta baddha koṇāsana Reclined bound angle pose or reclined cobbler's pose.

supta padāṅguṣṭhāsana Reclined big toe pose.

sūrya bhedana Translated as "sun piercing breath" and also called the "revitalizing breath," this *prāṇāyāma* technique is performed by inhaling through the right nostril and exhaling through the left nostril, thus amplifying the hot "solar" energy conducted through the *piṅgala nāḍī*, clearing and purifying the major energy channel on the right side of the body. It is said to increase physical energy, revitalize the body, improve one's ability to perform verbal tasks, and provide a boost for the sympathetic nervous system.

sūrya namaskāra A flowing sequence of *āsanas* known as Sun Salutations that link together breathing, movement, concentration, devotion, grace, exercise, worship, and meditation.

sūtra neti See *neti.*

svabhāva 1. Basic human character; self-nature.

2. Essence; essential quality or natural condition; a state of being, one's natural state or constitution, innate or inherent disposition.

svādhyāya One of the five *niyamas* or observances itemized in Patañjali's *Yoga Sūtra,* this personally motivated study traditionally includes repetitive recitation of key *sūtras* or epitome texts, as well as the practice of self-study, self-inquiry, and self-reflection.

svarūpa 1. Our own form or essential nature.

2. The power of pure awareness.

svāstha 1. This is "true health" or a sound state of well-being in body, mind, and soul.

2. Health, ease, comfort, contentment.

Svastha Yoga and Ayurveda *Svastha* is a state of holistic health and balance and literally means "to stay in oneself" or "to be oneself." This style of Yoga Therapy founded by the Mohan family is not a "style" of practicing Yoga, per se, rather it is doing Yoga in a way that helps lead the individual toward *svastha.* It carries on the work of Professor Tirumalai Krishnamacharya and his guiding principle that any teaching has to be modified for the individual to create and stay in a state of balanced health.

Svastha Yoga Therapy See Svastha Yoga and Ayurveda.

svasti mudrā Translated as "gesture of well-being," this hand gesture is for protection, from negative energy, optimum alignment of the spine, good fortune, prosperity, releasing muscular tension from the upper back and shoulder blades, and supporting the health of the endocrine and immune systems. It is performed by beginning with the hands in a prayer position and then crossing the forearms so that the backs of the hands are facing each other, about six inches apart, with the right arm closer to the chest and the fingers pointed upward.

Svatmarama Yogi A disciple of Gorakhnath, who lived around the mid-fourteenth century CE, he is the author of *The Haṭha Yoga Pradīpikā,* which is one of the primary texts of Haṭha Yoga and a possible starting point for the entire system of Yoga Therapy.

svedana One of the five classic purification methods of *pañca karma,* this is medicated sweating, perspiring, sudation, and/or any instrument or remedy that causes those effects.

Swami Kuvalayananda One of the most important figures in Yoga during his time, Swami Kuvalayananda was a Yoga researcher and educator, who pioneered the first scientific journal specifically devoted to studying Yoga, *Yoga Mīmāṁsa*. He was the founder of the Kaivalyadhama Health and Yoga Research Center in Lonvala, India, and paved the way for today's modern advancements in the field of Yoga Therapy.

Swami Rama Founder of the Himalayan Yoga Institute in Honesdale, Pennsylvania, and a pioneer in Yoga research, Swami Rama was one of the first yogis to be studied by Western scientists in the 1970s. He displayed the ability to voluntarily induce cardiac atrial fibrillation for seventeen seconds and increase the blood flow to one side of his right hand while decreasing the blood flow on the opposite side resulting in a 10 degrees Fahrenheit temperature change between the two sides of his hand, which prior to this time was considered impossible. He wrote many books including *Living with the Himalayan Masters* and *The Art of Joyful Living* and is largely considered one of the greatest adepts, teachers, proponents of Yoga nidra, writers, scholars, humanitarians, and Yoga researchers of the twentieth century.

Swami Satchidananda An Indian guru, philosopher, Yoga adept, and founder of Yogaville in Buckingham, Virginia, Swami Satchidananda is the creator and developer of Integral Yoga, a scientific system that integrates the classical four main paths of Yoga in order to bring about a complete and harmonious development of the individual. His name literally means "truth, consciousness, and bliss" and his disciples include many of today's most well-recognized Yoga Therapists including Dean Ornish, M.D., Michael Lerner, Ph.D., and Jnani Chapman, R.N., as well as poet Allen Ginsberg and musician Alice Coltrane. He is perhaps best known for giving the opening talk at Woodstock in 1969 and for authoring the most widely used commentary of Patañjali's *Yoga Sutras* in the United States.

Swami Sivananda One of the greatest spiritual figures in India's modern history, Swami Sivananda was the founder of the Divine Life Society and a physician, spiritual teacher, and proponent of Yoga, Yoga nidra, and Vedanta. He taught a full spectrum lifestyle approach to Yoga, authored over 200 books in the early to mid-twentieth century, inspired the creation of "Sivananda Yoga" by his disciple, Swami Vishnudevananda, and continues to have millions of followers all over the world through the Sivananda Yoga Vedanta Centers.

Swami Veda Bharati A sunnyasin and master Sanskrit grammarian, Swami Veda Bharati is a disciple of Swami Rama, founder of the Himalayan Institute, and was one of the twentieth century's chief proponents of the practice of Yoga nidrā.

Swami Vishnudevananda Founder of the Sivananda Yoga Vedanta Center and author of *The Complete Illustrated Book of Yoga*, Swami Vishnudevananda was a disciple of the Indian guru and doctor, Swami Sivananda and was one of the top authorities on Haṭha Yoga, Rāja Yoga, and Yoga nidra in the twentieth century.

Swami Vivekananda Founder of the Vedanta Society and the foremost disciple of the great nineteenth century Indian guru and saint, Śrī Paramahansa Ramakrishna, Swami Vivekananda was the first yogi to introduce Yoga, Vedanta, and Hinduism to the Western world at the Parliament of World Religions in Chicago in 1893. He wrote numerous books, poems, and letters throughout his life and even today his Vedanta Society continues to be one of the world's leaders in carrying out research on Yoga as a therapy.

T. K. V. Desikachar Son and student of famed Yoga master and innovator, Professor Tirumalai Krishnamacharya, and founder of the Krishnamacharya Yoga Mandiram in Chennai, India, T. K. V. Desikachar is the author of four books, *Health, Healing, and Beyond* and *The Heart of Yoga: Developing a Personal Practice* as well as *Vedic Chant Companion* and *Viniyoga of Yoga*, which were coauthored with his son, Kausthub Desikachar, Ph.D., M.Sc. He has devoted himself to teaching therapeutic Yoga for over forty-five years and his teaching method is based on Krishnamacharya's fundamental principle that Yoga must always be adapted to an individual's changing needs in order to derive the maximum therapeutic benefit of the practice.

T. Krishnamacharya See Krishnamacharya.

taḍāsana Mountain pose or palm tree pose.

Tae-Woo Yoo A Korean Acupuncturist and Doctor of Oriental Medicine, who developed a therapeutic method of hand acupuncture to awaken the body to health and wellness through stimulation of the meridian energy system, in miniature, on the hands.

Tai Chi Formally referred to as *tai chi chuan,* this is an internal martial arts technique that originated in China, which may relate to a variety of different traditions each designed to teach self-defense techniques and expand one's awareness, breath, confidence, skills in movement, and meditative abilities. It should be differentiated from Qi Gong, which is traditionally a Taoist Yoga and Chinese medicine practice designed to improve health, cultivate awareness, and balance the chi/qi (energy).

Taittirīya Upaniṣad One of the earliest of the principal Upaniṣads, c. sixth century BCE, possibly during the Buddha's lifetime (c. 563–483 BCE). This text is found within the *Āraṇyaka* (*Forest Text*) section of the *Taittirīya Yajurveda*. The classical metaphysical paradigm of the five *koṣas*—the sheaths or layers enclosing the *ātman* or spiritual self—is found in this *Upaniṣad.* Within this description is one of the earliest uses of the word *yoga* in a specifically spiritual context. Therein, *yoga* is understood as the "harnessing" or "yoking" of one's attention to that which is being investigated in order to gain understanding (*vijñāna*). The text states that as the body is to the person, so *yoga* is to the *vijñāna-maya-koṣa* or the "sheath made of understanding." It also describes the various degrees of happiness enjoyed by the different beings in creation, discusses techniques of Yoga nidrā, and introduces a variety of mantras and the importance of the holy syllable, *oṁ.*

tamas Part of the balance of the "trimurti of the three *gunas*,"and the three constituents of *prakṛti* (nature) along with *rājas* and *sattva*, this represents the qualities of heaviness, solidity, inertia, darkness, and dullness. In a psycho-spiritual context, when *tamas* is out of balance it is associated with lethargy, ignorance, negligence, and depression.

tantra 1. A science or "well-woven" system of knowledge, or a text detailing such a system or body of knowledge.

2. A general term referring to a non-Vedic, pan-Indic religious movement emerging in the early centuries of the Common Era, characterized, among other things, by the belief that the body and its physical sensations—including those of a sexual quality—are of divine nature and can thus be utilized, through skillful techniques, as the means of achieving spiritual realization and liberation. Yogic exploration of the divine forces naturally embedded within the psycho-physical structures of the human organism contributed to the development of esoteric *yogic* systems of practice during the middle to later centuries of the first millenium of the Common Era, such as Haṭha Yoga, Kundalini Yoga, and Vajrayāna Buddhism.

3. A type of religio-spiritual text centered around ritual enactments and/or visualization practices intended to weave a continuity between mundane human experience and direct realization of one's ultimately divine nature.

Tao (or Dao) Literally meaning, "way," "path," or "principle," this is a nondualistic philosophical system that has many commonalities with principles found in Chinese Medicine and Yoga, including harmonizing one's will with Nature to achieve "effortless action," finding balance within the phenomena of life and the Yin and the Yang, and that moderation in all areas of life leads one to longevity, health, and happiness.

tapas One of the five *niyamas,* this is the practice of austerity, asceticism, and self-discipline that brings about a transformative heat in the body, emotions, or spirit, burning off impurities and obstacles from the body and/or the subjective personality for spiritual growth.

Tapping Series for Lymphatic Circulation A *kriyā* in Kundalini Yoga Therapy designed to stimulate lymph circulation, detoxify the body, decrease stress, improve sleep and mood, increase vitality, and restore more comfort and ease in the body.

tattva* or *tattwas Lit. "thatness," this is the true nature of something. Reality or an essential ontological principle thereof. The Sāṁkhya metaphysical system is based on twenty-five *tattvas,* beginning with *puruṣa* (individual Spirit) and *prakṛti* (Nature). The remaining twenty-three *tattvas* lay out the fundamental evolutes of *prakṛti* in terms of the three inner components of the individual psyche (*antaḥkaraṇa*), the five gross elements (*mahābhūtas*), the five subtle perceptibilities (*tanmātras*), the five sensory organs (*buddhendriyas*), and the five organs of action (*karmendriyas*), serving as a philosophical foundation for explicating the relationship between Spirit and Matter.

teacher training manuals This is a manual, book, booklet, and/or binder created by the lead instructor(s) of a particular style, discipline, training, or school of Yoga, which is intended to be used as a study guide/aid and reference text by prospective teachers training to teach in that particular tradition.

team doctor The lead physician in charge of coordinating the medical staff and services for a sports team and/or Olympic team.

tejas 1. "Cellular digestion," "essence of life," and "flame of intelligence."

2. A refined form of *pitta dosha* said to create discernment, illumination, the desire to know truth, immunity, metabolic activity, and a higher functioning mind. When it is in balance, it directs the flow of energy in the body and mind and is the essence of the heat one absorbs through food and sunlight.

3. The sharp edge of a knife, tip of a flame, or ray.

4. Glow, splendor, radiance, brilliance, light, fire.

5. Clearness of the eyes; bright appearance of good health; beauty.

6. Fiery energy, ardor, vital power, spirit, efficacy, essence.

7. Heating and strengthening power of *pitta doṣa* (bile).

8. Semen, marrow, brain.

The Beatles Perhaps the most famous music band of all-time, the Beatles turned an entire generation of Westerners on to practices of Yoga, chanting, meditation, and Indian philosophy by studying with Maharishi Mahesh Yogi, Indian musician Ravi Shankar, and other Indian masters while at the height of their fame.

The Bill & Melinda Gates Foundation One of the largest private foundations in the world, this nonprofit organization seeks to end suffering and reduce extreme poverty and hunger by enhancing accessibility to vaccines and health care and providing monetary grants for educational opportunities and research.

The Heart of Yoga: Developing a Personal Practice Written by T. K. V. Desikachar, son of Professor Tirumalai Krishnamacharya, this book offers a refined, practical Yoga Therapy program for the spine at every level: physical, mental, and spiritual. It was one of the first Yoga texts to outline a step-by-step sequence for developing a complete personal therapeutic practice according to the age-old principles of Yoga and discusses all of the elements of Yoga from poses to counterposes, to conscious breathing, meditation, philosophy, and Patañjali's *Yoga Sutras*.

The Mother See Mira Alfassa (The Mother).

The Twelve Primary Meridians Also called the "twelve principle meridians" and grouped as Yin and Yang organ systems, the twelve meridians, or energy channels, consist of lung, large intestine, stomach, spleen, heart, small intestine, bladder, kidney, pericardium, thyroid/triple burner, gall bladder, and liver meridians, respectively. These channels are paired with the eight extraordinary channels as the main parts of the channel system in Chinese Medicine and are intended to be the primary channels or "rivers" of energy that regulate the change of life cycles.

The Twelve Principle Meridians See The Twelve Primary Meridians.

The Zone In Yoga Therapy and sports science, this is a steady stillness of the mind, a meditative ability, and/or an internal yogic trance state known as "samadhi" and "nirvana" that athletes can train, reinforce, and self-initiate when they work out, when they practice Yoga, when they study, when they are running, when they are jumping and throwing, when they prepare for competition, and when they are on the field of play actually competing.

TheraBand™ A rehabilitation-based company that specializes in elastic bands for resistance training as well as other therapeutic equipment like exercise balls, balance boards, rollers, educational videos, and other devices intended to create balance, stability, and/or flexibility.

Tibetan medicine A system of alternative medicine that originated in ancient Tibet, that treats illness as well as imbalances of the "three humors" and the five elements through techniques of diagnosis, pulse analysis, urinalysis, behavior and dietary modifications, herbal medicines, blood-letting, hot/cold therapy, cleansing techniques, massage, moxibustion, and golden needle acupuncture.

Tim McCall, M.D. A board-certified, Western-trained internist and medical editor for *Yoga Journal,* he is the author of the books, *Yoga as Medicine* and *Examining Your Doctor,* and is considered one of world's current leading scholars and teachers on integrating Yoga into the context and approach of Western medicine.

Tirumalai Krishnamacharya See Krishnamacharya.

TM See Transcendental Meditation.

Traditional Chinese Medicine See Chinese Medicine.

Transcendental Meditation (TM) Similar to Deepak Chopra's Primordial Sound meditation and The Art of Living's Sahaj Samadhi meditation, this meditation technique from the teachings of Maharishi Mahesh Yogi involves the use of a sound or mantra that helps in one's awareness to transcend the mind. It is practiced twice daily for at least 15–20 minutes per day and promotes deep relaxation, stress reduction, and self-development.

trataka One of the six shat karmas (cleansing techniques) mentioned in the *Haṭha Yoga Pradīpikā,* this is a practice for cleansing and strengthening the eye. It is performed by gazing at a point of focus like a candle flame, a star in the sky, a cloud, a leaf, a picture, or even another person's eyes where one is instructed to avoid blinking. By gazing without blinking, the cornea is exposed to the air, causing irritation to the eye and tears are formed producing a cleansing effect for the eyes. Once tears arise, the eyes are closed and the image of the object persists. Seeing this image will improve the function of *alochaka pitta* (the subdosha of *pitta* responsible for vision and color perception) and the optic nerve and the eyes will look more charming, attractive, and full of luster.

tri-dosha theory (three bodily humors) See *doṣa.*

Trika-Shāsana One of the classical source texts addressing the practice of *Yoga nidrā* along with the *Mahānirvāṇa,* the *Māṇḍūkya and Taittirīya Upaniṣads,* the *Tripura Rahasya,* the *Yogatārāvalī,* and Patañjali's *Yoga Sutras.*

trikoṇāsana Triangle pose.

Tripura Rahasya One of the classical source texts addressing the practice of *Yoga nidrā* along with the *Trika-Shāsana* (as found in the *Shiva Sutras*), the *Māṇḍūkya and Taittirīya Upaniṣads*, the *Yogatārāvalī*, the *Mahānirvāṇa*, and Patañjali's *Yoga Sūtra*.

True Self In Yoga philosophy, this is the sattvic (pure) form of atman (self) or the unification of jivatma (the living self) and paramatma (the supreme self). In modern psychology, this is the truest, best version of a person beyond his/her habits and patterns, which has a variety of characteristics: free will, reasoning, creativity, discernment, moment-to-moment awareness, compassionate, spirit-based, and loving.

Tui Na A hands-on massage and bodywork technique in Chinese Medicine where the practitioner brushes, kneads, rolls, presses on, and/or rubs the "eight gates" between each of the joints to open the body's wei chi (defensive chi) and move the energy in the meridians and muscles.

Turkish get-ups An exercise and complex movement pattern from rehabilitative medicine, sports science training, and Yoga Therapy that teaches the body to isolate, engage, and re-educate the serratus anterior muscles and further engages various other intrinsic muscles of the scapula and thorax, which have the tendency toward hypotonicity, weakness, not recruiting together as a unit, and/or inhibition. The exercise is performed by lying down supine while holding a weight in front of the chest in one arm and going through a series of specific steps to "get up" and stand up fully in an upright position. It is designed to teach the shoulder joints functional stability and has the appearance from start to finish of how a soldier with a spear would lunge at an approaching enemy if he/she was lying on his/her back.

type 2 diabetes Formerly known as noninsulin dependent or adult-onset diabetes, this is the most common form of diabetes in the world and is characterized by high blood sugar levels and a lack of insulin. Categorized as a "lifestyle disease," along with obesity and heart disease, this is a metabolic condition that can be largely prevented and treated by regulating one's diet, exercise, and lifestyle choices.

U.S. Olympic track and field trials A track and field competition held every four years to determine which athletes will be selected to represent the United States at the Olympics.

uddīyāna bandha Lit. "upward-flying lock," this refers to the abdominal retraction lock, the belly lock, or the abdominal hallowing procedure where the abdominal muscles are drawn inward and upward toward the spine. Energetically, it is often applied with the throat *jālandhāra bandha* (the neck lock) and *mūla bandha* (the root lock) to unify *prāṇa* and *apāna* within the *suṣumna*, or the central channel, to thus awaken *kuṇḍalinī* in the *yogin's* body.

udgīta prāṇāyāma One of the most traditional and simple prāṇāyāma exercises, this technique involves inhaling through the nose and exhaling out through the mouth while making the sound "Aum" or "*oṁ*." with a 6:1 or a 1:1 vowel to consonant ratio. The technique improves the quality of one's sleep, a lack of concentration, and bad dreams and is said to vibrate, awaken, and energize the mind.

ujjāyi Translated as "victorious breath," this *prāṇāyāma* technique involves oceanic, wave-like guttural breathing that maximizes the efficiency of the diaphragm and lungs and puffs the chest out like a proud conqueror. The technique highlights a small, soft hissing sound created in the back of the throat and cultivates an energetic quality that is energizing, calming, and balancing, improves oxygenation, creates an internal heat in the body, and increases one's focus when actively engaged in a Haṭha Yoga practice.

ujjāyi prāṇāyāma See *ujjāyi*.

Universal Intelligence An *a priori* vitalistic principle from chiropractic philosophy, similar to the concept of innate intelligence, which highlights that all matter is part of a universal creation and, as such, each individual organism contains the same intelligence, existence, and/or healing ability found innately within nature.

Upaniṣads Translated as "to sit down near" and referring to a student sitting down near a teaching while receiving esoteric, mystical, and/or spiritual knowledge, these are a collection of Indian Vedic texts that contain revealed truths describing the nature of Brahman (ultimate reality), The Self, and moksha (liberation).

Urban Zen Integrative Therapy (UZIT) An approach to Yoga Therapy and wellness founded in 2007 through the vision of Donna Karan, Colleen Saidman Yee, and Rodney Yee, UZIT is a methodology that pulls together five different modalities into a comprehensive integrative system that promotes relaxation and mindfulness. The modalities are Yoga Therapy, Reiki, essential oil therapy, nutrition, and contemplative care.

ūrdhva dhanurāsana Upward facing bow pose.

uṣṭrāsana Camel pose.

uttānāsana Stretched out pose or standing forward bend pose.

Uttara Mīmāṁsā *mīmāṁsā* = examination *uttara* = crossing over

One of the six *darśanas* or schools of orthodox Hindu philosophy, paired with Pūrva Mīmāṁsā. Commonly referred to as Vedānta (end of the Vedas), since the ideas are distilled through a close examination of the *Upaniṣads*, which form the final layer of the Vedas. While Pūrva Mīmāṁsā is concerned with conventional Vedic religious matters, Uttara Mīmāṁsā deals with ultimate spiritual matters, including the nature of Self and Reality, and *mokṣa* or the potential for spiritual liberation of a radical kind.

V. A. Devasenapathi A respected mystic/scholar in Chennai, India, and author of commentaries on the *Śaivite Siddhanta*, the *Śaivite Tantra* of south India, he was a teacher of Gary Kraftsow, founder of the American Viniyoga Institute.

vairāgya Dispassion, detachment, or an absence of worldly desires. According to the *Yoga Sūtra*, *vairagya* and *abhyāsa* (discipline) are the two principal requisites for the successful practice of *yoga*.

Vaiśeṣika* or *Vaisheshika One of the six darshans, or systems of Indian Vedic philosophy, this is a philosophy that says that all things that exist, can be cognized, and/or named are "objects of experience" and, in the physical universe, are reducible to a finite number of atoms that can only be taken as valid knowledge by the sources of perception and inference. Paired with Nyāya, it is an approach emphasizing an analysis and description of the world as a divine creation formed of atoms of earth, air, fire, and water, woven within the context of space, time, mind, and soul, and coexisting with the Creator.

vājī-karaṇa Ayurvedic therapy that improves virility for male sexual problems, including infertility, low libido, and erectile dysfunction, by applying a combination of detoxification, lifestyle and dietary changes, and medicinal protocols.

vajra-pradama mudrā Translated as "unshakable trust," this hand gesture is for balancing the *mano-maya-kośa,* cultivating a sense of inner faith, strength, confidence, openness, and trust in oneself and in life, releasing muscular tension from the chest and rib cage, creating ease and relaxation, improving mood, and opening the *anāhata* (heart) chakra. It is performed by placing the hands a hand's width away from the chest and interlacing the second through fifth fingers with the left little finger on bottom and the thumbs spreading upward and outward while keeping the shoulders relaxed.

vamana One of the *pañca karma* treatments of Ayurveda, this is emission, therapeutic vomiting, or applying an emetic intended to purge the system of excess or toxic *kapha.*

vāsanā 1. The impression of anything remaining unconscious in the mind.

2. Knowledge or present consciousness derived from memory.

3. A way of being; conditioned inclinations, desires, or expectations.

vāta One of the three *doshas,* along with *kapha* and *pitta, vāta* is located primarily in the colon and digestive system and represents the energy of movement (both voluntary and involuntary). It is characterized as light, cool, dry, and mobile and is associated with the energetic mobility of body and mind. Made up elementally of space/ether and air, it is responsible for breathing, blinking, coughing, muscle and tissue movement, yawning, pulsation of the heart, all movements in the cytoplasm and cell membranes, and the elimination of urine, feces, and sweat. In balance, vata promotes creativity and flexibility. Out of balance, *vata* produces fear, coughing/COPDs, and anxiety.

Vedānta One of the six darshans, or systems of Indian Vedic philosophy, and literally translated as "the end or conclusion of the Vedas," it is a system that is rooted in the interpretation of the Upaniṣads (circa eighth to second centuries BCE), along with the *Bhagavad Gītā* (c. second century BCE to second century CE) and the *Brahma Sūtras* (c. third century CE). The central doctrines of *Vedānta* are concerned with the ultimate nature of existence, largely in such terms as *brahman* (Divine Ground of Being), Īśvara (God), *jīva* or *cit* (individual conscious beings), *acit* (insentient matter), *māyā* (illusion), and *mokṣa* (spiritual liberation). An enduring point of dispute within Vedānta concerns the ontological relationship between *brahman* and *ātman* or *jīva*, the principal variations being *advaita* (nondualism), *dvaita* (dualism), and *viśiṣtād-vaita* (qualified nondualism). The latter two positions often serve as a philosophical support for the *bhakti* or devotional traditions. Vedānta features four main points: Brahman is the supreme cause of the entire universe and is all pervading and eternal; actions are subordinate to knowledge or devotion; bondage is subject to the cycle of birth and death; and liberation is the goal.

Vedantic Of, or referring to, the philosophy espoused by Vedanta.

Vedas Lit. "knowledge," the *Vedas* are the three or four literary collections constituting the holy scriptures of Hinduism. The *Ṛg Veda, Sāma Veda,* and *Yajur Veda* are related collections used extensively in traditional Brahmanical rituals, while the fourth (see *Atharva Veda*) is of independent origin and of distinctive character.

vicāra* or *vichara Inquiry, investigation.

vidyā Lit. "knowing," or knowledge, especially higher or spiritual knowledge; a specific science.

vijñāna darśana The art and science of subtle observation of a person's self-presentation (pulse, skin color, tone of voice, eye movements, etc.) in order to assess what is going on internally in making a reliable diagnosis.

vijñāna kosha See *vijñāna-maya-kośa.*

vijñāna-maya-kośa According to the *Taittirīya Upaniṣad,* this is the "sheath made of understanding" or one of the intermediate shells covering the *ātman* or individual self. *Vijñāna* in this context means the faculty of understanding and discrimination and serves as the support for the coarser sheath, which constitutes the thinking or instrumental mind (*mano-maya-koṣa*).

vikṛti* or *vikruti 1. In Ayurveda, an assessment of the current state of *doṣa* balance within the body, taking into account the person's basic physical constitution. (see *prakṛti*)

2. Deformed, disfigured, mutilated, maimed; sick, diseased, imbalanced.

Viniyogatherapy™ See American Viniyoga Institute.

vinyāsa As a term of practice, *vinyāsa* refers to movement, connecting, sequence, or placing one's attention on the breath and aligning it synchronistically and consciously with the body's movements.

Vinyasa Flow Yoga As a tradition of Haṭha Yoga, Vinyasa Flow Yoga is commonly referred to as Vinyasa Yoga and derived from the style of Ashtanga Vinyasa Yoga, which refers to a fitness-like style of Haṭha Yoga that incorporates breath-oriented flowing movements sequenced in an orderly way, as well as other physical yogic elements such as *bandhas* (locks), *dṛṣṭis* (eye gazing points), and the use of *ujjāyi prāṇāyāma.* There are many sub-styles of the tradition of Vinyasa Yoga, including Jivamukti Yoga, Forrest Yoga, Prana Flow Yoga, and the therapeutic traditions of Vinyasa Krama Yoga and Chikitsa Vinyasa Yoga.

viparita karani Legs up the wall pose or inverted action pose.

viparyaya Misapprehension, misperception, error, inverted, reversed, mistake.

vīrabhadrāsana Warrior pose. *vīra* = hero, warrior *bhadra* = good, auspicious

virecana* or *virechana One of the *pañca karma* treatments of Ayurveda, this is medicated purgative therapy for cleansing excess *pitta* from the body and purifying the blood.

vīrya 1. Strength, power, energy, valor, virility, manliness, heroism.

2. In Ayurveda, the potency or efficacy of a medicine.

vittam mudrā Translated as "gesture of vital energy," this hand gesture directs breath, awareness, and energy into the pelvis and abdomen and is for balancing the prāṇa-maya-kośa. It is performed by holding the hands about twelve inches apart with the palms facing each other, slightly cupped, in front of the lower abdomen. The hands are allowed to gently expand away from each other on the inhalation and to rest back toward each other on the exhalation.

viveka Discernment, discrimination; investigation; right judgment.

viyoga 1. Eliminating dysfunctional associations, habits, and activities.

2. Disjunction, separation; loss, absence; abstention; getting rid of.

vṛkśāsana Tree pose or balancing tree pose.

vṛtti Lit. "rolling," these are modifications of the mind, thought fluctuations, modes of being, character, disposition, state, and condition; behaviour, course of action, practice, general usage; process.

vṛttibheda Differences in mental modifications. Functional distinctions. For example, although *prāṇa* refers generically to the coursing of life force in the body, there are five major and five minor types of *prāṇa,* each identifiable in terms of their distinct functions. (see *pañca vāyu*)

vyāyāma 1. Dragging different ways, contest, strife, struggle.

2. Exertion, athletic or gymnastic exercise, considered in Ayurveda to be an essential component of preventative health care, rejuvenation, and longevity.

warm-ups The beginning exercises, breathing techniques, meditations, and/or āsanas (postures) that initiate a practice and make one more receptive to deeper experiences.

Water One of the five elements in each of the systems of Chinese Medicine, Ayurveda, and Yoga. Chinese Medicine lists the other four elements as fire, earth, metal, and wood; Ayurveda lists the other four elements as fire, earth, wind/air, and space; and Yoga lists the other four elements as fire, earth, ether, and air. In Yoga philosophy, water is represented by Varuna, the god of water and the celestial ocean, and symbolizes fluidity, adaptability, power, sensitivity, and, when out of balance, stagnation and passivity.

well-being A generic term that is intended to measure and assess the physical, emotional, social, economic, psychological, spiritual, and/or medical state for an individual or group.

wellness counselor See Ayurvedic Wellness Counselor.

Western Of, or relating to, the western world including any of the countries, people, approaches, and/or ideas from the Americas and Europe.

Western biomedicine A branch of Western medicine that applies biological, physiological, environmental, and other natural-science principles to clinical practice.

Williams flexion exercises Rehabilitation exercises and Yoga-like movements developed by orthopedic surgeon, Paul Williams, M.D., that focus on the flexion of the spine and include, but are not limited to, *paścimottanāsana* (seated forward bend pose), *uttānāsana* (standing forward bend pose), supine knees to chest, and core work, which reduce compression in the facet joints and also decrease the pressure in the spinal column in cases of spinal stenosis and spondylolisthesis when properly and appropriately applied.

world arts and culture A university department and/or degree that focuses on three concentrations: community-based, arts activism; studies of visual culture; and critical ethnographies.

World Health Organization (WHO) A special agency of the United Nations that focuses on international public health and the attainment of the highest possible level of health by all people. The organization is responsible for providing leadership on global health matters, shaping health research, setting norms and standards, articulating evidence-based policies, providing countries with technical support, and monitoring and assessing current health trends.

World Health Organization Quality of Life (WHOQOL) Scale A cross-cultural outcome measure comprised of twenty-six items, including physical health, psychological health, social relationships, and the environment, which are designed to quantify one's perceptions and quality of life in the context of his/her culture and value systems, personal goals, standards, and concerns.

Wu Qin Xi Until the discovery of the *Mawangdui* in 1973, these were the earliest-known written examples of Chinese Medicine exercises that are akin to Yoga āsanas (postures) for physical health.

Wu Xing Also known as the "five phases," "five elements," "five steps/stages," or "five agents," this refers to the five elements, not as basic constituents of Nature, but as five basic processes, qualities, phases of a cycle, and/or inherent capabilities of change of phenomena.

xian-tian-zhi-jing A source of Jing in Taoist Yoga and Chinese Medicine, this type of genetically-inherited constitution, literally defined as "Before Heaven Essence" or "Prenatal Essence," is "fixed at birth and, together with Original Qi, determines an individual's basic makeup and constitution."

Y-exercises Exercises from rehabilitative medicine and Yoga Therapy that can isolate, engage, and reeducate the posterior stabilizers of the scapula, which have the tendency toward hypotonicity, weakness, and/or inhibition. They are performed by placing the arms overhead in a "Y" position while lying on the stomach with the forehead on the floor. The hands are repetitively lifted off the floor in an attempt to initiate activity in the middle and lower trapezius, latissimus dorsi, and rhomboid muscles.

yamas Classically listed as the first component or limb of Patañjali's *rāja* or *aṣṭāṅga-yoga,* these are ethical restraints, moral observances, or qualities of "right living" that lead an individual to a healthier, more *sattvic* lifestyle and include *ahiṁsa* (nonviolence), *asteya* (nonstealing), *satya* (truthfulness), *brahmacarya* (divine awareness and energetic control), and *aparigraha* (non-greediness).

Yang Compared to the root word *Ha* in the Sanskrit word, *Haṭha,* this concept from the I Ching in Chinese Medicine represents the sun, brightness, daytime, summer, and masculine energy.

YCat Yoga Therapist This is a Yoga Therapist and/or health educator, who has completed the three-level, 300-hour YCat Yoga Therapy training given by Jnani Chapman, R.N., which introduces the effective and appropriate application of Yoga Therapy for patients undergoing cancer treatment and/or cardiovascular rehabilitation.

Yellow Emperor (Huang Di) One of the legendary cultural heroes of ancient China, he lived about 5,000 years ago and is credited as the initiator of Chinese civilization. In traditional Chinese Medicine, he is regarded as one of the two "legendary founders" along with Shen Nong and is the author of the foundational text, *Huang-di Nei-Jing.*

Yijing Also called the "I Ching," and the "Book of Changes," this book's Taoist and Chinese origins date back to the third and second millennia BCE and it highlights many wise aphorisms and divination concepts. It additionally outlines a philosophical system that says change and balance are created by the interplay of two 'forces,' *Yin* and *Yang,* which correspond in Haṭha Yoga to *Tha* and *Ha,* and are said to be "two faces of a single mountain."

Yin Compared to the root word *Tha* in the Sanskrit word, *Haṭha,* this concept from the I Ching in Chinese Medicine represents darkness, the moon, nighttime, winter, and feminine energy.

yoga 1. Yoking, harnessing, union, setting up, application.

2. In the *Upaniṣads,* the term ***yoga*** refers to the resolute binding of one's attention to the deepest levels of awareness to reveal the ultimate identity of *ātman* and *brahman.* Achievement of the *brahma* knowledge, through this one-pointed focus of attention, was considered to be the key to *mokṣa* or spiritual liberation from the cycle of birth, death, and reincarnation.

3. Any serious or focused discipline or relationship undertaken for spiritual, healing, or some other specific pragmatic purpose.

Yoga One of the six darshans, or systems of Indian Vedic philosophy, this is a dualistic philosophy that is rooted in the perspective of Samkhya and is based largely on the practices, techniques, and viewpoints most authoritatively and concisely described in Patañjali's *Yoga Sutras.* At its core, Yoga is a physio-psycho-emotiono-socio-spiritual system of self-care, which aims to improve the human condition and alleviate *duḥkha* (suffering) by transforming the habitual patterns of one's mind, one's body, and one's behavior, and can be universally adapted to a wide spectrum of individuals, situations, and other systems.

Yoga Alliance (YA) Currently, the largest nonprofit association representing the Yoga community internationally, their mission is "to spread the power of Yoga one person at a time" in a safe and responsible manner. YA provides credentialing and educational standards for four levels of Yoga instructors (RYT 200, RYT 500, E-RYT 200, E-RYT500) and a registry and directory of its members made up of certified Yoga instructors and Yoga schools.

Yoga Anatomy Written in 2007 by Yoga educators, Leslie Kaminoff and Amy Matthews, this bestselling book has wonderfully detailed anatomy illustrations and intelligent physiological, biomechanical, and clinical reflections about the most popular poses, movements, and practices found in the system of Haṭha Yoga.

Yoga and Health A book written by Indian-born Yoga teacher, Selvarajan Yesudian, and Elisabeth Haisch, in the 1950s and selling more than four million total copies, it features the lead author performing a variety of Yoga āsanas (poses) while sharing the health benefits of the practice of Haṭha Yoga.

Yoga as medicine A common phrase coined at the beginning of the twenty-first century that applies to Yoga being used as a therapy, intervention, prescription, treatment, and/or medical substitute for pharmatoxicology, traditional therapy, or more invasive procedures in any field of medicine or complementary and alternative medicine.

Yoga as Medicine Written by Western-trained internist and *Yoga Journal* medical editor, Tim McCall, M.D., this book focuses on Yoga from a Western medicine perspective and includes the yogic approaches, advice, and prescriptions for an assortment of physical and disease-oriented issues from a variety of master Yoga instructors. For readers challenged by illness, the book provides an overview of some of the most popular styles of Yoga and their suitability for various degrees of fitness; steps to finding a Yoga Therapist; what to expect from a session; and ways to make Yoga Therapy accessible to the public.

Yoga in Breast Cancer Treatment and Recovery Course A Yoga Therapy course or program that is specifically designed to be used in treatment and recovery from breast cancer.

Yoga nidrā The "yoga of sleep or dreams," which as a general term refers to maintanence of conscious awareness while the body is asleep, or what is elsewhere referred to as "lucid dreaming." As a more contemporary term, this yogic technique is designed to bring the mind to a condition between wakefulness and sleep, through a combination of establishing intention, awareness of breath, internal scanning of the body, visualization, etc. The practice purports to give the *yogin* access to deeper layers of consciousness. Reported benefits include deep relaxation, stress reduction, and heightened mastery over the autonomic nervous system. In recent years, Yoga nidrā has been shown to be helpful for returning soldiers suffering from posttraumatic stress disorder (PTSD).

Yoga Rx Written by Larry Payne, Ph.D., and Richard Usatine, M.D., this book offers readers Yoga-based treatments for a wide variety of diseases like allergies, arthritis, COPDs, common colds, constipation, chronic fatigue syndrome, depression, diabetes, headaches, hypertension, impotence, insomnia, lower back and neck complaints, menopause, multiple sclerosis, obesity, and substance abuse. In each chapter Richard Usatine, M.D., gives a Western medical point of view followed by Dr. Payne's Yoga Therapy perspective and recommended yogic treatments, which include *āsana* (postures), *prāṇāyāma* (breathing techniques), food choices, and Yoga nidra-based relaxation techniques.

Yoga Sūtra See Patañjali's *Yoga Sūtra.*

Yoga Therapist One who practices, evaluates, facilitates, and treats patients and/or clients using Yoga Therapy.

Yoga Therapy A modern approach to health and wellness with ancient roots, this discipline takes into consideration the complete state of one's health in terms of physical conditioning, mental and emotional state, energetic balance, attitude, dietary and behavioral patterns, personal associations and relationships, and the environment. It seeks the vital integration of the mind, body, and spirit to heal the whole person, promote health, and prevent disease and consists of therapeutically natured practices from Yoga that may or may not include *āsana* (postures), *prāṇāyāma* (breathing practices), *dhyāna* (meditation), *bhāvana* (imagery), philosophical training, lifestyle modification techniques, and experiential and foundational elements of Ayurveda.

Yoga Therapy: A Guide to the Therapeutic Use of Yoga and Ayurveda for Health and Fitness Written by A. G. Mohan, Indra Mohan, Ganesh Mohan, and Nitya Mohan, this is a book that describes the therapeutic use of Yoga and prescribes postures, breathing techniques, and basic Ayurvedic principles for a variety of common health problems, including asthma, back pain, constipation, hip pain, knee pain, menstrual problems, and scoliosis. It also details how to correctly move into, hold, and move out of poses, how to breathe during practice to achieve specific results, and how to customize a yoga practice by creating sequences of yoga poses for a particular person.

Yoga Therapy Rx Program Inspired by T. K. V. Desikachar and founded at Loyola Marymount University by Larry Payne, Ph.D., this is an approach to Yoga Therapy that is a marriage between Yoga and complementary medicine. It is designed to train Yoga teachers to be Yoga Therapists and applies classical applications of Yoga for use in clinical settings to help treat common ailments and conditions. It was the first Yoga Therapy program offered at a major University and is considered the "gold standard" by the International Association of Yoga Therapists. The program's diverse faculty of licensed healthcare professionals and Yoga Therapists focus on all of the systems of the body including the musculoskeletal, circulatory, respiratory, digestive, nervous, reproductive, and endocrine systems. The program also offers other concepts like mental health care, Yoga philosophy, spirituality, Ayurveda, and an opportunity to intern at the Venice Family Clinic in Venice, California, to get live, supervised clinical experience while working as part of an integrated healthcare team.

Yoga Vidyā 1. Known as the "knowledge of connection to life," this is the "living body" of yogic knowledge that can only be understood through the practice, application, and direct experience of yogic techniques and/or a yogic lifestyle.

2. Knowledge of *yoga;* science of *yoga.*

Yoga Yajñavalkya Considered by Professor Tirumalai Krishnamacharya to be one of the most important texts on Yoga, this book defines Yoga as "the union between jivatma (the living self) and paramatma (the supreme self)" and also opens up the practice to women, which was rare in Yoga before the twentieth century. As an important Haṭha Yoga text of twelve chapters and 504 verses, it was written in the style of a dialogue between the Vedic sage, Yajñavalkya, and the female philosopher, Gargi, who are also found in dialogue in the earliest of the principal Upaniṣads, the *Bṛhadāraṇyaka* (c. eighth century BCE). Although some would date the *Yoga Yajñavalkya* as early as the second century BCE to fourth century CE, its extensive discussion of *kuṇḍalinī* and *prāṇayāma*—along with potential therapeutic applications—suggests a much later date, perhaps as late as the thirteenth or fourteenth century CE.

yogāsana A Yoga posture or pose.

yogaścittavṛttinirodhaḥ The second aphorism of Patañjali's *Yoga Sūtra,* articulating the definition of *Yoga* according to the Yoga *darśana*: "*Yoga* is the arresting of the activities of the mind."

Yogatārāvalī One of the classical source texts addressing the practice of *Yoga nidrā* along with the *Trika-Shāsana* (as found in the *Shiva Sutras*), the *Māṇḍūkya and Taittirīya Upaniṣads,* the *Tripura Rahasya,* the *Mahānirvāṇa,* and Patañjali's *Yoga Sūtra.* This text is a Haṭha Yoga treatise attributed to the celebrated eighth century philosopher-saint Śaṅkara, which concisely discusses the spiritual purposes underlying the yogic practices of *prāṇāyāma* and the *bandhas,* and the arousal of *kuṇḍalinī.*

Yogavalli An interpretation of Patañjali's *Yoga Sutras* written by Professor Tirumalai Krishnamacharya, which suggests that the *Sutras* are "par excellence," or the only work that totally and concisely covers all aspects of the Yoga practice without any Hindu, Buddhist, and/or religious overtones, and that the four chapters of the Sutras were individual instructions given to four individual disciples, highlighting Krishnamacharya's insistence on the importance of Yoga being personalized to the needs of the individual.

Yogi Bhajan Born Harbhajan Singh Puri and an avid peacekeeper, a wonderful orator, and a master teacher of over 8,000 Yoga classes, he was the founder of the Happy, Healthy, Holy Organization (3HO) and the first teacher of Kundalini Yoga and Sikh Dharma in the Western world.

yogi/yogini/yogin/yogic These are general vocabulary terms that are universal in nature and have the following definitions and applications: a *yogi* is a male practitioner of Yoga; a *yogini* is a female practitioner of Yoga; a *yogin* is a nongender specific practitioner of Yoga; and *yogic* refers to the quality of or having an association with a practice, person, technique, philosophy, and/or feature of Yoga in all of its many forms, paths, limbs, philosophies, and manifestations.

yogins See yogi/yogini/yogin/yogic.

yukti Union, juncture, connection, combination. In Ayurveda, the concept that all conditions, including disease, come into being through the synergistic confluence of various factors.

INDEX

Abdominal bracing, 308–309
Abdominal hallowing. *See* *Uddīyāna bandha* (belly lock).
Abhiniveśa (fear of impermanence), 422
Abhyanga (oil massage), 57
Academic Consortium for Complementary and Alternative Healthcare (ACCAHC), 553
Acceptance, 187, 188, 382
Acetylcholine, 115
Activities of daily living (ADL), 284
Acupuncture
  points, 20–21, 23, 25, 27, 29
  popularity of, 33
  research studies on, 32
Adaptive competence, 378
Adhesive capsulitis, 134–136
Ādi mantra, 384
Advaita Vedānta, 173
Advent Lutheran Church, New York, 483
Affirmations, 342, 346, 349, 353, 354, 467
AGE (advanced glycosolated end-product), 229–230
Aggression, 332
Agni (digestive fire), 58, 61
Ahaṁkāra (individuation), 367
Ahiṁsa (nonviolence), 69, 99, 170, 178, 434
Alkalinity, 158
Allen, David R., 219–234
Allergies, food, 220, 228–229
Aluminum, 423
Alzheimer's disease, 119–120, 538
American Holistic Nurses Association (AHNA), 212–213, 215, 216
American Nurses Association (ANA), 207, 213
American Viniyoga Institute (AVI), 469–481
Ames, Donna, 170
Amygdala, 332–333
Anahāsana (heart opening pose), 301
Anand, B. K., 239
Ānanda (bliss), 341, 475, 486
Ānanda-maya-kośa (bliss body), 341, 345, 353–354, 358, 407
Anger, 89–90, 465
Ankles, 85
Anna-maya-kośa (physical body), 338–339, 344, 345–347, 356
Anterior head carriage, 79–80, 296, 297
Antidepressants, 171, 172
Antiperspirants, 423
Anxiety, 72, 88–89, 171, 198, 214, 278, 350–351, 499, 532
Apāna vāyu, 462–463
Apānāsana (supine knees to chest/abdominal breath pose), 310, 463
Aperture (journal), 191
Apology, 195
Ardha-añjaneyāsana (kneeling crescent pose), 132
Ardha kumbhakāsana (half plank pose), 301
Ardha salabhāsana (half locust pose), 253–254
Aromatherapy, 497, 502, 503
Arousal, physiological, 145
Artha (material prosperity), 50, 443
Āsanas (postures), 13, 60–63, 65, 100, 113, 149, 171, 176–177, 198–200, 268, 270–271, 276, 338–339, 342, 361, 370, 390, 410, 419, 420, 437, 445, 446, 456–459, 462–463, 478, 485, 521
  abdominal, 252–254, 283, 463
  animal names and, 63
  assisted, 410, 412
  back bending, 446, 448
  cardiovascular disease patients and, 244–256
  chair position, 198–199, 210, 256
  chest/heart opening, 301, 467
  core strength, 457, 458
  forward bending, 77, 310, 463, 468
  guidelines (Structural Yoga Therapy), 439
  hip opening, 426, 426, 463
  in-bed, 499–500, 507, 508
  inverted, 251–252, 298, 467
  length of, 365
  props for, 365, 501
  rehabilitation clients and, 276–277
  restorative, 500–501
  sequences of, 365, 397–399, 428–429, 456–459, 463, 467–468
  sitting, 198–199, 256, 446
  standing, 255–256
  supine, 250–251, 456
  tolerable edge and, 403–404, 406, 412
  twisted, 82, 250, 399, 446, 463, 468
  See also specific poses.
Ashwagandha, 460, 468
Ashwini mudrā (horse gesture), 307
Asmitā (ego/self-importance), 422
Aspartame, 230
Aṣṭāṅga Yoga, 113, 302
Asthma, 535
Atharva Veda, 11
Athletes, 156–169
  will of, 163–164
Ātman (consciousness/essential Self), 50, 113, 182, 473
Attention, 184–185
Aurobindo, Sri, 407, 417–418, 445
AVI. *See* American Viniyoga Institute (AVI)
AVI Viniyoga Therapist Training Program, 470, 477–478, 559
Avidyā (ignorance), 407, 422, 487
Avoidance, 186, 278, 284
Awareness, 187–188, 330, 342, 410, 414

CPSIA information can be obtained
at www.ICGtesting.com
Printed in the USA
FSOW03n0913051216

9 781591 203667